The GALE
ENCYCLOPEDIA of
PUBLIC HEALTH

The GALE ENCYCLOPEDIA of PUBLIC HEALTH

VOLUME

2

M–Z
ORGANIZATIONS
GLOSSARY
INDEX

LAURIE J. FUNDUKIAN, EDITOR

GALE
CENGAGE Learning

Detroit • New York • San Francisco • New Haven, Conn • Waterville, Maine • London

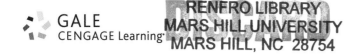

The Gale Encyclopedia of Public Health

Project Editor: Laurie J. Fundukian

Product Manager: Kate Hanley

Editorial Support Services: Andrea Lopeman

Indexing Services: Hawkeye Indexing

Rights Acquisition and Management:
    Sheila Spencer

Composition: Evi Abou-El-Seoud

Manufacturing: Wendy Blurton

Imaging: John Watkins

Product Design: Kristine Julien

For product information and technology assistance, contact us at
Gale Customer Support, 1-800-877-4253.
For permission to use material from this text or product,
submit all requests online at **www.cengage.com/permissions.**
Further permissions questions can be emailed to
permissionrequest@cengage.com

While every effort has been made to ensure the reliability of the information presented in this publication, Gale, a part of Cengage Learning, does not guarantee the accuracy of the data contained herein. Gale accepts no payment for listing; and inclusion in the publication of any organization, agency, institution, publication, service, or individual does not imply endorsement of the editors or publisher. Errors brought to the attention of the publisher and verified to the satisfaction of the publisher will be corrected in future editions.

LIBRARY OF CONGRESS CATALOGING-IN-PUBLICATION DATA

The Gale encyclopedia of public health / Laurie J. Fundukian, editor. – First edition.
    2 volumes ; cm
    Summary: "Alphabetically arranged encyclopedia contains approximately 257 entries pertaining to important Public Health concerns. Topics include diseases and conditions, health and wellness efforts, nutrition, ethics and law related topics and statistics, sanitation issues, everyday environmental effects and more. Contains images, tables, and illustrations"– Provided by publisher.
    Includes bibliographical references and index.
    ISBN-13: 978-1-4144-9876-8 (set : hardback)
    ISBN-10: 1-4144-9876-4 (set : hardback)
    ISBN-13: 978-1-4144-9877-5 (v. 1 : hardback)
    ISBN-10: 1-4144-9877-2 (v. 1 : hardback)
    [etc.]
    1. Public health–Encyclopedias.   I. Fundukian, Laurie J.
    RA423.G35 2013
    362.103–dc23
    2012051201

Gale
27500 Drake Rd.
Farmington Hills, MI, 48331-3535

ISBN-13: 978-1-4144-9876-8 (set)   ISBN-10: 1-4144-9876-4 (set)
ISBN-13: 978-1-4144-9877-5 (vol. 1)   ISBN-10: 1-4144-9877-2 (vol. 1)
ISBN-13: 978-1-4144-9878-2 (vol. 2)   ISBN-10: 1-4144-7878-0 (vol. 2)

This title is also available as an e-book.
ISBN-13: 978-1-4144-9879-9   ISBN-10: 1-4144-9879-9
Contact your Gale, a part of Cengage Learning sales representative for ordering information.

Printed in China
1 2 3 4 5 6 7 17 16 15 14 13

CONTENTS

ALPHABETICAL LIST OF ENTRIES

A

AARP
Abortion
Acrylamide
Addiction
Aging
AIDS/HIV
Air pollution
Alcoholism
Allergies
Alternative medicine
Amebiasis
American Public Health
    Organization
Anthrax
Antibiotics
Antimicrobial resistance
Asbestosis
Assessment Protocol for Excellence
    in Public Health
Association of State and Territorial
    Health Officers
Asthma
Autisim
Avian influenza

B

Bed bug infestation
Behavioral health
Birth defects
Bisphenol-A
Black lung disease
Bovine spongiform encephalopathy

Brucellosis
Bullying
Burns

C

Campylobacteriosis
Cancer
Car seats
Carbon monoxside poisoning
Centers for disease control and
    prevention (CDC)
Chagas disease
Chemical poisoning
Child abuse
Child labor laws
Childhood obesity
Children's health
Chlorination
Cholera
Clostridium
Common cold
Community development
    workers
Community health
Community health assessment
Community health improvement
    process
Community mental health
Concussion
Consumer safety
Contraception and birth
    control
Correctional health
Cytomegalovirus

D

Defibrillation
Dengue fever
Dental health
Department of Health and Human
    Services
Diabetes mellitis
Diphtheria
Distracted driving
Domestic abuse
Dracunculiasis infection
Drinking water
Drug resistance
Dysentery

E

Eating disorders
Ebola hemorrhagic fever
Economic and financial stress
Emergency health services
Emergency preparedness
Emerging diseases
Encephalitis
Environmental disasters
Environmental health
Environmental Protection Agency
Environmental toxins
Epidemiology
Epstein barr virus
Escherichia coli
Essential medicines
Ethics and legal issues of public health
Evidence-based policy

Public health administration
Public health engineers
Public Health Foundation
Public health nurses

Q

Q fever
Quarantine and isolation

R

Rabies
Radiation
Refugee health
Reproductive health
Ringworm
Risk factors and assessment
Road traffic safety
Rotavirus
Rubella
Rural health

S

Safe sex
Salmonella
Sanitation
Scarlet fever
Schistosomiasis
School health
Scurvy
Secondhand smoke

Senior health
Severe acute respiratory syndrome
  (SARS)
Sexual assault
Sexually transmitted diseases
Shigellosis
Shingles
Sick building syndrome
Sleep deprivation
Small pox
Smoking
Society for Public Health Educators
  (SOPHE)
Sociologists
Sodium
Staphylococcal infections
Stress
Stroke
Substance abuse and dependence
Suicide
Sun protection
Syphilis

T

Tetanus
Tobacco control
Trachoma
Travel health
Tuberculosis
Tularaemia
Typhoid fever
Typhus

U

United States Public Health
  Service

V

Vaccination
Variant Creutzfeldt-Jakob
  Disease
Veterinary medicine
Violence
Visual health
Vitamins

W

Water
West nile virus
Whooping cough
Women's health
Workplace safety
World Health Organization

Y

Yellow fever

Z

Zoonosis

PLEASE READ—IMPORTANT INFORMATION

The *Gale Encyclopedia of Public Health* is a health reference product designed to inform and educate readers about a wide variety of subjects pertaining to public health, such as diseases, related organizations, laws and industries, and practices and population. The Gale Group believes the product to be comprehensive, but not necessarily definitive. It is intended to supplement, not replace, consultation with a physician or other healthcare practitioners. While The Gale Group has made substantial efforts to provide information that is accurate, comprehensive, and up-to-date, The Gale Group makes no representations or warranties of any kind, including without limitation, warranties of merchantability or fitness for a particular purpose, nor does it guarantee the accuracy, comprehensiveness, or timeliness of the information contained in this product. Readers should be aware that the universe of medical knowledge is constantly growing and changing, and that differences of opinion exist among authorities. Readers are also advised to seek professional diagnosis and treatment for any medical condition, and to discuss information obtained from this book with their healthcare provider.

INTRODUCTION

The *Gale Encyclopedia of Public Health* is a source for readers who are looking to investigate health topics that effect the public. The encyclopedia minimizes medical jargon and uses language that any reader can understand, while still providing thorough coverage of each topic.

SCOPE

257 full-length articles are included in *The Gale Encyclopedia of Public Health*. Entries follow a standardized format that provides information at a glance. An example of such a format:

Diseases and conditions

• Definition
• Demographics
• Description
• Causes and symptoms
• Diagnosis
• Treatment
• Prognosis
• Prevention
• Effects on Public health
• Costs to Society

INCLUSION CRITERIA

A preliminary list of public health topics was compiled from a wide variety of sources, including professional medical guides and textbooks, as well as consumer guides and encyclopedias. An advisory board comprised of professionals in public health and medicine evaluated the topics and made suggestions for inclusion. The final selections were determined by Gale editors in conjunction with the advisory board.

ABOUT THE CONTRIBUTORS

The entries were written by experienced medical writers, including healthcare practitioners and educators, pharmacists, researchers, and other professionals. The essays were reviewed by advisors to ensure that they are appropriate, up-to-date, and accurate.

HOW TO USE THIS BOOK

The Gale Encyclopedia of Public Health has been designed with ready reference in mind:

• A timeline of historic events that were important within the scope and development of Public Health (which you'll find just before the entries begin)

• Straight **alphabetical arrangement** of topics allows users to locate information quickly.

• **Bold-faced terms** within entries direct the reader to related articles.

• Lists of **key terms** are provided where appropriate to define unfamiliar terms or concepts. A **glossary** of key terms is also included at the back of Volume 2.

• **Cross-references** placed throughout the *Encyclopedia* direct readers to primary entries from alternate names, drug brand names, and related topics.

• **Questions to Ask Your Doctor** sidebars provide sample questions that patients can ask their physicians.

• **Resources** at the end of every entry direct readers to additional sources of information on a topic.

• Valuable **contact information** for organizations and support groups is included with each entry and compiled in the back of Volume 2.

• A comprehensive **general index** at the back of Volume 2 allows users to easily find areas of interest.

GRAPHICS

The Gale Encyclopedia of Public Health is enhanced with approximately 200 full-color images, including photographs, tables, and custom illustrations.

ADVISORY BOARD

Thank you to the following experts in health for providing invaluable assistance in the formulation of this encyclopedia. Advisors listed have also acted as contributing advisors—writing various articles related to their fields of expertise and experience.

Tamra J. Fairchild
MPH Health Educator and Public Information Officer
Wood County Health District
Genoa, Ohio

L. Fleming Fallon, Jr.
Distinguished Professor; MD, Dr. PH
Public Health
Bowling Green University
Bowling Green, OH

Brenda Wilmoth Lerner
Infectious disease specialist; R.N.
L&L Publishing, LLC
Montrose, AL

CONTRIBUTORS

Margaret Alic, Ph.D.
Science Writer
Eastsound, Washington

William Arthur Atkins
Science Writer
Atkins Research and Consulting
Pekin, Illinois

Rosalyn Carson-DeWitt, M.D.
Medical Writer
Durham, NC

**Laura Jean Cataldo,
RN, Ed.D.**
Medical Writer
Myersville, MD

Rhonda Cloos, R.N.
Medical Writer
Austin, TX

Tish Davidson, A.M.
Medical Writer
Fremont, California

**L. Fleming Fallon Jr., M.D.,
Dr. PH**
*Associate Professor of Public
Health*
Bowling Green State University
Bowling Green, OH

Karl Finley
Medical Writer
West Bloomfield, MI

Rebecca Frey, Ph.D.
*Research and Administrative
Associate*
East Rock Institute
New Haven, Connecticut

Frances Hodgkins
Medical writer
Rockport, Maine

Sally J. Jacobs, Ed.D.
Medical Writer
Los Angeles, CA

Monique Laberge, PhD
Research Associate
Department of Biochemistry and
Biophysics
University of Pennsylvania
Philadelphia, Pennsylvania

Leslie Mertz, PhD
Medical writer
Kalkaska, Michigan

David E. Newton
Medical Writer
Ashland, Oregon

Andrea Nienstedt, M.A.
Medical Writer
Lake Orion, Michigan

**Melinda Granger Oberleitner,
RN, DNS**
*Acting Department Head and
Associate Professor*
Department of Nursing
University of Louisiana at
Lafayette
Lafayette, Louisiana

Teresa Odle
Medical Writer
Albuquerque, New Mexico

Judith Sims, M.S.
Medical Writer
Logan, UT

Carol Turkington
Medical Writer
Lancaster, PA

Samuel Uretsky, PharmD
Pharmacist and medical writer
Wantagh, New York

Ken Wells
Freelance Writer
Laguna Hills, California

CHRONOLOGY

Sample milestone world events involving public health throughout history.

1348: The Black Plague or Black Death, also known as the Bubonic Plague, reappeared in Europe after nearly a 1,000 year absence.

1700: Bernardino Ramazzini (1633–1714) published the first comprehensive occupational health treatise, which was the birth of occupational health.

1700–1800: In the United States, governmental agencies were created to address mounting health problems, sanitation and the protection of water supply, concerns that arose with the industrial revolution.

1761: World's first formal veterinary school was founded in Lyon, France.

1763: Smallpox infected blankets were distributed in the "New World" to Native Americans starting an epidemic that killed thousands.

1779: The first recognized Dengue epidemics occurred at about the same time in Asia, Africa, and North America in the 1780s.

1796: Edward Jenner (1749–1843) published his first paper on the potential for inoculation, which led to the development of the small pox vaccine.

1793: Yellow Fever appeared in the U.S. in the late 17th century. In 1793, Philadelphia was the scene of one of the worst outbreaks.

1799: The Lying-in Hospital of the City of New York is chartered, the first to provide obstetrical care for women in New York City.

1804: The first city water treatment plant was built in Scotland, initiating the idea that all people should have access to clean, safe drinking water.

1842: Social reformer Edwin Chadwick published his landmark report, "Report on the Inquiry into Sanitary Conditions of the Laboring Population of Great Britain", outlining the major public health challenges facing England at the time, leading to the beginnings of reform.

1831–1832: Cholera first came to Sunderland, England. Several epidemics appeared overtime throughout England, eventually killing more people than the Black Plague.

1840: The first dental college, the Baltimore College of Dental Surgery, was established.

1849: Swedish physician Magnus Huss (1807–1890) first coined the term alcoholism to systematically classify the damage that was attributable to the excessive consumption of alcohol.

1863: New York City conducted the first sanitation survey. New York's Association for the Improvement of the Condition of the Poor finds "dark, contracted, ill constructed, badly ventilated and disgustingly filthy" housing.

1869: Dr. Robert Dalton creates the world's first hospital ambulance, a horse-drawn carriage serving Bellevue Hospital in New York.

1872: The American Public Health Association was founded by American physician Stephen Smith, a pioneer in the U.S. public health movement.

1873: The nation's first nursing school based on Florence Nightingale's principles opens at Bellevue in New York City. Nursing students work on the hospital wards 12 hours a day, six days a week. By 1910, there are more than 1,000 nursing schools in the country.

1879: The National Board of Health was established.

1881: The first anthrax vaccine was perfected by Louis Pasteur.

1890: Naturopathy is recognized as a formal system of healthcare.

1891: Bisphenol A was first synthesized by Russian chemist Alexksandr Dianin.

1919: Methamphetamine was first synthesized in Japan.

1921: The Bureau of Indian Affairs Health Division was created.

1928: Scottish physician Alexander Fleming (1881–1955) inadvertently discovered Penicillin while studying moulds.

1938: Fair Labor Standards Act (FLSA) passed as part of President Roosevelt's New Deal, providing regulations for employers to improve conditions of workers.

1946: Centers for Disease Control and Prevention (CDC) was established in 1946 in Atlanta as the Communicable Disease Center.

1947: American cardiac surgeon Claude Schaeffer Beck (1894–1971) was the first to use a defibrillator on a human when he successfully applied it to a 14-year-old male during surgery.

1948: The World Health Organization (WHO) was established by the United Nations.

1949: National Institute of Mental Health is founded.

1950: Mass TB immunization with the bacille Calmette-Guerin (BCG) vaccine is under way to protect children from tuberculosis.

1960: G. D. Searle & Company receives FDA approval to sell Enovid as a birth control pill. The development of the first highly effective contraceptive transforms women's lives around the world and opens the door to the sexual revolution.

1962: President John F. Kennedy signed into law the Migrant Health Act, which provided for the establishment of health clinics across the nation designed to deal specifically with migrant health issues.

1962: Child abuse is formally acknowledged in the United States.

1963: Measles vaccine was developed.

1965: The Johnson Administration created Medicare and Medicaid.

1965: The first report on diabetes mellitus is issued.

1968: Noroviruses are named after the original strain that caused an outbreak of gastroenteritis in a Norwalk, Ohio school.

1969: Federal Coal Mine Health and Safety Act of 1969 is passed.

1970: Environmental Protection Agency (EPA) was established under the Nixon Administration.

1970: The Occupational Safety and Health Act of 1970 was passed, which requires employers to create a workplace free of known hazards.

1972: The Special Supplemental Nutrition Program for Women, Infants, and Children, commonly referred to as WIC, a federally funded nutrition-intervention program administered by the food and Nutrition Service of the U.S. Department of Agriculture, was founded.

1973: The American Psychiatric Association removed homosexuality from their list of mental disorders.

1973: Roe v. Wade is decided by the U.S. Supreme Court. The court rules that laws prohibiting abortions violate a constitutional right to privacy. Texas attorney Sarah Weddington argues the case on behalf of "Jane Roe."

1975: First cases of Lyme disease discovered in Lyme, Connecticut, where the disease got its name.

1977: The U.S. Consumer Product Safety Commission announces a ban on lead paint on toys and furniture, nearly 60 years after studies show that lead is dangerous to children and decades of opposition from the lead industry.

1980: The American Psychological Association adds Post Traumatic Stress Syndrome (PTSD) to its DSM-III (Diagnostic and Statistical Manual of Mental Disorders) classification system.

1981: A mysterious epidemic was identified as Acquired Immune Deficiency Syndrome (AIDS). It was found to be caused by the Human immunodeficiency virus (HIV).

1987: The F.D.A. approves Prozac, which becomes the most prescribed antidepressant drug worldwide.

1988: Congress passed the Medical Waste Tracking Act of 1988.

1990: The Nutrition Labeling Education Act was signed into law. The act required food manufacturers to disclose the fat (saturated and unsaturated), cholesterol, sodium, sugar, fiber, protein and carbohydrate content in their products.

1994: U.S. Congress passed the Violence Against Women Act, which established the Rape Prevention and Education(RPE) program at the CDC. It expired in 2012, but president Congress voted to renew it and president Obama signed the extension in March 2013.

2002: The Public Health Security and Bioterrorism Preparedness and Response Act of 2002 provided grants to improve hospitals' preparedness to respond to bioterrorism and other public health emergencies.

2003: Severe acute respiratory syndrome, or SARS, is a contagious and potentially fatal disease that first appeared in the form of a multi-country outbreak.

2005: The continued spread of a highly pathogenic avian influenza virus across eastern Asia and other countries raised concerns about a potential human pandemic.

Hurricane Katrina, one of the most destructive natural disasters in U.S. history, slams the Gulf Coast. Subsequent flooding from the failure of the New Orleans levee system adds to the crisis. Hospitals around the country respond by sending workers and supplies to the devasted areas.

2006: Two vaccines are introduced to protect against H.P.V. viruses that can cause cervical cancer and genital warts. H.P.V. is the most common sexually transmitted virus in the United States.

2009: President Barack Obama signs the Family Smoking Prevention and Tobacco Control Act, which gives the F.D.A. the power to regulate nicotine and ban tobacco advertising aimed at children.

2010: President Barack Obama signs the Affordable Health Care for America Act, with the intent of enabling millions of Americans to obtain health insurance.

2011: According to the WHO's 2011 Malaria Report, the global incidence of malaria dropped 17 percent since 2000 and by more than 50 percent in several endemic countries. Malaria-specific mortality rates fell by 26 percent worldwide. Much of this success is due to increased access to and use of insecticide-treated mosquito nets.

2012: On January 13th, India marks one year without any new polio cases diagnosed. This set the stage for India's removal from the list of polio endemic countries in February, leaving only Afghanistan, Nigeria and Pakistan as nations where transmission of the poliovirus has never been stopped.

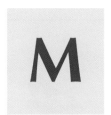

M

Mad cow disease *see* **Bovine spongiform encephalopathy**

Malaria

Definition

Malaria is a serious **infectious disease** caused by a parasite called plasmodium, which is transmitted via bites of infected mosquitoes. In the human body, the **parasites** multiply in the liver and then infect red blood cells. The disease is most common in tropical climates. It is characterized by recurrent symptoms of chills, fever, and an enlarged spleen. The disease can be treated with medication, but it often recurs. Malaria is endemic (occurs frequently in a particular locality) in many developing countries. Isolated, small outbreaks sometimes occur within the boundaries of the United States. There are concerns that climate change might allow the disease to be more widespread if suitable breeding areas for the mosquitoes are present.

Description

Malaria is a growing problem in the United States. The **Centers for Disease Control and Prevention (CDC)** continues to conduct malaria surveillance in order to detect locally acquired cases. Since the Anopheles mosquito that carries the malaria parasite exists in the United States, there is a constant risk that malaria could be reintroduced. In 2007, **CDC** reported 1,505 cases of malaria among persons in the United States. All but one of these cases were acquired outside the United States; one was acquired through a blood transfusion. More than half of the cases were reported by New York, Florida, California, Texas, New Jersey, and Maryland. Although malaria can be transmitted in blood, the U.S. blood supply is not screened for malaria. Widespread malarial epidemics are far less likely to occur in the United States,

but small localized epidemics could return to the Western world. As of 2012, primary care physicians were being advised to screen returning travelers with fever for malaria.

The picture is far more bleak, however, outside the territorial boundaries of the United States. In 2012, about 3.3 billion people, half of the world's **population**, were at risk of malaria, according to the **World Health Organization (WHO)**. Every year, this situation leads to about 250 million malaria cases and nearly one million deaths. People living in the poorest countries are the most vulnerable, including Africa, India, Southeast Asia, the Middle East, Oceania, and Central and South America. Malaria is a extremely serious problem in Africa, where one in every five childhood deaths is due to the effects of the disease. An African child has on average between 1.6 and 5.4 episodes of malaria fever each year, and a child in Africa dies every 30 seconds from the disease.

As many as 500 million people worldwide are left with chronic anemia due to malaria infection. In some parts of Africa, people battle up to 40 or more separate episodes of malaria in their lifetimes. The spread of malaria is becoming even more serious as the parasites that cause malaria develop resistance to the drugs used to treat the condition.

Causes and symptoms

Human malaria is caused by four different species of a parasite belonging to genus *Plasmodium*: *Plasmodium falciparum* (the most deadly), *Plasmodium vivax*, *Plasmodium malariae*, and *Plasmodium ovale*. The last two are fairly uncommon. Many animals can get malaria, but human malaria does not spread to animals. Similarly, animal malaria does not spread to humans.

Individuals get malaria when bitten by a female mosquito that is looking for a blood meal and is infected with the malaria parasite. The parasites enter the blood stream and travel to the liver, where they multiply. When they re-emerge in the blood, symptoms appear. By the

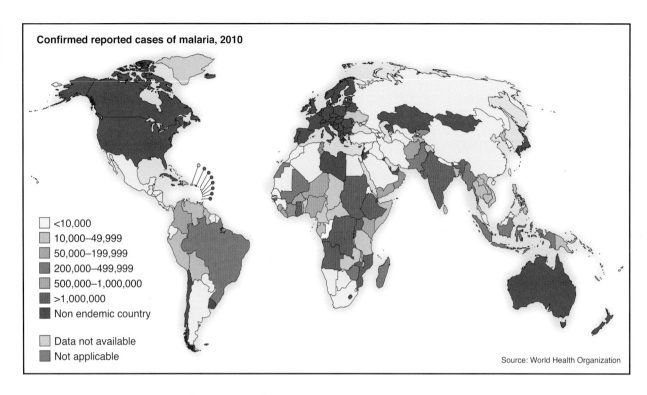

Confirmed reported cases of malaria, 2010

<10,000
10,000–49,999
50,000–199,999
200,000–499,999
500,000–1,000,000
>1,000,000
Non endemic country

Data not available
Not applicable

Source: World Health Organization

(Illustration by Electronic Illustrators Group. © 2013 Cengage Learning)

time patients show symptoms, the parasites have reproduced rapidly, clogging blood vessels and rupturing blood cells.

Malaria cannot be casually transmitted from one person to another. Instead, a mosquito bites an infected person and then passes the infection on to the next human it bites. Malaria also spreads via contaminated needles or in blood transfusions. Thus, all blood donors are carefully screened with questionnaires for possible exposure to malaria.

It is possible to contract malaria in nonendemic areas, although such cases are rare. Nevertheless, at least 89 cases of so-called airport malaria, in which travelers contract malaria while passing through crowded airport terminals, have been identified since 1969.

The amount of time between the mosquito bite and the appearance of symptoms varies, depending on the strain of parasite involved. The incubation period is usually between 8 and 12 days for falciparum malaria, but it can be as long as a month for the other types. Symptoms from some strains of *P.vivax* may not appear until 8–10 months after the mosquito bite occurred.

The primary symptom of all types of malaria is the malaria ague (chills and fever). In most cases, the fever has three stages, beginning with uncontrollable shivering for an hour or two, followed by a rapid spike in temperature (as high as 106°F), which lasts three to six

hours. Then, just as suddenly, the patient begins to sweat profusely, which will quickly bring down the fever. Other symptoms may appear, including fatigue, severe headache, and nausea and vomiting. As the sweating subsides, the patient typically feels exhausted and falls asleep. In many cases, this cycle of chills, fever, and sweating occurs every other day, or every third day, and may last for between a week and a month. Those with the chronic form of malaria may have a relapse as long as 50 years after the initial infection.

Falciparum malaria is far more severe than other types of malaria because the parasite attacks all red blood cells, not just the young or old cells, as do other types. It causes the red blood cells to become sticky. A patient with this type of malaria can die within hours of the first symptoms. The fever is prolonged. So many red blood cells are destroyed that they block the blood vessels in vital organs (especially the kidneys), and the spleen becomes enlarged. There may be brain damage, leading to coma and convulsions. The kidneys and liver may fail.

Malaria in pregnancy can lead to premature delivery, miscarriage, or stillbirth.

Certain kinds of mosquitoes (called anopheles) can pick up the parasite by biting infected humans. (The more common kinds of mosquitoes in the United States do not transmit the infection.) This is true for as long as those individuals have parasites in their blood. Since strains of

Malaria

Malaria caused an estimated 655,000 deaths in the world in 2010 (most recent year for which the World Health Organization [WHO] had statistics. These statistics represent a decline from 863,000 in 2008.

Estimated malaria cases and deaths by WHO Region, 2010

	Estimated cases	Estimated deaths
African Region	174 million	596,000
Americas Region	1 million	1,000
Eastern Mediterranean Region	10 million	15,000
European Region	200	0
South-East Asia Region	28 million	38,000
Western Pacific Region	2 million	5,000

(Table by PreMediaGlobal. © 2013 Cengage Learning)

malaria do not protect against each other, it is possible for individuals to be reinfected with the parasites repeatedly. It is also possible for individuals to develop a chronic infection without developing an effective immune response.

Diagnosis

Malaria is diagnosed by examining blood under a microscope. The parasite can be seen in the blood smears on a slide. These blood smears may need to be repeated over a 72-hour period in order to make a diagnosis. Antibody tests are not usually helpful because many people develop antibodies from past infections, and the tests may not be readily available. A laser test to detect the presence of malaria parasites in the blood was developed in 2002.

Two new techniques to speed the laboratory diagnosis of malaria show promise. The first is acridine orange (AO), a staining agent that works much faster (3–10 min) than the traditional Giemsa stain (45–60 min) in making the malaria parasites visible under a microscope. The second is a bioassay technique that measures the amount of histadine-rich protein II (HRP2) in the patient's blood. It allows for an accurate estimation of parasite development. A dip strip that tests for the presence of HRP2 in blood samples appears to be more accurate in diagnosing malaria than standard microscopic analysis.

Individuals who become ill with chills and fever after being in an area where malaria exists must see a doctor and mention their recent travel to endemic areas. Individuals with the above symptoms who have been in a high-risk area should insist on a blood test for malaria. The doctor may believe the symptoms are just the common flu virus. Malaria is often misdiagnosed by North American doctors who are not used to seeing the

disease. Delaying treatment of falciparum malaria can be fatal.

Treatment

Falciparum malaria is a medical emergency that must be treated in the hospital. The type of drugs, the method of giving them, and the length of the treatment depend on where the malaria was contracted and how sick the patient is.

For all strains except falciparum, the treatment for malaria is usually chloroquine (Aralen) by mouth for three days. Those falciparum strains suspected to be resistant to chloroquine are usually treated with a combination of quinine and tetracycline. In countries where quinine resistance is developing, other treatments may include clindamycin (Cleocin), mefloquin (Lariam), or sulfadoxone/pyrimethamine (Fansidar). Most patients receive an antibiotic for seven days. Those who are very ill may need intensive care and intravenous (IV) malaria treatment for the first three days.

Individuals who acquired falciparum malaria in the Dominican Republic, Haiti, Central America west of the Panama Canal, the Middle East, or Egypt can still be cured with chloroquine. Almost all strains of falciparum malaria in Africa, South Africa, India, and Southeast Asia are resistant to chloroquine. In Thailand and Cambodia, there are strains of falciparum malaria that have some resistance to almost all known drugs.

Patients with falciparum malaria need to be hospitalized and given antimalarial drugs in different combinations and doses depending on the resistance of the strain. Patients may need IV fluids, red blood cell transfusions, kidney dialysis, and assistance breathing.

The drug primaquine may prevent relapses after recovery from *P. vivax* or *P. ovale*. These relapses are caused by a form of the parasite that remains in the liver and can reactivate months or years later.

Another drug, halofantrine, is available abroad. While it is licensed in the United States, it is not marketed in the United States, and it is not recommended by the CDC.

Alternative treatments

The Chinese herb qiinghaosu (the Western name is artemisinin) has been used in China and Southeast Asia to fight severe malaria, and it became available in Europe in 1994. Because this treatment often fails, it is usually combined with another antimalarial drug (mefloquine) to boost its effectiveness. It is not available in the United States and other parts of the developed world due to fears of its toxicity, in addition to licensing and other issues.

KEY TERMS

Arteminisinins—A family of antimalarial products derived from an ancient Chinese herbal remedy. Two of the most popular varieties are artemether and artesunate, used mainly in Southeast Asia in combination with mefloquine.

Chloroquine—An antimalarial drug that began being used in the 1940s and stopped being used after evidence of quinine resistance appeared in the 1960s. In the early 2000s, it was considered ineffective against falciparum malaria almost everywhere. However, because it is inexpensive, it continued to be still the antimalarial drug most widely in Africa. Native individuals with partial immunity may have better results with chloroquine than travelers with no previous exposure.

Mefloquine—An antimalarial drug that was developed by the U.S. Army in the early 1980s. By the early 2000s, malaria resistance to this drug had become a problem in some parts of Asia (especially Thailand and Cambodia).

Quinine—One of the first treatments for malaria, a natural product made from the bark of the Cinchona tree. It was popular until being superseded by chloroquine in the 1940s. In the wake of widespread chloroquine resistance, however, it became popular again. Quinine, or its close relative quinidine, can be given intravenously to treat severe *Falciparum* malaria.

Sulfadoxone/pyrimethamine (Fansidar)—An antimalarial drug developed in the 1960s. It was the first drug tried in some parts of the world where chloroquine resistance is widespread. It has been associated with severe allergic reactions due to its sulfa component.

The Western herb wormwood (*Artemesia annua*) that is taken as a daily dose can be effective against malaria. Protecting the liver with herbs such as goldenseal (*Hydrastis canadensis*), Chinese goldenthread (*Coptis chinensis*), and milk thistle (*Silybum marianum*) can be used as preventive treatment. Taking precautions to prevent mosquitoes from biting is another possible way to avoid malaria.

Prognosis

If treated in the early stages, malaria can be cured. Those who live in areas where malaria is epidemic, however, can contract the disease repeatedly, never fully recovering between bouts of acute infection.

Prevention

Malaria is an especially difficult disease to prevent by vaccination because the parasite goes through several separate stages. One vaccine appeared to protect up to 60% of people exposed to malaria. This was evident during field trials for the drug that were conducted in South America and Africa.

The World Health Association (**WHO**) worked to eliminate malaria between 1970 and 2000 by controlling mosquitoes. Their efforts were successful as long as the pesticide DDT killed mosquitoes and antimalarial drugs cured those who were infected. In the early 2000s, however, the problem returned a hundredfold, especially in Africa. Because both the mosquito and parasite were extremely resistant to the insecticides designed to kill them, governments tried to teach people to take antimalarial drugs as a preventive medicine and avoid getting bitten by mosquitoes.

Those who use the following preventive measures get fewer infections than those who do not:

• Between dusk and dawn, remain indoors in well-screened areas.

• Sleep inside pyrethrin or permethrin repellent-soaked mosquito nets.

• Wear clothes over the entire body.

Individuals visiting endemic areas should take antimalarial drugs starting a day or two before they leave the United States. The drugs used are usually chloroquine or mefloquine. This treatment is continued through at least four weeks after leaving the endemic area. However, even those who take antimalarial drugs and are careful to avoid mosquito bites can still contract malaria.

International travelers are at risk for becoming infected. Most Americans who have acquired falciparum malaria visited sub-Saharan Africa; travelers in Asia and South America are less at risk. Travelers who stay in air conditioned hotels on tourist itineraries in urban or resort areas are at lower risk than backpackers, missionaries, and Peace Corps volunteers. Some people in western cities where malaria does not usually exist may acquire the infection from a mosquito carried onto a jet. This is called airport or runway malaria.

Resources

BOOKS

Ashraf A. "Malaria." In *Ferri's Clinical Advisor 2010.* Philadelphia: Mosby Elsevier, 2010.

Beers, Mark H., and Robert Berkow, eds. "Extraintestinal Protozoa: Malaria." *The Merck Manual of Diagnosis and*

Therapy. Whitehouse Station, NJ: Merck Research Laboratories, 2004.

Fairhurst, R. M., and T. E. Wellems. "Plasmodium Species (Malaria)." In *Principles and Practice of Infectious Diseases*, 7th ed. Edited by G. L. Mandell, J. E. Bennett, and R. Dolin. Philadelphia: Elsevier Churchill Livingstone, 2009.

Krogstad, D. J. "Malaria." In *Cecil Medicine*, 23rd ed. Edited by Lee Goldman, and D. Ausiello. Philadelphia: Saunders Elsevier, 2007.

Rocco, Fiammetta. *Quinine: Malaria and the Quest for a Cure That Changed the World.* New York: Harper Perennial, 2004.

World Health Organization. *World Malaria Report 2008.* Geneva: World Health Organization, 2008.

PERIODICALS

Van Lieshout, M., et al. "Climate Change and Malaria: Analysis of the SRES Climate and Socio-Economic Scenarios." *Global Environmental Change* 14 (2004): 87–99.

WEBSITES

Bill & Melinda Gates Foundation. "Malaria." http://www.gatesfoundation.org/GlobalHealth/Pri_Diseases/Malaria/ (accessed March 1, 2012).

Centers for Disease Control and Prevention (CDC). "Malaria." http://www.cdc.gov/malaria (accessed March 1, 2012)

World Health Organization (WHO). "Malaria: Global Malaria Programme (GMP)." WHO Programs and Projects. http://www.who.int/malaria (accessed March 1, 2012).

World Health Organization (WHO). "Malaria: Roll Back Malaria Partnership." WHO Programs and Projects. http://www.rbm.who.int/ (accessed March 1, 2012).

ORGANIZATIONS

Centers for Disease Control Malaria Hotline, (770) 332-4555

Centers for Disease Control Travelers Hotline, (770) 332-4559

Carol A. Turkington
Rebecca J. Frey, PhD
Karl Finley

Measles

Definition

Measles is an infection caused by a virus, which causes an illness displaying a characteristic skin rash known as an exanthem. Measles is also sometimes called rubeola, 5-day measles, red measles, or hard measles.

There are two types of measles, each caused by a different virus. Although both produce a rash and fever, they are different diseases. When most people use the

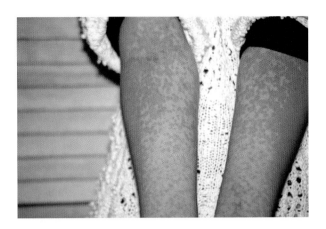

Measles rash on the arms of a female patient.
(© mediacolor's / Alamy)

term measles they are referring to rubeola. The rubeola virus causes red measles, also known as hard measles or measles. Although most people recover without problems, rubeola can lead to **pneumonia** or inflammation of the brain (**encephalitis**). The second type of measle is called the **rubella** virus or German measles, also known as three-day measles. This type of measle is usually a milder disease. However, this virus can cause significant **birth defects** if an infected pregnant woman passes the virus to her unborn child.

Description

Measles infections appear all over the world. Prior to the current effective **immunization** program, large-scale measles outbreaks occurred on a two to three-year cycle, usually in the winter and spring. Smaller outbreaks occurred during the off-years. Babies up to about eight months of age are usually protected from contracting measles, due to immune cells they receive from their mothers in the uterus. Once someone has had measles infection, he or she can never get it again.

Historically, one of the earliest known written descriptions of measles as a disease was provided by an Arab physician in the ninth century who described the differences between measles and **smallpox** in his medical notes. Later, a Scottish physician, Francis Home, demonstrated in 1757 that measles was caused by an infectious agent present in the blood of patients. In 1954 the virus that causes measles was isolated in Boston, Massachusetts, by John F. Enders and Thomas C. Peebles. Before measles vaccine was developed in 1963, nearly all children got measles by the time they were 15 years of age and about 450-500 people died because of measles, 48,000 were hospitalized, 7,000 had seizures, and about 1,000 suffered permanent brain damage or deafness. Today there are only about 50 cases a year reported in the United States, and most of these originate outside the country.

Demographics

As a result of widespread immunization, the measles virus does not circulate in the United States. All reported cases of measles in the United States have been brought in from other countries, usually Europe and Asia. Travelers leaving the United States should be immune to measles. Although measles is usually considered a childhood disease, it can be contracted at any age by a person who never had the disease or been vaccinated. Unvaccinated individuals are 22 times more likely to get measles than are who those who have two measles vaccines, usually given as measles, **mumps** and rubella vaccine (MMR).

Causes and symptoms

Measles is caused by a type of virus called a paramyxovirus. It is an extremely contagious infection, spread through the tiny droplets that may spray into the air when an individual carrying the virus sneezes or coughs. About 85% of those people exposed to the virus will become infected with it. About 95% of those people infected with the virus will develop the illness called measles. Once someone is infected with the virus, it takes about 7–18 days before he or she actually becomes ill. The most contagious time period is the three to five days before symptoms begin through about four days after the characteristic measles rash has begun to appear.

The first signs of measles infection are fever, extremely runny nose, a cough, and red, runny eyes. A few days later, a rash appears in the mouth, particularly on the mucous membrane which lines the cheeks. This rash consists of tiny white dots (like grains of salt or sand) on a reddish bump. These are called Koplik's spots, and are unique to measles infection. The throat becomes red, swollen, and sore.

A couple of days after the appearance of the Koplik's spots, the measles rash begins. It appears in a characteristic progression, from the head, face, and neck, to the trunk, then abdomen, and next out along the arms and legs. The rash starts out as flat, red patches, but eventually develops some bumps. The rash may be somewhat itchy. When the rash begins to appear, the fever usually climbs higher, sometimes reaching as high as 105°F (40.5°C). There may be nausea, vomiting, diarrhea, and multiple swollen lymph nodes. The cough is usually more problematic at this point, and the patient feels awful. The rash usually lasts about five days. As it fades, it turns a brownish color, and eventually the affected skin becomes dry and flaky.

Many patients (about 5–15%) develop other complications. Bacterial infections, such as ear infections, sinus infections, and pneumonia are common, especially in children. Other viral infections may also strike the patient, including croup, bronchitis, laryngitis, or viral pneumonia. Inflammation of the liver, appendix, intestine, or lymph nodes within the abdomen may cause other complications. Rarely, inflammations of the heart or kidneys, a drop in platelet count (causing episodes of difficult-to-control bleeding), or reactivation of an old **tuberculosis** infection can occur.

An extremely serious complication of measles infection is swelling of the brain. Called encephalitis, this can occur up to several weeks after the basic measles symptoms have resolved. About one out of every thousand patients develops this complication, and about 10-15% of these patients die. Symptoms include fever, headache, sleepiness, seizures, and coma. Long-term problems following recovery from measles encephalitis may include seizures and mental retardation.

A very rare complication of measles can occur up to 10 years following the initial infection. Called subacute sclerosing panencephalitis, this is a slowly progressing, smoldering swelling and destruction of the entire brain. It is most common among people who had measles infection prior to the age of two years. Symptoms include changes in personality, decreased intelligence with accompanying school problems, decreased coordination, involuntary jerks and movements of the body. The disease progresses so that the individual becomes increasingly dependent, ultimately becoming bedridden and unaware of his or her surroundings. Blindness may develop, and the temperature may spike (rise rapidly) and fall unpredictably as the brain structures responsible for temperature regulation are affected. Death is inevitable.

Measles during pregnancy is a serious disease, leading to increased risk of a miscarriage or stillbirth. In addition, the mother's illness may progress to pneumonia.

Risk factors

People who do not receive the vaccine for measles are much more likely to develop the disease. Unvaccinated people traveling to developing countries, where measles is more common, are also at higher risk of catching the disease, and people who do not have enough vitamin A in their diets are more likely to contract measles and to have more severe symptoms.

Diagnosis

Measles infection is almost always diagnosed based on its characteristic symptoms, including Koplik's spots, and a rash which spreads from central body structures out toward the arms and legs. If there is any doubt as to the diagnosis, then a specimen of body fluids (mucus, urine) can be collected and combined with fluorescent-tagged measles virus antibodies. Antibodies are produced by the body's immune cells that can recognize and bind to markers (antigens) on the outside of specific organisms, in this case the measles virus. Once the fluorescent antibodies have attached themselves to the measles antigens in the specimen, the specimen can be viewed under a special microscope to verify the presence of measles virus.

Treatment

There are no treatments available to stop measles infection. Treatment is primarily aimed at helping the patient to be as comfortable as possible, and watching carefully so that **antibiotics** can be started promptly if a bacterial infection develops. Fever and discomfort can be treated with acetaminophen. Children with measles should never be given aspirin, as this has caused the fatal disease Reye's syndrome in the past. A cool-mist vaporizer may help decrease the cough. Patients should be given a lot of liquids to drink, in order to avoid dehydration from the fever.

Some studies have shown that children with measles encephalitis benefit from relatively large doses of vitamin A.

Alternative treatment

Botanical immune enhancement (with echinacea, for example) can assist the body in working through this viral infection. Homeopathic support also can be effective throughout the course of the illness. Some specific alternative treatments to soothe patients with measles include the Chinese herbs bupleurum (*Bupleurum chinense*) and peppermint (*Mentha piperita*), as well as a preparation made from empty cicada (*Cryptotympana atrata*) shells. The itchiness of the rash can be relieved with witch hazel (*Hamamelis virginiana*), chickweed (*Stellaria media*), or oatmeal baths. The eyes can be soothed with an eyewash made from the herb eyebright (*Euphrasia officinalis*). Practitioners of ayurvedic medicine recommend ginger or clove tea.

Prognosis

The prognosis for an otherwise healthy, well-nourished child who contracts measles is usually quite good. In developing countries, however, death rates may reach 15–25%. Adolescents and adults usually have a more difficult course. Women who contract the disease while pregnant may give birth to a baby with hearing

---

KEY TERMS

Antibodies—Cells made by the immune system which have the ability to recognize foreign invaders (bacteria, viruses), and thus stimulate the immune system to kill them.

Antigens—Markers on the outside of such organisms as bacteria and viruses, which allow antibodies to recognize foreign invaders.

Encephalitis—Swelling, inflammation of the brain.

Exanthem (plural, exanthems or exanthemata)—A skin eruption regarded as a characteristic sign of such diseases as measles, German measles, and scarlet fever.

Koplik's spots—Tiny spots occurring inside the mouth, especially on the inside of the cheek. These spots consist of minuscule white dots (like grains of salt or sand) set onto a reddened bump. Unique to measles.

MMR vaccine—The standard measles, mumps, and rubella (MMR) vaccine that is given to prevent measles, mumps and rubella (German measles). The MMR vaccine is now given in two dosages. The first should be given at 12-15 months of age. The second vaccination should be given at 4-6 years. There are some exceptions depending on a person's health condition.

---

impairment. Although only 1 in 1,000 patients with measles will develop encephalitis, 10–15% of those who do will die, and about another 25% will be left with permanent brain damage.

Prevention

Measles is a highly preventable infection. A very effective vaccine exists, made of live measles viruses which have been treated so that they cannot cause actual infection. The important markers on the viruses are intact, however, which causes an individual's immune system to react. Immune cells called antibodies are produced, which in the event of a future infection with measles virus will quickly recognize the organism, and kill it off. Measles vaccines are usually given at about 15 months of age; because prior to that age, the baby's immune system is not mature enough to initiate a reaction strong enough to ensure long-term protection from the virus. A repeat injection should be given at about 10 or 11 years of age. Outbreaks on college campuses have occurred among unimmunized or incorrectly immunized students.

QUESTIONS TO ASK YOUR DOCTOR

- What are the indications that I may have measles?
- How contagious is this disease?
- What treatment options do you recommend for me?
- What kind of changes can I expect to see with the antibiotics you have prescribed for me?

Measles vaccine should not be given to a pregnant woman, however, in spite of the seriousness of gestational measles. The reason for not giving this particular vaccine during pregnancy is the risk of transmitting measles to the unborn child.

Surprisingly, new cases of measles began being reported in some countries—including Great Britain—in 2001 because of parents' fears about vaccine safety. The combined vaccine for measles, mumps, and rubella (MMR) was claimed to cause **autism** or bowel disorders in some children. However, the **World Health Organization (WHO)** says there is no scientific merit to these claims. The United Nations expressed concern that unwarranted fear of the vaccine would begin spreading the disease in developing countries, and ultimately in developed countries as well. Parents in Britain began demanding the measles vaccine as a separate dose and scientists were exploring that option as an alternative to the combined MMR vaccine. Unfortunately, several children died during an outbreak of measles in Dublin because they had not received the vaccine. Child mortality due to measles is considered largely preventable, and making the MMR vaccine widely available in developing countries is part of WHO's strategy to reduce child mortality by two-thirds by the year 2015.

Public health role and response

According to the Centers for Disease Control (**CDC**), worldwide, there are estimated to be 20 million cases and 164,000 deaths linked to measles each year. More than half of the deaths occur in India. In the United States, measles was declared eliminated in 2000 due to high **vaccination** coverage and effective public health response. That means measles no longer occurs year round in the United States. This effect is called "herd" immunity. But herd immunity may now be weakening a bit since some parents are choosing to not vaccinate their children. Measles is still common in some parts of Europe, Asia, the Pacific, and Africa. Travelers who have

not been vaccinated are at risk of getting the disease and spreading it to their friends and family members who may not be up to date with vaccinations. Because of this risk, all travelers should be up to date on their vaccinations, regardless of where they are going. Measles is one of the most contagious diseases, and even domestic travelers may be exposed on airplanes or in airports.

Resources

BOOKS

Corrales-Medina VF, et al.Viral and rickettsial infections. In: McPhee SJ, et al. *Current Medical Diagnosis & Treatment 2011*. 50th ed. New York, N.Y.: The McGraw-Hill Companies; 2011.

Justin L. Kaplan, and Robert S. Porter, eds. *The Merck Manual of Diagnosis and Therapy*. 19th ed. Whitehouse Station, NJ: Merck Research Laboratories, 2012.

Parker AA, et al. Measles (Rubeola). In: Brunette GW, et al. *CDC Health Information for International Travel 2010.* Philadelphia, Pa.: Mosby Elsevier; 2009.

PERIODICALS

Chiba, M. E., M. Saito, N. Suzuki, et al. "Measles Infection in Pregnancy." *Journal of Infection* 47 (July 2003): 40–44.

"Measles—United States, 2011. (From the Centers for Disease Control and Prevention)." *Journal of the American Medical Association* 2012;307(22):2363-2365.

Scott, L. A., and M. S. Stone. "Viral Exanthems." *Dermatology Online Journal* 9 (August 2003): 4.

Sur, D. K., D. H. Wallis, and T. X. O'Connell. "Vaccinations in Pregnancy." *American Family Physician* 68 (July 15, 2003): 299–304.

ORGANIZATIONS

American Academy of Pediatrics (AAP), 141 Northwest Point Boulevard, Elk Grove Village, IL 60007-1098, (847) 434-4000, Fax: (847) 424-8000, kidsdocs@aap.org, http://www.aap.org

Centers for Disease Control and Prevention (CDC), 1600 Clifton Road, Atlanta, GA 30333, (800) 232-4636, cdcinfo@cdc.gov, http://www.cdc.gov.

Rosalyn Carson-DeWitt, MD
Rebecca J. Frey, PhD
Karl Finley

Medicaid and Medicare

Definition

Medicaid is a federal-state entitlement program for low-income citizens of the United States. The Medicaid program is part of Title XIX of the Social Security Act Amendment that became law in 1965. Medicaid offers

Approximate percentage of persons under age 65 with private health insurance coverage, public health plan coverage, and uninsured, United States, 1997– March 2012

Year	Percent of persons with private health insurance coverage	Percent of persons with public health plan coverage	Percent uninsured[1]
1997	70.8	13.6	17.4
1998	72.0	12.7	16.5
1999	73.1	12.4	16.0
2000	71.8	12.9	16.8
2001	71.6	13.6	16.2
2002	69.8	15.2	16.5
2003	68.2	16.0	17.2
2004	68.6	16.1	16.6
2005	68.4	16.8	16.0
2006	66.5	18.1	16.8
2007	66.8	18.1	16.4
2008	65.4	19.3	16.7
2009	62.9	21.0	17.5
2010	61.2	22.0	18.2
2011	61.2	23.0	17.3
2012 (Jan. – Mar.)	60.2	23.5	17.6

[1] Includes Medicaid, Children's Health Insurance Program (CHIP), state-sponsored or other government-sponsored health plan, Medicare (disability), and military plans.

Source: Schiller J.S., Ward B.W., Freeman G. *Early Release of Selected Estimates Based on Data from the January–March 2012 National Health Interview Survey.* National Center for Health Statistics, September 2012. Available from: http://www.cdc.gov/nchs/nhis.htm

(Illustration by Electronic Illustrators Group. © 2013 Cengage Learning)

federal matching funds to states for costs incurred in paying health care providers for serving covered individuals. State participation is voluntary, but since 1982, all 50 states have chosen to participate in Medicaid.

Medicare is federal health insurance available to persons age 65 years and up, as well as to persons under age 65 who have certain types of disabilities and persons of any age who suffer from end-stage renal disease (ESRD) or Lou Gehrig's disease. Like Medicaid, Medicare laws were enacted in 1965.

Medicare coverage is determined by state and federal laws, national coverage decisions that Medicare makes, and local coverage decisions made by the companies in a state that process Medicare claims.

Description

Medicaid benefits

Medicaid benefits cover basic health care and long-term care services for eligible persons. About 58% of Medicaid spending covers hospital and other acute care services. The remaining 42% pays for nursing home and long-term care.

States that choose to participate in Medicaid must offer the following basic services:

• hospital care, both inpatient and outpatient

• nursing home care

• physician services

• laboratory and diagnostic x-ray services

• immunizations and other screening, diagnostic, and treatment services for children

• family planning

• health center and rural health clinic services

• nurse midwife and nurse practitioner services

• physician assistant services

Participating states may offer the following optional services and receive federal matching funds for them:

- prescription medications

- institutional care for the mentally retarded

- home- or community-based care for the elderly, including case management

- personal care for the disabled

- dental and vision care for eligible adults

Because participating states are allowed to design their own benefits packages as long as they meet federal minimum requirements, Medicaid benefits vary considerably from state to state. About half of all Medicaid spending covers groups of people and services above the federal minimum.

Medicare benefits

Medicare covers approximately 47 million American people. It has four parts, which offer different types of coverage:

- Part A—hospital insurance

- Part B—medical insurance

- Part C—Medicare Advantage Plans

- Part D—prescription drug coverage

A person may file for Medicare when filing for federal government retirement benefits (or a person may file for Medicare only and not retirement benefits) or when he or she files for disability benefits. The government notifies individuals of their eligibility for Medicare a few months before they become eligible, and automatically registers people for Medicare if they already receive Social Security. A Medicare identification card is sent to these individuals three months before they reach 65 years of age or when they reach their 25th month of disability.

Most individuals who purchase Part A must also have Part B and pay the monthly premiums for both parts. A person has the option of declining Part B by following the directions contained on the Medicare card. If Medicare Part B is declined, the person must return the Part B card. Medicare Part A covers care provided in a hospital, skilled nursing facility, nursing home, or hospice, or through a home health agency. Medicare Part B covers medically necessary services or supplies required to diagnose or treat a medical condition as well as preventive services designed to prevent illness or detect the presence of an illness at an early, more treatable, stage. These services are available at no cost if received from a health care provider who accepts payment directly from Medicare.

To sign up for Medicare Part A and Part B, a person may take one of these four steps:

- Apply online at the Social Security website (socialsecurity.gov/medicareonly).

- Apply in person at his or her Social Security office.

- Apply by phone, by calling 800-772-1213.

- Apply by calling the Railroad Retirement Board at 877-772-5772, if appropriate for that individual.

A plan that is offered by a private company, which contracts with Medicare to provide both Part A and Part B is a Medicare health plan. The types of Medicare health plans are:

- Medicare Advantage Plans—offered by a private company to provide Part A and Part B Medicare benefits. These types of plans may be Health Maintenance Organizations (HMOs); Preferred Provider Organizations (PPOs); Private Fee-for-Service Plans; Special Needs Plans; and Medicare Medical Savings Account Plans. Most of the Medicare Advantage Plans provide coverage for prescriptions drugs.

- Medicare Cost Plan—a type of HMO that is similar to a Medicare Advantage Plan. With this type of plan, services provided out of network are covered under Original Medicare, and the individual would pay coinsurance and deductibles for Medicare Part A and Part B.

- Demonstration/Pilot Programs—Restricted to a certain geographic area or to a certain group of people, these programs test improvements in Medicare coverage on a smaller scale.

- Programs of All-inclusive Care for the Elderly (PACE)—Community-based care and services for persons age 55 years and up who would require nursing home care if this program were not available to them. The program provides services that allow these people to continue to live in their communities.

Eligibility for Medicaid and Medicare

MEDICAID ELIGIBILITY. Medicaid covers three major groups of low-income Americans:

- All recipients. In 2010, Medicaid covered an estimated 53.9 million low-income persons in the United States. It is estimated that Medicaid will serve more than 85 million people in 2020.

- Parents and children. In 2010, 26.8 children were enrolled in Medicaid.

- The disabled. About 18% of Medicaid recipients are blind or disabled. Most of these persons are eligible for Medicaid because they receive assistance through the Supplemental Security Income (SSI) program. These individuals account for 45 % of Medicaid expenditures.

KEY TERMS

Categorically needy—A term that describes certain groups of Medicaid recipients who qualify for the basic mandatory package of Medicaid benefits. There are categorically needy groups whom states participating in Medicaid are required to cover, and other groups whom the states have the option to cover.

Department of Health and Human Service (DHHS)—A federal agency that houses the Centers for Medicare and Medicaid Services and distributes funds for Medicaid.

Entitlement—A program that creates a legal obligation by the federal government to any person, business, or government entity that meets the legally defined criteria. Medicaid is an entitlement both for eligible individuals and for the states that decide to participate in it.

Federal poverty level (FPL)—The definition of poverty provided by the federal government, used as the reference point to determine Medicaid eligibility for certain groups of beneficiaries. The FPL is adjusted every year to allow for inflation.

Health Care Financing Administration (HCFA)—A federal agency that provides guidelines for the Medicaid program.

Medically needy—A term that describes a group whose coverage is optional with the states because of high medical expenses. These persons meet category requirements of Medicaid (they are children or parents or elderly or disabled), but their income is too high to qualify them for coverage as categorically needy.

Supplemental Security Income (SSI)—A federal entitlement program that provides cash assistance to low-income blind, disabled, and elderly people. In most states, people receiving SSI benefits are eligible for Medicaid.

All Medicaid recipients must have incomes and resources below specified eligibility levels. These levels vary from state to state, depending on the local cost of living and other factors. For example, in 2006, the federal **poverty** level (FPL) was determined to be $16,600 for a family of three on the mainland of the United States, but $24,900 in Hawaii and $29,050 in Alaska.

In most cases, persons must be citizens of the United States to be eligible for Medicaid, although legal immigrants may qualify under some circumstances,

depending on their date of entry. Illegal aliens are not eligible for Medicaid, except for emergency care.

Persons must fit into an eligibility category to receive Medicaid, even if their income is low. Childless couples and single childless adults who are not disabled or elderly are not eligible for Medicaid.

MEDICARE ELIGIBILITY. Medicare Part A is available free to some persons; others may need to pay for it. It is free for persons age 65 who:

- already receive Social Security or Railroad Retirement Board benefits

- are eligible to receive Social Security or Railroad Retirement Boar benefits but have not filed for them

- had Medicare-covered government employment or had a spouse with such

Medicare is available free of charge to persons under age 65 who received Social Security or Railroad Retirement board disability benefits for 24 months or who have ESRD and meet the requirements.

Persons in higher income categories must pay a monthly premium for Medicare Part B and Part D.

Costs to society

Medicaid costs

From 1971 to 2010, the average growth in Medicaid expenditures was 11.5%.

Although more than half (54%) of all Medicaid beneficiaries are children, most of the money (more than 70%) goes for services for the elderly and disabled. The single largest portion of Medicaid money pays for long-term care for the elderly. Only 18% of Medicaid funds are spent on services for children.

There are several factors involved in the steep rise of Medicaid costs:

- The rise in the number of eligible individuals. As the lifespan of most Americans continues to increase, the number of elderly individuals eligible for Medicaid also rises. The fastest-growing age group in the United States is people over 85.

- The price of medical and long-term care. Advances in medical technology, including expensive diagnostic imaging tests, cause these costs to rise.

- The increased use of services covered by Medicaid.

- The expansion of state coverage from the minimum benefits package to include optional groups and optional services.

The need to contain Medicaid costs is considered one of the most problematic policy issues facing legislators. In addition, the complexity of the Medicaid system, its vulnerability to billing fraud and other abuses, the confusing variety of the benefits packages available in different states, and the time-consuming paperwork are other problems that disturb both taxpayers and legislators.

Medicaid has increased the demand for health care services in the United States without greatly impacting or improving the quality of health care for low-income Americans. Medicaid impacts the employment of several hundred thousand health care workers, including health care providers, administrators, and support staff. Participation in Medicaid is optional for physicians and nursing homes. Many do not participate in the program, because the reimbursement rates are low. As a result, many low-income people who are dependent on Medicaid must go to overcrowded facilities, where they often receive substandard health care.

Medicare costs

Medicare is the largest health insurance program in the United States. In 2010, Medicare expenditures totaled $524 million, or 15% of federal spending. By 2020, it is projected that Medicare will account for 17% of federal expenditures. Growth in Medicare spending averaged nearly 9% between 1985 and 2009. In 2006, the addition of pharmaceutical coverage contributed to the rise in expenditures. Growth in Medicare expenditures is predicted to fall because of decreases in reimbursements to physicians due to cuts in the fees that Medicare will pay to them.

The large increase in the number of Medicare enrollees between 1985 and 2009 was attributed to the large number of persons born during the Great Depression who had reached the age of eligibility for Medicare during that timeframe. In that period, more than 600,000 individuals became eligible for Medicare each year. Between 2010 and 2030, Medicare coverage is expected to grow at a rate of 1.6 million additional enrollees per year, reaching 80 million enrollees in 2030.

Resources

BOOKS

Atlantic Publishing Company. *The Complete Guide to Medicaid and Nursing Home Costs: How to Keep Your Family Assets Protected - Up to Date Medicaid Secrets You Need to Know*. Ocala, FL: Atlantic Publishing Company, 2008.

Engel, J. *Poor People's Medicine: Medicaid and American Charity Care Since 1965*. Durham, NC: Duke University Press, 2006.

Scott, S.W. *The Medicaid Handbook 2007: Protecting Your Assets From Nursing Home Costs*. 3rd ed. Largo, FL: Masveritas Publishing, 2007.

Smith, D., and J.D. Moore. *Medicaid Politics and Policy*. New Brunswick, NJ: Transaction Publishers, 2007.

Stewart, Marcia, Ed. *Social Security, Medicare and Government Pensions: Get the Most Out of Your Retirement*. Berkeley, CA: NOLO, 2012.

PERIODICALS

Bhuridej, P., KR. A. Kuthy, S.D. Flach, K.E. Keller, D.V. Dawson, M.J. Kanellis, and P.C. Damiano. "Four-year cost-utility analyses of sealed and nonsealed first permanent molars in Iowa Medicaid-enrolled children." *Journal of Public Health Dentistry* 67, no. 4 (2007): 191–198.

Churchill, S.S., B.J. Williams, and N.L. Villareale. "Characteristics of publicly insured children with high dental expenses." *Journal of Public Health Dentistry* 67, no. 4 (2007): 199–207.

Goetzel, R.Z., D. Schecter, R.J. Ozminkowski, D.C. Stapleton, P.J. Lapin, J.M. McGinnis, C.R. Gordon, and L. Breslow. "Can health promotion programs save Medicare money?." *Clinical Interventions in Aging 2*, no. 1 (2007): 117–122.

Grabowski, D.C. "Medicare and Medicaid: conflicting incentives for long-term care." *Milbank Quarterly* 85, no. 4 (2007): 579–610.

Perry, C.D., and G.M. Kenney. "Preventive care for children in low-income families: how well do Medicaid and state children's health insurance programs do?" *Pediatrics* 120, no. 6 (2007): e1393–e1401.

Potetz, Lisa, Juliette Cubanski, and Tricia Neuman. "Medicare Spending and Financing: A Primern. The Henry J. Kaiser Family Foundation" *Medicare Report February 2011*.

Truffer, Christopher J., F.S.A., John D. Klemm, Ph.D., A.S.A., M.A.A.A., Christian J. Wolfe, A.S.A., and Kathryn E. Rennie "Centers for Medicare and Medicaid Services." *2011 Actuarial Report on the Financial Outlook for Medicaid March 2012*.

WEBSITES

Centers for Medicare and Medicaid Services, U.S. Department of Health and Human Services. Information about Medicaid. 2007 [cited December 26, 2007 and September 24, 2012]. http://cms.hhs.gov/.

National Association of State Medicaid Directors. Information about Medicaid. 2007 [cited December 26, 2007]. http://www.nasmd.org/Home/home_news.asp.

National Governor's Association. Information about Medicaid. 2007 [cited December 26, 2007]. http://www.nga.org/portal/site/nga.

Social Security Administration. Information about Medicaid. 2007 [cited December 26, 2007]. http://www.ssa.gov/.

ORGANIZATIONS

Henry J. Kaiser Family Foundation, 2400 Sand Hill Road, Menlo Park, CA 94025, (650) 854-9400 Fax: (650) 854-4800, http://www.kff.org/

National Center for Policy Analysis, 12770 Coit Rd., Suite 800, Dallas, TX 75251-1339, (972) 386-6272 Fax: (972) 386-0924, http://www.ncpa.org

National Library of Medicine, http://www.nlm.nih.gov/medlineplus/medicaid.html

United States Department of Health and Human Services, 200 Independence Avenue SW, Washington, DC 20201, http://www.hhs.gov.

L. Fleming Fallon, Jr, MD, DrPH
Rhonda Cloos, RN

Medical waste

Definition

Medical waste is solid waste from medical or clinical uses at hospitals, clinics, physician offices, dental offices, blood banks, medical research facilities, and veterinary facilities. Medical waste is a form of hazardous waste that is stained or soaked with blood or includes body tissues or organs. Medical waste also can be deemed hazardous because it contains certain toxins or is radioactive.

Description

Waste from medical practices and facilities can include used needles, syringes, surgical gloves, surgical instruments, blood-soaked bandages, lab samples, or body parts. This type of waste can expose people who handle it, and in turn an entire community, to infection. Medical waste materials also can include toxic chemicals, pharmaceuticals, or radioactive materials that can cause health risks to people and pollute the environment.

The **Environmental Protection Agency (EPA)** began to define and control the tracking and disposal of medical waste in 1989 after Congress passed the Medical Waste Tracking Act of 1988. The act came about mostly because medical waste washed up on several East Coast beaches. Congress directed the **EPA** to gather data on the sources, associated health hazards, and current procedures and regulations for management and disposal of the waste. The EPA also was to evaluate the health hazards associated with transporting, incinerating, and burying medical waste materials in a landfill, and disposing of them in a sanitary sewer system. Under the act, the EPA gathered a lot of data, and most states subsequently controlled medical waste under local regulations.

Infection control practices in hospitals were emphasized and improved following the HIV/AIDS epidemic in the 1980s to better control the spread of the infection to healthcare workers or patients. This work included new hospital policies and government regulations regarding using and disposing of needles and other medical waste. New policies and regulations have been used around the world to better control the spread of many infections, most notably HIV and **hepatitis**.

Effects on public health

Careless handling of hazardous medical waste can have several detrimental effects on public health. Medical waste containing blood and other body fluids or body parts can spread diseases. Waste with needles and other sharp objects presents physical hazards, and toxic or radioactive waste can harm individuals or the environment.

Risk factors

Medical waste use and disposal is not regulated everywhere in the world, and little research on public health effects from medical waste has been conducted in developing countries. What is more, there can be hazards associated with small, scattered sources of medical waste. It also can be impossible to enforce all medical waste management in spite of best efforts. As recently as September 2012, Volusia County, Florida, authorities reported medical waste washing ashore at Ormond Beach. The waste included hypodermic needles and medicine bottles that spread over a mile. The source of the waste was unknown.

Demographics

An EPA study reported that approximately 3.2 million tons of medical waste are produced in the United States each year. Not surprisingly, hospitals, long-term health care facilities, and physicians' offices are the major producers of medical wastes, which account for about 0.3% by weight of all municipal solid waste. However, facilities that produce less than 50 lb (23 kg) of medical waste per month are exempt from most requirements. More people are being treated at home, and many people with diabetes treat themselves with daily injections. In short, it is difficult to adequately measure all of the medical waste in the United States or elsewhere in the world.

In addition to ongoing concerns about the potential for medical waste to spread HIV/AIDs and hepatitis, other disease outbreaks can be caused or intensified by medical waste. In 2009, **World Health Organization (WHO)** officially recognized the 2009 H1N1 virus as the cause of **influenza** and noted that a flu **pandemic** was underway. This announcement caused increased attention to the role medical waste can play in spreading the virus through contaminated tissues, gloves, masks, and other waste.

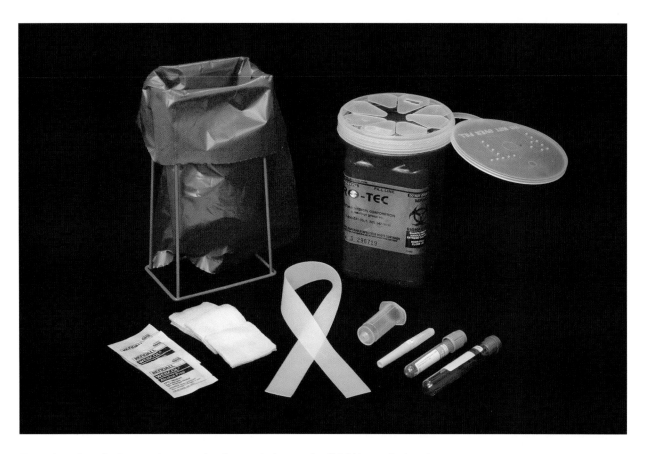

Examples of medical waste that must be disposed of properly. *(CDC/James Gathany)*

Costs to society

There are potential health, pollution, and esthetic effects of unregulated medical waste. It is expensive for medical facilities to control biohazardous waste and ensure infectious and toxic materials do not enter the general waste stream or pollute communities' air and **water**. Healthcare facilities can spend five to 10 times as much to dispose of regulated medical waste as they do their general solid waste.

Common health problems

If not managed properly, medical waste can spread disease from hospital and other clinical settings to the general public. Occupational safety also is a concern because healthcare workers can become infected with diseases their patients have if they do not follow infection control procedures. Infections such as HIV and hepatitis can spread from patients to workers. In addition, some medical waste is toxic to humans and animals and can cause or add to pollution of water if not controlled properly.

Infectious disease

Many diseases can be spread blood-borne pathogens, disease-causing microorganisms that exist in blood.

Certain body fluids also carry blood or transmit pathogens that cause disease. Hepatitis B and HIV/AIDS are serious diseases that receive the most attention in healthcare facilities and the media. HIV is a virus that affects the immune system and can lead to **AIDS** and many related conditions. Hepatitis B is an infection caused by the hepatitis B virus that affects the liver. The infection can be chronic and cause long-term damage to the liver. Other diseases that can spread through blood in medical waste are:

• brucellosis

• Creutzfeldt-Jakob disease

• malaria

• hepatitis C

Injuries

Certain types of medical waste can cause disease or injuries. For example, sharps, which include needles, scalpels, and other sharp medical instruments, can be coated with blood or fluids that spread disease but also can injure by cutting someone who comes in contact with them. Genotoxic waste includes highly toxic drugs and materials, such as chemotherapy medications used in

QUESTIONS TO ASK YOUR DOCTOR

- Does this facility follow sound infection control policies?
- How can I safely dispose of medical waste I use in my home?
- Are there any recent incidents of medical waste exposures in our community?

treating **cancer**. Even waste from patients undergoing certain treatments can be highly toxic. These toxins can potentially contaminate municipal wastewater systems. Heavy metals, such as mercury, also can make their way to the environment. Mercury is used in thermometers. Its toxic effects vary, but mercury can cause **poisoning** and death. Its toxins can be released into the air during incineration, adding to **air pollution**. Finally, radioactive materials are used in medical imaging and to treat cancer. **Ionizing radiation** causes cancers. Exposure to high levels of **radiation** has been linked to **birth defects**, and direct exposure can cause serious radiation **burns**. The biggest problem with radioactive waste is the long half-life of the materials. Special management and disposal strategies are required to ensure the radiation is contained.

Public health role and response

The Medical Waste Tracking Act of 1988 was perhaps the most formal large response to managing medical waste and potential spread of disease resulting from medical waste. As a result of the participation of four states (New York, New Jersey, Connecticut, and Rhode Island), along with Puerto Rico, in the voluntary program, the EPA gathered data on the disease-causing potential of medical waste. The data helped the agency determine that the highest potential danger from medical waste existed at the occupational level. The Occupational Safety and Health Administration oversees a number of activities aimed at protecting healthcare workers from needlestick injuries and spread of blood-borne pathogens. Infection control practices are developed and monitored at health care facilities, by accrediting organizations, and by states. Some states assess penalties for placing infectious waste materials into regular solid waste systems. These policies and regulations protect workers, patients, and communities.

WHO created the first comprehensive global publication to address the hazards and control of medical waste in 1999 and has since updated the information. The document addresses how countries can create

regulations, improve planning, and minimize waste. It also suggests strategies for handling medical waste, such as how best to store, transport, and dispose of materials.

Prevention

Developing and adhering to proper controls of medical waste can help prevent threats to public health and safety. These threats might come in the form of infections that spread through blood-borne pathogens or because of health risks introduced by environmental exposure to medical waste products and toxins. **Prevention** includes proper management practices and knowing how to respond should an unexpected exposure occur. Proper management means that healthcare workers follow infection control policies and procedures promoted by their facilities and all regulations regarding infection control and medical waste management that are enforced by their states.

Efforts and solutions

Healthcare facilities, with the help of their states and consulting companies or agencies, have learned how to reduce the amount of regulated medical waste they produce. Doing so saves the facilities money by only paying for special handling of materials that are hazardous through careful sorting of wastes as employees use and discard them. Preventing the release of toxins such as mercury or dioxins from plastics during incineration has improved somewhat by hospitals packaging waste and shipping it to companies that can control emissions from commercial incinerators. A better solution is to increase use of reusable containers that can be sterilized. An autoclave is equipment that uses steam heated to a temperature that destroys bacteria and pathogens. Materials then can be reused or added to general waste.

WHO asserts that awareness and training are the first steps toward creating change in many countries. The organization offers countries and facilities publications to help guide them in safe medical waste management on a daily basis or in emergencies.

Resources

WEBSITES

Centers for Disease Control and Prevention. "Biologic and Infectious Waste." http://www.cdc.gov/nceh/ehs/etp/biological.htm (accessed September 24, 2012).

Greenpeace International. "Alternatives to Incineration." http://www.greenpeace.org/international/en/campaigns/toxics/incineration/alternatives-to-incineration/ (accessed September 25, 2012).

HealthCare Waste Management. "The 10 Categories of HCRW." http://www.healthcarewaste.org/basics/categories/ (accessed September 25, 2012).

Miami Herald. "Medical Waste Washes Ashore in Ormond Beach." http://www.miamiherald.com/2012/09/15/3004081/medical-waste-washes-ashore-in.html (accessed September 25, 2012).

ORGANIZATIONS

Environmental Protection Agency, 1200 Pennsylvania Ave. NW, Washington, DC 20460, http://www.epa.gov/waste/comments.htm

World Health Organization, Avenue Appia 20, 1211 Geneva 27, Switzerland, 41 22 ( ) 791-2111, Fax: 41 22 791-3111, publications@who.int, http://www.who.int.

Teresa G. Odle

Melamine

Definition

Melamine is an organic compound whose systematic name is 1,3,5-triazine-2,4,6-triamine. It is also known by a number of other names, including 2,4,6-triamino-s-triazine, cyanurotriamide, cyanurotriamine, and cyanuramide. Melamine has no etymological or other connection with the pigment known as melanin or the hormone called melatonin.

Description

Melamine is a derivative of cyanamide, CH_2N_2, an important chemical feedstock used in the preparation of other chemicals. It occurs as a fine white crystalline powder with a melting point of about 345°C that is soluble in **water**. Like cyanamide, it is am important chemical feedstock used in the production of many commercial and industrial products. It reacts with formaldehyde to produce a thermosetting plastic known as melamine resin which is used primarily in the manufacture of Formica™. Formica™, in turn, is used to make countertops, flame retardants, kitchenware, fabrics, acoustic foam paneling, dry erase boards, and a host of other household and commercial products. Melamine is also used commercially in the form of melamine polysulfonate, a compound added to concrete to increase its strength and durability. At one time, melamine was promoted as a fertilizer because of its high nitrogen content. However, it never achieved much popularity for that purpose because melamine decomposes and releases its nitrogen only very slowly, and the cost of producing melamine fertilizers was too great compared to that of other synthetic fertilizers. Addition of melamine to any food product for use by humans or other animals in the United States is prohibited. The United Nations *Codex Alimentarius*, which establishes voluntary worldwide food standards, permits the addition of 2.5 mg/kg of melamine in most human and nonhuman animal foods, but only 1 mg/kg in infant formula.

Toxicity

The acute toxicity (LD50) of melamine by oral ingestion is reported to be 3151 mg/kg, based on rat studies (comparable to the acute toxicity of table salt) and more than 1000 mg/kg by dermal absorption based on rabbit studies. Exposure to melamine is thought to produce a variety of non-lethal symptoms, such as skin irritation, irritation of the respiratory system, irritation of the eyes, and irritation of the digestive and urinary systems that may result in nausea and vomiting. Melamine's chronic toxicity is classified at level 3 by the U.S. National Toxicology Program, meaning that it may have carcinogenic effects, although the evidence is not entirely clear at this point. Melamine is also classified as a mutagen for protokaryotic organisms such as bacteria and yeast, although comparable data for eukaryotes are not available. Acute toxic effects of melamine are thought to result in part from their tendency to form tiny crystals that may block and damage renal cells of the kidneys, causing the kidneys to malfunction or fail.

Effects on public health

The addition of melamine to human and/or nonhuman animal foods has been recommended in the past primarily because of the high nitrogen content of the compound. For this reason, melamine-treated foods score high when standard tests of nitrogen content in food are conducted. These tests tend to measure the amount of nitrogen present in a food, not necessarily the nutritional value it provides a consumer. Thus, high scores from melamine-treated foods suggest to consumers that foods may be more nutritious than they actually are. A scheme

KEY TERMS

Acute toxicity—Health problems that occur shortly after exposure and last a relatively short period of time.

Carcinogenic—Having a tendency to cause cancer.

Chronic toxicity—Health problems that occur over a long period of time and that last for an extended period.

Feedstock—A chemical that is used in the commercial or industrial preparation of other chemicals.

Mutagenic—Having a tendency to cause genetic mutations.

Systemic name—The official chemical name of a compound.

Thermosetting plastic—A polymer that, once formed, can not be reheated, melted, or reformed. Also known as a resin.

for adding melamine to cattle feed in the late twentieth century turned out to be unsatisfactory since the release of nitrogen from melamine occurred too slowly to be of practical value to cattle nutritional needs.

Two incidents involving the contamination of foods by melamine were reported in 2007 and 2008. In both cases, the contamination occurred as the result of improperly prepared foods imported from China for use in North America, Europe, and South Africa. In the first instance, a number of pets in North America became ill as the result of eating pet foods manufactured primarily (but not exclusively) by the Menu Foods company of Canada. On March 16, 2007, the company issued a recall notice for a wide range of its products based on studies conducted in its own laboratories. Those studies showed that food products imported from China used in the production of Menu Foods products contained high levels of melamine and were responsible for the development of kidney problems in animals who ate the foods. No specific numbers are available for the extent of the problem, with the range from 14 confirmed deaths of pets in the United States (from the **Centers for Disease Control and Prevention**) to an estimated 3,600 deaths (based on an Internet survey of the extent of the problem). Investigations by scientific, governmental, and journalistic groups eventually revealed that the use of melamine as a food additive in China was widespread and routine, and that a number of companies simply ignored national and international regulations about the use of melamine in foods intended for both nonhuman animals and animals.

The second instance of melamine contamination involved its use in milk products in 2008. In this case, a number of companies operating in China had first added water to milk products to reduce their cost, and then added melamine to raise their nitrogen content. The adulterated milk products were eventually found to be responsible for more than 300,000 cases of illness among children, 860 of whom had to be hospitalized, and six of whom eventually died from kidney-related problems. An extended investigation of the scandal by the Chinese government resulted in the conviction of 15 individuals involved in the scheme, two of whom were executed, one given a suspended death sentence, three sentenced to life imprisonment, two given 15-year sentences, and the remaining number fired from their government positions. In response to the events in China, almost every country in the world (with 11 exceptions) ordered a ban on the import of dairy imports from that country. As a result, the number of illnesses and deaths was very low in other parts of the world. In the United States, for example, there were no confirmed illnesses or deaths attributable to contaminated food products from China. The activities of the U.S. Food and Drug Administration, the Centers for Disease Control and **Prevention** and other public health agencies in monitoring the progress of the Chinese event, enforcing existing importation regulations, and informing the general public about the melamine problem prevented the development of a health crisis in the United States.

Resources

BOOKS

Nestle, Marion. *Pet Food Politics: The Chihuahua in the Coal Mine.* Berkeley: University of California Press, 2008.

Perrett, Heli. *The Safe Food Handbook: How to Make Smart Choices about Risky Food.* New York: Experiment, 2011.

Wiwanitkit, Viroj. *Melamine and Other Problematic Food Carcinogens.* New York: Nova Science Publishers, 2009.

PERIODICALS

Bischoff, K., and W. K. Rumbeiha. "Pet Food Recalls and Pet Food Contaminants in Small Animals." *The Veterinary clinics of North America. Small Animal Practice* 42. 2. (2012): 237–50.

Chang, H., et al. "Characterization of Melamine-associated Urinary Stones in Children with Consumption of Melamine-contaminated Infant Formula." *Clinica Chimica Acta; International Journal of Clinical Chemistry* 413. 11-12. (2012): 985–91.

Mo, D., et al. "Checking into China's Cow Hotels: Have Policies Following the Milk Scandal Changed the Structure of the Dairy Sector?" *Journal of Dairy Science* 95. 5. (2012): 2282–98.

Pei, X., et al. "The China Melamine Milk Scandal and its Implications for Food Safety Regulation." *Food Policy* 36. 3. (2011: 412–20.

WEBSITES

China Seizes 22 Companies with Contaminated Baby Milk Powder. China View. http://news.xinhuanet.com/english/2008-09/17/content_10046949.htm. Accessed on September 18, 2012.

Crisis Management Helps China's Dairy Industry Recover. China View. http://news.xinhuanet.com/english/2008-09/25/content_10112354.htm. Accessed on September 18, 2012.

Melamine Contamination in China. U.S. Food and Drug Administration. http://www.fda.gov/NewsEvents/Public HealthFocus/ucm179005.htm. Accessed on September 18, 2012.

Statement of EFSA on Risks for Public Health due to the Presence of Melamine in Infant Milk and Other Milk Products in China. European Food Safety Authority. http://www.efsa.europa.eu/en/efsajournal/doc/807.pdf. Accessed on September 18, 2012.

ORGANIZATIONS

U.S. Food and Drug Administration (FDA), 10903 New Hampshire Ave., Silver Spring, MD USA 20993, (888) 463–6332, http://www.fda.gov/AboutFDA/ContactFDA/default.htm, http://www.fda.gov/.

David E. Newton, Ed.D.

Meningitis

Definition

Meningitis is a potentially fatal inflammation of the meninges, the membranes that encase the brain and spinal cord. Meningitis is most commonly caused by viruses, but also may be caused by a bacterial, or less commonly, a fungal infection. Non-infective causes of meningitis include certain drug **allergies**, some cancers, and systemic lupus erythematosus (SLE). Inflammation causes swelling of the brain. As the brain swells, fragile brain tissues are pressed against the skull. Brain cells in these areas can become damaged and eventually die.

Demographics

According to the **Centers for Disease Control and Prevention (CDC)**, there are about 4 to 10 cases of meningitis per every 100,000 persons in the United States each year. The introduction of Hib vaccine against *Haemophilus influenzae* in 1990 has changed the demographics of bacterial meningitis in North America, shifting the median age of this type of meningitis from less than 2 years of age to 39 years. In addition, in the 2000s, there was an increase in cases among adults over age 60. According to the **CDC**, adults over the age of 60 account for between 1,000 and 3,000 cases of acute bacterial meningitis and more than 50% of all meningitis fatalities annually in the U.S.

People of any race can get meningitis; however, African Americans are more likely to get meningitis than either Caucasian or Hispanic Americans. Infant males in the United States are three times more likely to develop meningitis than infant females; the rates are similar for both genders in adults.

The rates of meningitis in developing countries are thought to be at least 10 times as high as those in the United States and Canada. The lack of vaccines in these countries is the major factor in the difference between statistics. Periodic epidemics occur in sub-Saharan Africa and parts of India.

Description

Doctors sometimes divide cases of meningitis into three categories according to the speed of symptom development. Acute meningitis develops in less than 24 hours and is caused by one of several species of bacteria; it is considered a medical emergency. Subacute meningitis takes between 1 and 7 days for symptoms to appear; it may be caused by bacteria or viruses. Chronic meningitis develops over a period of more than a week and may result from an infection or a noninfectious cause.

Structure of the brain

In order to understand why meningitis can be so dangerous, it is important to have a basic understanding of the anatomy of the brain. The meninges are three separate membranes, layered together, which encase the brain and spinal cord:

- The dura mater is the toughest, outermost layer and is closely attached to the inside of the skull.
- The middle layer, the arachnoid mater, is important because of its involvement in the normal flow of the cerebrospinal fluid (CSF), a lubricating and nutritive fluid that bathes both the brain and the spinal cord.
- The innermost layer, the pia mater, helps direct blood vessels into the brain.
- The space between the arachnoid mater and the pia mater contains CSF, which helps insulate the brain from trauma. Many blood vessels, as well as peripheral and cranial nerves, pass through this space.

CSF, produced in specialized chambers deep inside the brain, flows over the surface of the brain and spinal

HATTIE ALEXANDER (1901–1968)

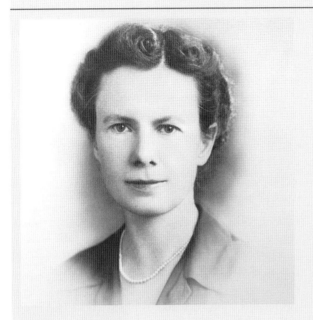

(© Bettmann/CORBIS)

Hattie Alexander, a dedicated pediatrician, medical educator, and researcher in microbiology, won international recognition for deriving a serum to combat influenzal meningitis, a common disease that previously had been nearly always fatal to infants and young children. Alexander subsequently investigated microbiological genetics and the processes whereby bacteria, through genetic mutation, acquire resistance to antibiotics. In 1964, as president of the American Pediatric Society, she became one of the first women to head a national medical association.

As an intern at the Harriet Lane Home of Johns Hopkins Hospital from 1930 to 1931, Alexander became interested in influenzal meningitis. The source of the disease was *Hemophilus influenzae*, a bacteria that causes inflammation of the meninges, the membranes surrounding the brain and spinal cord. In 1931, Alexander began a second internship at the Babies Hospital of the Columbia-Presbyterian Medical Center in New York City. There, she witnessed first-hand the futility of medical efforts to save babies who had contracted influenzal meningitis.

Alexander's early research focused on deriving a serum (the liquid component of blood, in which antibodies are contained) that would be effective against influenzal meningitis. Serums derived from animals that have been exposed to a specific disease-producing bacterium often contain antibodies against the disease and can be developed for use in immunizing humans against it. Alexander knew that the Rockefeller Institute in New York City, however, had been able to prepare a rabbit serum for the treatment of pneumonia, another bacterial disease. Alexander therefore experimented with rabbit serums, and by 1939 was able to announce the development of a rabbit serum effective in curing infants of influenzal meningitis.

In the early 1940s, Alexander experimented with the use of drugs in combination with rabbit serum in the treatment of influenzal meningitis. Within the next two years, she saw infant deaths due to the disease drop by eighty percent.

cord. This fluid serves to cushion these relatively delicate structures, as well as supplying important nutrients for brain cells. CSF is reabsorbed by blood vessels located within the meninges. A careful balance between CSF production and reabsorption is important to avoid the accumulation of too much CSF.

Because the brain is enclosed in the hard, bony case of the skull, any disease that produces swelling will be damaging to the brain. The skull cannot expand at all, so when the swollen brain tissue pushes up against the skull's hard bone, the brain tissue becomes damaged and the blood supply is compromised, and this tissue may ultimately die. Furthermore, swelling on the right side of the brain will not only cause pressure and damage to that side of the brain, but by taking up precious space within the tight confines of the skull, the left side of the brain will also be pushed up against the hard surface of the skull, causing damage to the left side of the brain as well.

Types of meningitis

Viral meningitis, which is also called "aseptic meningitis," is the most common type of meningitis. It is a less severe infection than bacterial meningitis, is rarely fatal, and may not require any specific treatment. Viral meningitis is caused by one or more enteroviruses, which are viruses that normally live in the digestive tract. Viral meningitis usually develops in the late summer and early fall and is most likely to affect children and adults under age 30. Most viral infections occur in children under the age of 5. Enteroviruses are present in saliva, throat mucus, and feces; they can be transmitted through direct contact with an infected person or an infected object or surface. Viral meningitis can also be caused by the viruses that cause chickenpox, **mumps**, HIV infection, **West Nile virus** infection, and genital **herpes**.

Bacterial meningitis is a medical emergency and has a high mortality rate if untreated. The origin of a bacterial infection leading to meningitis varies according to an individual's age, habits, geographical location, and health status. In newborns, the most common agents of meningitis are those contracted from the mother during labor and delivery, including the bacteria Group B streptococci, *Escherichia coli*, and *Listeria monocytogenes*. Older children are more frequently infected by *Haemophilus influenzae*, *Neisseria meningitidis*, and *Streptococcus pneumoniae* bacteria, while adults are infected by *S. pneumoniae* and *N. meningitidis*. Persons who have had pneumococcal meningitis may be left with lifelong damage to their nervous system that includes deafness and brain damage. *N. meningitidis* is highly contagious and can cause epidemics. Epidemics of meningitis most often occur under crowded conditions, such as day care centers, college residence halls, or military barracks. Meningococcal meningitis has a mortality rate of 10–15 %.

Meningitis caused by fungi is rare in the general population but is a fairly common opportunistic infection in patients with HIV infection.

Risk factors

Risk factors for meningitis include:

- Age. Since the introduction of childhood vaccines, bacterial meningitis is now more common in young adults.
- Group living situations. These may include military bases, college dormitories, and child care centers.
- Having a weakened immune system. People with AIDS or diabetes are at increased risk of meningitis.
- Working with animals. Farmers and others who work with animals have an increased risk of *Listeria* infections.
- Pregnancy.
- Spleen removal. People who have had their spleen (a part of the immune system) removed have weaker immune systems.
- Gender. Among newborns, boys are three times more likely than girls to get meningitis.
- Lifestyle. Unsafe sexual practices and having a large number of sexual partners increases the risk of viral meningitis.

Causes and symptoms

Meningitis occurs when disease organisms that have entered the body and multiplied in the nose, mouth, and throat get into the bloodstream and are carried to the brain and the meninges. In some cases, meningitis can develop when the bacteria gain entrance to the body through a surgical incision or an injury to the head or neck. A few cases of meningitis result from inflammatory diseases like lupus or certain cancers.

Organisms causing meningitis

About 90% of cases of viral meningitis is caused by viruses from the enterovirus family. Viruses from this family also cause viral gastritis (stomach flu). However, viruses that cause mumps, **measles**, and **polio** can also cause viral meningitis. Although these diseases are uncommon in developed countries, they are still prevalent in the developing world and may be of concern to travelers.

Bacterial meningitis is caused primarily by four types of bacteria.

- *Streptococcus pneumoniae*. This is also called "pneumococcal meningitis." This bacterium also causes pneumonia and ear and sinus infections. It is a leading cause of bacterial meningitis in young children.
- *Neisseria meningitidis*. Also called "meningococcal meningitis," this bacterium is highly contagious and is often responsible for outbreaks of meningitis among young adults.
- *Haemophilus influenzae*. Routine childhood vaccinations against Haemophilus bacteria have been available since the 1990s and in the developed world have substantially reduced this cause of meningitis.
- *Listeria monocytogenes*. Pregnant women and older adults are at higher risk than other groups for contracting listeria meningitis. Listeria can cross the placenta and kill a developing fetus.

Methods of disease transmission

Bacterial meningitis can be passed from person to person through coughing, sneezing, or kissing, but the disease does not spread as easily as the **common cold**. Once in the body, the bacteria are carried to the brain through the blood. However, in some cases, a person may have another type of infection (for instance, infection of the lungs, throat, or tissues of the heart) caused by an organism that can also cause meningitis. If this initial infection is not properly treated, the organism will continue to multiply, find its way into the blood stream, and be delivered in sufficient quantities to invade past the blood-brain barrier. Direct spread occurs when an organism spreads to the meninges from infected tissue next to or very near the meninges. This can occur, for example, with a severe and poorly treated ear or sinus infection. Insect and pet bites can also deliver disease organisms directly into the bloodstream.

Patients who experience skull fractures have abnormal openings to the sinuses, nasal passages, and middle ears. Organisms that usually live in the human respiratory system without causing disease can pass through openings caused by such fractures, reach the meninges, and cause infection. Similarly, patients who undergo surgical procedures or who have had foreign bodies surgically placed within their skulls (such as tubes to drain abnormal amounts of accumulated CSF) have an increased risk of meningitis.

Disease organisms can also reach the meninges via an uncommon method called "intraneural spread." Intraneural spread involves an organism invading the body at a considerable distance away from the head, spreading along a nerve, and using that nerve as a pathway into the skull, where the organism can multiply and cause meningitis. Herpes simplex virus is known to use this type of spread, as is the **rabies** virus.

Symptoms

The most important symptoms used to diagnose meningitis are a high fever, stiff neck, and severe headache, which may come on in less than a day after infection. Other symptoms in adults may include:

• nausea and vomiting

• extreme sensitivity to light (photophobia)

• confusion and difficulty concentrating

• seizures

• loss of appetite

• drowsiness or difficulty waking up

• skin rash (more common with meningococcal meningitis)

Infants and small children may have somewhat different symptoms:

• bulging of the soft spot (fontanelle) at the top of an infant's skull

• constant crying

• poor feeding

• unusual sleepiness

• stiffness in the baby's body as well as neck

It is important to note that very young infants might not show the classic signs of meningitis. Early in infancy, a baby's immune system is not yet developed enough to mount a fever in response to infection, so fever may be absent. In some infants with meningitis, seizures are the only identifiable symptom. Similarly, debilitated elderly people might not have fever or other clearly identifiable symptoms of meningitis.

Diagnosis

Diagnosis of the cause of meningitis is essential to proper treatment, as the **antibiotics** used to treat bacterial

meningitis are not useful in treating viral meningitis. A patient who has acute bacterial meningitis will usually have treatment started as soon as the doctor obtains a sample of cerebrospinal fluid for testing. The CSF is obtained by performing a lumbar puncture, also known as a "spinal tap." This is a procedure in which a needle is inserted into an area in the lower back where the doctor can easily obtain a sample of cerebrospinal fluid (CSF).

Examination

An examination of a patient with suspected meningitis will include a recent history of the patient's activities to indicate possible exposure to disease agents, such as recent travel, contact with infected persons, or contact with animals or insects. The season of the year may be an important diagnostic clue; enterovirus infections are more common in North America in late summer and early fall, while insect-borne infections are more common in late spring and summer. The doctor will also perform a neurological examination, which includes testing of the patient's hearing and speech, vision, coordination and balance, reflexes, mental status, and recent changes in mood or behavior. In addition, certain manipulations of the patient's head (lowering the head, chin toward chest, for example) are difficult to perform and painful for a person with meningitis.

A patient with subacute meningitis may be given an examination to check for an ear, throat, or sinus infection. In addition to moving the patient's head, the doctor may also perform two other maneuvers to see whether the patient's meninges are inflamed. In one test, the doctor raises the patient's leg at the hip to a right angle from the examining table and tries to straighten the lower leg. If the leg cannot be straightened or if the patient experiences neck **pain**, he or she most likely has meningitis. The other maneuver involves bending the patient's neck forward as they lie on the table. If the knees and hips flex upward, the patient probably has meningitis.

Tests

If a sample of CSF is taken, it is sent to a laboratory for analysis. The CSF is then examined under a microscope to look for bacteria or fungi. Normal CSF contains set percentages of glucose and protein. These percentages will vary with bacterial, viral, or other causes of meningitis. For example, bacterial meningitis causes a smaller-than-normal percentage of glucose to be present in CSF, as the bacteria are essentially "eating" the host's glucose and using it for their own **nutrition** and energy production. Normal CSF should contain no infection-fighting cells (white blood cells), so the presence of white blood cells in CSF is another indication of meningitis. Some of the withdrawn CSF is also put into special lab dishes to allow growth of the suspected infecting organism, which can then be identified more easily.

Identification of the specific bacterium can take as long as a week; meanwhile, the doctor can begin to treat the patient with a broad-spectrum antibiotic until the test results come back. In some cases the doctor will swab the patient's throat to obtain a sample of mucus and saliva for culture. The sample can be sent to a local or state laboratory or to the CDC for analysis. Throat cultures usually take between two and three days to yield results.

In March 2007, the Food and Drug Administration (FDA) approved a rapid CSF test that identifies virus particles in CSF called the "Xpert EV test." Using a sample of CSF, this test can accurately identify about 90% of viral meningitis cases in less than three hours. Since bacterial meningitis is often fatal, if no virus is found in the CSF, the disease is treated as if it is caused by bacteria until proven otherwise. This test allows doctors to distinguish fairly quickly between viral and bacterial meningitis and avoid giving unnecessary antibiotics to patients with viral meningitis.

The doctor may also order such imaging tests as a computed tomography (CT) scan or magnetic resonance imaging (MRI). A CT scan may detect signs of inflammation of the meninges. Imaging tests can also be used to rule out head trauma, **stroke**, tumors, and blood clots in the brain.

Treatment

Traditional

Meningitis is a medical emergency. Individuals with the symptoms of meningitis must get to a hospital as quickly as possible, particularly if the symptoms have developed in less than one day. People who are acutely ill and are taken to a hospital are usually treated within 30 minutes of their arrival, as emergency room doctors assume that the patient has bacterial meningitis and do not want to delay treatment until the specific organism is identified. A sample of cerebrospinal fluid is taken by a spinal tap for analysis; then the patient is given intravenous penicillin or another broad-spectrum antibiotic, intravenous fluids, and pure oxygen to assist breathing. The patient may also need to be treated for seizures, or to have fluid drained from the sinuses or from the space between the meninges and the brain. After the specific bacterium has been identified, the doctor can adjust the type and dosage of the antibiotics given to the patient. People with bacterial meningitis may need additional treatment for shock, seizures, dehydration, and brain swelling. Serious cases of bacterial meningitis may require treatment in an intensive care unit (ICU) and life support.

Viral meningitis cannot be treated with antibiotics. Patients are usually advised to stay home and rest in bed for a few weeks. They can take over-the-counter pain relievers for muscle aches and pains and to bring down fever. If the viral meningitis is caused by the herpes virus, the doctor may also prescribe acyclovir or gancyclovir, antiviral drugs used to treat herpes.

Drugs

Bacterial meningitis is usually treated with a combination of intravenous antibiotics. The specific combination depends on the patient's age and immune status; however, most antibiotic combinations consist of ampicillin (Marcillin, Omnipen) plus cefotaxime (Claforan) or ceftriaxone (Rocephin) plus vancomycin (Vancocin). Treatment is given for 7–10 days for less severe infections to 14–21 days for severe infections. In some cases, the patient may also be given steroids, most commonly dexamethasone, to reduce inflammation caused by the bacteria.

Alternative

Because meningitis is a potentially deadly condition, traditional medical doctors should be contacted immediately for diagnosis and treatment. Alternative treatments should be used only to support the recovery process following appropriate antibiotic treatments, or used concurrently with antibiotic treatments.

Alternative therapies, such as homeopathy, traditional Chinese medicine, and Western herbal medicine may help patients regain their health and build up their immune systems. The recovering individual, under the direction of a professional alternative therapist, may opt to include mushrooms in his or her diet to stimulate immune function. The patient should contact an experienced herbalist or homeopathic practitioner for specific remedies.

Prognosis

The patient's prognosis depends on the type of meningitis that they have as well as their overall health. Patients who experience only headache, fever, and stiff neck may recover in 2–4 weeks. Patients with bacterial meningitis typically show some relief within 48 to 72 hours following initial treatment; however, they are more likely to experience complications caused by the disease. Acute bacterial meningitis has a mortality rate of 10–15 percent even with treatment. The reported mortality rates for each specific organism are 19–26% for *S. pneumoniae* meningitis, 3–6% for *H. influenzae* meningitis, 3–13% for *N. meningitidis* meningitis, and 15–29% for *L. monocytogenes* meningitis. Pneumococcal meningitis may have a mortality rate as high as 21 percent. Of the patients who survive bacterial meningitis, between 10 and 20 percent will suffer such complications as blindness, hydrocephalus, **hearing loss**, learning

disorders, or even paralysis. Scarring of the meninges may result in obstruction of the normal flow of CSF, causing abnormal accumulation of CSF. This may be a chronic problem for some people, requiring the installation of shunt tubes to drain the accumulation on a regular basis.

Viral meningitis is usually a much milder disease than bacterial meningitis. Patients receiving treatment for viral meningitis and **encephalitis** usually see some relief in 24–48 hours. Some patients may need to be hospitalized for supportive care for a week or so, but most can recover at home within two to four weeks. Complications are rare with viral meningitis; the mortality rate is less than 1%.

Efforts and solutions

As of 2012, several vaccines can be used to prevent meningitis. As has already been mentioned, the rates of *Haemophilus influenzae* meningitis among young children dropped dramatically after the Hib vaccine was added to childhood **immunization** schedules in the 1990s. Other vaccines have been developed to protect adults as well as children from pneumococcal and meningococcal meningitis. There is one type of pneumococcal vaccine known as PCV7, recommended for children between 2 and 5 years of age who are at high risk of infection.

A different vaccine, known as "PPV," is recommended for adults at risk of pneumococcal meningitis: those over 65, those with weakened immune systems, those with diabetes or **heart disease**, and those whose spleen has been removed. The vaccine that protects against the meningococcus is known as "Menactra T" or "MCV4." It is recommended for all children at 11–12 and for college students who were not vaccinated at that age. MCV4 can also be used to protect people exposed to meningitis during an outbreak or who must travel to countries with high rates of meningococcal meningitis. Adults over 55 should be immunized with a similar vaccine called "MPSV4," a meningococcal polysaccharide vaccine known as Menomune.

Other preventive measures that people can take include:

- Keeping the immune system strong by getting enough sleep, exercising regularly, and eating a healthy diet.
- Washing the hands regularly, particularly when living in a dormitory or similar shared housing situation.
- Avoiding sharing glasses, drinking cups, food utensils, and similar items with others who may be infected or exposed to infection.
- Covering the mouth or nose before sneezing or coughing.

• Taking any antibiotics that may be prescribed during a meningitis outbreak in one's school or workplace.

• Asking the doctor about vaccination against meningitis before traveling abroad.

Resources

BOOKS

Goldman, Lee, and Dennis Ausiello., eds. *Cecil Textbook of Medicine*, 23rd ed. Philadelphia Saunders Elsevier, 2008.

Goldsmith, Connie. *Meningitis*. Minneapolis, MN: Twenty-First Century Books, 2008.

Klosterman, Lorrie. *Meningitis*. New York: Marshall Cavendish Benchmark, 2007.

PERIODICALS

Black, S. "Pneumococcal Vaccine Reduces the Rates of Pneumococcal Meningitis in Children." *Journal of Pediatrics* 155 (July 2009): 149–50.

Jolobe, O. M. "We Ought to Perform Blood Cultures on Admission in All Cases of Suspected Meningitis." *Journal of the American Geriatrics Society* 57 (June 2009): 1131–2.

Kim, K. S. "Treatment Strategies for Central Nervous System Infections." *Expert Opinion on Pharmacotherapy* 10 (June 2009): 1307–17.

Pelton, S. I., and G. P. Gilmet. "Expanding Prevention of Invasive Meningococcal Disease." *Expert Review of Vaccines* 8 (June 2009): 717–27.

Verma, R., and M. C. Fisher. "Bacterial Meningitis Vaccines: Not Just for Kids." *Current Infectious Disease Reports* 11 (July 2009): 302–08.

WEBSITES

Meningitis. Mayo Foundation for Education and Research. August 8, 2008. http://www.mayoclinic.com/health/meningitis/DS00118

Meningitis. MedlinePlus. June 15, 2012. http://www.nlm.nih.gov/medlineplus/meningitis.html. Accessed August 19, 2012.

Meningitis and Encephalitis Fact Sheet. National Institute of Neurological Disorders and Stroke (NINDS). February 16, 2011. http://www.ninds.nih.gov/disorders/encephalitis_meningitis/encephalitis_meningitis.htm. Accessed August 19, 2012.

Meningitis: Questions and Answers. United States Centers for Disease Control and Prevention. March 15, 2012. http://www.cdc.gov/meningococcal/about/index.html. Accessed August 19, 2012.

ORGANIZATIONS

Immunization Action Coalition (IAC), 1573 Selby Avenue, Suite 234, Saint Paul, MN 55104, (651)647-9009, Fax: (651)647-9131, admin@immunize.org, http://www.immunize.org

Infectious Diseases Society of America (IDSA), 1300 Wilson Boulevard, Suite 300, Arlington, VA 22209, (703) 299-0200, Fax: (703) 299-0204, info@idsociety.org, http://www.idsociety.org

Meningitis Research Foundation, Midland Way, Thornbury-BristolUnited Kingdom BS25 2BS, 01454 281811, Fax: 01454 281094, info@meningitis.org, http://www.meningitis.org

National Institute of Allergy and Infectious Diseases Office of Communications and Government Relations, 6610 Rockledge Drive, MSC 6612, Bethesda, MD 20892-6612, (301) 496-5717, (866) 284-4107 or TDD: (800)877-8339 (for hearing impaired), Fax: (301) 402-3573, http://www3.niaid.nih.gov

National Institute of Neurological Disorders and Stroke (NINDS), P.O. Box 5801, Bethesda, MD 20828, (301) 496-5751. TTY: (301) 468-5981, (800) 352-9424, http://www.ninds.nih.gov

United States Centers for Disease Control and Prevention (CDC), 1600 Clifton Road, Atlanta, GA 30333, (404) 639-3534, 800-CDC-INFO (800-232-4636). TTY: (888) 232-6348, inquiry@cdc.gov, http://www.cdc.gov

World Health Organization (WHO), Avenue Appia 20, 1211 Geneva 27, Switzerland, + 41 22 791 21 11, Fax: + 41 22 791 31 11, info@who.int, http://www.who.int/en.

Helen Colby, MS
Tish Davidson, A.M.
Andrea Nienstedt, MA

Men's health

Definition

Men's health is concerned with identifying, preventing, and treating conditions that are most common or specific to men.

Description

On average, men do not live as long as women; **life expectancy** in the United States in 2010 was 75.7 years for men and 80.8 years for women. The reasons for this discrepancy are not completely understood. Men may have some genetic predisposition for lower life expectancy, as women tend to outlive men in most areas throughout the world, but men also have different lifestyle patterns that may increase the wear and tear on their bodies and promote the development of specific diseases. Studies have shown that as a group, men drink more alcohol, use more illicit drugs, use more tobacco products, and have more sexual partners than women. Men seek medical care less frequently than women, and men generally have more stressful and violent habits. Health professionals believe that men can benefit from increased knowledge of male medical issues and by understanding how lifestyle choices impact health.

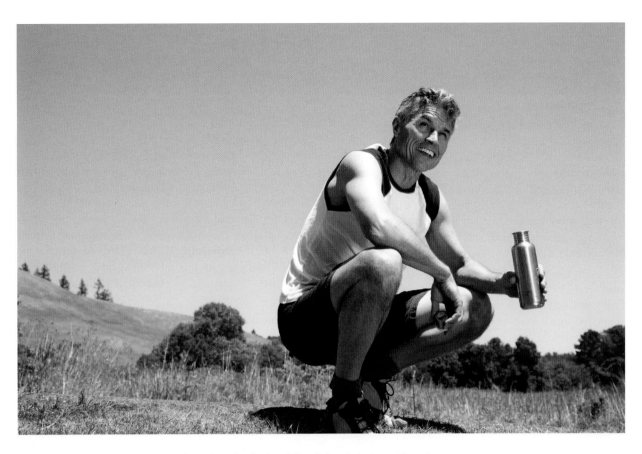

A healthy man stretching and resting after physical activity. *(©istockphoto.com/jonya)*

According to the Centers for Disease Control (**CDC**), the 10 leading causes of death for men in the United States in 2007 were (in order):

• heart disease

• cancer

• unintentional injury

• stroke

• chronic lower respiratory disease

• diabetes

• suicide

• influenza and pneumonia

• kidney disease

• Alzheimer's disease

Men also regularly develop health problems as diverse as **sexually transmitted diseases** (STDs), mental illness, arthritis, urinary tract infections, athletic injuries, hair and skin problems, and digestive disorders. The field of men's health strives to reduce the risks and incidence of men's conditions by researching preventive practices, designing testing procedures for early disease detection, and recommending specialized courses of treatment.

Prevention

DIET. Preventive practices for men's health empha-size diet, exercise, and **stress** management, as well as the elimination of risky behaviors such as **smoking**, exces-sive alcohol use, illicit drug use, and unprotected sex. Four of the leading causes of death for American men are related to diet—heart disease, **cancer**, **stroke**, and diabetes. In addition, men are more likely than women to develop diet-related conditions including high choles-terol, high blood pressure, and **obesity**, that predispose them to certain diseases and premature death.

For American men, dietary problems often arise from consuming too much fat, sugar, salt, and overall calories. The dietary change most likely to improve the health of males is reduced intake of calories and fats, particularly saturated fats. Cholesterol and saturated fats are found mainly in meat and dairy products. Current recommendations are that calories from fat should amount to no more than 30% of total daily calories.

Eating adequate protein is generally not a problem for American men, so replacing some dairy and meat consumption with high fiber vegetable proteins such as beans and soy would be beneficial in reducing fat and cholesterol intake. Complex carbohydrates such as those from whole grains and legumes should provide the bulk of daily calories. Sugar and "empty" (low nutritional) calories from foods such as soft drinks, desserts, and processed foods, should be reduced. Increasing dietary fiber by eating plenty of fresh fruits, vegetables, whole grains, and legumes is strongly recommended.

Other principles of a healthy diet are eating food that is as fresh and unprocessed as possible, drinking plenty of **water**, and avoiding hydrogenated or partially hydrogenated oils that contain trans-fats. Overeating should be avoided and snacking between meals limited. Alcohol intake should be limited to one drink per day. Reading food labels provides information about how much fat, cholesterol, salt, and calories processed foods contain and can help men make better dietary decisions.

EXERCISE. The health of men has been affected as work patterns have shifted. Many jobs once involving heavy physical labor are now done by machines. In 2011, about 70% of all American men were overweight or obese according to their body mass index (BMI). Obesity poses many risks, including increased risk of developing **heart disease**, diabetes, and some cancers. Effective exercise programs help men control weight, reduce stress, increase energy levels, improve self-esteem, and improve sleep. A balanced exercise program will emphasize stretching for flexibility, aerobic activities for stamina, and resistance training for strength. A well-rounded program will exercise all parts of the body and help to burn excess calories. Routines should begin with warm-ups to reduce the chances of injuries and end with cool-down exercises to speed recovery.

STRESS REDUCTION. Chronic (long-term) stress is a risk factor in many of the major diseases affecting men's mortality rates. Prolonged stress may also cause sleep disorders, addictions, depression, anxiety, and other conditions. Reduction of stress may require changes in both activities and attitudes. Regular exercise is a good stress reducer, as is reducing dependence on alcohol and nicotine. Men with serious job-related stress may need to commit to spending more time with their loved ones and in enjoyable leisure activities in order to relieve stress. Men with high stress levels that lead to destructive behaviors may need to pursue psychotherapy or significant lifestyle changes. Good **nutrition**, social support, and healthy sleep patterns also reduce stress.

Alternative therapies often are used to help with stress reduction. Biofeedback allows men to monitor their stress levels as a way of learning to control them. Meditation, massage, yoga, and various mind/body techniques can be taught to facilitate the relaxation response to rid the body of stress.

TESTING. Routine physical examinations performed by physicians are recommended at least every three years for men in their twenties and thirties, every two years for men in their forties, and every year for men over 50. Physicians may order several screening tests as well, depending on the age and condition of the patient. Blood tests screen for diabetes, high cholesterol, infections, and HIV. As of 2012, there was debate within the medical community about the value of the prostate-specific antigen (PSA) blood test as a useful tool for screening for prostate cancer. The digital rectal exam is used to manually check the prostate gland for enlargement or irregularities. Urine tests check for infections, kidney problems, and diabetes. The fecal occult blood test examines the stool for indications of ulcers or cancer. A sigmoidoscopy checks the health of the rectum and lower colon. Electrocardiograms (ECGs) check the status of the heart. Older men may consult an ophthalmologist (eye specialist) at least every two years for vision and glaucoma testing.

Men may perform self-tests as preventative measures. During a skin cancer self-exam, the entire skin is checked closely for irregular or changing moles, lesions, or blemishes, usually red, white, or blue in color. Abnormal findings should be reported to a physician. Like some forms of skin cancer, testicular cancer tends to spread rapidly and early detection is crucial. The testicular self-exam is best performed in the shower or bath, because warm water relaxes the scrotum. The testicles are gently rolled and massaged between the fingers and thumb to feel for bumps, swelling, tenderness, or irregularities. Some self-test kits are available in pharmacies, including kits for blood pressure, high cholesterol, colorectal cancer, and blood glucose (diabetes). These do not replace proper preventative medical care. Any abnormal results should immediately be followed up with a visit to a physician.

Specific diseases

HEART DISEASE. About 34% of all American men have some type of cardiovascular disease, which is the leading cause of death among American men. According to the American Heart Association, in 2008, about 392,000 men died of cardiovascular disease. The death rate was 287 per 100,000 **population** for white males and 390 for black males, a significant difference. Cardiovascular disease was the primary diagnosis of 3,230,000 males discharged after short hospital stays in 2009. Risk factors for heart disease include male gender, race, **aging**, family history of the disease, smoking, high cholesterol levels, high blood pressure, diabetes, **alcoholism**, obesity, physical inactivity, and stress. Lifestyle habits such as diet, exercise, and stress control play major roles in the development or **prevention** of heart disease in men.

Heart disease can take many forms, but one of the most common is coronary artery disease. In 2008, the American Heart Association estimated that 8.8 million American men over age 20 had this disease. Coronary artery disease is an inflammatory disease in which cellular debris, cholesterol, and other fatty substances build up in the blood vessels (coronary arteries) that supply the heart with blood and oxygen, causing blood flow to be reduced or blocked. Hypertension (high blood pressure) accelerates this process and also poses major risks for both heart disease and stroke. When blockage of blood supply to the heart is severe, a myocardial infarction (heart attack) is likely to occur. Angina pectoris is the chest **pain** associated with the early stages of heart disease; about 3.5% of American men have angina.

CANCER. The American Cancer Society (ACS) estimated that more than 577,000 Americans died from cancer in 2012. Men have a slightly higher risk for cancer than women. The top five cancers responsible for deaths in men in 2011 were lung, prostate, colorectal (colon and rectum), pancreas, and liver cancers. The ACS lists seven warning signs of cancer:

- unusual bleeding or discharge
- changes in bowel or bladder patterns
- persistent sores
- lumps or irregularities on the body
- difficulty swallowing or indigestion
- changes in warts or moles
- persistent cough or hoarseness in the throat

Although the causes of cancer are incompletely understood, there are several general risk factors that increase its chances: family history of cancer, smoking, poor diet (e.g., high in fat, low in fiber), excessive alcohol consumption, skin damage from sunlight, and exposure to **radiation**, chemicals, and environmental pollutants.

Prostate cancer is of concern exclusively to men. The prostate gland is a walnut-sized organ in the male reproductive system, located near the rectum below the bladder. The ACS estimated that 242,000 new cases of prostate cancer were diagnosed in the United States in 2012 and about 28,200 men would die from the disease. Looked at another way, 1 in 6 men will get prostate cancer at some time in their life, while 1 in 36 will die from the disease.

With early detection, about 98% of men with prostate cancer survive for five years. Symptoms of prostate cancer include difficulty in stopping or starting urination, frequent nighttime urination (nocturia), weak urine flow, and blood in the urine or semen. Many older men will develop another prostate problem, benign prostatic hyperplasia (BPH). This is a non–cancerous enlargement of the prostate gland that may make urination difficult or painful.

Testicular cancer is most common in men between the ages of 15 and 34. The ACS estimated that there would be about 8,600 new cases of testicular cancer in 2012 in the United States. However, the success rate in curing testicular cancer is very high, and only 1 of every 5,000 die from the disease.

STROKE. Strokes occur when the blood supply to the brain is interrupted and brain function becomes impaired due to lack of oxygen. Ischemic strokes occur due to blood vessels becoming blocked while hemorrhagic strokes are the result of broken blood vessels in or near the brain. Ischemic strokes account for about 80% of all strokes. The American Heart Association estimates that more than 600,000 Americans experience a stroke each year. Men have a higher risk of having a stroke, although more women die from strokes. African American men are at particularly high risk. Other risk factors for stroke include hypertension, previous heart attack, old age (three-fourths of all strokes occur in people over age 55), family history, high cholesterol levels, smoking, obesity, alcoholism, and physical inactivity.

Symptoms of strokes include sudden weakness or numbness, blurring or loss of vision, difficulty speaking or understanding, sudden severe headache, and dizziness or falling. Individuals showing symptoms of stroke need immediate emergency medical care.

MALE URINARY TRACT PROBLEMS. The urinary system includes the kidneys and bladder, the ureters between the kidneys and bladder, and the urethra, the tube through which urine flows from the bladder. Symptoms of urinary tract problems include frequent urination, excessive urination at night, painful or burning urination, weak urination, blood in the urine, or incontinence (involuntary loss of urine). Urethritis is an infection of the urethra, which is a major symptom of sexually transmitted diseases (STDs). Kidney stones (nephrolithiasis) are the most common urinary tract problems. About 12% of American men and 7% of American women will develop kidney stones during their lifetimes. The higher the socioeconomic class, the more likely the individual is to develop a kidney stone. Kidney stones can cause extreme pain when they move from the kidneys into the ureters. Often they will pass on their own or can be broken up into smaller pieces using ultrasound waves; a few require surgery. The best prevention for kidney stones is drinking plenty of fluids daily.

THE MALE REPRODUCTIVE SYSTEM. The male reproductive system includes the penis, testicles, scrotum, prostate, and other organs. Problems include **infertility**, orchitis (infection of the testicles), and hydrocele, the buildup of fluid on the testicles. Epididymitis is inflammation of the tube that transports sperm from the testicles, and can cause severe pain, swelling, and fever. A varicocele is a group of varicose veins in the scrotum that can cause swelling and damage sperm. Peyronie's disease is the abnormal curvature of the penis caused by accumulated scar tissue. Testicular torsion, a medical emergency, occurs when a testicle becomes twisted and the blood supply is cut off. This condition can lead to permanent damage if not treated quickly. It is most common in males between the ages of 12 and 18. Prostatitis is infection or inflammation of the prostate gland.

Sexually transmitted diseases include genital warts, chlamydia, gonorrhea, **syphilis**, genital **herpes**, **hepatitis**, and HIV (human immunodeficiency virus)/AIDS. Symptoms of STDs include discharge of fluid from the penis; painful urination; sores, lesions, itching, or rashes in the genital area; and swelling of the lymph nodes in the groin. Prevention of STDs begins with safer sexual behavior: wearing condoms, limiting the number of sexual partners, not mixing sexual encounters with alcohol, avoiding anal intercourse, and avoiding sexual contact with infected people, prostitutes, and intravenous drug users. Men who engage in risky behaviors should have frequent HIV tests and medical examinations.

MALE SEXUAL HEALTH. Erectile dysfunction (ED), also called impotence, is a man's inability to maintain an erection for sexual intercourse. It affects nearly 1 in every 10 American men. Incidence of ED increases with age, but the problem can occur at any age. Up to 80% of ED is caused by physical problems, while 20% of cases are psychogenic, or psychological in origin. Causes of ED include hormonal problems, injuries, nerve damage, diseases, infections, diabetes, stress, depression, anxiety, drug abuse, and interactions of certain prescription drugs. ED also may be the first indication of circulation problems due to diabetes, high blood pressure, or coronary artery disease.

A self-test men can perform to determine whether ED is physical or psychological is the stamp test, or nocturnal penile tumescence test. Physically healthy men experience several prolonged erections during sleep. The stamp test is done by attaching a strip of stamps around the penis before bedtime; if the stamps are torn in the morning, it generally indicates that nocturnal (nighttime) erections have occurred, and thus ED is not of physiological origin. Men with ED should see a urologist for further diagnosis and discussion of the treatment options available, including drug therapy, hormone injections, and surgical repair or implants.

Infertility is the inability to conceive a child after 12 months or unprotected sex. By this definition, 1 in 25 men are infertile, although an additional 25% conceive within 2 years. The most common causes of infertility in men are low sperm counts, poor semen quality, or both. Injuries, **birth defects**, infections, environmental pollutants, chronic stress, drug abuse, and hormonal problems account for the majority of male infertility cases, while about 15% of infertility cases for both men and women have no apparent cause (idiopathic infertility).

Declining sperm counts have been observed in industrialized countries, and possible explanations for this decrease are as diverse as increased environmental pollutants to the use of plastic diapers, which a German study claims damages infant testicles by keeping in excess heat. Male infertility can be diagnosed by sperm analysis, blood tests, and radiographic scans of the testicles.

Other types of sexual dysfunction include premature ejaculation, in which men cannot sustain intercourse long enough to bring their partners to climax, and retarded ejaculation (also called male orgasmic disorder) when male orgasm becomes difficult. Some men have periods of inadequate sexual desire (hypoactive sexual desire disorder), while sexual aversion disorder is fear and repulsion of sexual activity. Dyspareunia is painful intercourse and should be reported to physicians, as it may indicate STDs or infections. In addition to medical care, sexual dysfunction may be treated by sex therapy or psychotherapy depending on its causes.

Vasectomy, a permanent form of male birth control, is an outpatient operation that severs the tubes that transport sperm from the testicles. Men continue to produce male hormones and sperm and can have erections and ejaculations, but the sperm cannot enter the ejaculate, thus the man cannot father a child. Occasionally vasectomies can be reversed, but in making the decision whether to have this operation performed, the man should consider it permanent. Circumcision is the surgical removal of the foreskin of the penis, for religious and medical reasons. Increasing controversy surrounds this procedure. Advocates of circumcision claim it prevents infections (called balanitis) on the head of the penis, reduces chances of penile cancer, and reduces the risk of HIV transmission from infected men to women. Opponents of circumcision claim that the outdated procedure affords no medical benefits, that it causes unnecessary pain for infants, and that the lack of a foreskin may reduce sexual pleasure and performance.

MEN'S EMOTIONAL HEALTH. Men are far less likely to seek professional help for mood, emotional, and psychological problems than women. Depression is a mood disorder marked by continuing sadness, emotional pain, and the inability to enjoy formerly pleasurable activities. At least 12% of men will experience an episode of major depression at least once in their lives.

More women attempt **suicide**, but completion of suicide occurs far more frequently in men than in women. As a result, suicide in 2007 was the seventh leading cause of death in males, but the 15th leading cause in females. The Men's Health Network reports that 15–19-year-old boys were five times more likely than girls to commit suicide. The rate increases to seven times more likely in men ages 20–24. Some men experience depression and emotional problems between the ages of 50 and 65 as they face the major transition into retirement and older age. In men over age 65, the suicide rate is almost seven times higher in men than in women.

Panic attacks have symptoms of overwhelming fear, chest pain, shortness of breath, numbness, and increased heart rate. Men may mistake them as heart attacks. Men also are subject to dependence on nicotine, alcohol, and other drugs. This dependence is often a sign of an unhealthy attempt to escape from deeper emotional issues. Men can improve their health by seeking professional help for emotional and psychological problems before these problems become entrenched in their lives.

Mental illness can be particularly difficult for men because in our society men are taught to withhold rather than express emotions and feelings. Emotional problems can be strong signals for men to communicate and confront deeper issues. Help can be found from physicians, psychotherapists, and spiritual or religious counselors.

OSTEOPOROSIS. According the National Osteoporosis Foundation, 10 million Americans have osteoporosis with another 30 million at risk of developing the disease. Although osteoporosis is four times more prevalent in women than in men, a substantial number of men are affected. After age 40, the risk for osteoporosis increases five-fold for each decade of life, however, osteoporosis tends to develops about 10 to 15 years later in men than in women. Early osteoporosis in men may be associated with alcoholism and hormonal imbalances. Men can decrease their risk by increasing calcium and vitamin D.

Costs to society

As of 2009, there were 151.4 million men living in the United States. Of these, about 15% of men over age 18 were considered to be in poor health. Much of their poor health was related to the fact that approximately one-third of men over age 20 were obese, one-third had hypertension (high blood pressure), and one-third had consumed five or more alcoholic drinks in a single occasion within the past year. In addition, 21% smoked.

KEY TERMS

Benign—Not malignant, noncancerous.

Body Mass Index (BMI)—A measurement of fatness that compares height to weight.

Depression—A mental condition in which a person feels extremely sad and loses interest in life. A person with depression may also have sleep problems and loss of appetite and may have trouble concentrating and carrying out everyday activities. Severe depression may instigate a suicide attempt.

Osteoporosis—A condition found in older individuals in which bones decrease in density and become fragile and more likely to break. It can be caused by lack of vitamin D and/or calcium in the diet.

Sigmoidoscopy—Test procedure using an optical instrument to view the internal rectum and colon.

Stroke—Irreversible damage to the brain caused by insufficient blood flow to the brain as the result of a blocked artery. Damage can include loss of speech or vision, paralysis, cognitive impairment, and death.

Urologist—Physician specializing in male reproductive and urinary systems.

According to the Centers for Disease Control 2011 National Health Interview Survey, 45.9 million Americans or 17.3% of the population under age 65 lacked any type of medical insurance, and men were more likely than women to be without insurance. The same survey indicated that approximately 7% of men ages 18–64 failed to receive medical care due to costs during the preceding 12 months, and about 20% of men in this age group had no specific place to go for medical care.

The lack of insurance and lack of a usual place to receive medical care suggest that there is a twofold cost to society for men's health. First, health care for uninsured men and women is frequently paid for through taxpayer dollars, often through emergency room services because emergency rooms, by law, cannot turn away individuals because of inability to pay. Second, a substantial percentage of men do not establish a regular relationship with physicians or other healthcare professionals. Thus, they miss out on preventive care and screening tests that could prevent or detect illness. Finally, because men, on average, die before women, a certain percentage of older women who do not have their own independent pensions are left in financial distress and need to turn to charitable and government social services and their relatives for financial support.

Resources

BOOKS

Simon, Harvey B. *The Harvard Medical School Guide to Men's Health: Lessons from the Harvard Men's Health Studies.* New York: Free Press, 2004.

WEBSITES

Agency for Healthcare Research and Quality. "Healthy Men." http://www.ahrq.gov/healthymen/index.html (accessed October 21, 2012).
MedlinePlus. "Men's Health." http://www.nlm.nih.gov/medlineplus/menshealth.html (accessed October 21, 2012).
Men's Health Network. "Blueprint for Men's Health." http://www.menshealthnetwork.org/blueprint/index.htm (accessed October 21, 2012).

ORGANIZATIONS

Men's Health Network, PO Box 75972, Washington, DC 20013, (202) 543-6462, info@menshealthnetwork.org, http://www.menshealthnetwork.org.

Douglas Dupler, MA
Teresa G. Odle
Tish Davidson, AM

Mental health *see* **Community mental health**

Methamphetamine

Definition

Methamphetamine, or "meth," is an addictive central nervous system (CNS) stimulant with limited medical value. The United States Drug Enforcement Administration (DEA) lists methamphetamine as a Schedule II drug, which means it has high abuse potential and must be prescribed by a prescription that cannot be refilled.

Demographics

The national Monitoring the Future survey of 2008 found that in 2007, about 1.3 million Americans had used methamphetamine, a decrease from 1.9 million in 2006. This survey found that 2.3% of 8th graders, 2.4% of 10th graders, and 2.8% of 12th graders had tried methamphetamine at some time in their lives.

In the United States, methamphetamine use peaks in white men 30–40 years old; however, according to the Monitoring the Future survey, the average age of first use in 2007 was 19.1 years. In addition, methamphetamine use is highest in western states. Internationally, methamphetamine use is highest in Eastern Europe and Southeast Asia.

Description

Methamphetamine was first synthesized in Japan in 1919 and was used as a drug therapy in **asthma** inhalers in the 1930s. Amphetamines of all kinds were used during World War II by both sides to increase the alertness and prolong wakefulness of soldiers. After the war, the government developed stricter regulations for the manufacture and use of amphetamines, but they remained popular among people who wanted to stay awake for long periods (e.g., students, long-haul truck drivers) and were commonly used by people who wanted to lose weight. In 1970, more restrictions were put on methamphetamine, so that today it is a Schedule II drug. Despite this, methamphetamine remains a popular drug of abuse.

Methamphetamine is produced illegally in many countries, including the United States, and can be synthesized with readily available materials. The drug's misuse is deemed to be a major societal problem. Methamphetamine is addictive. It goes by the street names of "ice," "chalk," "crystal," "crystal meth," "speed," "crank," and "glass."

Methamphetamine is similar to other CNS stimulants, such as amphetamine (its parent drug), methylphenidate, and cocaine, in that it stimulates dopamine reward pathways in the brain. Consistent with its stimulant profile, methamphetamine causes increased activity and talkativeness, decreased appetite and fatigue, and a general sense of well-being. Compared to amphetamine, methamphetamine is more potent and longer-lasting, and it has more harmful effects on the brain. In animals, a single high dose of methamphetamine has been shown to damage nerve terminals in the dopamine-containing regions of the brain.

Methamphetamine

Short-term effects:

• Increased alertness
• Rapid and irregular heartbeat
• Rise in blood pressure and body temperature

Long-term effects:

• Anxiety and feelings of confusion
• Dental problems
• Increased risk of contracting diseases such as HIV/AIDS and hepatitis
• Insomnia
• Mood disturbances
• Violent behavior

In 2008, 850,000 Americans aged 12 and older had abused methamphetamine at least once in the past year, 11% of whom were younger than 18.

SOURCE: National Institutes of Health, National Institute on Drug Abuse, "Methamphetamine." Available online at: http://www.drugabuse.gov/drugpages/methamphetamine.html; also Substance Abuse and Mental Health Services Administration, *Results from the 2008 National Survey on Drug Use and Health: National Findings.* Available online at: http://www.oas.samhsa.gov/nsduh/2k8nsduh/2k8Results.cfm (accessed August 19, 2010).

Consequences of methamphetamine abuse. *(Table by PreMediaGlobal. Reproduced by permission of Gale, a part of Cengage Learning.)*

Methamphetamine is a white, odorless, bitter-tasting crystalline powder that easily dissolves in **water** or alcohol. Misuse occurs in many forms, as methamphetamine can be smoked, snorted, injected, or taken orally. When smoked or injected, methamphetamine enters the brain very rapidly and immediately produces an intense, but short-lived, rush that many abusers find extremely pleasurable. Snorting or oral ingestion produces euphoria—a feeling of being high—within minutes. As with other abused stimulants, methamphetamine is most often used in a binge-and-crash pattern. A "run" of repeated doses may be continued over the course of days (binge) before stopping (crash). Exhaustion occurs with repeated use of methamphetamine, involving intense fatigue and need for sleep after the stimulation phase.

Approved medical indications for the drug are the sleep disorder narcolepsy, attention deficit hyperactivity disorder (ADHD), and extreme **obesity**, but in each case methamphetamine is a second-line drug at best and is used only after other, less harmful drugs have failed to be effective.

A prescription form of methamphetamine (brand name Desoxyn) is used to treat ADHD. Desoxyn comes in the form of a small, white tablet, which is orally ingested. Dosing begins at 5 mg once or twice a day and is increased weekly until the lowest effective dose is attained. Desoxyn should not be taken with other stimulants (including caffeine and decongestants) or antidepressant drugs (especially monoamine oxidase inhibitors [MAOs], but also tricyclic antidepressants). Desoxyn should not be taken by patients with glaucoma, cardiovascular disease (including hypertension and arteriosclerosis), or hyperthyroidism.

Meth labs

Around the United States are homemade methamphetamine-producing operations, or "meth labs," of various sizes. Meth labs are often run in residential dwellings like apartments, houses, and mobile homes. Often, meth labs are discovered when the volatile chemicals used in making methamphetamine combust unexpectedly, resulting in a fire, to which firefighters and other emergency personnel respond. The persons actually making the methamphetamine are obviously at great risk for health problems due to inhaling the toxic chemical vapors emitted by the methamphetamine creation process, however, those who live with or around them are also at risk. In addition to the danger of explosion, serious health problems can occur from exposure to chemicals produced during the manufacture of methamphetamine. When looking for a home or apartment, particularly in rural or western areas where meth use is prevalent, it is important for prospective buyers to have the home and property inspected.

Causes and symptoms

Short-term effects of methamphetamine relate to its stimulation of the brain and the cardiovascular system. Euphoria and rush, alertness, increased **physical activity**, and decreased sleep and appetite occur from an increase in available dopamine in the brain. Any or all of these effects can lead to compulsive use of the drug that characterizes **addiction**. In addition, methamphetamine causes rapid heart beat (tachycardia), increased respiration, and increased blood pressure (hypertension), and with very high doses, increased body temperature (hyperthermia) and convulsions can occur.

Chronic use of methamphetamine can result in two hallmark features of addiction: tolerance and dependence. Tolerance to the euphoric effects in particular can prompt abusers to take higher or more frequent doses of the drug. Withdrawal symptoms in chronic users include depression, anxiety, fatigue, and an intense craving for the drug. Users who inject methamphetamine risk contracting life-threatening viruses such as HIV and **hepatitis** through the use of dirty needles.

With repeated use, methamphetamine can cause anxiety, insomnia, mood disturbances, confusion, hallucinations, psychosis, and violent behavior. Psychotic features sometimes emerge, such as paranoia,

KEY TERMS

Central nervous system (CNS)—Part of the nervous system consisting of the brain, cranial nerves, and spinal cord. The brain is the center of higher processes, such as thought and emotion, and is responsible for the coordination and control of bodily activities and the interpretation of information from the senses. The cranial nerves and spinal cord link the brain to the peripheral nervous system, that is the nerves present in the rest of body.

Dopamine—A neurochemical made in the brain that is involved in many brain activities, including movement and emotion.

Hallucination—A false or distorted perception of objects, sounds, or events that seems real. Hallucinations usually result from drugs or mental disorders.

Psychosis—A serious mental disorder characterized by defective or lost contact with reality often with hallucinations or delusions.

hallucinations, and delusions, and can last well after methamphetamine use has stopped. **Stroke** and weight loss are other long-term effects.

Other symptoms experienced by methamphetamine addicts include:

- Increased body temperature—methamphetamine can cause an individual's body temperature to rise, leading to unconsciousness or death.

- "Crank bugs"—a sensation that bugs or something similar are crawling on or under an individual's skin.

- "Meth mouth"—ongoing methamphetamine use causes the user's teeth to become stained, rotten, and even broken. This is aggravated by the tendency of meth addicts to consume sweet foods and drinks, grind their teeth, and have dry mouth.

- Aged appearance—meth addicts tend to age rapidly. Addicts' highly agitated and active state, poor nutrition, and drastic weight loss tend to make them look sick and/or old. Addicts often have shaky hands, a dulled sunken appearance, and the presence of sores on their bodies.

Diagnosis

Methamphetamine use may be suspected by the symptoms described previously and confirmed with a urine drug screening test.

Treatment

For acute intoxication accompanied by psychosis, patients may be calmed by reassurance and a quiet setting, but sometimes antipsychotic drugs or sedatives are administered. Substances that prevent absorption from the gastrointestinal tract (e.g., activated charcoal) may be used if the drug was taken orally. Additional care is given as needed (e.g., keeping the airways open, treatment of seizures.) Individuals with methamphetamine intoxication may be violent, agitated, and a danger to themselves and others.

The most effective treatment for methamphetamine addiction is cognitive-behavioral intervention, such as counseling, but may also include family education, drug testing, and group support in a twelve-step program. The goal of these modalities is to modify the patient's thinking, expectancies, and behaviors to increase coping skills in the face of life's stressors. Contingent management is a promising behavioral intervention, where incentives are provided in exchange for staying clean and for participating in treatment. Residential programs and therapeutic communities may be helpful, particularly in more severe cases.

Antidepressant drugs such as bupropion (Wellbutrin) can be a useful treatment aid, but as of 2012, there are no FDA-approved medications specifically for the treatment of stimulant addiction.

Prognosis

Addiction is a complex disorder, and prospects for individual addicts vary widely. Chronic methamphetamine use causes changes in brain and mental function. While some effects are reversible, others are very long-lasting and perhaps permanent. Methamphetamine is addictive. Relapses are common, and cravings may continue for a long time after drug use has stopped.

Efforts and solutions

Methamphetamine use became a national epidemic starting in the 1990s, particularly in western and rural areas. Many teens experiment with meth, sometimes overdosing on their first use. As a result of the widespread problem of methamphetamine abuse, many government and social institutions have implemented **prevention** programs.

Teenagers and schools

Teenagers are a target group for prevention strategies as adolescence and young adulthood are associated with exposure to, and an inclination to experiment with, drugs. Drug education and prevention programs should begin early, and parents and teachers should be alert to the possibility of methamphetamine abuse. Many states have such programs or task forces in place, such as the Illinois Attorney General's office, which hosts "Meth Net," a website with resources and strategies for fighting meth use, especially in schools.

Methamphetamine ingredients

Due to the relative ease with which methamphetamine can be produced, and the prevalence of dangerous home "meth labs," ongoing efforts are being made to increase the difficulty of acquiring methamphetamine ingredients. One of the main ingredients in homemade varieties of meth is found in common over-the-counter cold medicines that contain pseduoephedrine or ephedrine. Someone planning to make methamphetamine might buy large quantities of such cold medicines. Though state laws vary, many states and retailers require photo identification to purchase such over-the-counter medicines, or limit and record the quantities that can be purchased, and some states input buyer information into a statewide database to help prevent abuse.

The Meth Project

In 2005, businessman Thomas M. Siebel founded the Meth Project, which is currently funded by the Thomas and Stacey Sibel Foundation. The Meth Project funds separate Meth Project programs in eight states. It attempts to reduce the meth epidemic through confrontational, research-based public service messages, as well as education and legislative advocacy. The Meth Project is known for its blunt and even graphic public service ads, which show the effects of methamphetamine abuse on the human body and brain, as well as social, sexual, familial, and legal effects. The Meth Project also hosts a website that contains public service messages, resources for addicts looking for help, resources for family and friends of addicts, and interactive modules demonstrating the effects of meth use.

Faces of meth

In 2004, the Multnomah County Sheriff's Office started a program, which eventually became Faces of Meth. Multnomah County is in Oregon, which is a state that has been hit especially hard by the methamphetamine epidemic. The program, which is used as an educational tool, compares mug shots of detainees, usually one from before or early on in their methamphetamine use, and one from later. Sometimes the time span between the two photos is not great, but the subject's change in appearance is usually drastic, sometimes

making him or her unrecognizable. The pictures on the Faces of Meth websites are free and available for educational purposes. Due to the success and popularity of the Faces of Meth project, the Multnomah County Sheriff's Office developed a film *From Drugs To Mugs*, designed for educational use, that is available through its website.

Resources

BOOKS

Lee, Steven J. *Overcoming Crystal Meth Addiction: An Essential Guide to Getting Clean.* New York: Marlowe & Co., 2006.

Weisheit, Ralph A. and William White. *Methamphetamine: Its History, Pharmacology, and Treatment.* Center City, MN: Hazelden, 2009.

PERIODICALS

Derlet, Robert W., Timothy E. Albertson and John J. Richards. *Toxicity.* "Methamphetamine." http://emedicine.medscape.com/article/820918-overview. Accessed December 4, 2009.

WEBSITES

Faces of Meth. http://www.facesofmeth.us/. Accessed August 20, 2012.

Faces of Meth. "Drugs To Mugs." http://www.facesofmeth.us/drugs_to_mugs.html. Accessed August 20, 2012.

Illinois Attorney General "Methamphetamine Prevention in Schools." http://illinoisattorneygeneral.gov/methnet/fightmeth/schools.html. Accessed August 20, 2012.

Meth Project. http://www.methproject.org/. Accessed August 20, 2012.

MedlinePlus. "Methamphetamine." http://www.nlm.nih.gov/medlineplus/methamphetamine.html. Accessed December 15, 2009.

National Institute on Drug Abuse. "Methamphetamine Abuse and Addiction." http://www.nida.nih.gov/ResearchReports/methamph/methamph.html. July 2009.

National Institute on Drug Abuse "Effects of Meth on Bodies and Brains." http://www.drugabuse.gov/infofacts/methamphetamine.html

Partnership for a Drug-Free America. "Warning Signs: Is Your Child Using Meth?" http://www.drugfree.org/Portal/DrugIssue/MethResources/is_my_child.html. Accessed March 2, 2010.

ORGANIZATIONS

National Clearinghouse on Alcohol and Drug Information, P. O. Box 2345, Rockville, MD 20847, (877) SAMHSA-7; Hablamos español: (877) 767-8432; TDD: (800) 487-4889, Fax: (240) 221-4292, http://ncadi.samhsa.gov

National Council on Alcohol and Drug Dependence, 244 East 58th Street 4th Floor, New York, NY 10022, (212) 269-7797, 24-hour help line: (800) NCA-CALL, Fax: (212) 269-7510, national@mcadd.org, http://www.ncadd.org

Partnership for a Drug-free America, 405 Lexington Avenue, Ste 1601, New York, NY 10174, (212) 922-1560, Fax: (212) 922-1570, http://www.drugfree.org.

Jill U. Adams
Tish Davidson, AM
Andrea Nienstedt, MA

Miasma

Definition

According to a now-disproven theory, miasma is foul air that can cause outbreaks of disease.

Description

Miasma was once thought to be the cause of many major disease outbreaks, such as the epidemics of **cholera** and the Black Death. Miasma was defined as air that became malignant due to contamination with suspended particles of rotting organic matter. This belief in miasma-caused disease was popular for several centuries, beginning at least as early as the Middle Ages, but has since been disproven.

Origins

Before scientists, medical doctors, and others understood that pathogens, such as bacteria and viruses, caused disease, the general hypothesis was that vapors or mists were responsible for many illnesses. This belief stemmed from a faulty correlation. People noticed high rates of illness in poorer, more congested areas of cities that were often visibly dirty and carried a noticeable, foul odor attributable to decaying organic matter. They also recognized that cleaner, wealthier neighborhoods carried lower rates of illness. This led to the so-called theory of miasma, or the miasmatic theory: Bad air, and particularly airborne particles of decaying matter, was causing illnesses, including plagues and epidemics. Miasmas could be associated with small areas, such as neighborhoods within a city, or larger areas, such as major geographic regions of a country. Miasmas could be temporary, lasting only as long as the illness remained in that community, or permanent. The designation of a permanent miasma was sometimes enough to cause people to avoid that location for many years.

Many cultures from Europe to Asia shared this notion that miasma in a particular location caused illness. In other words, all a person had to do to acquire an illness was to set foot in a place that had this "bad air." When cholera epidemics swept through Paris and London in the 1850s, authorities of the day blamed miasma. English

medical doctor William Farr (1807–1883) suspected that miasma originated in the mist above the heavily polluted River Thames, because he had documented that the closer individuals lived to the **water** or the nearer they worked to the water, the higher their risk of contracting the disease. Eventually, however, English medical doctor John Snow (1813–1858) correctly suggested that it was not the air, but the water that was causing cholera. Specifically, he identified the culprit as water that was distributed from a public water pump.

During the 1700s and 1800s, scientists were also beginning to use newly developed microscopes to notice small organisms with which humans shared the planet, and some of these scientists were suggesting that the organisms could be the cause of certain diseases. By the late 1800s, scientists confirmed that microorganisms were the cause of many diseases, and developed what is known as the **germ theory** of disease. With this theory in place, the concept of miasma was discounted once and for all.

Effects on public health

Before the scientific and medical community were aware that bacteria and viruses existed, and before they learned that these microorganisms could cause disease, they based much of their understanding of illnesses on observations. They noted that many disease outbreaks occurred in neighborhoods that had filthy living conditions and bad-smelling air, and made the assumption that the air was the root of the illnesses. As a result, at the first signs of an outbreak, neighborhood residents would flee the area. Many of these disease outbreaks, such as the Black Death, were actually a result of infections with pathogens that could be spread from one person to another, and therefore the movement of infected individuals from the original site often allowed the disease to spread from one area to another.

Costs to society

Millions of people died as a result of the Black Death, cholera, and other illnesses that were mistakenly associated with miasma. (Today, the term miasma is used to describe any unpleasant, unwholesome, oppressive or corrupting atmosphere.) In addition, the belief in miasma prevented the economic and agricultural development of certain geographic regions where "bad air" was deemed to be present. This was especially the case around swamps or in areas with depressed economic conditions, where miasma was believed to be a permanent regional condition.

Efforts and solutions

The belief in miasma was already waning when the scientific and medical community accepted the germ theory, and had solid evidence that microorganisms were indeed the cause of many diseases formerly attributed to miasma. This paradigm shift allowed researchers to begin finding

Cholera—A bacterial infection of the small intestine that causes profuse watery diarrhea. Left untreated, this can lead to severe dehydration and death.

Black Death—Also known as The Plague, the Black Death is a bacterial infection that caused millions of deaths in Europe during the 14th century.

methods to fight the pathogens and medical professionals to more successfully treat disease. In addition, it gave public health officials and others the understanding they needed to help contain outbreaks and prevent the spread of infection, and also allowed them to begin to eliminate the source of many pathogens through such efforts as:

• providing clean drinking water to citizens

• constructing better sanitation systems

• promoting proper food-safety and food-handling measures to prevent infections

• improving sanitary conditions in hospitals and care facilities

Resources

WEBSITES

"Brief History During the Snow Era." The Glaucoma Foundation. http://www.ph.ucla.edu/epi/snow/1859map/cholera_prevailingtheories_a2.html (accessed October 8, 2012).

"Concepts of Contagion and Epidemics." Contagion: Historical Views of Diseases and Epidemics. Harvard University Library Open Collections Program. http://ocp.hul.harvard.edu/contagion/concepts.html (accessed October 8, 2012).

"Disease Theories: Miasma v. Microbes." St. Francis of Assisi Parish. http://www.stfrancisparish.com/history/chapter4b.pdf (accessed October 8, 2012).

"Competing Theories of Cholera." Department of Epidemiology, School of Public Health, University of California Los Angeles. http://www.ph.ucla.edu/epi/snow/cholera theories.html (accessed October 8, 2012).

"Miasma." Science Museum, London. http://www.science museum.org.uk/broughttolife/techniques/miasmatheory.aspx (accessed October 8, 2012).

Leslie Mertz, Ph.D.

Migrant farm workers

Definition

The term *migrant worker* has a variety of meanings in various parts of the world. The United Nations uses the term to describe any person who works outside her or his home country. In some regions, the term may be used for individuals who travel to other parts of their own country to find employment. In the United States, the term usually applies to men, women, and children who come from other nations to this country to find work. In many cases, these individuals are seasonal workers, individuals who come to the United States for only a certain part of the year when crops are ready for harvesting. Although the term *migrant worker* may apply in principle to people who are looking for any type of employment, in reality the vast majority of such individuals end up working in the agricultural sector.

The situation is very different in other parts of the world. In China, for example, people tend to migrate from the countryside to urban areas, where opportunities for gainful employment are much greater than in their home communities. By some estimates, more than 230 million Chinese had moved from rural to urban settings by the early 2010s, with the possibility of that number doubling by 2025. This essay focuses on the U.S., rather than the Chinese, pattern of migration and health problems associated with that pattern.

Demographics

According to the most recent statistics available, about three million people in the United States can be classified as migrant or seasonal farmworkers. About three-quarters of that number are from Mexico and about 29% from the United States. The latter individuals move from one part of the country to take advantage of farm work opportunities and may or may not be documented residents. Nearly 30% of migrant farm workers in the United States have been here 20 years or more, with an almost equal number having been resident for less than four years. The median age of migrant farm workers in 2011 was 36 years, with more than three-quarters of the **population** older than 25 years. A plurality of migrant farm workers (45%) had six years of education or less, with the average level of schooling completed being eighth grade. About a third of migrants reported that they spoke English "well," with a slightly larger percentage saying that they spoke English "not at all."

About a third of all migrant farm workers are U.S. citizens, but nearly half (48%) are undocumented aliens. The remaining number live in the United States under green card status. Most migrant workers are employed for less than a full year, with 35 weeks being the average period of employment. Average annual personal income for workers in 2009 (the last year for which data are available) was between $15,000 and $17,500, while the average for a family was slightly more, at about $17,500 to $20,000. About a quarter of all families were classified as living below the national **poverty** level in 2009, a significant drop from 56% in 1997. About 43% of all

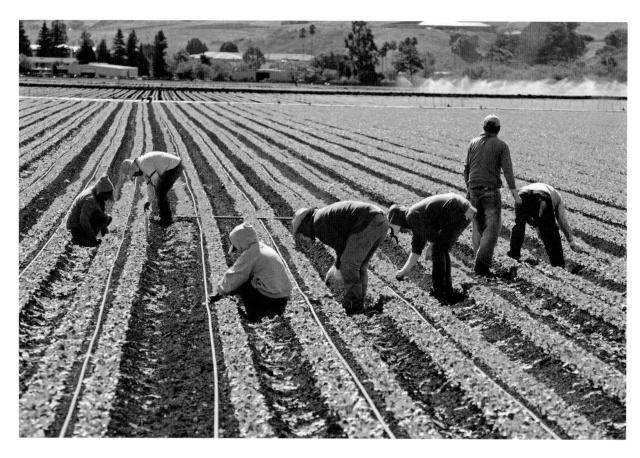

Migrant farm workers tending to a spinach crop. *(© iStockphoto.com/Nancy Nehring)*

workers received some type of public assistance, either need- or contribution-based, or both.

Health issues

Migrant farm workers face many of the same health and safety issues encountered by all workers in the United States, especially those employed in the field of agriculture. In addition, their risk for injury or death is likely to be exacerbated by the lack of healthcare facilities and opportunities available to other works in agriculture or other occupations. The United States Department of Labor (DOL) and other federal agencies consistently rank farming as one of the most dangerous occupations in the nation. In 2009, for example, 440 farm workers died of work-related injuries. Fatality rate for the occupation was seven times that of workers in private industry in general. Injury rate among farm workers was also far above that of workers in other fields, 20% greater than the average of all fields of employment. According to the DOL, an average of 243 agricultural workers every day sustain some type of injury that requires their absence from the fields, with about five percent of those injuries developing into a permanent disability.

Children and youth are at special risk in the field of agriculture. They are often assigned jobs not that different from adult workers, but with physical skills unable to tolerate the **stress** created in the fields. As a result, a disporportionate number of farm-related injuries and deaths occur among boys and girls under the age of 18. The fatality rate on farms among this age group in 2009, for examples, was 21.3 children per 100,000 fulltime employees, making agriculture the most dangerous occupation for American youth under the age of 18. In the same year, the Child Labor Coalition estimated that 16,100 children and adolescents were injured while performing farm work.

Risks

Migrant farm workers, along with agricultural employees, face a number of risks unique to their field of employment. These include:

• The number one cause of fatalities in agriculture is events involving tractors. These events include overturns (the major cause of injury and death), run-overs by tractors, collisions with other vehicles, tractors being ensnared in other agricultural equipment, and a variety of other tractor-use-related events.

- The most common types of injuries are sprains, strains, and torn ligaments (22% of all injuries), fractures (15%), and cuts (13%). These injuries result from a variety of causes, most commonly some type of interaction with animals, falls, or tractor-related incidents.

- Infectious diseases are especially common among farm workers. The rate of tuberculosis is six times greater than that among the general population with nearly half of all farm workers having positive skin tests for the disease. Parasitic infections are also common, with the rate of such diseases reaching almost 60 times that of the general population in some instances.

- Pesticide and fertilizer poisoning is also widespread because of the close contact farm workers have with these chemicals. The U.S. Environmental Protection Agency (EPA) has estimated that upwards of 300,000 farm workers may experience acute pesticide poisoning each year on American farms. A number of farm chemicals are known or thought to be carcinogenic, mutagenic, and/or teratogenic.

- Farm workers are also at high risk for dermatitis from exposure not only to pesticides and fertilizers, but also to other chemicals used in the fields and to allergenic plants themselves. Exposure to sun and wind may also result in dermatitis.

- Exposure to a wide variety of airborne chemicals, such as ammonia, hydrogen sulfide, carbon monoxide, and methane, may result in a host of respiratory disorders, including allergies, asthma, hypersensitivity pneumonitis, (so-called farmer's lung), pulmonary fibrosis, chronic bronchitis, pulmonary edema, tracheobronchitis, emphysema, and asphyxiation.

- Chronic muscular disorders are likely to result also from routine farming activities, such as bending, stooping, reaching, lifting, and carrying.

- Farm workers also tend to have a disproportionately high rate of dental problems, up to three times the rate among the general population in some studies.

- A number of social and mental issues are also associated with farm work, such as stress, depression, anxiety, thoughts of suicide, relationship problems, alcoholism, substance abuse, and child and spousal abuse.

Not only do migrant farm workers face an unusually heavy burden of health risks, but also they tend to lack many of the basic skills and tools with which to attack their health issues. Some of their greatest handicaps are poor or non-existent English language skills, limited financial resources, lack of transportation, lack of health care insurance, fear of deportation, fear of loss of income or employment, and lack of sick leave for dealing with

---

KEY TERMS

Contribution-based assistance—Financial or other type of aid to a person or a family for which the individual or family has made some type of contribution, such as payments toward Social Security or Medicare.

Migration—Movement of an individual or group of individuals from one geographic region to another geographic region within a single nation or across international boundaries.

Need-based assistance—Financial or other type of aid to a person or a family that is determined entirely by that person's or family's needs.

---

health issues. Even when workers are able to obtain medical services, those services are often directed at acute problems, with more serious chronic issues ignored because of time, financial, or other constraints.

Treatment

The U.S. government has understood and acknowledged the important of migrant farm worker health issues for more than 50 years. In 1962, President John F. Kennedy signed into law the Migrant Health Act, which provided for the establishment of health clinics across the nation designed to deal specifically with migrant health issues. Funding legislation for these clinics has been adopted on a regular basis ever since, and in 2012 there were 159 federally funded migrant worker health centers throughout the United States. Virtually all of these clinics have satellite operations that focus on one or another specific health issues, resulting in a total of more than 700 health care units in all for migrant workers. The system is designed to provide all migrant workers with basic health care regardless of their citizenship or their ability to pay for such services.

The problem that remains is that only a very low percentage of migrant farm workers—less than 15% according to some estimates—take advantage of these services. A number of reasons have been posited for this fact, such as fear of penalties and/or deportation among undocumented workers, lack of adequate employment and payment records, lack of knowledge and/or understanding about the program, and failure to meet state residency requirements for attendance at the clinics. Experts in migrant worker health issues suggest that improvements in the efficiency with which the national migrant health clinic system operates could be a major step forward in dealing with this complex and persistent public health issue.

Resources

BOOKS

Chavez, Leo R. *Shadowed Lives: Undocumented Immigrants in American Society.* Belmont, CA: Wadsworth, Cengage Learning, 2013.

Holmes, Seth M. *Fresh Fruit, Broken Bodies: Migrant Farmworkers in the United States.* Berkeley: University of California Press, 2013.

PERIODICALS

Garcia, D., et al. "The Migrant Clinicians Network: Connecting Practice to Need and Patients to Care." *Journal of Agromedicine* 17, 1. (2012): 5–14.

Holmes, Seth M. "The Clinical Gaze in the Practice of Migrant Health: Mexican Migrants in the United States." *Social Science & Medicine* 74, 6. (2012): 873–81.

Luque, J. S., et al. "Mobile Farm Clinic Outreach to Address Health Conditions among Latino Migrant Farmworkers in Georgia." *Journal of Agromedicine* 17, 4. (2012): 386–97.

Quesada, James, Laurie Kain Hart, and Philippe Bourgois. "Structural Vulnerability and Health: Latino Migrant Laborers in the United States." *Medical Anthropology* 30, 4. (2011): 339–62.

WEBSITES

Carroll, Daniel, Annie George, and Russell Saltz. "2011 Changing Characteristics of U.S. Farm Workers:21 Years of Findings from the National Agricultural Workers Survey." http://migration.ucdavis.edu/cf/files/2011-may/carroll-changing-characteristics.pdf. Accessed on December 4, 2012.

"Farmworkers in the United States." Migrant Health Promotion. http://www.migranthealth.org/index.php?option=com_content&view=article&id=38&Itemid=30. Accessed on December 4, 2012.

"Migrant Health. Rural Assistance Center."http://www.raconline.org/topics/public_health/migrant.php. Accessed on December 4, 2012.

Moyer, Christine S. "Migrant Farmworkers: Medical Care for an Invisible Population." amednews.com. http://www.ama-assn.org/amednews/2012/06/11/hlsa0611.htm. Accessed on December 4, 2012.

ORGANIZATIONS

National Center for Farmworker Health, Inc., 1770 FM 967, Buda, TX USA 78610, 1 (512) 312–2700, (800) 531–5120, Fax: 1 (512) 312–2600, info@ncfh.org, http://www.ncfh.org/.

David E. Newton, Ed.D.

Military health

Definition

The term *military health* refers to the range of physical and mental health and medical care available to

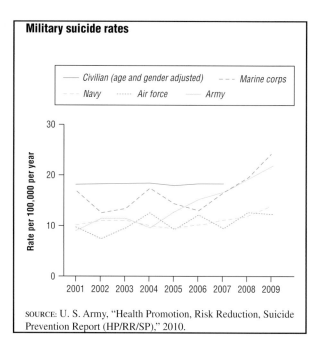

Military suicide rates

SOURCE: U. S. Army, "Health Promotion, Risk Reduction, Suicide Prevention Report (HP/RR/SP)," 2010.

(Graph by PreMediaGlobal. © 2013 Cengage Learning.)

members of the military service and, often, their dependents. Since military health programs vary from country to country, this entry focuses on military health policies and practices in the United States.

Purpose

The purpose of military health programs in the United States is to provide appropriate medical care to service members at or near the field of battle, at care facilities more remote from the battlefield itself, and in long-term healthcare facilities located throughout the nations. Additional health and medical care is also offered to veterans of military service and their dependents, as well, under certain circumstances, as to members of the reserve corps.

Description

Origins

The character of military health care has evolved throughout the nation's history. During Colonial and Revolutionary times, medical care was restricted almost entirely to battlefield injuries and illness, often focusing on efforts to keep military personnel alive after injuries or bouts of disease. The primary focus of treatment was often getting personnel well enough to return to battle as soon as possible. Treatment was usually a local practice, with no centralized policies or programs to act as guidelines for individual medical practitioners. Given the primitive state of medical care in general, battlefield treatments were often no more than moderately successful in saving lives and promoting the recuperation of the sick and injured.

This situation began to change during the Civil War, when specialized facilities were developed both at the battlefield and at nearby locations, where somewhat standardized treatment procedures were sometimes available. Again, the main emphasis of such programs was to help personnel recover well enough and rapidly enough to return to battle.

Until the second half of the twentieth century, there were essentially no formal provisions for health and medical care for dependents of military personnel or for retirees from the military service. As early as 1884, the U.S. Congress instructed the military services to provide health and medical care to dependents on a "space-available" basis, resulting in a policy that varied widely in its application from time to time and location to location. In some places and at some times, dependents could receive a level of healthcare equivalent to the best available anywhere in the country; at other times and places, little or no care was available.

During World War II and the Korean War, U.S. military facilities were so severely stressed by wartime demands that they were unable to keep pace with the health and medical demands of dependents also. Thus, over time, the U.S. Congress expanded programs designed to serve the needs of dependents as well as of active personnel. For example, the Congress passed the Emergency Maternal and Infant Care Program (EMIC) in 1943, making available maternity care and the care of infants up to the age of one year for wives and children of service members in the lower four pay grades. The program was actually administered by state **health departments**, relieving the military of having to deal with this issue. In 1956 and 1966, Congress also adopted legislation leading to the most ambitious healthcare program of all for military dependents, the Dependents Medical Care Act of 1956 and the Military Medical Benefits Amendments of 1966. The program produced by this legislation was called the Civilian Health and Medical Program of the Uniformed Services (CHAMPUS). CHAMPUS provided for a comprehensive program of health and medical care for military dependents operated by civilian providers. In the late 1980s, a number of revisions in CHAMPUS were mandated by Congress, resulting in today's version of the program, TRICARE. TRICARE is a healthcare program available to active military personnel and their dependents and to retired personnel. It comes in three forms with different levels of service and types of providers, called Tricare Standard, Tricare Extra, and Tricare Prime. Other

variations of the standard program are Tricare Reserve Select, available to active members of the Reserves and National Guard; Tricare Reserve Retired, for retired members of the Reserves and National Guard; Tricare for Life, intended as back-up medical insurance for retirees covered by Medicare; and Tricare Young Adult, for dependents who are no longer covered by their parents' other Tricare policies.

Coverage

Injuries incurred during military combat include virtually every type of damage to the human body that can be imagined. Most injuries occur when a person is struck by a projectile (such as a bullet) or by the blast of an explosion. Those injuries include, but are not limited to:

- damage to one or both ears, resulting in temporary or permanent deafness
- damage to one or both eyes, causing temporary or permanent blindness or other eye problems
- damage to the respiratory system, causing hemorrhaging or perforation of the lungs, injury to the airways, formation of clots, or pneumonitis
- damage to the digestive system, causing rupture of the spleen or liver, perforation of the bowel, or hemorrhaging of the gut
- damage to the circulatory system, resulting in myocardial infarction, production of embolisms, or shock
- damage to the central nervous system, causing concussion, spinal injury, stroke, or brain injury
- damage to the kidneys, resulting in acute renal failure or other kidney problems
- Damage to the extremities, resulting in loss of hands, feet, arms, or legs, as well as burns, cuts, lacerations, and fractures.

Each of these problems must be treated at first on the battlefield itself, and eventually at facilities with increasingly extensive and sophisticated technology and personnel.

In recent years, an increasingly important cause of battlefield injuries has been relatively simple home-made devices known as improvised explosive devices (IEDs). These devices have been responsible for a significant increase in the number of injuries to fingers, toes, arms, and legs that have required amputations. The total number of such injuries in the Iraq and Afghan wars between 2001 and 2010 was 1,621, with more than three quarters resulting in the loss of an arm or a leg. These injuries represent a challenge both to the individual who has suffered the loss and the military and civilian medical profession because of the dramatic change in lifestyle occasioned by such injuries and the long-term care they will require for the injured individual.

The military medical system is confronted not only with having to deal with traumatic battlefield wounds like those listed, but with a host of other health and medical problems. For example, many military personnel are injured or killed in behind-the-front events, such as simply traveling to a battle area or delivering supplies to personnel at the front. One study of military personnel evacuated from Iraq between 2003 and 2007 found that more than 77 percent were being treated for non-combat injuries and health problems, such as sore knees, bad backs, respiratory illnesses, kidney stones, hypertension, and arthritis. **Infectious disease** continues to be a battlefield problem for many military personnel also. A 2004 epidemic of **leishmaniasis** in Iraq resulted in hospitalizations of up to 140 personnel per month until a spraying program for mosquitoes responsible for the disease ended the epidemic.

Yet another health problem encountered by military personnel is exposure to chemical and biological agents and a variety of environmental hazards. These exposures vary from time to time and location to location. They include a range of hazards, such as sand and dust, fog, garbage, industrial pollutants, ionizing **radiation**, a variety of fuels, metal fragments, toxic chemicals, everyday chemicals such as ammonia and formaldehyde, paint fumes, pesticides, microwaves, smoke from burning trash or oil fires, solvents, vaccines, and vehicle exhaust fumes.

Military personnel who have served in battle zones are also at risk for a variety of mental and emotional disorders. Perhaps the best known of these conditions today is post-traumatic stess disorder (PTSD), an anxiety disorder that may develop after a person is exposed to a severe psychological trauma. The condition has been associated with military service for centuries and has been known by a variety of names, including combat fatigue and shell shock. The symptoms and signs of PTSD include flashbacks and nightmares, anger, restlessness, tendencies toward confusion, fatigue, reduced reaction times, headaches, impulsivity, and thoughts of **suicide**. According to some studies, as many as 30 percent of returned combat veterans have experienced PTSD at one time or another in their lives and more than 20 percent of military personnel who have been deployed to combat zones over the last six years have experienced PTSD signs and symptoms. Other data suggest that between 12 and 20 percent of men and women who served in the Iraq war experienced PTSD at one time or another, and 6 to 11 percent of Afghan war veterans reported experiencing PTSD.

KEY TERMS

Leishmaniasis—An infection of the respiratory tract transmitted by the female sandfly.

Post-traumatic stress disorder (PTSD)—A severe anxiety disorder caused by exposure to a very stressful event or experience.

TRICARE—A healthcare program provided by the federal government to active military personnel and their dependents and to retired personnel.

Demographics

The U.S. Military Health Service (MHS) is responsible for the health and medical care of all active members of the armed forces, as well as that of retired personnel and dependents of both active and retired personnel. As of early 2013, the MHS employed more than 137,000 men and women in 65 hospitals, 412 medical clinics, and 414 dental clinics throughout the world. They were responsible for an estimated 9.6 million men and women with an annual budget of about $50 billion. As with many health and medical organizations, MHS has constantly been looking for ways to rein in financing for health care, particularly at a time when costs of medical services are continuing to climb. In 2012, the MHS announced a number of administrative changes in its health program designed to deal with the rising costs of health care, such as centralizing all health care services within a single new Defense Health Agency and the consolidation and transfer of health care in the Washington, D.C. area to a single central location.

Veteran services

Men and women who meet certain eligibility requirements qualify for a wide variety of health, medical, and related services from the U.S. Department of Veterans Affairs (DVA). In general, the minimum requirement is that a person entered active duty after October 1, 1981, and served a minimum of 24 months of active duty. Under those conditions, a person is eligible for a host of benefits that include health care, pensions, support for education and training programs, home loan guarantees, life insurance, transition assistance, dependent and survivors health care, burial and memorial benefits, and other special benefits available only or primarily to military veterans. Among the special health benefits provided by the DVA are special care programs for veterans who are more than 50 percent disabled, victims of sexual trauma, veterans with spinal cord injuries, and members of special health registries, such as the Gulf War Registry, Depleted Uranium Registries, Agent Orange Registry, and **Ionizing Radiation** Registry. The DVA also offers a number of counseling programs, such as readjustment counseling for recently discharged service members and bereavement counseling for family members. The department also provides special medical equipment, such as prosthetic and sensory aids, and specialized services for blind and visually impaired veterans.

Resources

BOOKS

Amara, Jomana, and Ann M. Hendricks, eds. *Military Health Care: From Pre-deployment to Post-separation.* London: Routledge, 2013.

Barton, Phoebe L. *Understanding the U.S. Health Services System*, 4th ed. Chicago: Health Administration Press, 2009.

Finley, Erin P. *Fields of Combat: Understanding PTSD among Veterans of Iraq and Afghanistan.* Ithaca, NY: ILR Press, 2011.

Morrison, Marjorie. *The Inside Battle: Our Military Mental Health Crisis.* Washington, D.C.: Military Psychology Press, 2012.

PERIODICALS

Gibbons, S. W., S. D. Barnett, and E. J. Hickling. "Family Stress and Posttraumatic Stress: The Impact of Military Operations on Military Health Care Providers." *Archives of Psychiatric Nursing* 26, 4. (2012): e31–9X.

Harris, G. L. "Reducing Healthcare Disparities in the Military through Cultural Competence." *Journal of Health and Human Services Administration* 34, 2. (2011): 145–81.

Meyer, K. S., et al. "Combat-related Traumatic Brain Injury and Its Implications to Military Healthcare." *Psychiatric Clinics of North America* 33, 4. (2010): 783–96.

WEBSITES

"Center for Military Health Policy Research." The Rand Corporation. http://www.rand.org/multi/military.html. Accessed on October 14, 2012.

"Federal Benefits for Veterans Dependents and Survivors." Department of Veterans Affairs. http://www.va.gov/opa/publications/benefits_book/2012_Federal_benefits_ebook_final.pdf. Accessed on October 14, 2012.

"Health." Army Times. http://www.armytimes.com/benefits/health/. Accessed on October 14, 2012.

"Veterans and Military Health." Medline Plus. http://www.nlm.nih.gov/medlineplus/veteransandmilitaryhealth.html#cat42. Accessed on October 14, 2012.

ORGANIZATIONS

Department of Defense (DOD), 1400 Defense Pentagon, Washington, DC USA 20301–1400, 1 (703) 571–3343, http://www.defense.gov/landing/comment.aspx, http://www.defense.gov/

Department of Veterans Affairs (DVA), 810 Vermont Ave., N.W., Washington, DC USA 20420.http://www.va.gov/landing2_contact.htm, http://www.va.gov/.

David E. Newton, Ed.D.

Millennium Development Goals

Definition

The Millennium Development Goals are a set of eight objectives established by the United Nations to be achieved by the year 2015.

Purpose

The purpose of the Millennium Development Goals (MDG) is to improve social and economic conditions in the world's poorest countries.

Description

The MDG were adopted in 2000 at a United Nations (UN) meeting known as the Millennium Summit. The Summit was the final step in a series of conferences and other meetings sponsored by the UN to consider the issue of improving the life of people living in developing countries. The New York meeting concluded with the adoption of the United Nations Millennium Declaration, which set forward the following eight goals:

• eradicating extreme poverty and hunger
• achieving universal primary education
• promoting gender equality and empowering women
• reducing by two-thirds the mortality rate of children under the age of five
• reducing by three-quarters the maternal mortality rate
• halting and then beginning to reduce the rate of HIV infection
• integrating the concept of sustainable development in the policies of all nations
• developing an open, rule-based, predictable, non-discriminatory trading and financial system

The New York meeting was followed by a number of conferences aimed at putting the MDG plan into action. Perhaps the most important of these conferences was the 2005 World Summit held in New York with 170 heads of state in attendance. The agenda for this meeting was a document prepared by Secretary-General Kofi Annan, in which specific actions for the achievement of

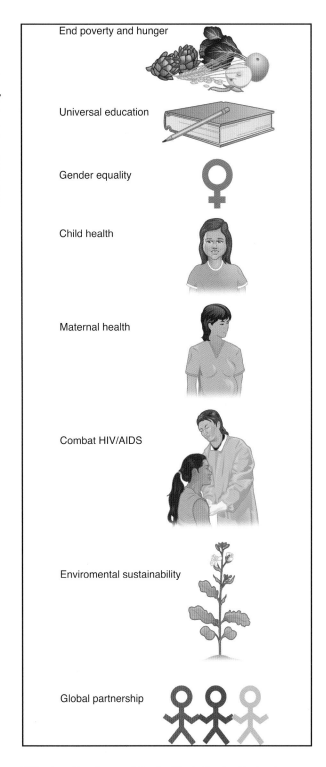

End poverty and hunger

Universal education

Gender equality

Child health

Maternal health

Combat HIV/AIDS

Enviromental sustainability

Global partnership

Millenium Development Goals *(Illustration by Electronic Illustrators Group. © 2013 Cengage Learning)*

the MDG program were proposed. At about the same time, the eight countries that make up the G8 group of nations devised a financing program that made available funds from the World Bank, the International Monetary Fund, and the African Development Bank to make possible the cancellation of up to $50 billion in debts owed by developing countries to entities in developed countries. The plan proposed that instead of spending this money on debt service, the world's poorest countries would be able to invest in programs aimed at achieving the MDG.

The MDG is obviously a very large and complex program that uses a wide range of activities to achieve its objectives. Some examples of the actions taken to reach these objectives are as follows. Governmental agencies and private businesses in developed countries:

- Post skilled personnel in governmental agencies in developing nations to teach them ways of improving the efficiency and extent of their operations.
- Work with individual farmers and farm cooperatives to teach them more efficient agricultural procedures.
- Provide teachers and other educational specialists to help countries improve their own educational systems.
- Develop mechanisms by which larger numbers of girls and women are incorporated into the educational system.
- Provide funds, material, and personnel with which to improve the infrastructure of a nation's education system.
- Help nations develop policies that will bring more women into the political and economic structure of the country.
- Devise new businesses and new products that extend a nation's market potential and, hence, its gross domestic product.
- Develop and implement health programs that teach children the basics of good nutrition and health practices.
- Aid countries in building and/or reforming their health services to provide a larger range of citizens with better basic health care.
- Help nations find ways of attacking fundamental problems that lead to widespread health issues, such as youth unemployment, abuse of children in the workplace, and trafficking in children and women.
- Provide nations with both the training and therapeutic materials needed to reduce the rate of HIV infection.

The question as to how successful the MDG program has been is one of great interest and concern to everyone involved with the project. Clearly, expectations have been high for its success, but there are a number of challenges that stand in the way of its success. Many countries lack either the will or the resources (or both) with which to attack the eight challenges listed in the MDG. A number of evaluative studies have found varying degrees of success, with some countries moving forward with all or at least some of the eight goals, and other countries making only minimal progress, or none at all, on all or many of the goals. In 2010, a major conference on the progress of the program was held in New York to consider the status of the MDG. That conference concluded with the adoption of a new position statement that outlined challenges that remained to be met and action programs designed to meet these challenges. The topics of **poverty**, hunger, disease, and women's and **children's health** received special attention in the conference's concluding document.

Another topic of the 2010 summit meeting in New York was the future of the MGD program beyond 2015. Participants acknowledged that most, if not all of the original MGD goals were too ambitious to be accomplished by the date specified, and that an extension of that time line would be necessary. As a consequence, the conference established a framework through which member nations of the UN, individual nations and groups of nations, nongovernmental agencies, and independent corporations and companies would continue meeting and talking about a program similar to MGD that would extend well beyond the original target date. A general meeting to codify this program has not yet been scheduled.

Professional publications

The primary source for information on the Millennium Development Goals is the UN website We Can End Poverty 2015 Millennium Development Goals at http://www.un.org/millenniumgoals/. That site provides access to all reports of conferences and other publications dealing with the MDG, including regular annual reports on the progress of the program. Other reports on specific topics are also available, such as *Trends in Maternal Mortality, MDG Good Practices 2010, Tourism and the MDGs, Energy for a Sustainable Future, WHO Publications on Weather, Climate, and Water*, and *Towards More Coherent United Nations Support to Africa*.

Resources

BOOKS

McGillivray, Mark, ed. *Achieving the Millennium Development Goals*. Basingstoke, UK: Palgrave Macmillan, 2008.
The Millennium Development Goals Report 2011. New York: United Nations, 2011.
Stijns, Jean–Philippe. *Can We Still Achieve the Millennium Development Goals?: From Costs to Policies*. Paris: OECD Development Centre, 2012.

PERIODICALS

Amieva, S., and S. Ferguson. "Moving Forward: Nurses Are Key to Achieving the United Nations Development Program's Millennium Development Goals." *International Nursing Review* 59. 1. (2012): 55–58.
Everett, Bryony, Erika Wagner, and Christopher Barnett. "Using Innovation Prizes to Achieve the Millennium Development Goals." *Innovations* 7. 1. (2012): 107–114.
Pienaar–Steyn, Sunette. "The Millennium Development Goals as a Conceptual Framework for Enabling and Evaluating Community Engagement." *South African Review of Sociology* 43. 2. (2012): 40–57

WEBSITES

Keeping the Promise: United to Achieve the Millennium Development Goals. United Nations, October 19, 2010. http://www.un.org/en/mdg/summit2010/pdf/outcome_documentN1051260.pdf (accessed October 11, 2012).
We Can End Poverty. 2015 Millennium Development Goals. United Nations. http://www.un.org/millenniumgoals/bkgd.shtml (accessed October 11, 2012).

ORGANIZATIONS

Information Centres Service. Strategic Communications Division. Department of Public Information. United Nations, New York, NY 10017, dpi_dis_unit@un.org, http://www.un.org/en/.

David E. Newton, EdD

Minority health

Definition

Minority health addresses the special medical and/or health needs associated with specific ethnic and racial groups—those who are included in the minority populations within the United States.

Demographics

The specific ethnic and racial groups in the United States who are included within minority populations, as stated by the Office of Minority Health (part of the U.S. **Department of Health and Human Services**), include Native Americans and Alaska Natives, Asian Americans, African Americans, Hispanics and Latinos, Native Hawaiians, and other Pacific Islanders.

Description

The United States, as well as many other countries, experiences cultural diversity. This poses health issues that are specific to ethnic groups. Additionally, the propensity for certain diseases or illnesses is of concern in certain minority groups. These specific health issues include infant mortality rates, **cancer**, cardiovascular disease, diabetes, HIV (human immunodeficiency virus) infection, and **immunization.**

Infant mortality rates

Infant mortality rates (IMRs) in the United States and in all countries worldwide are an accurate indicator of health status. They provide information concerning programs about pregnancy education and counseling, technological advances, and procedures and aftercare. IMRs vary among racial groups. The IMR in the United States, in 2012, was estimated at 5.98 per 1,000 live births, according to the Central Intelligence Agency. Males have an IMR of 6.64, while females have an IMR of 5.30.

African Americans have an IMR of 13.31 per 1,000 live births, nearly 2.5 times higher than that of whites. The IMRs among American Native Indian groups vary greatly, with some communities possessing IMRs about two times more than national rates. Overall, Native Americans had an IMR of 9.2. Hispanic Americans' IMRs (7.6 per 1,000 live births, overall) are also diverse for separate groups, since the IMR, for example, among Puerto Rican Americans is higher (8.3 per 1,000 live births), while with Mexican Americans it is lower (5.5 per 1,000 live births). Asian- and Pacific Islander Americans came in at 4.9, Central Americans and South Americans at 4.7, and Cuban Americans at 4.4 per 1,000 live births. (Statistics for the various minority groups were provided by the U.S. Centers for Disease Control and Prevention.)

Cancer

Cancer is a serious national, worldwide, and minority health concern, and is the second leading cause of death in the United States. In 2009, it was estimated that more than 12.5 million living adults had been diagnosed with cancer at some point in their lives. An estimated 848,170 new cases were diagnosed in 2012. Each year, cancer claims over half a million lives in the United States (approximately 572,000 in 2011, according to the American Cancer Society). Approximately 50% of persons who develop cancer will die from it.

There is great disparity among the cancer rates in minority groups. Across genders, cancer death rates for African Americans are 35% higher when compared to statistics for white Americans. The death rates for prostate cancer (two times more) and lung cancer (27 times more) are disproportionately higher when compared to whites. In addition, Hispanic men and women have higher incidence and mortality rates for stomach and liver cancer than non-Hispanics.

Alaskan Native men and women have a greater propensity for cancers in the rectum and colon than do Caucasians. Native American and Alaska Native men are more at risk for liver and stomach cancer than are non-Hispanic white men. Asian American men are more prone to stomach cancer than are non-Hispanic white men. At the same time, Asian and Pacific Islander American women will develop stomach cancer more often than non-Hispanic American white women.

Cancer is the leading cause of death for Hispanic Americans, according to the American Cancer Society. In 2009, 29,935 Hispanic Americans died as a result of the disease.

There are also gender differences among ethnic groups and specific cancers. Lung cancers in African American and Hawaiian men are higher when compared with Caucasian males. Vietnamese females who live in the United States have five times more new cases of cervical cancer when compared to Caucasian women. Hispanic females also have a greater incidence of cervical cancer than Caucasian females, and they are more likely than non-Hispanic white women to have kidney cancer.

Cardiovascular disease

Cardiovascular disease is the leading cause of disability and death rates in the United States. African Americans are more likely to have high blood pressure than other ethnic groups in the United States. However, African Americans and non-Hispanic white Americans have similar rates of **heart disease**. Unfortunately, African American males are three times more likely to die from heart disease than are white males.

Stroke is the leading cause of cardiovascular-related death, which occurs in higher numbers for Asian American males than for Caucasian men. Mexican American men and women and African American males have a higher incidence of hypertension. African American women have higher rates of overweight, which is a major risk factor of cardiovascular disease. Mexican Americans, African Americans, Native Hawaiian/Pacific Islanders, and Native Americans/Alaskan Natives also have higher rates of **obesity** than do other groups.

Diabetes

Diabetes—a serious health problem—is the seventh leading cause of death in the United States. More than 25 million people in the United States have diabetes; about 40% of all American adults have pre-diabetes. Racial and ethnic minorities are especially at risk for diabetes. American Hispanic/Latino persons are 66% more at risk for developing diabetes than non–Hispanic whites. At 77%, the risk is even higher for African Americans. The elderly within the African American population are especially at risk for diabetes, particularly women over 65. Diabetes is also common in older Hispanics. Native Americans and Alaska Natives have approximately double the risk for diabetes than do non-Hispanic whites.

HIV

HIV infection/AIDS (acquired immune deficiency syndrome) is the most common cause of death for all persons age 25 to 44 years old. More than one million people in the United States have HIV. Ethnic groups account for about 25% of the United States population and nearly two-thirds of all recently diagnosed **AIDS** cases, according to the Office of Minority Health. In addition, about 75% of all babies born with HIV/AIDS are members of one of the minority groups in the United States. Besides an increase of sexual transmission of HIV/AIDS within the minority communities, there is an increase in HIV among ethnic groups related to intravenous drug usage. Specifically, African Americans, both men and women, are more likely to die from AIDS than are non-Hispanic white men. An African American male is 6.5 times more likely to develop AIDS than a non-Hispanic caucasian male in the United States. A Hispanic male is more than two times more likely to contract the disease than is a non-Hispanic caucasian male.

Immunizations

The gap among immunizations, the reduction of preventable disease by **vaccination**, between minority groups and whites has narrowed. However, there are still smaller percentages of minority adults being immunized when compared to white adults. Overall, immunization rates among all groups are much higher than compared to adults. In 2009, the Office of Minority Health reported that 64% of older non-Hispanic whites received the **influenza** (flu) vaccination, while only 51% of older African Americans and Hispanics received it.

Tuberculosis is a disease that is controlled by immunizations. However, Asian and Pacific Islander Americans were 24 times more at risk for contracting tuberculosis (TB) than were non-Hispanic whites. **Hepatitis** B is another disease controlled with vaccines. Even though rates of hepatitis B continue to decline in the United States in the twenty-first century, its rate is twice as high for non-Hispanic blacks than for non-Hispanic whites. The Office of Minority Health also reports that, in 2010, older Asian Americans and Hispanic Americans (those over 65 years of age) were less likely to have received a **pneumonia** vaccine as compared to older non-Hispanic whites.

The Office of Minority Health and Health Disparities (OMHHD) stated that, in 2000, children living below the **poverty** level in the United States had lower immunization levels overall than did those above the poverty level. Disparities still exist, in 2010, concerning immunization rates among racial and ethnic groups in the United States. During the 2010s, the OMHHD hopes to be able to achieve and maintain a 90% rate of childhood immunization and to achieve a 60% rate in flu and pneumonia vaccinations in the United States. Such rates would help to eliminate disparities among minority groups with regard to immunizations.

Causes and symptoms

IMRs are correlated with prenatal care. Women who receive adequate prenatal care tend to have better pregnancy outcomes than those with little or no care. Women who receive inadequate prenatal care also have increased chances of delivering a very low birth weight (VLBW) infant, which is linked to risk of early death.

Cancer is related to several preventable lifestyle choices. Tobacco use, diet, and exposure to the sun (skin cancer) can be prevented by lifestyle modifications. Additionally, many cancers can occur due to lack of interest and/or lack of availability for screening and educational programs.

Cardiovascular diseases are higher among persons with high blood cholesterol and high blood pressure. Certain lifestyle choices may increase the chance for heart disease, including lack of exercise, overweight, and cigarette **smoking**. Cardiovascular disease is responsible for over 50% of the deaths in persons with diabetes.

HIV occurs at a higher frequency among homosexuals. (The number of African American males who contract HIV through sex with men has increased.) Additionally, unprotected sexual intercourse and sharing used needles for IV drug injection are strongly correlated with infection.

Vaccinations are an effective method of preventing certain disease such as **polio**, **tetanus**, pertussis, **diphtheria**, influenza, hepatitis b, and pneumococcal infections. Approximately 90% of influenza-related mortality is associated with persons aged 65 and older. This is mostly due to neglect of vaccinations. About 45,000 adults each year die of diseases related to hepatitis B, pneumococcal, and influenza infections.

Diagnosis

The diagnosis of VLBW is made by weight. Infants who weigh 1,500 grams (1.5 kilograms, or 3.3 pounds) at birth are at high risk for death. For cancer, the diagnosis can be made through screening procedures such as mammography (for breast cancer), Pap smears ("Pap" comes from the surname of Georgios Papanicolaou, the Greek physician who invented the test), and lifestyle modifications such as avoidance of ultraviolet rays from the sun (and artificially produced **radiation**, such as from tanning beds) and cigarette smoking, as well as balanced diets and adequate **nutrition**. Other specific screening tests (e.g., PSA, or "prostate surface antigen") are helpful for diagnosing prostate cancer.

Cardiovascular diseases can be detected by medical check-ups. Blood pressure and cholesterol levels can be measured. Obesity can be diagnosed by assessing a person's weight relative to their height (what is called BMI, or "body mass index"). Diabetes and its complications can be detected by blood tests, in-depth eye examinations, and studies that assess the flow of blood through blood vessels in legs. HIV can be detected through a careful history and physical examination and analysis of blood using a special test called a "western blot." Infections caused by lack of immunizations can be detected by careful physical examination and culturing the specific micro-organism in the laboratory.

Treatment

Treatment is directed at the primary reason(s) why minorities have increased chances of developing disease(s). Cancer may require treatment utilizing surgery, radiotherapy, or chemotherapy. Cardiovascular diseases may require invasive or surgical procedures for establishing a diagnosis and initiating treatment. Depending on the extent of disease, cardiovascular management can become complicated, requiring medications and daily lifestyle modifications. Treatment usually includes medications, dietary modifications, and—if complications arise—specific interventions tailored to alleviating the problem. HIV can be treated with specific medications and, more often than not, with symptomatic treatment as reported complications arise. Diseases caused by lack of immunization are treated based on the primary disease. The best methods of treatment are through **prevention** and generating public awareness through education.

Alternative treatment

Alternative therapies do exist, but more research is needed to substantiate present data. The diseases that relate to minority health are best treated with nationally accepted standards of care.

Prognosis

Generally, the prognosis is related to the diagnosis and the patient's state of health, age, and any other disease

or complication in addition to the presenting problem. The course for IMRs is related to educational programs and prenatal care, which includes medical and psychological treatments. The prognosis for chronic diseases such as cardiovascular problems, high blood pressure, cancer, and diabetes is variable. These diseases are not cured, and control is achieved by standardized treatment options. Eventually, complications can occur, even with treatment. For HIV, the clinical course at present is death, even though this process may take years. Educational programs with an emphasis on disease prevention can improve outcomes concerning pediatric and geriatric diseases.

Prevention

Prevention is accomplished best through educational programs specific to target populations. IMRs can be prevented by increasing awareness, interest, and accessibility for prenatal care that address a comprehensive approach for the needs of each patient. Regular physicals and special screening tests can prevent certain cancers in high-risk groups. Educational programs concerning lifestyle modifications, diet, exercise, and testing may prevent the development of cardiovascular disease and diabetes. Educational programs made available to illicit IV drug abusers and persons who engage in unprotected sexual intercourse may decrease the incidence of HIV infection.

All adults in the United States should be proactive, making sure to get information on those preventable diseases they are at most risk for acquiring and for which vaccines are available. Parents and other caregivers should make sure that their children have been fully vaccinated by the age of two years. Sons and daughters of **aging** parents should ensure that their parents are receiving the necessary vaccines, such as pneumococcal vaccines (for pneumonia), which will help them stay healthy and minimize the risk of premature death.

The importance of diagnosing, treating, and preventing minority health programs over the next decade will become increasingly important. The U.S. Census Bureau estimates that by 2100, only about 40% of the U.S. population will consist of non-Hispanic whites. As minority groups grow more rapidly, their health will become a larger factor in the overall health of all Americans. Hopefully, the disparities in health issue with minorities, when compared to whites, will dissipate, especially with regard to preventable diseases, disabilities, and mortality.

Costs to society

Cancer

In 2010, the National Cancer Institute estimated the direct cost of cancer at more than $120 billion. Expenditures for cancer care are on the rise, primarily because of new treatments that are available. It is estimated that the cost for cancer care will reach $158 billion in 2020. In addition to the direct costs, cancer results in indirect costs, such as time lost from work.

Cardiovascular disease

The cost of health care for the treatment of cardiovascular disease is expected to increase from $273 billion in 2008 to $818 billion in 2030. According to a report in the *Journal of the American Heart Association*, more than 40% of Americans will have cardiovascular disease by that year. In 2010, lost productivity due to cardiovascular disease cost approximately $172 billion. That number is expected to rise to $276 billion in 2030.

Diabetes

Total annual costs for diabetes in the United States (as of 2007) are estimated at $174 billion, with direct medical costs accounting for $116 million of that figure. The other $58 million is due to indirect costs, such as loss of work, disability, and early death. Individuals with diabetes have medical costs that are twice the costs for persons who do not have the disease.

HIV

In 2010, the cost of treating HIV infection throughout a person's life was estimated at $379,668. Depending on the health care setting and testing performed, the cost to diagnose the disease ranged from $1,900 to $10,000, as of 2010.

Resources

BOOKS

Gilman, Sander L. *Diseases and Diagnoses: The Second Age of Biology.* New Brunswick, NJ: Transaction, 2010.

Hofrichter, Richard, and Rajiv Bhatia, editors. *Tackling Health Inequities Through Public Health Practice: Theory to Action.* Oxford, UK: Oxford University Press, 2010.

Liburd, Leandris C., editor. *Diabetes and Health Disparities: Community-Based Approaches for Racial and Ethnic Populations.* New York: Springer, 2010.

Stanhope, Marcia, and Jeanette Lancaster. *Public Health Nursing: Population-Centered Health Care in the Community.* Maryland Heights, MO: Elsevier Mosby, 2012.

PERIODICALS

Heidenreich, Paul, M.D., M.S., F.A.H.A., et al. "Forecasting the Future of Cardiovascular Disease in the United States." *Circulation: Journal of the American Heart Association* 123: 933-44 (January 24, 2011).

WEBSITES

"Cancer."Centers for Disease Control and Prevention. http://www.cdc.gov/nchs/fastats/cancer.htm (accessed September 16, 2010).

"Cancer Death Rate down but 565, 650 Seen in 2008." Reuters. http://www.reuters.com/article/idUSN1926392720080220 (accessed September 16, 2010).

"Cancer Facts & Figures 2011." Reuters. http://www.cancer.org/acs/groups/content/@epidemiologysurveilance/documents/document/acspc-029771.pdf (accessed September 25, 2012).

"Country Comparison: Infant mortality rate." Central Intelligence Agency. https://www.cia.gov/library/publications/the-world-factbook/rankorder/2091rank.html (accessed September 16, 2010).

"Eliminate Disparities in Adult and Child Immunization Rates." Office of Minority Health and Health Disparities, Centers for Disease Control and Prevention. http://www.cdc.gov/omhd/amh/factsheets/immunization.htm (accessed September 16, 2010).

"HIV Cost-Effectiveness." Centers for Disease Control and Prevention. http://www.cdc.gov/hiv/topics/prevention-programs/ce/#Overview (accessed September 25, 2012).

"HIV in the United States." AIDS.gov. http://aids.gov/hiv-aids-basics/hiv-aids-101/statistics/ (accessed September 25, 2012).

"Immunizations Data/Statistics." Office of Minority Health, Department of Health and Human Services. http://minorityhealth.hhs.gov/templates/browse.aspx?lvl=3&lvlid=60 (accessed September 25, 2012).

"Learn About Cancer." American Cancer Society. http://www.cancer.org/Cancer/news/report-cancer-now-leading-cause-of-death-among-hispanic-americans (accessed September 25, 2012).

"Minority Health." Wychoff Heights Medical Center. http://www.wyckoffhospital.org/body.cfm?id=587 (accessed September 16, 2010).

"Surveillance Epidemiology and End Results." National Cancer Institute. http://seer.cancer.gov/statfacts/html/all.html (accessed September 25, 2012).

"National Diabetes Fact Sheet, 2011." Centers for Disease Control and Prevention. http://www.cdc.gov/diabetes/pubs/pdf/ndfs_2011.pdf (accessed September 25, 2012).

National Diabetes Information Clearinghouse. U.S. Department of Health and Human Services. http://diabetes.niddk.nih.

gov/dm/pubs/statistics/#fast (accessed September 25, 2012).

"The Cost of Cancer." National Cancer Institute.http://www .cancer.gov/aboutnci/servingpeople/cancer-statistics/cost-ofcancer (accessed September 25, 2012).

"Recent Trends in Infant Mortality in the United States." Centers for Disease Control and Prevention. http://www .cdc.gov/nchs/data/databriefs/db09.htm (accessed September 16, 2010).

ORGANIZATIONS

Office of Minority Health, Post Office Box 37337, Washington, DC 20013-7337, 800-444-6472, http://minorityhealth.hhs .gov/

Office of Minority Health and Health Disparities, 1600 Clifton Road, Atlanta, GA 30333, 800-232-4636, http://www.cdc .gov/omhd/.

Laith Farid Gulli, M.D.
Nicole Mallory, M.S.
Rhonda Cloos, RN

Mobilizing for Action through Planning and Partnerships (MAPP)

Definition

Mobilizing for Action through Planning and Partnerships (MAPP) is a planning process designed to improve **community health** programs.

Purpose

The purpose of MAPP is to make use of all available community health resources to identify and prioritize community public health issues and then to identify resources that are available to deal with those issues.

Description

In 1991, the National Association of County and City Health Officials (**NACCHO**) and the U.S. Centers for Disease Control (now the **Centers for Disease Control and Prevention**; **CDC**) collaborated to develop a program through which local public **health departments** could improve their organizational structure and leadership role in a community in a three–stage process that involved assessing their internal capacity, identifying essential community health issues, and developing action plans to deal with those issues. That program was called the **Assessment Protocol for Excellence in Public Health (APEX-PH)**. Although **APEX-PH** has become a

useful tool for public health agencies, it lacked some important elements, one of which was a mechanism for strategic planning for the agency. To remedy this deficiency, NACCHO and CDC developed a supplementary program in 2001, called Mobilizing for Action through Planning and Partnerships (MAPP). MAPP is a more sophisticated and more powerful version of APEX-PH that has been used by many state and local public health departments to improve their planning for the future.

MAPP has nine underlying principles and six phases of operation. The underlying principles are:

• MAPP is a strategic planning program, one that takes a long–term view of community needs and resources in the field of health.

• MAPP makes use of a systems approach to its planning, taking into consideration the interaction of all elements involved in the community's relationship with public health issues.

• MAPP encourages community members to become involved in the determination of public health policies and practices.

• MAPP promotes the philosophy that public health issues are a shared concern and opportunity for both professionals in the field and the general community.

• MAPP relies on objective data at all stages of its operation.

• MAPP builds on previous experiences in the development of new policies and practices.

• MAPP depends on partnerships formed between public health professionals and individuals with all types of knowledge and skills in the community.

• MAPP makes use of dialogue between public health professionals and other members of the community to develop policies and make decisions.

• MAPP encourages stakeholders to be aware of and to celebrate specific accomplishments in their work.

The six steps involved in carrying out the MAPP agenda are as follows:

• Organization, which consists of determining the reasons an agency might consider implementing MAPP, selecting participants in the program, identifying resources available in the community and in the agency, designing the planning process, conducting a readiness session at which the program is explained, and determining the readiness of personnel and resources.

• Vision, which involves developing a vision statement that describes what participants imagine the agency should look like at some point in the future, five or ten years down the road.

- Assessment, which means identifying the strengths and resources available to the public health effort from all possible sources, including the agency itself and the general community, with particular attention to forces that are expected to impact the future of the public health system, such as legislative and administrative rules and regulations.

- Strategizing issues, which involves identifying probable long-term issues that will impact health care, determining possible interactions among those issues, and arranging the issues in order of priority.

- Goals and strategies, which requires a selection of goals that are consistent with the vision statement that has been adopted and the strategic issues with which the agency is expected to deal. Goal selection should also include potential problems that might prevent realization of those goals, as well as specific actions that will be necessary to achieve the goals. At this stage, participants should produce a first draft of their final report of the MAPP process for the agency.

- Action cycle, which involves putting into practice all of the theoretical planning that has been done up to this point. The action cycle consists of three stages itself: planning for specific actions to achieve outcomes identified in the MAPP process, implementation of those plans, and final evaluation of the outcome of the actions.

Professional publications

The primary source of information about MAPP is the NACCHO website, which has a variety of print and online resources about the program. A useful starting point in learning about the program is the September 2005 issue of the *Journal of Public Health Management and Practice*, which is devoted almost exclusively to the topic. The issue is available for purchase online from the NACCHO website (https://eweb.naccho.org/eweb/DynamicPage.aspx?webcode=NACCHOPubHome). Other publications available from NACCHO include the MAPP Handbook, the MAPP Field Guide, and a MAPP brochure, all of which can be downloaded at no cost from the organization's website at http://www.naccho.org/topics/infrastructure/mapp/framework/mapppubs.cfm.

Resources

BOOKS

Healey, Bernard J., and Robert S. Zimmerman. *The New World of Health Promotion: New Program Development, Implementation, and Evaluation.* Sudbury, MA: Jones and Bartlett Publishers, 2010.

MAPP Community Health Action Plan: Charting a New Course for Our Healthy Future. Pasadena (CS) Public Health Dept. [Pasadena, CA: City of Pasadena], 2007.

PERIODICALS

Boyd, Rita Arras, and Mark Peters. "Using MAPP to Connect Communities: One County's Story."*Health Educator* 41. 2. (2009): 77–84.

Corso, L. C., P. J. Wiesner, and P. Lenihan. "Developing the MAPP Community Health Improvement Tool." *Journal of Public Health Management and Practice* 11. 5. (2005): 387–92

Lenihan, P. "MAPP and the Evolution of Planning in Public Health Practice." *Journal of Public Health Management and Practice* 11. 5. (2005): 381–88

WEBSITES

MAPP: Mobilizing for Action through Planning and Partnerships. The Community Tool Box. http://ctb.ku.edu/en/tablecontents/chapter2_section13_main.aspx (accessed October 11, 2012).

Mobilizing for Action through Planning and Partnerships. National Association of County & City Health Officials. http://www.naccho.org/topics/infrastructure/mapp/ (accessed October 11, 2012).

ORGANIZATIONS

National Association of County and City Health Officials (NACCHO), 1100 17th St., N.W., 17th floor, Washington, DC 20036, (202) 783-5550, Fax: (202) 783-1583, info@naccho.org, www.naccho.org/.

David E. Newton, EdD

Mold

Definition

Mold refers to a large, diverse group of fungal organisms that grow in filaments, resulting in a cottony, fuzzy appearance, and reproduce by forming spores. They grow on organic substances and other surfaces where moisture is present. They especially thrive in damp, warm, and humid environments. Molds that grow in shower stalls and bathrooms and that are white or gray in color are sometimes referred to as mildew.

Tiny mold spores are not visible to the naked eye. They are persistent, can be transported through the air, and can survive in conditions that molds cannot grow, such as dry environments. When mold spores land on a surface where moisture is present, the mold then starts to grow.

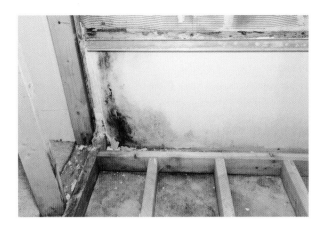

Mold that developed around a poorly installed bathtub and shower. (© iStockphoto.com/Wildroze)

Molds are found both outdoors and indoors. Outdoors molds aid in the decomposition of organic matter such as dead trees, compost, and leaves. The most common types of indoor household mold include *Cladosporium, Penicillium, Stachybotrys, Alternaria,* and *Aspergillus.*

There are several diseases of animals and humans that can be caused by molds due to allergic sensitivity to their spores. In addition, molds can produce mycotoxins, which are toxic compounds that are produced as some types of molds grow. At this time there is not convincing evidence to link health effects to indoor exposure to airborne mycotoxins, although ingestion of moldy food with mycotoxins has been shown to result in illness.

Indoor molds can also destroy surfaces and objects on which they grow.

Description

Molds (fungi) are present almost everywhere. Molds can be many different colors and produce a musty odor. In an indoor environment hundreds of different kinds of mold are able to grow wherever there is moisture and an organic substrate, which serves as a food source. They can grow on building and other materials, including: the paper on gypsum wallboard (drywall), ceiling tiles, wood products, paint, wallpaper, carpeting, some furnishings, books/papers, clothes, and other fabrics. Mold can also grow on moist, dirty surfaces such as concrete, fiberglass insulation, heating and air conditioning ducts, and ceramic tiles. It is not possible to eliminate the presence of all indoor fungal spores and fragments; however, mold growth indoors can and should be prevented and removed as much as possible, for molds have been associated with human health effects in persons allergic to molds. Molds produce irritating

substances that may act as allergens, and some molds produce toxic substances called mycotoxins.

Moisture in a building may come from a variety of sources, such as leakage or seepage through basement floors, showering, and cooking. The amount of moisture that air can hold is dependent on the temperature of the air, with colder air being able to hold less moisture than warmer air. This moisture can cause mold to grow. Mold can especially be troublesome after a building has been exposed to flooding.

Demographics

The prevalence of indoor dampness varies widely within and among countries, continents and climate zones. It is estimated to affect 10-50% of indoor environments in Europe, North America, Australia, India and Japan. In some areas, such as river valleys and coastal areas, the conditions of dampness can be substantially more severe.

Most people are not adversely affected by the presence of molds and other fungi. It has been estimated that about 10% of the **population** is allergic to one or more types of mold. Many of these people are affected by outdoor as well as indoor exposures to mold.

Except in buildings with extensive mold growth, the amount of mold found in indoor air is usually much less than what is found outdoors. For people with **allergies** to mold however, there may be no practical level of exposure, either indoors or outdoors, that would not create discomfort or harm. It is therefore wise to remove and prevent indoor mold growth.

Causes and symptoms

For persons who are sensitive to molds, exposure may result in nasal stuffiness and sneezing, eye irritation, wheezing, coughing, sinus problems, fatigue, skin irritation, and headaches or migraines. Exposure to molds can trigger **asthma** episodes in persons with asthma. Allergic individuals vary in their degree of susceptibility to mold, with the severity of an allergic response depending on the extent and type of mold that is present.

Persons with chronic lung illnesses, such as obstructive lung disease, or persons with severely weakened immune systems, including those with transplants, chemotherapy, **AIDS**, and newborn infants, may develop other diseases such as allergic bronchopulmonary aspergillosis, an allergic lung reaction to a type of fungus (most commonly Aspergillus fumigatus) that occurs in some people with asthma or cystic fibrosis, and hypersensitivity pneumonitis, an inflammation of the lung (usually of the very small airways) caused by the body's immune reaction to small air-borne particles, including molds and resulting in fever, chills, coughing, shortness of breath, and body aches.

There is no consensus on how significant a threat that inhalation of molds in residential, school, or office settings are to human health, except to persons who are allergic to mold. Building-related illnesses are often difficult to diagnose and interpret, for symptoms are non-specific and often allergy-related, and it is difficult to make conclusive links to environmental factors.

Diagnosis

Diagnosis of mold infestations

The U.S. Environmental Protection Association (**EPA**) has stated that if visible mold is present, testing is usually unnecessary. No standards have been established for mold or mold spore levels, since tolerable or acceptable limits of mold exposure for humans have not been defined. Individuals vary in their susceptibility to mold, so testing and measurement of mold presence is not effective in predicting the degree of health risks from an occurrence of mold.

Therefore, a mold infestation is determined primarily on visual assessment, knowledge of the building structure, and the history of **water** damage in the building.

Diagnosis of diseases associated with mold infestations

To diagnose an allergy to mold or fungi, the medical practitioner will take a complete medical history. If mold allergy is suspected, the doctor may do skin tests, where extracts of different types of fungi will be used to scratch or prick the skin. If there is no reaction, allergy is not likely. In some people with allergy, irritation alone can cause a reaction, so it may not actually be an allergic reaction. Therefore the medical practitioner combines the patient's medical history, the skin testing results, and a physical examination to diagnose a mold allergy.

Treatment

Treatment of a mold infestation

Visible fungal growth represents unnecessary exposure and should not be present in indoor spaces. Visible fungus indicates improper moisture management in the building.

The first step in treatment of mold is to identify and repair the moisture problem. Mold will not grow unless sufficient moisture is present. Small amounts of mold growing on visible surfaces can usually be easily cleaned without professional assistance. Larger amounts of mold

may require more extensive evaluation, repair or replacement, and dust control by professionals.

There are several methods available to clean up mold, depending on the size and type of surfaces affected. The work area can be cleaned using wet methods such as wet wiping with a detergent solution. In some cases, a dilute solution of chlorine bleach (no stronger than 1 cup of bleach in 1 gallon of water) or stronger commercial cleaners may be needed to kill the mold, for moldy surfaces should not be touched with bare hands. When washing with detergent and water, the use of rubber gloves is recommended. For bleach or harsher cleaning agents, nonporous gloves such as neoprene, nitrile, polyurethane, or PVC, should be worn along with protective eyewear. An N-95 respirator is recommended to limit exposure to airborne mold or spores during the cleaning process.

It is important to control dust associated with the clean-up activity. Dust should be controlled using damp cleaning methods and by using HEPA vacuuming. HEPA (High Efficiency Particulate Air) means that the vacuum filter is capable of removing particles that are 0.3 microns (one millionth of a meter) in diameter at 99.97% efficiency. Typical vacuum filters will not capture spores as efficiently and may disperse them in air. When the size of the area with visible mold growth is large or when sensitive people are present, the work area should be enclosed in plastic enclosure. The air inside the enclosure should be actively exhausted to the outdoors by placing the enclosed environment under negative pressure with respect to the rest of the room or building. If there are any leaks in the enclosure, that air will move from the cleaner areas outside the enclosure into the enclosure, and minimize air movement in the opposite direction.

When porous, cellulose-containing items such as drywall, clothing, carpets and carpet pads, textiles, upholstered furniture, leather, paper goods, and many types of artwork or decorative items get wet, they should be dried and disinfected within 48 hours or discarded. If sewage or gray water is involved, the materials should be discarded. These types of damp materials are usually the determining factor, rather than indoor humidity, are usually the primary determining factor whether mold growth will be excessive. Care should be taken to avoid that items not discarded become sources of re-infestation.

Treatment of diseases associated with mold

Since molds are common and it is difficult to avoid exposure, there are medications that may be used to alleviate allergic symptoms. These include:

• nasal corticosteroid sprays to aid in the prevention and treatment of inflammation caused by an upper respiratory mold allergy.

Allergen—A substance, such as mold, that causes an allergy.

Allergy—Extra sensitivity of the body to certain substances, such as pollens, foods, molds, or microorganisms, that produces an immune responses and that results in symptoms such as sneezing, itching, and skin rashes.

Alternaria—a group of fungi known as major plant pathogens and as common allergens in humans. They grow indoors and can cause hay fever or extra sensitive reactions that can lead to asthma. They can also cause infections in persons who are immuno-compromised.

Aspergillus—A group of several hundred mold species found in various climates worldwide, some of which are important medically and commercially while others cause infection in humans and other animals.

Asthma—A chronic long-lasting inflammatory disease of the lung airways, where the inflammation causes the airways to spasm and swell periodically so that the airways narrow. The individual wheezes or gasp for airs until the obstruction to air flow either resolves spontaneously or responds to a wide range of treatments. Continuing inflammation makes the airways extra sensitive to stimuli such as cold air, exercise, dust mites, molds, pollutants in the air, and even stress and anxiety.

Cladosporium—a group of fungi that includes some of the most common indoor and outdoor molds. Their spores are wind-dispersed and are often extremely abundant in outdoor airs. They can grow on surfaces when moisture is present. The airborne spores are significant allergens and in large amounts they can severely affect asthmatics and people with

respiratory diseases. Prolonged exposure may weaken the immune system.

Fungi—A group of organisms with a membrane-bound nucleus that derive their nourishment from dead or decaying organic matter. The group includes mushrooms, yeasts, mildew, and molds. They have rigid cell walls but lack chlorophyll.

Immunocompromised—Incapable of developing a normal immune response, usually as a result of disease, malnutrition, or immunosuppressive therapy.

Immunoglobulin E—A class of antibodies produced in the lungs, skin, and mucous membranes that are responsible for allergic reactions.

N-95 respirator—Most common of the types of particulate filtering face piece respirators. It filters at least 95 percent of airborne particles but is not resistant to oil.

Penicillium—A group of fungi of major importance in the natural environment as well as in food and drug production. Members of the genus produce penicillin, which is used as an antibiotic to kill or stop the growth of certain kinds of bacteria in the body. *Penicillium* is a common indoor mold, and its spores can cause mold allergy.

Stachybotrys—A group of molds with widespread distribution that inhabit materials high in cellulose. Certain species are known as "black mold" or "toxic black mold" in the U.S. and are frequently associated with poor indoor air quality arising from fungal growth on water-damaged building materials. Some species produce mycotoxins that are known to produce health symptoms, but it is not scientifically clear whether these mycotoxins affect human health during a mold infestation in a building.

• antihistamines to help with itching, sneezing and runny nose by blocking histamine, an inflammatory chemical released by the immune system during an allergic reaction.

• decongestants to relieve nasal congestion in the upper respiratory tract.

• montelukast to block the action of leukotrienes, which are immune system chemicals that cause allergy symptoms such as excess mucus

Other treatments for mold allergy include immunotherapy to eliminate allergies through a series of allergy

shots, although this therapy is only partially effective against mold allergies, and nasal rinses to soothe nasal symptoms. Your doctor may recommend additional treatments if you have mold-induced allergic bronchopulmonary aspergillosis and hypersensitivity pneumonitis.

Public health role and response

The public health community in most cases does not recommend evacuation in response to a mold infestation. There is no established level of airborne mold that is

QUESTIONS TO ASK YOUR DOCTOR

- Could my allergic symptoms be caused by molds?
- What treatments are available to help alleviate symptoms?
- What should I do to remediate the mold infestation in my home?
- Should I stay in my home or should I evacuate during the remediation process?

accepted as unsafe for the general population. However evacuation may be warranted for sensitive populations, such as infants, elderly, the immune-suppressed, and those with medically confirmed symptoms related to mold exposure.

The presence of mold in a building does not in itself constitute a health threat. Although control of indoor mold growth is usually preferred, a health-based assessment of the indoor environment and its occupants is required to identify the extent of the health threat. Such a determination is especially critical in deciding upon an expensive course of action in a large commercial or public building. The health assessment should include:

- Potential for exposure: an assessment of both the quantity and types of fungi present in bulk and air samples.

- Diagnosis of exposure: a symptom survey of building occupants to determine if there are health complaints consistent with mold exposure. The pattern of symptom expression should be investigated, such as determining when did the symptoms start, end, and when were they the worst, and are most of the complaints confined to occupants of specific rooms.

- Verification of exposure: an exposure assessment (for example, an immuno-assay for immunoglobulin E (IgE) specific to molds present) to establish a link between the presence of molds with potential health effects and building occupants' health complaints. Strict criteria should be established for the diagnosis of mold exposure by qualified health professionals in order to make accurate health recommendations and to avoid unnecessary building remedies.

It is important that public health officials effectively communicate the effects of indoor mold exposure to the public. The key messages that should be conveyed are:

the ubiquitous nature of fungi in the environment, the relative community of fungi found indoors compared to outdoors, the relative risk posed by the molds detected, and the range of options available to confront the problem.

Recent years have seen increased attention placed on mold-infested schools. Mold infestation in schools presents a special case in risk management and a challenge for public health officials, for parents usually have a low tolerance for either actual or perceived risk and are often organized and active in school issues.

Prognosis

Because people vary greatly in their immune response to environmental allergens, and because fungi are always present in the environment, it may not be possible to manage airborne fungal particles at a level protective of those individuals most sensitive to their allergenic effects. Therefore, molds are categorized with pollen, dander, and mite excrement as allergens to be managed but cannot be eliminated. When people present with allergic hypersensitivity, health effects due to mold are due more to individual sensitivity than to the presence or absence of exposure. However, to reduce exposure, mold **infestations** should be treated.

Prevention

There is no practical way to eliminate mold and mold spores from an indoor environment. Therefore, to control or prevent the growth of mold, moisture levels within the building must be controlled. Methods of control include:

- fix leaks and seepage
- put plastic covers over dirt in crawl spaces
- direct ground water drainage away from a house
- use exhaust fans in kitchens and bathrooms to vent moisture to the outside
- vent clothes dryer to the outside
- scour sinks and tubs at least monthly
- clean garbage pails frequently
- clean refrigerator door gaskets and drip pans
- throw away or recycle old books, newspapers, clothing or bedding
- turn off humidifiers if moisture is condensing on windows
- use dehumidifiers and air conditioners, especially in hot, humid climates, but be sure to maintain them so mold does not grow in them

- raise the temperature of cold surfaces where moisture condenses by installing insulation or storm windows and by increasing air circulation in the home (opening doors, using fans, and moving furniture from wall corners

- use area rugs over concrete that can be taken up and washed frequently. If permanent carpet is installed on a concrete floor, consider using plastic sheeting as a vapor barrier and cover it with subflooring made of insulation covered with plywood

- use paints that contain mold inhibitors

After moisture control has been completed, it may be necessary to remove and discard the materials that were affected by the mold.

Resources

BOOKS

Billings, Kurt and Lee Ann Billings. *Mold: The War Within.* Knoxville, TN: Partners Publishing LLC, 2010.

May, Jeffrey C. and Connie L. May. *The Mold Survival Guide: For Your Home and For Your Health.* Baltimore, MD: The Johns Hopkins University Press, 2004.

Rosen, Gary. *Environmentally Friendly Mold Remediation Techniques that Significantly Reduce Childhood Asthma.* Naples, FL: Hope Academic Press, 2007.

Schaller, James, and Gary Rosen. *Mold Illness and Mold Remediation Made Simple.* Naples, FL: Hope Academic Press, 2006.

WEBSITES

Mold. http://www.cdc.gov/mold/

Dampness and Mould - World Health Organization. www.euro.who.int/document/e92645.pdf

ORGANIZATIONS

Allergy and Asthma Foundation of America, 8201 Corporate Drive, Suite 1000, Landover, Maryland USA 20785, (800) 727-8462, Info@aafa.org, aafa.org.

Judith L. Sims

Mononucleosis *see* **Epstein-Barr disease**

Mortality and morbidity

Definition

Mortality refers to the rate of death (in general, or from a specific cause) in a given **population**. Morbidity refers to the rate of disease (in general, or a specific disease) in a given population.

Leading causes of death in persons 65 and older

Cause of death	Number of deaths	Percentage of all deaths in age group (65+)
Heart disease	496,095	28.3%
Malignant neoplasms (Cancer)	389,730	22.2%
Cerebrovascular diseases	115,961	6.6%
Chronic lower respiratory diseases	109,562	6.2%
Alzheimer's disease	73,797	4.2%
Diabetes mellitus	51,528	2.9%
Influenza and pneumonia	45,941	2.6%
Nephritis	38,484	2.2%
Unintentional injury	38,292	2.2%
Septicemia	26,362	1.5%

SOURCE: Centers for Disease Control and Prevention, National Center for Injury Prevention and Control.

(Table by PreMediaGlobal. © 2013 Cengage Learning)

Description

The terms mortality and morbidity are used to track and measure the trends of disease and death within or across populations. One use of mortality and morbidity statistics is to measure the quality of life that a population has—developed countries can examine their mortality and morbidity rates against those of developing nations, urban areas can measure their rates against rural areas, etc. Lower mortality and morbidity rates suggest a better quality of life. Mortality rates—often closely related to **life expectancy**—are usually grouped per 1,000 persons, and are usually sorted by gender and age group. Generally speaking, as an area experiences developments in municipal infrastructures and increases in access to medical care, its inhabitants experience higher quality of life and life expectancies, and lower mortality and morbidity rates. Often, this decline in mortality is accompanied by a shift in causes—as societies develop, problems change from those of **sanitation** and malnutrition to issues like **smoking**, alcohol abuse, **obesity**, and **cancer**.

Tracking rates of mortality and morbidity helps government and public health officials plan and revise legislation, treatment, and other measures to protect citizens and improve future rates. This data can also be used to track the progress and efficiency of implemented measures.

In the United States, according to the **Centers for Disease Control and Prevention (CDC)**, the leading causes of death are: **heart disease**, cancer, chronic lower respiratory diseases, **stroke**, accidents, Alzheimer's disease, and diabetes. The most recent data from the **CDC** estimates the death rate in the

United States at 793.8 deaths per 100,000 members of the population.

Infant mortality

Infant mortality measures the mortality rates of children under one year of age, and represents the number of deaths per 1,000 live births in a specific population. Given the specific challenges faced by newborns shortly after birth, infant mortality is usually split into two categories: neonatal (27 days old and younger) and postneonatal (28 days to 12 months old). Like other mortality data, infant mortality rates have varied over time and geography. According to the most recent data from the CDC, the approximate infant mortality rate in the United States is 6.39 deaths per 1,000 live births.

Infant mortality rates in the United States have been generally decreasing over the past few decades. Despite this decrease, however, as of the most recent data available from the Central Intelligence Agency (CIA) World Factbook, the U.S. is rated 49th among nations that have reliable data available. There is dispute as to the reason for this low ranking—one potential causes are disparity in prenatal and medical care among racial and ethnic groups. Proponents of alternative and natural birthing often point to the increase in U.S. rates of cesarean section and other interventions in the birthing process, because many higher-ranking nations have more nationally-diversified birthing cultures that utilize both midwives and obstetricians, and avoid interventions in the birthing process.

Despite the overall decrease in American infant mortality rates, the burden of these rates is not borne equally across the population. The infant mortality rate for African American babies in recent years has been more than two times higher than the rate for Caucasian babies. Low birthweight is the number one cause of death among African American babies. Puerto Rican American babies have a 40% higher mortality rate than Caucasian babies. Despite some overall trends across racial backgrounds, racial and socioeconomic differences are unable to fully account for disparities in American infant mortality rates.

Common causes for infant mortality include: preterm birth, infections, **birth defects**, **tetanus**, diarrhea, asphyxia, and abuse. These factors can be exacerbated or reduced by access to adequate medical care—this is especially true for many neonatal mortality causes.

Maternal mortality

Maternal mortality rates have similar statistical benefits to infant mortality rates, but international statistics usually follow United Nations standards and

measure the deaths of women during pregnancy and childbirth per 100,000 births. Despite advances in overall healthcare technology and accessibility, for a number of years, maternal mortality rates have stalled (have not declined) globally.

There are a number of factors that typically contribute to maternal mortality, including: age, economic resources, access to healthcare, access to effective family planning, access to adequate healthcare, and the power of women to make decisions regarding their own gynecological care.

In America, mortality rates are higher among certain ethnic groups. Around the world, certain regions have consistently high maternal mortality rates. Africa is particularly plagued by high maternal mortality rates. According to the United Nations (UN), one-third of sub-Saharan African countries have maternal mortality rates higher than 1,000 deaths per 100,000 live deaths. Additionally, 1 out of 11 women in sub-Saharan Africa die in pregnancy or childbirth, compared to 1 out of 30,000 women in Sweden. The maternal mortality rates in Asia account for one-third of the maternal mortality rates of the entire world.

Among the Asian rates of maternal mortality, 34% are attributed to hemorrhaging.

Effects on public health

Mortality and morbidity rates are public health concerns on local, national, and international levels. Other than the immediate and peripheral effects of the individual deaths, these statistics often indicate systemic issues of abuse, disease, health habits, medical care, and legislation. The data gathered in the compiling of mortality and morbidity statistics, and the inferences that can be made from this data, can contribute to general improvements in quality of life, life expectancy, and broader improvements in legislation, health care availability and practices, and cultural attitudes.

Costs to Society

The data used to compile mortality and morbidity statistics in the United States is gathered by cities and states and collected and organized by the CDC. The collection of this data is not a cost to society, however, the loss of life and peripheral effects that the data represents are significant costs to society. The financial burden of these deaths and often the emergency care required—particularly after illness or death subsequent to inadequate medical care—falls to society. Additionally, illnesses and death cause additional losses in work productivity and income, as well as lasting effects on the financial viability and mental health of survivors, and their families and communities.

Efforts and solutions

The CDC tracks the statistics for a number of diseases across the 50 states and numerous major U.S. cities. Provisional data is published by the CDC weekly and revised reports are published annually.

The **World Health Organization (WHO)** started a program called the Integrated Management of Childhood Illness (IMCI). IMCI is an effort aiming to improve the health and well-being of children under five years old. IMCI deals with both preventative and curative components of health care. According to **WHO**, IMCI seeks to improve three major facets affecting a child's well-being: case management skills of health care providers, general health care systems, and the health practices of communities and individual families.

The United Nations **Millennium Development Goals** (MDG) seeks to reduce global maternal mortality rates by 75% by 2015. MDG seeks to make these changes by implementing programs that improve maternal conditions with initiatives including: reducing teen pregnancies and family size, diagnosing high-risk pregnancies, and increasing the time between births.

Resources

BOOKS

Frost, Caren J. "Maternal Mortality." *Cultural Sociology of the Middle East, Asia, & Africa: An Encyclopedia. Vol. 2: Africa.* Thousand Oaks, CA: Sage Reference, 2012. 321-323.

Gurr, Barbara. "Infant Mortality." *Encyclopedia of Motherhood.* Ed. Andrea O'Reilly. Vol. 2. Thousand Oaks, CA: Sage Reference, 2010. 562-564.

Kulkarni, Vani S. "Maternal Mortality." *Cultural Sociology of the Middle East, Asia, & Africa: An Encyclopedia.* Vol. 4: South, Central, and West Asia. Thousand Oaks, CA: Sage Reference, 2012. 245-248.

McCormick, Marie C. "Infant Mortality." *Encyclopedia of Global Studies.* Ed. Helmut K. Anheier, Mark Juergensmeyer, and Victor Faessel. Vol. 2. Thousand Oaks, CA: Sage Reference, 2012. 910-913.

Warf, Barney. "Mortality Rate." *Encyclopedia of Geography.* Ed. Barney Warf. Vol. 4. Sage Reference, 2010.

WEBSITES

Centers for Disease Control and Prevention. "Morbidity and Mortality Weekly Report (MMWR)." http://www.cdc.gov/mmwr/. Accessed September 10, 2012.

Central Intelligence Agency. "The World Fact Book." https://www.cia.gov/library/publications/the-world-factbook/fields/2119.html. Accessed September 10, 2012.

United Nations. "Least Developed Countries: About LDCs." http://www.unohrlls.org/en/ldc/25/. Accessed September 10, 2012.

United Nations. "Millennium Development Goals." http://www.un.org/millenniumgoals/. Accessed September 10, 2012.

World Health Organization. "Integrated Management of Childhood Illness (IMCI)." http://www.who.int/maternal_child_adolescent/topics/child/imci/en/index.html. Accessed September 10, 2012.

ORGANIZATIONS

Centers for Diseae Control and Prevention, 1600 Clifton Rd., Atlanta, GA USA 30333, (800) 232-4636, cdcinfo@cdc.gov, www.cdc.goc.

Andrea Nienstedt, MA

Mumps

Definition

Mumps is a relatively mild short-term viral infection of the salivary glands that usually occurs

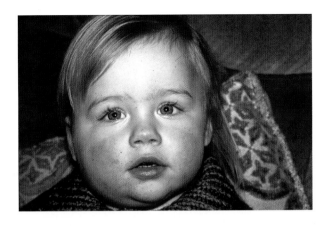

A child with an accute case of Mumps. *(c SPL/Photo Researchers, Inc. Reproduced by permission)*

during childhood. Typically, mumps is characterized by a painful swelling of both cheek areas, although the person could have swelling on one side or no perceivable swelling at all. The salivary glands are also called the parotid glands, therefore, mumps is sometimes referred to as an inflammation of the parotid glands (epidemic parotitis). The word mumps comes from an old English dialect, meaning lumps or bumps within the cheeks.

Description

Mumps is a very contagious infection that spreads easily in such highly populated areas as day care centers and schools. Although not as contagious as **measles** or chickenpox, mumps was once quite common. Prior to the release of a mumps vaccine in the United States in 1967, approximately 92% of all children had been exposed to mumps by the age of 15. In these pre-vaccine years, most children contracted mumps between the ages of four and seven. Mumps epidemics came in two to five year cycles. The greatest mumps epidemic was in 1941 when approximately 250 cases were reported for every 100,000 people. In 1968, the year after the live mumps vaccine was released, only 76 cases were reported for every 100,000 people. By 1985, fewer than 3,000 cases of mumps were reported throughout the entire United States, which works out to about 1 case per 100,000 people. The reason for the decline in mumps was the increased usage of the mumps vaccine. However, 1987 noted a five-fold increase in the incidence of the disease because of the reluctance of some states to adopt comprehensive school **immunization** laws. Since then, state-enforced school entry requirements have achieved student immunization rates of nearly 100% in kindergarten and first grade. In 1996, the **Centers for Disease Control and Prevention (CDC)** reported only 751 cases of mumps nationwide, or, in other words, about one case

for every five million people. Between 2000 and 2005, fewer than 350 cases of mumps were reported in the United States annually. Since that time, the number of mumps cases has increased significantly, largely because of the decision by many parents not to have their children immunized against the disease.

Causes and symptoms

The paramyxovirus that causes mumps is harbored in the saliva and is spread by sneezing, coughing, and other direct contact with another person's infected saliva. Once the person is exposed to the virus, symptoms generally occur in 14-24 days. Initial symptoms include chills, headache, loss of appetite, and a lack of energy. However, an infected person may not experience these initial symptoms. Swelling of the salivary glands in the face (parotitis) generally occurs within 12-24 hours of the above symptoms. Accompanying the swollen glands is **pain** on chewing or swallowing, especially with acidic beverages, such as lemonade. A fever as high as 104°F (40°C) is also common. Swelling of the glands reaches a maximum on about the second day and usually disappears by the seventh day. Once a person has contracted mumps, they become immune to the disease, despite how mild or severe their symptoms may have been.

While the majority of cases of mumps are uncomplicated and pass without incident, some complications can occur. Complications are, however, more noticeable in adults who get the infection. In 15% of cases, the covering of the brain and spinal cord becomes inflamed (**meningitis**). Symptoms of meningitis usually develop within four or five days after the first signs of mumps. These symptoms include a stiff neck, headache, vomiting, and a lack of energy. Mumps meningitis is usually resolved within seven days, and damage to the brain is exceedingly rare.

The mumps infection can spread into the brain causing inflammation of the brain (**encephalitis**). Symptoms of mumps encephalitis include the inability to feel pain, seizures, and high fever. Encephalitis can occur during the parotitis stage or one to two weeks later. Recovery from mumps encephalitis is usually complete, although complications, such as seizure disorders, have been noted. Only about one person in 100 with mumps encephalitis dies from the complication.

About one-quarter of all post-pubertal males who contract mumps can develop a swelling of the scrotum (orchitis) about seven days after the parotitis stage. Symptoms include marked swelling of one or both testicles, severe pain, fever, nausea, and headache. Pain and swelling usually subside after five to seven days, although the testicles can remain tender for weeks.

Girls occasionally suffer an inflammation of the ovaries, or oophoritis, as a complication of mumps, but this condition is far less painful than orchitis in boys.

Diagnosis

When mumps reaches epidemic proportions, diagnosis is relatively easy on the basis of the physical symptoms. The doctor will take the child's temperature, gently palpate (touch) the skin over the parotid glands, and look inside the child's mouth. If the child has mumps, the openings to the ducts inside the mouth will be slightly inflamed and have a "pouty" appearance. With so many people vaccinated today, a case of mumps must be properly diagnosed in the event the salivary glands are swollen for reasons other than viral infection. For example, in persons with poor oral **hygiene**, the salivary glands can be infected with bacteria. In these cases, **antibiotics** are necessary. Also in rare cases, the salivary glands can become blocked, develop tumors, or swell due to the use of certain drugs, such as iodine. A test can be performed to determine whether the person with swelling of the salivary glands actually has the mumps virus.

As of late 2002, researchers in London have reported the development of a bioassay for measuring mumps-specific IgG. This test would allow a doctor to check whether an individual patient is immune to mumps, and allow researchers to measure the susceptibility of a local population to mumps in areas with low rates of **vaccination**.

Public health response

Public health agencies most commonly become involved in dealing with mumps after they receive notice of one or more infected individuals from primary care physicians or other medical professionals. In such cases, the next step for a public health agency is to confirm the diagnosis of mumps, often by culturing the causative agent or by sending a sample taken from the patient to the U.S **Centers for Disease Control and Prevention (CDC)** in Atlanta, Georgia. Confirmation of the presence of the mumps virus, local public health agencies then initiate a surveillance program in which they seek out other individuals who may have contracted the disease, the source from which the disease originated, and the pattern by which the disease has been spread throughout the community. Agencies then provide whatever palliative and therapeutic treatments as may be necessary for infected patients for whom treatment is not available from private physicians. An important part of this program consists of educational activities that make

---

KEY TERMS

Asymptomatic—Persons who carry a disease and may be capable of transmitting the disease but who do not exhibit symptoms of the disease are said to be asymptomatic.

Encephalitis—Inflammation of the brain.

Epidemic parotitis—The medical name for mumps.

Immunoglobulin G (IgG)—A group of antibodies against certain viral infections that circulate in the bloodstream. One type of IgG is specific against the mumps paramyxovirus.

Meningitis—Inflammation of the membranes covering the brain and spinal cord.

Orchitis—Inflammation or swelling of the scrotal sac containing the testicles.

Paramyxovirus—A genus of viruses that includes the causative agent of mumps.

Parotitis—Inflammation and swelling of the salivary glands.

---

children and adults aware of the nature of mumps and efforts that can be exerted to avoid contracting the disease and treating it if and when it occurs. The role of immunization in reducing the risk of mumps for both individuals and the overall community is a critical part of such educational programs, both in the short- and long-term.

Treatment

When mumps does occurs, the illness is usually allowed to run its course. The symptoms, however, are treatable. Because of difficulty swallowing, the most important challenge is to keep the patient fed and hydrated. The individual should be provided a soft diet, consisting of cooked cereals, mashed potatoes, broth-based soups, prepared baby foods, or foods put through a home food processor. Aspirin, acetaminophen, or ibuprofen can relieve some of the pain due to swelling, headache, and fever. Avoid fruit juices and other acidic foods or beverages that can irritate the salivary glands. Avoid dairy products that can be hard to digest. In the event of complications, a physician should be contacted at once. For example, if orchitis occurs, a physician should be called. Also, supporting the scrotum in a cotton bed on an adhesive-tape bridge between the thighs can minimize tension. Ice packs are also helpful.

Alternative treatment

Acupressure can be used effectively to relieve pain caused by swollen glands. The patient can, by using the middle fingers, gently press the area between the jawbone and the ear for two minutes while breathing deeply.

A number of homeopathic remedies can be used for the treatment of mumps. For example, belladonna may be useful for flushing, redness, and swelling. Bryonia (wild hops) may be useful for irritability, lack of energy, or thirst. Phytolacca (poke root) may be prescribed for extremely swollen glands. A homeopathic physician should always be consulted for appropriate doses for children, and remedies that do not work within one day should be stopped. A homeopathic preparation of the mumps virus can also be used prophylactically or as a treatment for the disease.

Several herbal remedies may be useful in helping the body recover from the infection or may help alleviate the discomfort associated with the disease. Echinacea (*Echinacea* spp.) can be used to boost the immune system and help the body fight the infection. Other herbs taken internally, such as cleavers (*Galium aparine*), calendula (*Calendula officinalis*), and phytolacca (poke root), target the lymphatic system and may help to enhance the activity of the body's internal filtration system. Since phytolacca can be toxic, it should only be used by patients under the care of a skilled practitioner. Topical applications are also useful in relieving the discomfort of mumps. A cloth dipped in a heated mixture of vinegar and cayenne (*Capsicum frutescens*) can be wrapped around the neck several times a day. Cleavers or calendula can also be combined with vinegar, heated, and applied in a similar manner.

Prognosis

When mumps is uncomplicated, prognosis is excellent. However, in rare cases, a relapse occurs after about two weeks. Complications can also delay complete recovery. Scientific evidence for the safety and efficacy of most alternative treatments is often not available, so they should be used with caution.

Prevention

A vaccine exists to protect against mumps. The vaccine preparation (MMR) is usually given as part of a combination injection that helps protect against measles, mumps, and **rubella**. MMR is a live vaccine administered in one dose between the ages of 12-15 months, 4-6 years, or 11-12 years. Persons who are unsure of their mumps history and/or mumps vaccination history should be vaccinated. Susceptible health

QUESTIONS TO ASK YOUR DOCTOR

- My children have all been vaccinated against mumps. Are they at risk for the disease if our neighbors' children have NOT been vaccinated?

- What information can I provide to friends who are convinced that being vaccinated against mumps raises the risk of autism in their children?

- In what regions of the world is mumps still a common disease? Are my vaccinated children safe in traveling to these areas?

- What print or electronic resources can you recommend for getting more detailed information about mumps?

care workers, especially those who work in hospitals, should be vaccinated. Because mumps is still prevalent throughout the world, susceptible persons over age one who are traveling abroad would benefit from receiving the mumps vaccine.

The mumps vaccine is extremely effective, and virtually everyone should be vaccinated against this disease. There are, however, a few reasons why people should *not* be vaccinated against mumps:

- Pregnant women who contract mumps during pregnancy have an increased rate of miscarriage, but not birth defects. As a result, pregnant women should not receive the mumps vaccine because of the possibility of damage to the fetus. Women who have had the vaccine should postpone pregnancy for three months after vaccination.

- Unvaccinated persons who have been exposed to mumps should not get the vaccine, as it may not provide protection. The person should, however, be vaccinated if no symptoms result from the exposure to mumps.

- Persons with minor fever-producing illnesses, such as an upper respiratory infection, should not get the vaccine until the illness has subsided.

- Because mumps vaccine is produced using eggs, individuals who develop hives, swelling of the mouth or throat, dizziness, or breathing difficulties after eating eggs should not receive the mumps vaccine.

- Persons with immune deficiency diseases and/or those whose immunity has been suppressed with anti-cancer drugs, corticosteroids, or radiation should not receive the vaccine. Family members of immunocompromised people, however, should get vaccinated to reduce the risk of mumps.

- The CDC recommends that all children infected with human immunodeficiency disease (HIV) who are asymptomatic should receive an the MMR vaccine at 15 months of age.

The mumps vaccine has been controversial in recent years because of concern that its use was linked to a rise in the rate of childhood **autism**. The negative publicity given to the vaccine in the mass media led some parents to refuse to immunize their children with the MMR vaccine. One result has been an increase in the number of mumps outbreaks in several European countries, including Italy and the United Kingdom.

In the fall of 2002, the *New England Journal of Medicine* published a major Danish study disproving the hypothesis of a connection between the MMR vaccine and autism. A second study in Finland showed that the vaccine is not associated with aseptic meningitis or encephalitis as well as autism. Since these studies were published, American primary care physicians have once again reminded parents of the importance of immunizing their children against mumps and other childhood diseases. At this point, there appears to be no valid scientific basis for an association between the mumps vaccine and autism or other behavioral disorders.

Resources

BOOKS

Hawker, Jeremy, et al. *Communicable Disease Control and Health Protection Handbook*, 3rd ed. Chichester, West Sussex, UK: Wiley-Blackwell, 2012.

Stratton, Kathleen R. *Adverse Effects of Vaccines: Evidence and Causality*. Washington, D.C.: National Academies Press, 2012.

PERIODICALS

Berry, J. G., et al. "Public Perspectives on Consent for the Linkage of Data to Evaluate Vaccine Safety." *Vaccine* 30, 8. (2012): 4167–74.

Hahne, S., et al. "Mumps Vaccine Effectiveness against Orchitis." *Emerging Infectious Diseases* 18, 1. (2012): 191–93.

Holton, A., et al. "The Blame Frame: Media Attribution of Culpability About the MMR-Autism Vaccination Scare." *Health Communication* 27, 7. (2012): 690–701.

Rubin, S. A., et al. "Recent Mumps Outbreaks in Vaccinated Populations: No Evidence of Immune Escape." *Journal of Virology* 86, 1. (2012): 651–20.

White, Sarah J., et al. "Measles, Mumps, and Rubella." *Clinical Obstetrics and Gynecology* 55, 2. (2012): 550–59.

ORGANIZATIONS

American Academy of Pediatrics (AAP), 141 Northwest Point Blvd., Elk Grove Village, IL, 60007-1098. (847) 434-4000; Fax: (847) 424-8000. kidsdocs@aap.org. http://www.aap.org.

Centers for Disease Control and Prevention. 1600 Clifton Rd., NE, Atlanta, GA 30333. (800) CDC-INFO (800 232-4636) or (404) 639-3534. cdcinfo@cdc.gov. www.cdc.gov.

Ron Gasbarro, PharmD
Rebecca J. Frey, PhD

▌Mycobacterium

Definition

Mycobacterium describes a bacterial genus. The species that fall under this genus are varied and responsible for a number of diseases affecting humans and other animals.

Description

Species of mycobacterium tend to be rod-shaped and are often found in a variety of environments, including soil and **water**. Some species only survive on or in animals. Because there are so many species of mycobacterium, many specific qualities vary based on the type of mycobacterium. Mycobacteria are pathogens that are transmitted through ingestion or inhalation.

M. tuberculosis, a species of mycobacterium, causes most cases of **tuberculosis** in humans. Other species of mycobacterium—known as the tuberculosis complex—including *M. bovis*, *M. africanum*, *M. canetti*, *M. caprae*, and *M. microti* can also cause tuberculosis or similar disease in humans. When inhaled, these species of mycobacterium settle in the lungs, where they spread. When these cells become surrounded by healthy macrophages, the macrophages fuse, causing a granuloma. The granuloma then becomes a bump or tubercle in the lung, which can last as long as the person lives. These tubercles are large masses with the consistency of cheese that cause lung tissues to break down. The result of this breakdown is cavities in the lungs, and sometimes in the surrounding blood vessels.

Tuberculosis was the leading cause of death from the 18th century into the 20th century. Those who were not killed by the disease required years of treatment, including isolation in special facilities called sanitariums. Medical advances of the 20th century, including vaccinations and **antibiotics**, have drastically reduced the number of cases of tuberculosis as well as the treatment time. Instances of HIV/AIDS are connected with one out of four present-day tuberculosis deaths. Tuberculosis is now more common in underdeveloped countries with high populations and poor **sanitation**.

Two other mycobacteria, *M. leprae* and *M. lepromatosis* cause **leprosy**, also known as Hansen's disease. Like tuberculosis, leprosy results in granulomas in the peripheral nervous system and the respiratory tract. The external manifestations of leprosy are lesions on the skin.

Instances of leprosy have also declined in recent years and continue to decline globally. The **World Health Organization (WHO)** started an initiative to eliminate leprosy in 1991. Since that time, the rate of leprosy infections has dropped by 90%. The **WHO** identifies Brazil, Indonesia, the Philippines, the Democratic Republic of Congo, India, Madagascar, Mozambique, Nepal, and the United Republic of Tanzania as countries that still have areas with high occurrences of leprosy. According to the United States **Department of Health and Human Services** (HHS), there are currently approximately 6,500 cases in the U.S., and approximately 3,300 of these require current medical treatment. HHS also estimates that approximately 95% of the general population is not susceptible to *M. leprae*. Despite the traditional notion that leprosy is a disease affecting only humans, approximately 15% of the wild armadillos in Louisiana and southern Texas are infected with *M. leprae*.

Nontuberculous mycobacteria

Environmental or atypical mycobacteria—also known as nontuberculous mycobacteria (NTM)—do not cause leprosy or tuberculosis; however, NTM do cause other diseases of the lungs, infections of the lymph nodes, infections of the skin and other soft tissues, as well as disseminated disease in people suffering from HIV or **AIDS**. NTM are sometimes referred to as "mycobacteria other than tuberculosis," or MOTT. There are multiple types of NTM or MOTT infections, including *Mycobacterium avium complex*, *Mycobacterium marinum*, *Mycobacterium ulcerans*, and *Mycobacterium kansasii*.

The *Mycobacterium avium complex (MAC)* is a grouping that includes both *Mycobacterium avium* and *Mycobacterium intracellulare*. Infections associated with

---

KEY TERMS

Macrophage—Cells that aid in the immunity responses of vertebrates. Macrophages engulf and process both pathogens and debris.

Granuloma—A group of macrophages. This is a mass that forms when macrophages have grouped together to attempt the digestion of a potential threat but are unable to eliminate the threat.

Surface Plasmon Resonance (SPR)—describes the use of light to cause the oscillation of valence electrons in a solid. SPR can be used to measure absorption of material.

MAC are most often in the lymph nodes and lungs, though they often spread to other areas of the body, including the blood, bone marrow, intestines, liver, lungs, and spleen.

Infection of *Mycobacterium marinum* is very rare and causes lesions on the skin, which are often called "swimming pool" or "fish tank" granuloma. The infection is so called because it is usually found in persons with compromised immune systems who come in contact with contaminated fish, aquarium water, or swimming water.

Mycobacterium ulcerans infection occurs primarily in West Africa, though it has been known to occur in areas of Asia, the Western Pacific, and Latin America. This infection results in lesions on the skin—the ulcers release a toxin, causing damage to the skin and tissue. Though not necessarily painful, this infection can cause excessive damage to skin and bone.

Infections from *Mycobacterium kansasii* cause symptoms similar to tuberculosis, though not as severe. This infection is uncommon in the United States but poses a larger threat to those with chronic lung conditions. If untreated, this infection can be fatal.

Demographics

Second only to HIV/AIDS, tuberculosis causes the most deaths by a single infectious agent.

Though the global tuberculosis death rate dropped 41% between 1990 and 2011, in 2011 alone, 8.7 million contracted tuberculosis, and 1.4 million were killed by it.

Globally, tuberculosis is one of the three leading causes of death for women between the ages of 15 and 44.

Since 1991, the global prevalence of leprosy has dropped from 21.1 cases per 10,000 people to fewer than 1 case per 10,000 people.

Since 1985, leprosy has been eliminated from 119 of the 122 countries that considered it a public health problem.

Diagnosis

In most types of mycobacterial infections, the first symptoms that present include fatigue, fever, joint and bone **pain**, cough, weight loss, diarrhea, swollen lymph nodes, shortness of breath, and skin lesions. To diagnose a mycobacterial infection, doctors take a sample of blood, saliva, bone marrow, or fecal matter and culture it in a lab. This culture is used to isolate the specific species of mycobacteria involved. Depending on the strain, x rays, endoscopy, or other body scans can help identify areas of diseased tissue. It is critical to diagnose mycobacterial infections quickly, as treatments are long, and the infections can be highly damaging or fatal if left untreated for too long.

Treatment

Mycobacteria are resistant to the antibiotics usually employed to treat bacterial infections, and therefore, multiple drugs are usually required to treat mycobacterial infections.

The so-called first-line medications for pulmonary tuberculosis include isoniazid, rifampin, ethambutol, and pyrazinamide, administered in particular alternating cycles for roughly six months. Second-line medications (used when first-line treatments do not work or cannot be tolerated) include cycloserine, ethionamide, fluoroquinolones, p-aminosalicyclic acid, aminoglycosides, and capreomycin.

When treating extrapulmonary tuberculosis, many of the first-line pulmonary tuberculosis medications are used, though the treatment cycles and lengths are different. Treatment for extrapulmonary tuberculosis usually involves added use of steroids to reduce inflammation.

Some mycobacteria do not respond desirably to medication. Mycobacteria that resist isoniazid and rifampicin are called multi-drug-resistant (MDR). Mycobacteria that resist isoniazid, rifampin, fluoroquinolone, kanamycin, capreomycin, or amikacin are called extensively drug-resistant (XDR). When dealing with MDR-tuberculosis or XDR-tuberculosis, a laboratory test is needed to isolate the specific *Mycobacterium*. After this test, five drugs are combined to weaken the *Mycobacterium*.

Treatment of leprosy involves a year-long treatment of rifampin, dapsone, and clofazimine. NTM infections are treated with macrolides, ethambutol, and rifamycin.

Treating NTM or MOTT infections involves similar combinations of antibiotics and other medications for a period ranging from six months to two years.

Prognosis

The prognosis for mycobacterial infections depends on multiple factors, including the species of *Mycobacterium* involved, how far advanced the infection is, and the availability of medical care. Leprosy is curable; however, depending on the level of nerve damage and deformity before treatment, these effects are often irreversible. Rehabilitation and reconstructive surgery are sometimes able to help with this damage. Patients often need assistance learning to care for themselves, especially when treating lesions and any areas of the body with significant nerve damage.

Efforts and solutions

The WHO initiative to end leprosy has made the disease nearly extinct. Though the deadline the WHO set of eradicating leprosy by 2005 was not met, projections estimate that leprosy will continue to decline and could be eliminated by 2020.

In 2012, Chinese researchers announced a surface plasmon resonance (SPR) biosensor, which has the potential to offer real-time tuberculosis detection, instead of waiting weeks for cultures to isolate the specific strain a patient has.

Resources

BOOKS

Buratovich, Michael A. "Mycobacterium." *Infectious Diseases & Condictions.* Ed. H. Bradford Hawley. Vol. 2. Ipswich, MA: Salem Press, 2012. 717-720.

Cherath, Lata, and Rebecca J. Frey. "Leprosy." *The Gale Encyclopedia of Medicine.* Ed. Laurie J. Fundukian. 4th ed. Vol. 4. Detroit: Gale, 2011. 2566-2570.

"Mycobacterial Infections, Atypical." *Human Diseases and Conditions.* Ed. Miranda Herbert Ferrara. 2nd ed. Vol. 3. Detroit: Charles Scriber's Sons, 2010. 1150-1153.

"Tuberculosis." *Infectious Diseases.* Ed. Kara Rogers. New York: Britannica Educational Publishing with Rosen Educational Services, 2011. 35-37. Health and Disease in Society.

PERIODICALS

Chang, Chia-Chen, et al. "Rapid identification of Mycobacterium tuberculosis infection by a new array format-based surface plasmon resonance method." *Nanoscale Research Letters.* 7.1 (2012) 1+.

WEBSITES

U.S. Department of Health and Human Services. "National Hansen's Disease (Leprosy) Program." http://www.hrsa .gov/hansensdisease/Accessed November 14, 2012.

World Health Organization. "Leprosy." http://www.who.int/ mediacentre/factsheets/fs101/en/Accessed November 14, 2012.

World Health Organization. "Tuberculosis." http://www.who .int/mediacentre/factsheets/fs104/en/Accessed November 14, 2012.

ORGANIZATIONS

U.S. Department of Health & Human Services, 200 Independence Avenue, S.W., Washington, DC USA 20201, (877) 696-6775, www.hhs.gov.

Andrea Nienstedt, MA

National Association of City and County Health Officials (NACCHO)

Definition

The National Association of City and County Health Officials (NACCHO) is the national professional organization representing 2,700 local **health departments** in the 50 states and the District of Columbia.

Purpose

The purpose of NACCHO is to be a voice for local health departments with decision-makers at the federal, state, and local level (as well as the general public), and to serve as a resource for individual health departments in the United States.

Description

NACCHO was formed in 1994 through the merger of two preexisting groups, the National Association of County Health Officers and the U.S. Conference of Local Health Officers. In 2001, the Association expanded its scope to include health offices in tribal communities. It is governed by a 27–member board of directors that meets four times a year. NACCHO policies and programs are established largely on the basis of suggestions made by 41 advisory committees made up of local health deparment members from around the nation. Its day-to-day operations are carried out through a number of committees, such as: health equity and social justice, **community health**, **environmental health**, public health preparedness, public health infrastructure and systems, and workgroups such as access and integrated services, disability, **epidemiology**, HIV/STI, **food safety**, global climate change, biosurveillance, public health informatics, and **pandemic** flu.

Much of the organization's structure is divided into four major programs: Public Health Infrastructure and Systems, Community Health, Environmental Health, and Public Health Preparedness. As an example, the first of these programs assists local health agencies in developing and carrying out as effectively as possible their core functions and services. The last of these programs aims to assist local health departments in the development and utilization of programs and activities required for disaster preparedness. In addition to the broad, general progams, NACCHO also sponsors and operates a number of programs focused on more specific topics of interest to local health departments, such as: adolescent health, biosurveillance, **birth defects** and developmental disabilities, chronic disease **prevention**, climate change, cultural uses of mercury, diabetes, environmental justice, H1N1, **immunization**, injury prevention, mental health, performance standards, public health law, **radiation**, Superfund sites, traffic safety, and wastewater.

NACCHO is particularly active in the field of advocacy, presenting the needs of local health departments before legislative and administrative groups and other decision makers and relaying information about new and proposed laws and regulations to its members. For example, it has developed a number of position papers on topics of concern to local health departments on topics ranging from border and immigrant health and health and disability to climate change and food safety. It presents its views both through position papers and by letters to Congress on issues of significance to local health departments, testimony before Congressional committees, endorsements of actions by other health groups, and participation in coalitions of health groups. The organization maintains a Legislative Action Center on its website through which local health departments can stay in touch with legislative actions that are likely to have impact on local operations and through which local health departments can express their views on such potential actions.

Professional publications

NACCHO produces and distributes a large number of books, booklets, pamphlets, brochures, fact sheets, and other print and online materials on topics of interest to local health departments. Some of the topics included in its publications list are: A Compendium of Local Health Department Home Visitation Program Case Studies; Big Cities Health Inventory, 2007: The Health of Urban USA; Core Public Health Functions; **Drinking Water**, Pollution Prevention and Public Health; **Emergency Preparedness** Checklist for Case Management and Home Care Services; Impaired Driving Prevention in Rural Communities; Information Technology Capacity and Local Public Health Agencies; Medical Mass Care During an **Influenza** Pandemic; Overcoming Financial Barriers to Create and Sustain Local Mosquito Programs; Preconception Care—Healthy Women Today, Healthy Babies Tomorrow; and Report on **West Nile Virus**.

Resources

BOOKS

Hofrichter, Richard, and Rajiv Bhatia. *Tackling Health Inequities through Public Health Practice: Theory to Action: A Project of the National Association of County and City Health Officials.* Oxford; New York: Oxford University Press, 2010.

Stahl, Michael J. *Encyclopedia of Health Care Management.* Thousand Oaks, CA: Sage Publications, 2004.

PERIODICALS

Leep, C. J., and G. H. Shah. "NACCHO's National Profile of Local Health Departments Study: The Premier Source of Data on Local Health Departments for Surveillance, Research, and Policymaking." *Journal of Public Health Management and Practice* 18. 2. (2012): 186–9.

"Workforce Development at the Local Level: The NACCHO Perspective." *Journal of Public Health Management and Practice* 9. 6. (2003): 440–2.

WEBSITES

Operational Definition of a Functional Local Health Department. NACCHO. http://chfs.ky.gov/NR/rdonlyres/6C8BE6B2-A6B7-43E2-AB91-F2D6A2F50422/278155/OperationalDefinitionBrochure2.pdf (accessed October 11, 2012).

National Association of County and City Health Officials. Centers for Disease Control and Prevention. http://www.cdc.gov/stltpublichealth/partnerships/naccho.html (accessed October 11, 2012).

ORGANIZATIONS

National Association of County and City Health Officials (NACCHO), 1100 17th St., N.W., 17th floor, Washington, DC 20036, (202) 783-5550, Fax: (202) 783-1583, info@naccho.org, www.naccho.org/.

David E. Newton, EdD

▌National Association of Local Boards of Health (NALBOH)

Definition

The National Association of Local Boards of Health (NALBOH) acts as the voice for local boards of health on a national level and works to strengthen local boards of health by providing expert advice on governance, leadership, **health policy**, and health priorities.

Purpose

The purpose of the NALBOH is to provide education and training for local boards of health as a way of helping them to achieve maximum possible efficiency in carrying out their public health mandates. The association also acts at a national level to bring to decision makers the problems faced by local boards of health and potential solutions available for solving these problems. It acts overall as a liaison among national, state, and local organizations concerned with public health issues.

Description

The NALBOH was formed in 1992 when 37 local boards of health joined together to form the new organization. It has grown over the years to include 220 members in 1997, 627 members in 2000, 718 members in 2004, and 840 members in 2007 (the last year for which numbers are reported). In 1991, NALBOH expanded its mission to include state boards of health by forming the State Associations of Local Boards of Health (SALBOH) division of the organization. That division began with six members, Georgia (which later withdrew), Illinois, Massachusetts, North Carolina, Ohio, and Utah, and has since added seven more members, Colorado, Idaho, Indiana, Kentucky, Michigan, Missouri, Nebraska, and Wisconsin. Members of the SALBOH act as links between the national organization and local boards of health. The NALBOH is governed by a board of directors of 15 members whose policies are implemented by a full–time staff of ten.

Much of the day-to-day work at NALBOH is carried out by about a dozen standing committees that deal with topics such as board governance, finance, membership, education and training, chronic disease and tobacco use **prevention**, performance standards and accreditation, and **environmental health**.

An important NALBOH function is the development and distribution of position statements on public health issues for decision makers at all levels of government and the general public. Some of the topics on which the association has taken prominent positions are health care reform; climate change; raw sewage overflows; **influenza** vaccines; **nutrition**, **physical activity**, and **obesity**; San Francisco menu labeling; e-cigarettes; and workforce development. The organization has also developed and made available to its members information about and suggestions for the process by which individuals and local boards of health can influence the legislative process. These resources are available on the Association's Internet home pages. The website also contains a number of useful links to other organizations that advocate for public health issues, such as the **American Public Health Association**, the Council of State Governments, the National Conference of State Legislatures, and the Coalition for Health Funding. Some of the events sponsored by the NALBOH are conferences, symposia, and other meetings and webinars on topics of interest to local boards of health.

Professional publications

In addition to its free online newsletter, NEWS-ALERTS, the organization offers a long list of useful publications, such as: Accreditation Decision Making Tools for Local Boards; Being an Effective Local Board of Health Member; Community Guide Factsheets: **Tobacco Control**; **Emergency Preparedness** Including Bioterrorism: An All Hazards Approach for Local Boards of Health; Guide to Developing Effective Environmental Health Policies for Boards of Health; Oral Health Guide for Local Boards of Health: **Water** Fluoridation; State Statutory Authority for Local Boards of Health; and Tobacco Use Prevention and Control Tool Kit. A complete list of available print and electronic publications is available on the NALBOH website at http://www.nalboh.org/pdffiles/resource_list_w_orderform_Mar2012.pdf.

Resources

BOOKS

Kirch, Wilhelm, ed. *Encyclopedia of Public Health*. New York: Springer, 2008.

Stahl, Michael J. *Encyclopedia of Health Care Management*. Thousand Oaks, CA: Sage Publications, 2004.

PERIODICALS

Fenton, G. D. "The Status of State Boards of Health in 2010." *Journal of Public Health Management and Practice* 17. 6. (2011): 554–9

Patton, D., C. E. Moon, and J. Jones. "Describing Local Boards of Health: Insights from the 2008 National Association of Local Boards of Health Survey." *Public Health Reports* 126. 3. (2011): 410–19

WEBSITES

National Association of Local Boards of Health. Centers for Disease Control and Prevention. http://www.cdc.gov/

stltpublichealth/partnerships/nalboh.html (accessed October 11, 2012).

Local Boards of Health: A New Public Health Q&A With Marie Fallon. New Public Health. http://blog.rwjf.org/publichealth/2011/09/02/local-boards-of-health-a-newpublichealth-qa-with-marie-fallon/ (accessed October 11, 2012).

ORGANIZATIONS

National Association of Local Boards of Health (NALBOH), 1840 East Gypsy Lane Rd., Bowling Green, OH 43402, (419) 353-7714, Fax: (419) 352-6278, http://www.nalboh.org/Staff.htm, http://www.nalboh.org/.

David E. Newton, EdD

▎National Institute of Mental Health

Definition

The National Institute of Mental Health (NIMH) is the U.S. government agency that conducts and supports research on mental illness and mental health. The NIMH is a component of the National Institutes of Health (NIH) and was one of the first four institutes created. Proposed by the National Mental Health Act in 1946, the institute was formally established in 1949. Specific areas of research include the brain, behavior, and mental health services.

Purpose

The NIMH is dedicated to improving the mental health of the American people, fostering better understanding, diagnosis, treatment, rehabilitation, and **prevention** of mental and brain disorders. The NIMH's mission is "to transform the understanding and treatment of mental illnesses through basic and clinical research, paving the way for prevention, recovery, and cure."

Description

In order to carry out its mission, the NIMH supports research by awarding more than 2,000 research grants to scientists working in universities or other research facilities. Grants support the study of all aspects of mental illness, from biological to social, and they also help identify specific areas where research is needed. The NIMH also supports a large in-house research program, consisting of more than 500 scientists, that studies the causes of and new treatments for mental illnesses. In addition, the NIMH collects and disseminates statistical information to scientists and researchers, conducts training and career development programs, supports small business research programs, sponsors clinical trials, and prepares and distributes a wide variety of educational materials.

Among the key areas of research interest for NIMH are neuroscience and behavioral science, including sciences basic to the understanding of the anatomical and chemical basis of brain disorders, and the most prevalent mental disorders and their causes and prevention, such as schizophrenia, mood disorders, anxiety disorders, **eating disorders**, and Alzheimer's disease. Specific outside research divisions include the Division of Neuroscience and Basic Behavioral Science (DNBBS), the Division of Adult Translational Research and Treatment Development (DATR), the Division of Developmental Translational Research (DDTR), the Division of **AIDS** Research (DAR), and the Division of Services and Intervention Research (DSIR). Additional research efforts include the NIMH Professional Coalition for Research Progress and the NIMH Alliance for Research Progress.

The NIMH operates under the Office of the NIMH Director. Outside of the five research divisions, additional divisions include the Division of Extramural Activities (DEA) and the Division of Intramural Research Programs (DIRP). Advisory boards and groups include the National Advisory Mental Health Council (NAMHC), peer review committees, a board of scientific counselors (BSC), and the NIMH Outreach Partnership Program, which focuses on improving access to mental health information within communities.

Professional publications

The National Institute of Mental Health communicates current research, diagnosis, and treatment information to professionals and the public through conferences, symposia, and meetings, and works closely with professional and voluntary organizations and other federal agencies. The institute produces a number of publications, including booklets, brochures, and fact sheets, available in both English and Spanish. The NIMH also produces videos and podcasts on mental health topics, which are available on the NIMH website at http://www.nimh.nih.gov/news/index.shtml.

ORGANIZATIONS

National Institute of Mental Health, 6001 Executive Blvd., Rm. 8184, MSC 9663, Bethesda, MD 20892-9663, (301) 433-4513; TTY: (301) 443-8431, (866) 615-6464; TTY: (866) 415-8051, Fax: (301) 443-4279, nimhinfo@nih.gov, http://www.nimh.nih.gov.

Natural disasters

Definition

A natural disaster is an event caused by a natural force, such as an earthquake, volcanic eruption, tidal wave, flood, hurricane, or landslide, with devastating effects on human life and property and the natural environment.

Description

As their name suggests, natural disasters have two primary components. First, they are the result of natural forces occurring within the Earth. For example, earthquakes and volcanic eruptions occur because tectonic plates that underlie the Earth's crust are constantly in motion. When these plates collide with each other, they produce massive movements of the crust (earthquakes) with the release of molten magma from the Earth's interior. Second, natural disasters produce catastrophic loss of human life and property, causing profound challenges to public health agencies in regions where they occur. The worst earthquake in the world since 1900, for example, occurred in Haiti in January 2010, resulting in the loss of an estimated 316,000 lives. In addition, more than 97,000 houses were completely destroyed in the area of Port-au-Prince and 1.3 million residents were displaced.

No part of the Earth is immune from possible natural disasters. In many cases, those disasters occur without warning, although technological developments have made it possible to provide early warning for some types of disasters, such as hurricanes and typhoons, tsunamis, floods, and wildfires. General, long-term warnings of other disasters, such as earthquakes and volcanic eruptions, are also available, although they tend to be less reliable. The major types of natural disasters for which public health agencies should be prepared include:

• avalanches and other types of landslides

• earthquakes

• volcanic eruptions

• tsunamis

• floods

• droughts

• heat waves

• tornadoes

• hurricanes and typhoons

• blizzards

• wildfires

• epidemics

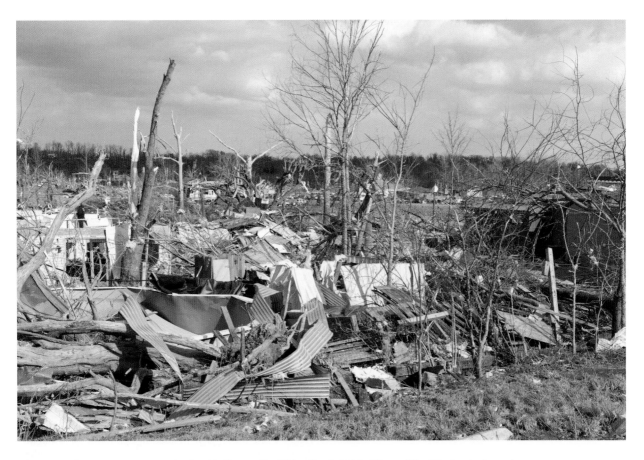

Aftermath of a category 4 tornado that hit Henryville, IN in March 2012. *(Alexey Stiop/Shutterstock.com)*

- solar magnetic storms, gamma ray bursts, impact events, and other types of so-called "space disasters"

Effects on public health

Natural disasters can have a devastating effect on public health systems. They can flood public health providers with a massive number of casualties that may greatly exceed the system's ability to respond normally and efficiently. The disaster can also disrupt the normal functions of a public health agency, leaving its clients in distress. The elderly who depend on nutritional or nursing services, for example, may have to find other resources when public health agencies are stretched beyond their normal capabilities. Public health facilities and assets themselves may also be destroyed or damaged during an emergency as, for example, when a hospital is damaged and unable to continue its normal operations. Roads may also be blocked or destroyed, making transportation into and out of care facilities difficult or impossible.

The activities of public health agencies with regard to natural disasters are sometimes divided into three major categories: preparation, response, and recovery.

Preparation for a natural disaster generally consists of two elements, the first of which involves the steps a public health office itself can take in preparation for an emergency. These steps may include:

- Ensuring that the physical materials needed to respond to the emergency, such as drugs and medical supplies, are on hand or readily available.

- Training staff in specific actions that may be necessary in any particular type of emergency; this may include trial "run-throughs" that educate staff members as to various scenarios to which they may be asked to respond.

- Maintaining a list of individual and organizational resources needed to deal with an emergency, with up-to-date contact information for each such person or agency.

- Providing training or re-training in Standard Precautions and other medical procedures that might be needed in case of an emergency.

- Ensuring that plans are in place and facilities are available for housing individuals who need care after an emergency.

- Understanding the procedures by which individuals are to be transferred to health care facilities (such as hospitals) after initial treatment by public health professionals.
- Arranging for procedures by which those who have been killed in the emergency are transported to morgues or other facilities.
- Carrying out public education programs for a natural disaster.

The last item on this list constitutes the second major element in preparing for a natural disaster. Public health agencies are the logical and ideal resource for helping members of the community prepare for natural disasters that may be imminent or that may occur at some unknown time in the future. A number of recommendations are valid for almost any type of emergency, such as ensuring that a household has an adequate supply of food and **water** for a possible emergency, that family members have a specific plan for remaining in touch with each other after an emergency, that households develop an emergency escape plan from their home, and that other essential supplies, such as a flashlight and battery-operated radio are available and ready to use at any time. More specific recommendations can also be made for certain types of natural disasters. For example, homeowners at risk for wildfires can be cautioned to prepare for an emergency by:

- Becoming familiar with local fire laws and recommendations.
- Ensuring that fire vehicles and firefighter teams have access to one's property.
- Reporting, repairing or removing hazardous conditions that might cause or contribute to a fire.
- Posting fire and other emergency telephone numbers in easily accessible locations.
- Removing all dead and flammable materials from around the house.
- Maintaining a 10-foot fire break around barbecues, propane tanks, and other sources of flames.
- Removing all limbs less than 15 feet above the ground from trees near the house.
- Stacking firewood at least 100 feet from the house.
- Asking the power company to remove any branches in contact with or near power lines.
- Removing leaves and rubbish from around trees and bushes.

The second phase of public health involvement in natural disasters involves responses that occur after the disaster has passed. The primary objective of this response effort is to identify the type and extent of damage that has occurred during the disaster, the types of

KEY TERMS

Space disaster—Events that follow accidents that occur in space or as the result of space materials, such as the collision of an asteroid with the surface of the Earth.

Standard precautions—A set of minimum infection prevention practices used in all types of patient care, regardless of suspected or confirmed infection status of any patients, in any setting where healthcare is delivered.

Tectonic plates—A rigid rocky plate within the lithosphere that moves horizontally below the Earth's surface.

aid that will be needed by survivors, and the resources available to provide that aid. A number of agencies have developed response programs that outline the ways in which this process can take place. One such program is the Community Assessment for Public Health Emergency Response (CASPER) Toolkit, developed by the **Centers for Disease Control and Prevention (CDC)**. The toolkit was first published in 2009 and then updated in 2012. It describes a detailed process by which a public health agency can determine the health status and basic needs of a community immediately after a natural disaster has occurred. This information makes it possible for public health officials to quickly draw up a program for prioritizing health care actions and distribution of resources in the most efficient way possible. The specific objectives of CASPER are to:

- Determine the critical health needs and assess the impact of the disaster.
- Characterize the population residing in the affected area.
- Produce household-based information and estimates for decision-makers.
- Evaluate the effectiveness of relief efforts through conducting a follow-up CASPER.

The recovery phase of public health activities after a natural disaster involves a number of elements, one of the most important of which is providing or arranging ongoing medical care for individuals who have been injured in the event. In general, this involves arranging for the transport of such individuals to facilities capable of providing the needed care, such as hospitals, clinics, or nursing homes. Public health teams may also be involved in surveys and evaluating homes and other physical

QUESTIONS TO ASK YOUR DOCTOR

- What emergency supplies do you recommend that we keep in our household at all times?
- In case of a natural disaster, what public health agency should we contact for assistance?
- Where can we learn about the city or county's program for emergency assistance in case of a natural disaster?
- How can we reach you in case of an emergency?

structures to determine how suitable they are for continued occupancy. Individuals displaced by the disaster may need counseling as to other housing and work options. Public health can also assume a crucial role in helping to protect workers involved in the cleanup after a natural disaster. Those workers are commonly exposed to a host of hazards, including carbon monoxide and other toxic gases, electrical hazards, damaged structures that can cause falls and other accidents, heat and cold **stress**, and exposure to confined spaces. Both survivors and cleanup workers may also need psychological counseling in order to deal with the extreme stress and fatigue to which they have been exposed as a result of the disaster. Public health workers may also be asked to provide counseling in a number of non-medical fields, such as economics and financing, for individuals who have lost everything they owned as a result of the natural disaster.

Costs to society

The financial and human costs of natural disasters around the world each year are high, but variable. For example, the total economic impact of all natural disasters in 2011 was estimated to be the highest in recorded history, some $380 billion, more than double the amount for the previous year. The earthquake and tsunami that hit Japan in March of 2011 cost somewhere between $35 billion and $40 billion, the most expensive single natural disaster in history. But an earthquake in New Zealand a month earlier was also costly, with an estimated value of lost property at $13 billion. Insurance researchers have noted that the economic costs of natural disasters have been rising regularly over the last century, although not because of worse disasters so much as the cost of replacing lost structures.

At the same time, the cost in human lives has been decreasing over the same period. Only 27,000 lives were lost worldwide to natural disasters in 2011, the vast majority in the Japanese earthquake and tsunami (15,840), a decrease from 296,000 deaths in the preceding year. This trend can partially be attributed to improved methods of disaster predictions and preparation, but it also reflects to some extent the variability in the times, places, and severity of natural disasters that do occur.

Resources

BOOKS

Brebbia, C. A., A. J. Kassab, and E. Divo, eds. *Disaster Management and Human Health Risk II*. Southampton, UK: WIT Press, 2011.

Brennan, Virginia M., ed. *Natural Disasters and Public Health: Hurricanes Katrina, Rita, and Wilma*. Baltimore: The Johns Hopkins University Press, 2009.

Duncan, K., and C. A. Brebbia. *Disaster Management and Human Health Risk: Reducing Risk, Improving Outcomes*. Southampton, UK: WIT Press, 2009.

Katz, Rebecca. *Essentials Of Public Health Preparedness*. Sudbury, MA: Jones & Bartlett Learning, 2011.

PERIODICALS

Chen, V., D. Banerjee, and L. Liu. "Do People Become Better Prepared in the Aftermath of a Natural Disaster? The Hurricane Ike Experience in Houston, Texas." *Journal of Public Health Management and Practice* 18, 3. (2012): 241–9.

Davis, J. S., et al. "Optimal Emergency Personnel Allocation after a Natural Disaster." *American Journal of Disaster Medicine* 7, 1. (2012): 31–6.

Montealegre, Jane R., et al. "An Innovative Public Health Preparedness Training Program for Graduate Students." *Public Health Reports* 126, 3. (2011): 441–6.

Rathore, F. A., et al. "Medical Rehabilitation after Natural Disasters: Why, When, and How?" *Archives of Physical Medicine and Rehabilitation* 93, 10. (2012): 1875–81.

WEBSITES

"Natural Disaster." United States Army Public Health Command. http://phc.amedd.army.mil/topics/emergency response/nd/Pages/default.aspx. Accessed on October 6, 2012.

"Natural Disasters: Coping with the Health Impact." Disease Control Priorities Project. http://www.dcp2.org/file/121/. Accessed on October 6, 2012.

"Natural Disasters and Severe Weather." Centers for Disease Control and Prevention. http://emergency.cdc.gov/disasters/. Accessed on October 6, 2012.

Shoaf, Kimberley I., et al. "Public Health Impact of Disasters." http://www.eird.org/isdr-biblio/PDF/Public%20health%20impact%20of%20disasters.pdf. Accessed on October 6, 2012.

ORGANIZATIONS

Centers for Disease Control and Prevention, 1600 Clifton Rd., N.E., Atlanta, GA USA 30333, 1 (800) 232–4636, cdcinfo@cdc.gov., www.cdc.gov.

David E. Newton, Ed.D.

Needle exchange programs *see* **Needles and syringes**

Needles and syringes

Definition

Syringes and needles are sterile devices used to inject solutions into or withdraw secretions from the body. The syringe is a calibrated glass or plastic cylinder with a plunger at one end, and an opening to which the needle attaches.

Purpose

This method is used to administer drugs when a small amount of fluid is to be injected, the patient is unable to take the drug orally, or intestinal secretions destroy the drug. It is also used to withdraw various types of bodily fluids, most commonly blood.

Description

There are different types and sizes of syringes used for a variety of purposes. Syringe sizes may vary from 0.25–450 ml, and can be made from glass or assorted plastics. Latex-free syringes eliminate the exposure of the health care professional and the patient to an allergen to which he or she may be sensitive. The most common type of syringe is the piston syringe. The pen, cartridge, and dispensing syringes are also extensively used.

A syringe consists of a hollow barrel with a piston at one end and a nozzle at the other end that connects to a needle. Other syringes have a needle already attached. These devices are often used for subcutaneous injections of insulin and are single-use (i.e., disposable). Syringes have markings etched or printed on their sides, showing the graduations (i.e., in milliliters) for accurate dispensing of drugs or removal of body fluids. Cartridge syringes are for multiple use, and are often sold in kits where a prefilled drug cartridge with a needle is inserted into the piston syringe. Syringes may also have anti-needlestick features, as well as positive stops that prevent accidental pullouts.

There are three types of nozzles:

• Luer-lock, which locks the needle onto the nozzle of the syringe.

• Slip tip, which secures the needle by compressing the hub onto the syringe nozzle.

• Eccentric, which secures with a connection that is almost flush with the side of the syringe.

The hypodermic needle is a hollow, metal tube, usually made of stainless steel and sharpened at one end. It has a female connector end that fits into the male connector of a syringe or intravascular administration set. The size of the diameter of the needle ranges from the largest gauge (13) to the smallest (27). The needle's length extends to 3.5 inches (8 cm) for the 13 gauge, and from 0.25–1 inch (0.6–2.5 cm) for the 27 gauge. The needle consists of a hub with a female connector at one end that connects to a syringe, and to the other end, where the bevel is located. The bevel is a flat aperture on one side of a needle's tip.

Needles are almost always disposable, but reusable ones are available for home use by a single patient.

Operation

Syringes and needles are used for injecting or withdrawing fluids from a patient. The most common procedure for removing fluids from a patient is the venipuncture, or blood drawing. In this procedure, the syringe and appropriate needle are used with a vacutainer, which is used to collect the blood as it is drawn. The syringe and needle can be left in place while the vacutainer is changed, allowing for multiple samples to be drawn.

Fluids can be injected into a patient by intradermal injection, subcutaneous injection, intramuscular injection, or Z-track injection. In all types of injections, the size of syringe should be chosen based on the amount of fluid being delivered, and the gauge and length of needle should be chosen based on the size of the patient and the type of medication. A needle with a larger gauge may be chosen for drawing up the medication into the syringe, and a smaller gauge needle will replace the previous one for injection into the patient. In all injections, proper procedures for **infection control** should be strictly followed.

Maintenance

Syringes and needles are normally sterile products and should be stored in appropriate containers. Care should be taken prior to using them. One should ensure that the needles are not blunt and that the packets are not torn; this would expose the contents to air and allow contamination by microorganisms.

Health care team roles

All personnel must be offered vaccines against blood-borne infections, such as **hepatitis** B. This is the responsibility of medical staff.

Used syringes and needles should be disposed of quickly in appropriate containers.

If a needlestick injury occurs, it is important that it is reported immediately and that proper treatment is administered to the injured person.

Training

Those responsible for training should ensure staff is skilled at up-to-date methods of aseptic technique and correct handling/use of syringes and needles.

Teaching the correct use of syringes and needles, as well as their disposal, is important to protect medical staff and patients from needlestick injuries and contamination from blood-borne infections. Presently, some of the more serious infections are human immunodeficiency virus (HIV), hepatitis B (HBV), and hepatitis C (HCV).

The staff should be aware of current methods of infection **prevention**.

Risk management

Protection of both patients and healthcare workers is of primary importance in the design and use of needles and syringes. Research over the last decade has resulted in the invention of at least four types of so-called safety syringes designed to reduce the risk of spreading disease during needle use. Those four designs have the following features:

- The auto-disabling syringe contains a device that blocks the plunger after one use, preventing the syringe from being used a second time by a healthcare worker or a patient.

- The breaking plunger syringe is also designed to prevent a second use by releasing an internal device that actually breaks the plunger, preventing it from being depressed more than once.

- A needle stick prevention syringe contains a cap that slides into place over the needle after a single use, preventing an accidental needle stick by healthcare worker or patient.

- A retractable syringe is designed so that the needle is retracted into the body of the syringe after a single use, again preventing a possible needle stick.

KEY TERMS

Bevel—The flat aperture on one side of a needle at the tip.

Piston—The plunger that slides up and down the inside barrel of a syringe.

Sterile—Free from living microorganisms.

Subcutaneous—Beneath the skin.

Needle exchange programs

Another approach to reducing the spread of disease through multiple needle use has been the development of needle exchange programs. A needle exchange program is a system whereby an individual who uses drugs for some (usually illegal) purpose, and who does so multiple times, is allowed to turn in used needles in exchange for new needles. The exchange usually takes place through the auspices of some public health agency or its representative. The logic behind needle exchange programs is that, if an individual is committed to the use of needles for drug injection, his or her risk of infection will be dramatically reduced if a new needle is used on each such occasion. The **Centers for Disease Control and Prevention (CDC)** estimates, for example, that about one-fifth of all new cases of hepatitis C infection result from the re-use of needles. A needle exchange program could in theory, then, dramatically reduce the number of new infections of hepatitis C among substance abusers.

The first needle exchange programs were instituted in the 1970s, primarily for the purpose of reducing the spread of hepatitis C among substance abusers. With the occurrence of the HIV/AIDS **pandemic** in the 1980s, however, the goal of needle exchange programs expanded to include that disease, which soon became the primary target of such programs. As of 2011, 221 legally authorized needle exchange programs were in existence in the United States. The largest fraction of these programs was funded by state governments, followed by city funding, foundation grants, county funding, the federal government, and individual donations. According to one estimate, about 37 million needles and syringes were exchanged by these programs in the United States in 2011. Needle exchange programs are also in operation in almost 90 other countries around the world, with vastly differing magnitudes of service and measurable results.

Resources

BOOKS

Rosdahl, Caroline Bunker, and Mary T. Kowalski. *Textbook of Basic Nursing*, 10th ed. Philadelphia: Wolters Kluwer Health/Lippincott Williams & Wilkins, 2012.

PERIODICALS

Sibbitt, W. L., Jr., et al. "Safety Syringes and Anti-needlestick Devices in Orthopaedic Surgery." *Journal of Bone and Joint Surgery* 93, 17. (2012): 1641–9.

WEBSITES

"Needle Exhange and Harm Reduction. Avert." http://www.avert.org/needle-exchange.htm. Accessed on December 4, 2012.

"Sharps Safety. Minnesota Department of Environmental Health & Safety." http://www.dehs.umn.edu/bio_pracprin_su_ss.htm. Accessed on December 4, 2012.

"What Every Worker Should Know: How to Protect Yourself From Needlestick Injuries." Centers for Disease Control and Prevention. http://www.cdc.gov/niosh/docs/2000-135/. Accessed on December 4, 2012.

Margaret A. Stockley, R.N.

Noise pollution

Definition

Noise pollution can be defined as any sound or combination of sounds that is annoying and/or physiologically harmful. The U.S. **Environmental Protection Agency (EPA)** further describes noise pollution as any sound that "either interferes with normal activities such as sleeping [or] conversation, or disrupts or diminishes one's quality of life."

Description

Sound is any vibration in the air or some other medium that reaches the ear of an animal and can be heard by that animal. It is characterized by three fundamental properties: wavelength, frequency, and amplitude. The wavelength of a sound wave is the distance between two consecutive peaks or troughs in the wave, while its frequency is the number of waves that pass a given point in some period of time, such as every second. Wavelength and frequency are inversely proportional to each other. The greater the wavelength, the lower the frequency, and the shorter the wavelength, the higher the frequency. Sound waves are most frequently measured in terms of their frequency. The unit of frequency most frequently used for sound waves is the hertz (Hz), the number of cycles per second for the wave.

The amplitude of a wave is a measure of the energy carried by the sound wave. The greater the amplitude of the sound wave, the louder the sound, and the lesser the amplitude, the quieter the sound. The most common unit used for expressing the intensity of a sound wave is the decibel (db). A decibel is a unit of measure comparing the intensity of two sounds (or other forms of energy) with each other. It is a logarithmic unit (compared to base 10), which means that every increase in one decibel unit represents an increase of ten times in the intensity of a sound. A sound with a rating of 4 db, for example, is 10 times louder than a sound with a rating of 3 db, and 100 times louder than a sound with a rating of 2 db. The intensity (loudness) of some common sounds is as follows:

- the threshhold of detectable sounds for humans: 0 db
- normal conversation: 50 db
- background noise in a typical surburban setting: 50 db
- typical vaccum cleaner: 70 db
- background noise on a busy city street: 80 db
- interior of a jet airplane during takeoff: 80 db
- power tool, such as a chain saw or jack hammer, at a distance of one meter: 100-110 db
- front rows of a rock concert: 110 db
- threshhold of pain: 130 db
- sound of a jet airplane during takeoff from outside the plane: 150 db
- perforation of the eardrum: 160 db

As this list illustrates, very loud noises can cause damage to the ear and, hence, to hearing. A second factor is involved in the possible damage caused by sound: time of exposure. Thus, the damage caused to hearing is a result of not only the intensity of a sound, but also the length of time to which one is exposed to that sound. The International Electrotechnical Commission (IEC) has prepared guidelines for the recommended maximum period of time for which a person should be exposed to sounds of various intensity. Some of those recommendations are as follows:

- for a loudness of 80 db, an exposure of 24 hours
- for a loudness of 85 db, an exposure of 8 hours
- for a loudness of 94 db, an exposure of 1 hour
- for a loudness of 97 db, an exposure of 30 minutes
- for a loudness of 100 db, an exposure of 15 minutes
- for a loudness of 106 db, an exposure of 3.75 minutes
- for a loudness of 112 db, an exposure of 0.94 minutes
- for a loudness of 115 db, an exposure of 28.12 seconds
- for a loudness of 121 db, an exposure of 7.03 seconds
- for a loudness of 130 db, an exposure of 0.88 second
- for a loudness of 139 db, an exposure of 0.11 second

Individuals differ as to what constitutes "sound" and what constitutes "noise." A listener may prefer to listen

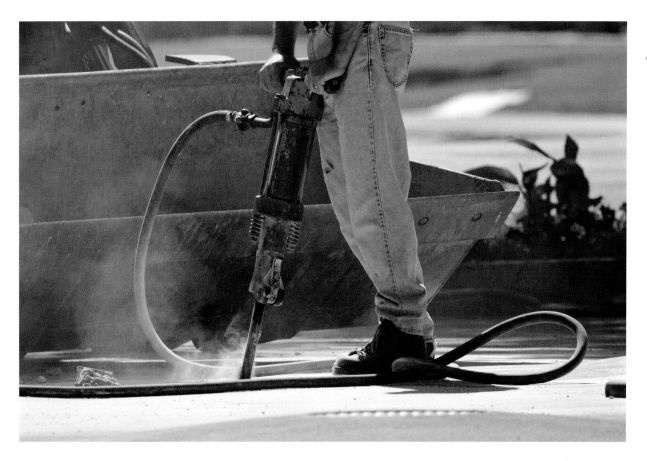

Using a Jack-hammer, which is a source of noise pollution. *(©iStockphoto.com/BirdofPrey)*

to hard rock, but find the sounds of an opera offensive, or vice versa. People also differ as to which sounds are "too loud," and which are "not loud enough." In spite of these differences in personal preferences, scientists now have relatively reliable data on the kinds of anatomical and physiological changes that occur in the human ear that has been exposed to a variety of sounds with different frequencies and intensities.

Humans detect sound by means of a set of sensory cells in the inner ear. These cells have tiny projections (called microvilli and kinocilia) on their surface. As sound waves pass through the fluid-filled chamber within which these cells are suspended, the microvilli rub against a flexible membrane lying on top of them. Bending of fibers inside the microvilli sets off a mechanico-chemical process that results in a nerve signal being sent through the auditory nerve to the brain where the signal is analyzed and interpreted.

The sensory cell's microvilli are flexible and resilient, but only up to a point. They can bend and then spring back up, but they die if they are smashed down too hard or too often. Prolonged exposure to sounds above about 90 decibels can flatten some of the microvilli

permanently and their function will be lost. By age 30, most Americans have lost five decibels of sensitivity and cannot hear anything above 16,000 Hz; by age 65, the sensitivity reduction is 40 decibels for most people, and all sounds above 8,000 Hz are lost. By contrast, in environments that are very quiet, such as a quiet countryside, even 70-year-olds tend to have no significant **hearing loss**.

Extremely loud sounds—above 130 decibels—actually can rip out the sensory microvilli, causing aberrant nerve signals that the brain interprets as a high-pitched whine or whistle. Many people experience a ringing in the ears after exposure to very loud noises called tinnitus. Coffee, aspirin, certain **antibiotics**, and fever can produce a similar effect. For most people, the ringing is noticeable only in a very quiet environment, and they rarely are in a place that is quiet enough to hear it. About 35 out of 1,000 people have tinnitus severe enough to the point where it interferes with their lives. Sometimes the ringing becomes so loud that it is unendurable, such as shrieking brakes on a subway train. Unfortunately, there is not yet a treatment for this distressing disorder.

Effects on public health

Although damage to one's hearing is an obvious effect of noise pollution, a variety of public health problems is possible also. Some of the additional issues associated with exposure to loud noises are the following:

• Interference with normal communication between individuals.

• Physiological effects, such as increased stress, increased cardiovascular and respiratory responses, and disruptions of the gastrointestinal system.

• Sleep problems, such as the inability to fall or stay asleep, arousal during sleep, and interrupted sleep patterns.

• Disruption of normal personal performance, such as the inability to focus or concentrate on a task, an increase in the number of errors produced during exposure to loud noises, and an increase in injury rates among those exposed to loud noises.

• Interference with normal interpersonal behavior, such as an increase in antisocial behavior and decrease in helping behaviors towards others.

• Disruption of community values, such as an interference with the normal interpersonal behaviors that make up a healthy and well-functioning community of individuals.

Demographics

One of the most extensive and complete studies of the health burden caused by noise pollution was a report published in 2011 by the **World Health Organization (WHO)** and the European Union (EU). The report summarized research that attempted to quantify the health effects caused by traffic noise in member states of the EU. The results were expressed in terms of the disability-adjusted life-years (DALYs) characteristic of various health effects resulting from noise pollution. DALYs are defined as the sum of the potential years of life lost due to premature death and the equivalent years of healthy life lost by virtue of being in states of poor health or disability, in this case because of exposure to loud sounds. Researchers found that noise pollution was responsible annually for 61,000 years lost as a result of ischemic **heart disease**, 45,000 years because of cognitive impairment of children, 903,000 years for sleep disturbance, 22,000 years for tinnitus, and 654,000 years for annoyance (which corresponds to a state that might be described as "psychological dissatisfaction." that causes severe **stress**). As a consequence, the report concluded, "at least one million healthy life years are lost every year from traffic-related noise in the western part of Europe."

KEY TERMS

Ambient conditions—Conditions in the surrounding environment.

Amplitude—A measure of the amount of energy carried by a wave.

Decibel—A logarithmic unit of measure comparing the intensity of two sounds (or other forms of energy) with each other.

Disability-adjusted life-years (DALYs)—A term used to describe the health effects of some environmental factor, defined as the sum of the potential years of life lost due to premature death and the equivalent years of healthy life lost by virtue of being in states of poor health or disability.

Frequency—The number of wave fronts that pass a given point in space in some specified period of time, such as one second.

Wavelength—The distance between two adjacent peaks or troughs of a wave.

White noise—Sound that contains a mixture of many frequencies and amplitudes, often used to mask competing unpleasant or distracting noises.

Hearing loss resulting from exposure to noise pollution is a particular problem of younger people, who often prefer to listen to loud music, often in enclosed spaces. Current research suggests that the rate of hearing loss among adolescents in the United States is about 2.5 times that of older people and that, as a result, by the year 2050, there may be as many as 50 million people in the United States with measurable hearing deficiencies. Hearing loss is also a special problem for workers in a variety of industries with high levels of ambient noise, such as steel mills. The U.S. Bureau of Labor Statistics (BLS) has estimated that noisy work conditions are responsible for about 21,000 new cases of hearing loss each year as a result of such conditions, with a total of more than 125,000 workers having become disabled over the past decade for such reasons.

Prevention

A number of options are available for individuals who wish to reduce their exposure to excessive noise. Some devices and procedures are suitable for personal use under normal everyday conditions, while others are more suitable for workplaces where noise can be much higher than average. Others can be used under either conditions. These noise-protection systems include:

- Soundproofing: Homes, offices, factories, and other structures can be soundproofed so as to reduce the amount of noise detected within the structure. Some types of soundproofing include sound-absorbing materials for the construction of walls, floors, and ceilings; sound curtains; and shrubs, trees, and other plantings to reduce exterior noise.

- Hearing protection devices: Devices that fit into or over the ears can help reduce ambient sound. Ear plugs and ear muffs are perhaps the most common examples of such devices.

- Noise cancellation and isolation devices: Some types of earphones and headphones are available that use electronic systems to cancel out or reduce ambient sounds, thus reducing the amount of noise that actually reaches a person's brain.

- White noise: White noise is a type of sound generated for the purpose of competing with and overcoming undesirable ambient sounds. White noise can take the form of gentle wave action, winds blowing through the trees, falling rain, or other sounds that are pleasant to listen to. They distract a person from more offensive and annoying sounds, such as car traffic and industrial sounds.

- Quieter products: Manufacturers have made great strides in making products—such as refrigerators, washing machines, dryers, and dishwashers—that operate with less noise production. Installing them in a house reduces the ambient noise level in the house. Manufacturers of industrial machinery have used similar technology to produce large-scale machines that are also better insulated and make less noise.

Efforts and solutions

Another approach to reducing noise pollution is the adoption of legislation and regulations that limit the amount of noise permitted in a neighborhood, city, or other locale. These laws and regulations vary widely from governmental unit to governmental unit. The first comprehensive urban noise control program was instituted in Portland, Oregon, in 1975, with support from the U.S. Enviromental Protection Agency (**EPA**). That law now covers a wide range of noise sources, such as motor vehicles, home equipment and power tools, leaf blowers, watercraft, motor racing events, construction projects, and parking lot sweepers. Legislation establishes certain permissable noise levels for each category and for special areas, such as residential, commercial, industrial, and open space locations. As an example, the maximum permitted noise level for a residential area in Portland between 7 a.m. and 10 p.m. is 55 db. For evening hours, this restriction is reduced by 5 db, as are all other noise regulations in the city.

QUESTIONS TO ASK YOUR DOCTOR

- Is there a way you can determine whether my children's hearing has been affected by their listening to loud music?

- My children claim that they can learn better while doing their homework if they also have loud music playing. Is that claim true?

- We live only a block from a very noisy freeway. What steps can we take to reduce the effect of freeway noise on our lives?

- Is there a way to measure actual physical damage to a person's ears as a consequence of noise pollution?

- Is there any reason our family should be concerned about the effects of loud noises in our neighborhood on our circulatory system or other body systems?

- Are there any local or state laws dealing with the amount of noise permitted in our neighborhood?

- How can I find out more about noise regulation in our community?

The federal government has a number of laws on the books dealing with noise pollution, as provided for primarily in the Clean Air Act of 1970 (Title IV), the Noise Control Act of 1972, and the Quiet Communities Act of 1978. In 1982, however, the federal government decided that noise pollution was a problem better handled by the state, and it closed the EPA Office of Noise Abatement and Control and has discontinued funding for federal noise pollution projects.

Resources

BOOKS

Kumar, Arvind. *Noise Pollution and Its Control*. New Delhi: Shree Publishers & Distributors, 2011.

Parpworth, Neil. *Noise Control: The Law and Its Enforcement*. London: Sweet & Maxwell, 2013.

Pinch, T.J., and Karen Bijsterveld. *The Oxford Handbook of Sound Studies*. New York: Oxford University Press, 2012.

Stewart, John, et al. *Why Noise Matters: A Worldwide Perspective on the Problems, Policies and Solutions*. Abingdon, Oxon; New York: Earthscan, 2011.

PERIODICALS

Gan, Wen Qi, et al. "Association of Long-term Exposure to Community Noise and Traffic-related Air Pollution With Coronary Heart Disease Mortality." *American Journal of Epidemiology* 175, 9. (2012): 898–906.

Hsu, T., et al. "Noise Pollution in Hospitals: Impact on Patients." *Journal of Clinical Outcomes Management* 19, 7. (2012): 301–9.

Hume, K.I. "Noise Pollution: A Ubiquitous Unrecognized Disruptor of Sleep?" *Sleep* 34, 1. (2011): 7–8.

Van Kempen, Elise, et al. "Neurobehavioral Effects of Exposure to Traffic-related Air Pollution and Transportation Noise in Primary Schoolchildren." *Environmental Research* 115, 5. (2012): 18–25.

WEBSITES

Goines, Lisa, and Louis Hagler. "Noise Pollution: A Modern Plague." http://www.nonoise.org/library/smj/smj.htm. Accessed on November 2, 2012.

"Noise!." http://www.noisehelp.com/. Accessed on November 2, 2012.

"Noise Pollution Clearing House." http://www.nonoise.org/. Accessed on November 2, 2012.

Weiss, Rick. "Noise Pollution Takes Toll on Health and Happiness."http://www.washingtonpost.com/wp-dyn/content/article/2007/06/04/AR2007060401430.html. Accessed on November 2, 2012.

ORGANIZATIONS

The Noise Pollution Clearinghouse, P.O. Box 1137, Montpelier, VT USA 05601–1137, (888) 200–8332, http://www.nonoise.org/cgi-bin/info-request.cgi, http://www.nonoise.org/.

David E. Newton, Ed.D.

Noroviruses

Definition

Noroviruses are a group of related, single-stranded RNA (ribonucleic acid) viruses that cause infection resulting in acute gastroenteritis in humans. Gastroenteritis, also commonly called stomach flu, involves an inflammation of the gastrointestinal tract, which results in diarrhea, abdominal **pain**, and vomiting. The infection caused by noroviruses is very highly contagious, being commonly spread through **water** or food that has been contaminated with fecal matter; or through contact with an infected person. Norovirus infections occur frequently in closed, and often times crowded, environments where the viruses can quickly spread. Such places include hospitals and medical facilities, schools, nursing/retirement homes and day-care facilities, and cruise ships.

Demographics

Anyone can become infected with a norovirus. During norovirus outbreaks there are high rates of infection among people of all ages. There are a large number of genetically distinct strains of noroviruses. Immunity appears to be specific for the norovirus strain and lasts for only a few months. Therefore, norovirus infection can recur throughout a person's lifetime. Because of genetic (inherited) differences among humans, some people appear to be more susceptible to norovirus infection and may suffer more severe illness. People with type O blood are at the highest risk for severe infection.

Description

Norovirus infection is caused by a variety of viruses. All such viruses cause acute gastroenteritis, an inflammation of the stomach and intestines. The illness is highly contagious, and usually requires professional medical care to treat the most serious of the symptoms, which often times include dehydration, bloody stool, abdominal pain, and vomiting. Noroviruses are difficult to eliminate in the environment because they can withstand very high and low temperatures, along with being able to resist most disinfectants.

Noroviral infection

Noroviruses are a major cause of viral gastroenteritis—an inflammation of the linings of the stomach and small and large intestines that causes vomiting and diarrhea. Viruses are responsible for 30 to 40% of all cases of infectious diarrhea, and viral gastroenteritis is the second most common illness in the United States, exceeded only by the **common cold**.

Infected individuals are contagious from the first onset of symptoms until at least three days after full recovery. Some people may remain contagious for as long as two weeks after recovery.

Gastroenteritis

Gastroenteritis often is referred to as the stomach flu even though the flu is a respiratory illness caused by an **influenza** virus. Other common names for viral gastroenteritis include:

• food poisoning

• winter-vomiting disease

• non-bacterial gastroenteritis

• calicivirus infection

The U.S. **Centers for Disease Control and Prevention (CDC)** estimate, in 2012, that noroviruses are responsible for some 20 million cases of acute gastroenteritis in the United States every year. Epidemiologists estimate that about 50,000 Americans are

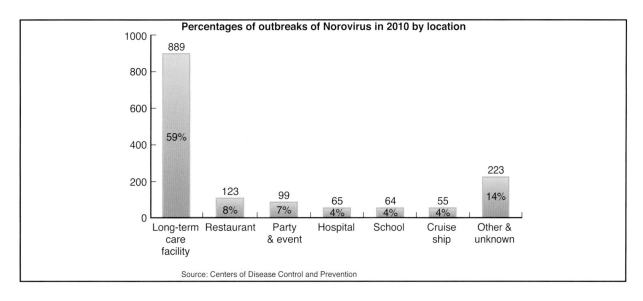

Percentages of outbreaks of Norovirus in 2010 by location

Source: Centers of Disease Control and Prevention

(Illustration by Electronic Illustrators Group. © 2013 Cengage Learning)

hospitalized annually and about 400 people die each year because of norovirus infection. However, the **CDC** points out that many cases of acute gastroenteritis go unreported. Consequently, the U.S. health organization suggests that up to 300,000 hospitalizations occur annually and about 5,000 deaths occur each year, all due to noroviruses. In developing countries, noroviruses are a major cause of human illness. The CDC estimate that about 900,000 visits to clinics and other medical facilities by children in developed countries of the world result in about 64,000 hospitalizations. Even worse, about 200,000 children under the age of five years die from noroviruses each year in developing countries of the world.

Gastroenteritis caused by infection with a norovirus is rarely a serious illness. Typically an infected person suddenly feels very ill and may vomit many times in a single day. The symptoms, although quite unpleasant, usually last only 24 to 60 hours.

Transmission

Noroviruses are ubiquitous in the environment. They are highly contagious and are considered to be among the most infectious of viruses. The reasons for this include:

• Only a small number of viral particles—as few as 10—are required for infection.

• Although noroviruses cannot reproduce outside of their human hosts, they can remain viable for weeks or even months on objects and surfaces.

• Human immunity to norovirus is short-lived and strain-specific.

Noroviruses are transmitted among people by a fecal-oral route, either by ingestion of food or water contaminated with feces or by contact with the vomit or feces of an infected person. Norovirus infection can occur by:

• consuming contaminated food or liquids

• hand contact with contaminated objects or surfaces, followed by hand contact with the mouth

• contact with an infected person, including caring for the sick person or sharing food or utensils

• aerosolized vomit that is swallowed or that contaminates surfaces

Environmental contamination or contact with infected clothing or linen also may be a source of transmission. Although evidence is not available that norovirus infection can occur via the respiratory system, the sudden and violent vomiting of noroviral gastroenteritis can lead to contamination of the surroundings and of public areas. Particles laden with virus can be suspended in the air and swallowed.

FOODBORNE TRANSMISSION. Noroviruses account for at least 50% of food-related outbreaks of gastroenteritis. A European study, published in 2010, showed that 21% of all norovirus outbreaks are caused by foodborne transmission. In addition, 25% of the outbreaks were initially reported to be "food handler-associated." This was later found to be caused from contamination of the food source. In addition, restaurant or catered foods are common sources of norovirus transmission, with subsequent infection of household members. The majority of norovirus outbreaks occur via contamination by a food handler immediately before the food is consumed.

Foods that frequently are associated with norovirus outbreaks include:

• foods that are eaten without further cooking, including sandwiches, salads, and bakery products

• liquids such as salad dressing or cake icing in which the virus becomes evenly distributed

• food that is contaminated at its source, including oysters and clams from contaminated waters and raspberries irrigated with sewage-contaminated water

• food that becomes contaminated before distribution, including salads and frozen fruit

Shellfish, including oysters and clams, concentrate norovirus from contaminated water in their tissues. Steaming shellfish may not completely inactivate the virus.

WATERBORNE TRANSMISSION. There is widespread norovirus contamination of rivers and seas, often with more than one strain of the virus. Waterborne outbreaks of norovirus have been associated with:

• sewage-contaminated wells

• contaminated municipal water systems

• stream and lake water

• swimming pools and spas

• commercial ice

Outbreaks

Norovirus infection can spread rapidly through day-care centers, schools, prisons, hospitals, nursing homes, camps, and other confined spaces. Norovirus is responsible for about 40% of group- or institution-related outbreaks of diarrhea. Outbreaks usually peak during the winter months.

In 2008, it was reported that outbreaks of the norovirus occurred on several university campuses in California, Michigan, and Wisconsin. The CDC, along with state and local **health departments**, found that approximately 1,000 cases of illness resulted from these outbreaks, including 10 hospitalizations. In addition, one college campus was closed temporarily due to an outbreak. In February 2012, an outbreak of norovirus at a basketball tournament in Kentucky was responsible for 242 cases of acute gastroenteritis, although no source for the disease was ever identified.

Cruise ships have become notorious for norovirus outbreaks among passengers and staff, and though they do happen, the media sensationalizes them to the point that the public thinks they happen more frequently than they really do. Cruise ships and naval vessels are at increased risk for contamination when docking in regions that lack adequate **sanitation** and where contaminated

food or water may be brought onboard. Close living quarters and the arrival of new, susceptible passengers every one to two weeks exacerbate outbreaks on cruise ships. Norovirus outbreaks have been reported to continue through more than 12 successive cruises on a single ship.

Noroviruses are relatively rare on cruise ships but they do happen. In 2006, the CDC reported that 34 cases of norovirus were reported, while 27 were reported in 2007, 15 in 2008, and 13 in 2009—all from cruises originating from U.S. ports. In 2010, for instance, the Celebrity Cruises company reported that 15% of its passengers come down with norovirus-like symptoms on its cruise ship that departed from Charleston, South Carolina, on February 15, 2010. A year before the incident, a paper published in the medical journal *Clinical Infectious Diseases* found that a large number of norovirus outbreaks on cruise ships were the result of dirty public restroom facilities. However, in 2010, the CDC reported that the trend was down for contracting a norovirus on a cruise ship sailing from a U.S. port. In fact, the incidence of noroviruses on a cruise ship was at a decade-long low as of January 2010. The International Council of Cruise Lines reported that less than 1% of passengers become infected with norovirus each year. As reported by the CDC the outbreaks on cruise ships during the 2000s were on the decline. However, it is too early in the 2010s to tell if the trend will continue.

Generally, outbreaks of norovirus appear on the increase. Near the end of the 2000s, the CDC reported that norovirus outbreaks were increasing in many closed, crowded facilities across the country.

Risk factors

Humans are at increased risk from contracting noroviruses if they:

• travel frequently on cruise ships or stay at lodging establishments where many people are living in close surroundings

• live with children that attend school or day care

• have a weakened immune system

• live in nursing homes, retirement centers, or other such facilities

Causes and symptoms

Norovirus strains

Noroviruses lack outer envelopes and their genetic material is carried as single-stranded RNA rather than DNA (deoxyribonucleic acid). Although noroviruses are not new, the extent of norovirus infection was not recognized until the 1990s. This has led to increased research on noroviruses and more monitoring of outbreaks.

Until 2004 noroviruses were commonly referred to as:

• Norwalk virus

• Norwalk-like viruses (NLVs)

• caliciviruses

• small, round-structured viruses (SRSVs).

Noroviruses are named after the original strain—the Norwalk virus—that caused an outbreak of gastroenteritis in a Norwalk, Ohio, school in 1968. The virus was identified in 1972. Since then many related viruses have been identified. In 2004, these viruses were grouped together in the genus *Norovirus* within the Caliciviridae family of viruses. Eight to 10 distinct genogroups of norovirus have been found in various parts of the world. There are five common genogroups and, of those, three (GI, GII, and GIV) affect humans. Each of these groups can be further differentiated into at least 20 genetic clusters. Evidence suggests that noroviruses in different genetic clusters can recombine to form new, genetically distinct noroviruses. As of 2012, GII strains, especially GII4, are the most prevalent, and have caused the most norovirus outbreaks since 2002. However the most common method of identifying noroviruses—the reverse transcription-polymerase chain reaction (RT-PCR)—may not always identify GII genetic clusters correctly.

The increased number of norovirus outbreaks in European countries in the early 2000s—occurring in the spring and summer rather than in winter—were found to be associated with the emergence of a new variant of the GII4 strain. Increased international outbreaks in 2003 and 2004 also were caused by a GII4-related norovirus that was found to mutate rapidly. Mutations in the viral capsid—the virus' outer protective layer—were used to determine the predominant routes of norovirus transmission.

Then, in the first quarter of 2010, 334 cases of norovirus were reported at 65 different locations within the United Kingdom, Norway, France, Sweden, and Denmark. All of the cases were associated with the eating of raw oysters. The International Society of Infectious Diseases reports that the Rapid Alert System for Food and Feed (RASFF) database contained 19 reports of norovirus in oysters between March 2006 and March 2010—all within the European Union.

Symptoms

Symptoms of norovirus infection usually appear within 24–48 hours after exposure, with a median incubation period during outbreaks of 33–36 hours. However symptoms can occur as early as 12 hours or less after exposure.

Typical symptoms of norovirus infection are:

• nausea

• vomiting

• fever

• malaise (general feeling of sickness)

• watery or loose diarrhea without blood

• abdominal cramping and pain

• bloody stool

• dehydration

• weight loss

Among children, vomiting is the predominant symptom, whereas diarrhea is more common in adults. Vomiting can be frequent and violent and may occur without warning.

Additional symptoms of norovirus infection may include:

• low-grade fever

• chills

• headache

• muscle aches

• fatigue

Dehydration is the major risk from gastroenteritis caused by norovirus, particularly among infants, young children, the elderly, and those with underlying health conditions. Symptoms of dehydration include:

• dry mouth

• increased or excessive thirst

• low urine output

• nausea

• dizziness or faintness

• sunken eyes

• sunken fontanelle—the soft spot on an infant's head

• confusion

As many as 30–50% of norovirus infections do not produce symptoms. It is not known whether individuals with asymptomatic infections can transmit the virus.

Diagnosis

Identifying noroviruses

Viral gastroenteritis usually is diagnosed on the basis of the symptoms. Many types of viruses cause gastroenteritis. Rotoviruses are a leading cause of gastroenteritis in children who then transmit the virus to adults. In addition to noroviruses, viral gastroenteritis in humans can be caused by another genus of viruses within the Caliciviridae family. Formerly known as the Sapporo-like virus, or classic or typical calicivirus, these now are

Norovirus

grouped in the genus *Sapovirus*. Other genera in the Caliciviridae family are not pathogenic in humans. Some bacteria and **parasites** also cause illnesses that are similar to norovirus infection.

The cloning and sequencing of noroviruses in the early 1990s made it easier to identify norovirus outbreaks. RT-PCR is the most commonly used method for identifying norovirus. With this technique the virus' RNA is used as the template for transcribing the corresponding DNA using the enzyme reverse transcriptase. The DNA is amplified into many copies using the polymerase chain reaction. Many state public health laboratories use this method to detect norovirus in vomit and stools. The best identification usually comes from stool samples taken within 48–72 hours after the onset of symptoms; however norovirus can be detected in stool samples taken five days after the onset of symptoms and sometimes even in samples taken up to two weeks after recovery.

Norovirus from fecal samples can be visualized using electron microscopy. With immune electron microscopy (IEM), antibodies against norovirus are collected from blood serum and used to trap and visualize the virus from fecal samples. However these methods require high concentrations of norovirus in the stool, as well as a fourfold increase in norovirus-specific antibodies in blood samples taken during the acute or recovery phases of gastroenteritis.

Enzyme-linked immunosorbent assays may be used to detect noroviruses in fecal samples. In these assays noroviral-specific antibodies bound to the virus are detected by the reaction of an enzyme that is attached to the antibody. Nucleic acid probes that hybridize with noroviral RNA also can be used for virus detection in feces.

Research continues on commercial devices for detecting norovirsuses. For example, scientists at the Department of Infectious Diseases, Osaka Prefectural Institute of Public Health (Osaka, Japan) are developing modified reagent kits for norovirus genogroups I and II. They reported their advancement in the *Journal of Medical Virology* (December 2009).

Investigating outbreaks

Epidemiological studies often involve sequencing the norovirus RNA. This can help to determine whether outbreaks in different geographical locations are connected to each other and can help trace the source of the norovirus to contaminated food or water. CaliciNet is a database that stores the RNA sequences of all norovirus strains that cause gastroenteritis in the United States.

Criteria that are sometimes used to determine whether an outbreak of gastroenteritis is caused by a norovirus include:

- a mean incubation period of 24–48 hours
- a mean duration time for illness of 12–60 hours
- vomiting in more than 50% of patients
- failure to find a bacterial cause for the illness

During investigations of norovirus outbreaks, food handlers may be asked to provide a stool sample and possibly a blood sample. Food rarely is tested for norovirus since each type of food requires a specific assay. However, tests are used to detect the virus in shellfish. When large amounts—1–25 gallons (5–100 liters)—of water are processed through specially designed filters, the norovirus can be concentrated and assayed by RT-PCR.

Treatment

Gastroenteritis caused by noroviruses usually resolves itself without treatment within a very few days. As of 2012, medications or vaccines are not available that are effective against the norovirus. Viruses are not affected by **antibiotics** and antidiarrheal medications may prolong the infection.

Norovirus infections should be treated by:

- drinking plenty of fluids, such as water and juice, to prevent dehydration caused by vomiting and diarrhea
- intravenous fluids if severe nausea prevents drinking, particularly in small children
- drinking oral rehydration fluids (ORFs) to prevent dehydration and to replace electrolytes (salt and minerals) and glucose
- avoiding alcohol and caffeine which can increase urination

Commercially available ORFs include Naturalyte, Pedialyte, Infalyte, and Rehydralyte.

Juice, soda, and water do not replace lost electrolytes; nor do sports drinks replace nutrients and minerals lost through vomiting and diarrhea. In fact, drinks containing sugar may make diarrhea worse. Those taking diuretics should ask their healthcare provider whether to stop taking the medication during acute diarrhea.

Since the risk of dehydration is higher for infants and young children, the number of wet diapers per day should be closely monitored. Severely dehydrated children may receive rapid intravenous rehydration in a hospital or emergency-room setting.

A health care provider should be consulted if:

- symptoms of dehydration appear
- diarrhea persists for longer than a few days
- there is blood in the stool

Alternative treatment

An infusion of meadowsweet (*Filipendula ulmaria*) may reduce nausea. Once the symptoms are reduced, slippery elm (*Ulmus fulva*) may calm the digestive system. Castor oil packs placed on the abdomen can reduce inflammation and discomfort.

Homeopathic remedies for gastroenteritis include *Arsenicum album*, ipecac, and *Nux vomica*. Chinese patent herbal remedies include Po Chai and Pill Curing.

During recovery from viral gastroenteritis, live cultures of *Lactobacillus acidophilus*, found in live-culture yogurt or as powder or capsules, may be useful for restoring the native flora of the digestive tract. Scientific evidence for the safety and efficacy of most herbal, Chinese, alternative and other complementary medicines is often lacking, so they should be used only with caution.

Public health response

Public health responses to norovirus outbreaks pose distinctly difficult problems for public health agencies. Since the virus can not be cultured in the laboratory, a great deal of basic information is not readily available about the virus or the diseases it causes. Thus far, most guidelines for public health responses to outbreaks of gastroenteritis caused by noroviruses have been developed based on experiences in hospitals, cruise ships, and adult care facilities. The first step in the public health response to a suspected norovirus outbreak consists of data collection on reported cases, which includes information such as the number of individuals affected, the time at which the outbreak occurred, the environmental conditions involved, especially the type of food that may have been involved, and the results of any laboratory tests that may have been conducted. These items of information allow a public health agency to develop a plan of action which focuses on identifying and eliminating the suspected cause of the epidemic (such as the type of food involved) and initiate clean-up programs to eliminate that causative agent. Efforts to provide palliative care for those affected by the epidemic are also initiated. On a long term basis, information obtained about any specific outbreak of norovirus infection can be used to bolster and improve existing programs of education for the general public as well as for professionals in the field or, if such programs do not exist, to plan, develop, and implement such programs.

Prognosis

Norovirus infection is usually followed by complete recovery. Any long-term health effects are not known. Infected persons do not become long-term carriers of the

virus. However, in some cases dehydration can become a very serious possible consequence of noroviral infection and can be fatal, particularly among young children, older people, and anyone with debilitating medical conditions or impaired immune systems.

Prevention

Noroviruses are difficult to destroy. They can survive freezing as well as temperatures as high as 140°F (60°C). Noroviruses can survive chlorine levels as high as 10 parts per million (ppm), far higher than the levels present in most public water systems. A 2004 study from the Netherlands found that inactivation of norovirus with 70% ethanol was inefficient and that **sodium** hypochlorite solutions were effective only at concentrations above 300 ppm.

The best **prevention** against noroviral infection is frequent, thorough hand washing with soap and water. All soaped hand surfaces should be rubbed vigorously for at least 10 seconds. The hands should be thoroughly rinsed under a stream of water. In particular hands always should be washed before handling food and after using the toilet or changing diapers.

Other important measures for preventing norovirus infection include:

• proper handling of cold foods

• careful washing of fruits and vegetables

- steaming oysters before eating, although even this may be insufficient for destroying norovirus

- taking particular care when handing the diapers of children with diarrhea

- properly disposing of sewage and diapers

- excluding sick infants and children from food preparation areas

To prevent further transmission of norovirus:

- All surfaces exposed to vomit or otherwise contaminated should be immediately cleaned and disinfected with a solution of between 5 to 10% bleach, followed by rinsing.

- Contaminated clothing and linens should be removed immediately and washed with hot water and detergent on the maximum machine cycle and with a minimum of handling, followed by machine drying.

- Vomit and feces should be discarded or flushed immediately and the toilet area should be kept clean.

- Exposed or contaminated food should be discarded.

- Masks may be worn while cleaning areas that have been badly contaminated with vomit or feces, such as in hospitals or nursing homes.

- Stay home and do not go to work or school in order to prevent further passing on of the virus.

Scientific studies have found that detergent-based cleaning with a cloth consistently fails to eliminate norovirus contamination. With fecal contamination, detergent-based cleaning, followed by cleaning with a combination hypochlorite/detergent formula containing 5,000 ppm of available chlorine significantly reduced contamination. However, norovirus still could be detected on as much as 28% of the surfaces. When this procedure failed to eliminate contamination, the virus was transmitted to the cleaner's hands. Contaminated fingers consistently transferred norovirus to up to seven different surfaces including doorknobs and telephones. However the contamination was diluted during secondary transmission and treatment with the combined bleach/detergent eliminated the virus without prior cleaning.

In situations where there is a periodic renewal of susceptible people, such as on cruise ships and at camps, the facility may have to be closed until cleaning is complete. Although many state and local health departments require that food handlers with gastroenteritis not return to work until two to three days following recovery, this may not be an adequate length of time to prevent noroviral transmission.

The prevention of norovirus outbreaks include reducing contamination of water supplies with human waste and using high-level chlorination—at least 10 ppm

QUESTIONS TO ASK YOUR DOCTOR

- If we are planning to take a cruise, are there steps we can follow to reduce our risk of being infected with a norovirus?

- What can we do to reduce the risk of our children's being infected by a norovirus in the school environment?

- What types of palliative care can we provide to elderly parents in a nursing home who have contracted a noroviral infection?

for more than 30 minutes. Surveillance of shorelines for potential sources of fecal contamination and for boats that are dumping human waste may help prevent shellfish-associated norovirus outbreaks.

In 2004, researchers at Washington University (St. Louis, Missouri) became the first to grow a norovirus in a laboratory setting. They grew a mouse norovirus, with the goal of studying the virus and developing a vaccine against it. Research is ongoing in the early 2010s. New surveillance systems also are being developed to detect norovirus outbreaks at an early stage.

Resources

BOOKS

Hall, Aron J. *Updated Norovirus Outbreak Management and Disease Prevention Guidelines.* Atlanta, GA: Centers for Disease Control and Prevention, 2011.

Vildevall, Malin. *The Norovirus Puzzle: Characterization of Human and Bovine Norovirus Susceptibility Patterns.* Linköping: Linköping University, Faculty of Health Sciences, 2011.

PERIODICALS

Verhoef, L., et al. "Use of Norovirus Genotype Profiles to Differentiate Origins of Foodborne Outbreaks." Emerging Infectious Diseases 16 4 (2010): 610-24.

OTHER

Manning, Anita. *Nasty, Contagious Norovirus Is 'Everywhere' Now.* USA Today. http://www.usatoday.com/news/health/story/health/story/2012-02-22/Nasty-contagious-norovirus-is-everywhere-now/53211908/1 (accessed August 23, 2012).

Norovirus. Centers for Disease Control and Prevention. http://www.cdc.gov/norovirus/ (accessed August 23, 2012).

Norovirus Infection. Mayo Clinic. http://www.mayoclinic.com/health/norovirus/DS00942 (accessed August 23, 2012).

Purdy, Michael C. *Scientists Grow Norovirus in Lab.* http://news.wustl.edu/news/Pages/4418.aspx (accessed August 23, 2012).

Norovirus: Symptoms and Treatment. WebMD. http://children .webmd.com/norovirus-symptoms-and-treatment (accessed August 23, 2012).

ORGANIZATIONS

Centers for Disease Control and Prevention, 1600 Clifton Rd., NE, Atlanta, GA 30333, (800) CDC-INFO (800 232-4636) or (404) 639-3534, cdcinfo@cdc.gov, www.cdc.gov.

National Health Information Center, Office of Disease Prevention and Health Promotion, U.S. Department of Health and Human Services, P. O. Box 1133, Washington, D.C., 20013-1133, (847) 434-4000, http://www.health .gov/nhic/.

Margaret Alic, Ph.D.

Nutrition

Definition

Nutrition is the sum of all the processes by which food enters and is utilized by the body. Nutrients include protein, carbohydrates, fats, **vitamins**, minerals, and water. Fiber in foods is not a nutrient in the strict sense but helps to prevent disease and control weight.

Description

The human body absorbs many different nutrients from food. A good nutrition plan includes a variety of foods from the different food groups, with adequate amounts of the nutrients in each group. Keys to good nutrition include:

- fruits, vegetables, and whole grains

- protein, fiber, calcium, iron, magnesium, potassium, and vitamins A, C, and E

- low-fat dairy products, lean meats, poultry, fish, and beans

- no more than 20–35% of total calories from fat, mostly from polyunsaturated and monounsaturated fats

- plenty of water

- more fluids and carbohydrates from fruits and whole grains for athletes and other physically active individuals

- additional vitamin D from fortified foods and/or supplements for older adults, those with darker skin, and people with insufficient exposure to sunlight

- limited salt (less than about one teaspoon daily for most people), added sugar, saturated fat, trans fat, cholesterol, and alcohol (no more than one drink per day for women and two for men)

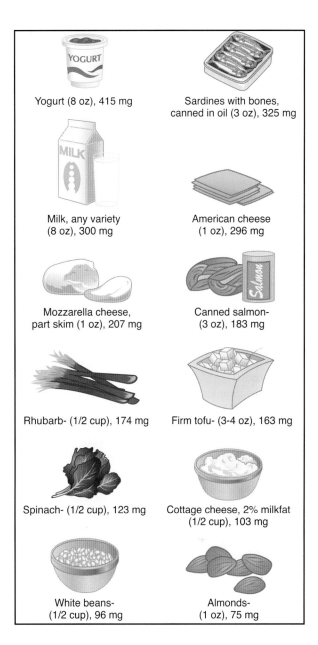

Yogurt (8 oz), 415 mg

Sardines with bones, canned in oil (3 oz), 325 mg

Milk, any variety (8 oz), 300 mg

American cheese (1 oz), 296 mg

Mozzarella cheese, part skim (1 oz), 207 mg

Canned salmon- (3 oz), 183 mg

Rhubarb- (1/2 cup), 174 mg

Firm tofu- (3-4 oz), 163 mg

Spinach- (1/2 cup), 123 mg

Cottage cheese, 2% milkfat (1/2 cup), 103 mg

White beans- (1/2 cup), 96 mg

Almonds- (1 oz), 75 mg

Food sources for calcium. *(Illustration by Electronic Illustrators Group. © 2013 Cengage Learning)*

Vitamins are required for regulating metabolism and maintaining normal growth and functioning. Minerals are vital for building tissue, muscles, and bones, and for many life-supporting systems, including hormones, oxygen transport, and enzyme function. Although foods are the preferred source of these nutrients, they can also be obtained from nutritional supplements.

Nutritional supplements

Nutritional supplements include vitamins, minerals, herbs, meal supplements, sports nutrition products, natural food supplements, and other related products that

Tips to avoid drug interactions

- Carefully read all drug and supplement labels.
- Research interaction warnings before taking any new drugs or supplements.
- Keep all medications in their original containers so they can be easily identified.
- Ask your doctor what to avoid when starting a new medication (including foods and drinks, supplements, and other drugs).
- Check with your doctor or pharmacist before taking a dietary supplement or an OTC drug.
- Use one pharmacy.
- Keep a record of all the prescription drugs, OTC drugs, and dietary supplements (including herbs) that you take and share it with your doctor and other healthcare professionals.

SOURCE: U.S. Food and Drug Administration.

Dietary supplements, some foods, and herbs can interact with medication. *(Table by PreMediaGlobal. © 2013 Cengage Learning)*

are used to boost the nutritional content of the diet. Considering average dietary needs and the prevalence of certain health conditions, some basic guidelines may provide the foundation for the effective use of nutritional supplements. First, a high quality, broad-spectrum multivitamin and mineral supplement, taken once per day, may be recommended for some people. This should contain the B-complex vitamins B_6, B_{12}, and folic acid, which may help prevent **heart disease**, and the minerals zinc and copper, which aid the immune system.

In addition to a multivitamin, antioxidants can be added to a supplementation regimen. These include vitamin A (or beta-carotene), vitamin C, and vitamin E, and the mineral selenium. Antioxidants are popularly believed have several positive effects on the body, such as slowing the **aging** process, reducing the risks of **cancer** and heart disease, and reducing the risks of illness and infection by supporting the immune system. Coenzyme Q_{10} is another antioxidant in wide usage, as studies have shown it may improve the health of the heart and reduce the effects of heart disease. Essential fatty acids, particularly omega-3, are also recommended as they are involved in many important processes in the body, including brain function. Calcium supplementation is recommended for the elderly and for women to support bone strength. Calcium supplements that are balanced with magnesium have a less constipating effect and are better absorbed.

After basic nutritional requirements are supported, supplements may be used to target specific needs and health conditions. For instance, athletes, men, women, children, the elderly, and vegetarians have differing needs for nutrients, and an informed use of supplements would take these differences into account. People suffering from health conditions and diseases may use specific supplements to target their condition and to support the body's healing capacity by providing optimal amounts of nutrients.

MyPlate

In June 2011 the U.S. Department of Agriculture (USDA) replaced its longstanding food pyramid nutrition guides and diagrams with MyPlate, a food guide icon that displays a plate divided into four segments of slightly unequal size, with a circle representing dairy products at the upper right. The four differently colored segments on the plate represent the USDA's recommendations for a healthful diet: approximately 30 percent grains, 30 percent vegetables, 20 percent fruits, and 20 percent protein foods. The MyPlate icon has been praised for its relative simplicity compared to the older food pyramid diagrams, and for its emphasis on a high intake of fruits and vegetables.

The MyPlate icon is supplemented with additional recommendations on the ChooseMyPlate website, such as:

- Make half the plate fruits and vegetables.
- Use low-fat or fat-free milk rather than whole milk.
- Choose whole grains for at least half of the day's grain products.
- Vary the protein choices; have seafood twice a week.
- Lower calorie intake by cutting back on solid fats or drinks and desserts with added sugar.
- Enjoy food but eat less of it.
- Exercise regularly: 60 minutes a day for children and teens, 2.5 hours a week for adults. Additional information about food choices, weight management, and physical exercise is available on the ChooseMyPlate website.

2010 Dietary Guidelines for Americans

In January 2011 the USDA's Center for Nutrition Policy and Promotion (CNPP) released the seventh edition of the government's official nutrition guide, titled *Dietary Guidelines for Americans, 2010*. The updated guidelines continue to incorporate the 2006 DASH (Dietary Approaches to Stop Hypertension) Eating Plan developed by the U.S. National Heart, Lung, and Blood Institute. The 2010 guidelines are divided into five chapters following the introduction: balancing calories to manage weight; foods and food components to reduce; foods and nutrients to increase; building healthy eating patterns; and helping Americans make healthy choices. One significant difference between the 2010 guidelines and the previous 2005 edition is the growing recognition of the influence of cultural and environmental factors on food choices and

Calorie[1] requirements by age, gender, and activity level[2]

Age (years)	Male, sedentary	Male, moderately active	Male, active	Female, sedentary	Female, moderately active	Female, active
18	2,400	2,800	3,200	1,800	2,000	2,400
19–20	2,600	2,800	3,000	2,000	2,200	2,400
21–25	2,400	2,800	3,000	2,000	2,200	2,400
26–30	2,400	2,600	3,000	1,800	2,000	2,400
31–35	2,400	2,600	3,000	1,800	2,000	2,200
36–40	2,400	2,600	2,800	1,800	2,000	2,200
41–45	2,200	2,600	2,800	1,800	2,000	2,200
46–50	2,200	2,400	2,800	1,800	2,000	2,200
51–55	2,200	2,400	2,800	1,600	1,800	2,200
56–60	2,200	2,400	2,600	1,600	1,800	2,200
61–65	2,000	2,400	2,600	1,600	1,800	2,000
66–70	2,000	2,200	2,600	1,600	1,800	2,000
71–75	2,000	2,200	2,600	1,600	1,800	2,000
76+	2,000	2,200	2,400	1,600	1,800	2,000

[1]Calories determined using a 5'10", 154 lb. man and a 5'4", 126 lb. woman. Estimates for females do not include women who are pregnant or breastfeeding.
[2]Sedentary refers to participating only in the light physical activity associated with day-to-day tasks. Moderately active refers to engaging in physical activity equivalent to walking about 1.5–3 miles per day at a 3–4 miles-per-hour (MPH) pace, in addition to everyday tasks. Active refers to daily physical activity equivalent to walking more than 3 miles per day at 3–4 MPH, in addition to routine tasks.

SOURCE: U.S. Department of Agriculture and U.S. Department of Health and Human Services, *Dietary Guidelines for Americans, 2010*, 7th ed., Washington, DC: U.S. Government Printing Office, December 2010.

(Table by PreMediaGlobal. © 2013 Cengage Learning)

eating patterns, and the need to take these factors into account when advising individuals about weight management and regular exercise. The full CNPP document and the DASH eating plan can be downloaded from each organization's website.

DASH recommendations for a 2,000-calorie daily diet for adults include:

- fruit group: 2–2.5 cups (4–5 servings) of fresh, frozen, canned, or dried fruit, with only limited juice
- vegetable group: 2–2.5 cups (4–5 servings)
- grain group: 6–8 ounce-equivalents of cereal, bread, crackers, rice, or pasta; with at least 50% whole grain
- meat and beans group: 5.5–6 ounce-equivalents of baked, broiled, or grilled lean meat, poultry, or fish, eggs, nuts, seeds, beans, peas, or tofu
- milk group: 2–3 cups low-fat/fat-free milk, yogurt, or cheese, or lactose-free, calcium-fortified products
- oils: 2–6 teaspoons
- discretionary: 267 calories; for example, solid fats (saturated fat such as butter, margarine, shortening, or lard) or added sugar

The vegetable group includes:

- dark greens, such as broccoli and leafy greens: three cups per week
- orange vegetables, such as carrots and sweet potatoes: two cups per week
- legumes, such as pinto or kidney beans, split peas, or lentils: three cups per week
- starchy vegetables: three cups per week
- other vegetables: 6.5 cups per week

Role of dietitians in nutrition

Dietitians are healthcare professionals with specialized training in nutrition. They work in a variety of settings ranging from the food service industry and health maintenance organizations to hospitals, educational institutions, and public health facilities. There are several different categories of dietitians who practice in the United States and Canada:

- Clinical dietitians. Clinical dietitians work in hospitals, nursing homes, and similar facilities to provide nutrition therapy or provide consultations about diet to patients and their families. They work closely with other members of hospital healthcare teams and may provide tube feedings or parenteral (intravenous) feedings as well as standard hospital meals.
- Community dietitians. Community dietitians work in public health agencies, home healthcare agencies, health maintenance organizations, and other wellness programs. They provide information about food and nutrition to groups as well as individuals. Some community dietitians concentrate on special populations, such as the elderly, children, or other individuals

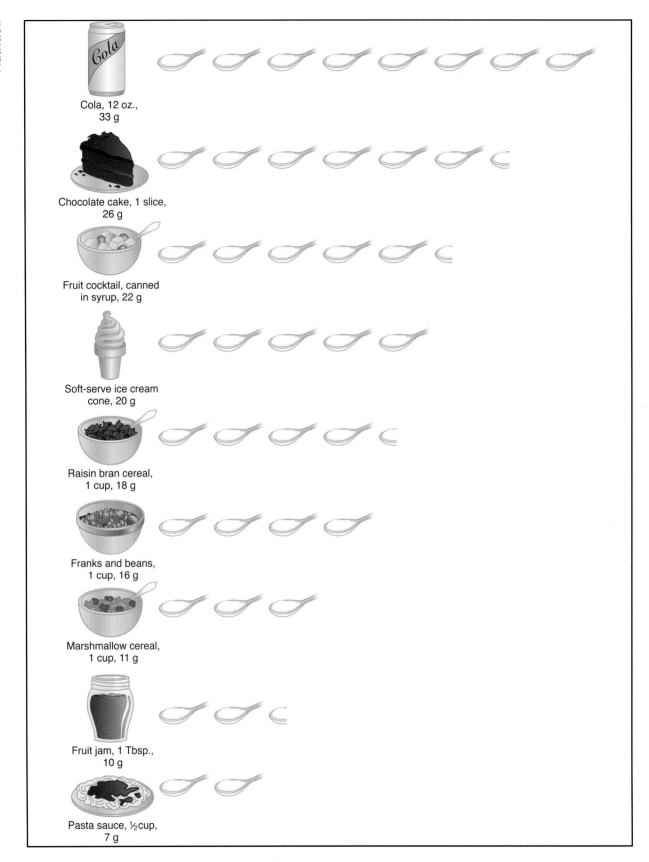

Cola, 12 oz.,
33 g

Chocolate cake, 1 slice,
26 g

Fruit cocktail, canned
in syrup, 22 g

Soft-serve ice cream
cone, 20 g

Raisin bran cereal,
1 cup, 18 g

Franks and beans,
1 cup, 16 g

Marshmallow cereal,
1 cup, 11 g

Fruit jam, 1 Tbsp.,
10 g

Pasta sauce, ½ cup,
7 g

Sugar content of various foods. *(Illustration by Electronic Illustrators Group. © 2013 Cengage Learning)*

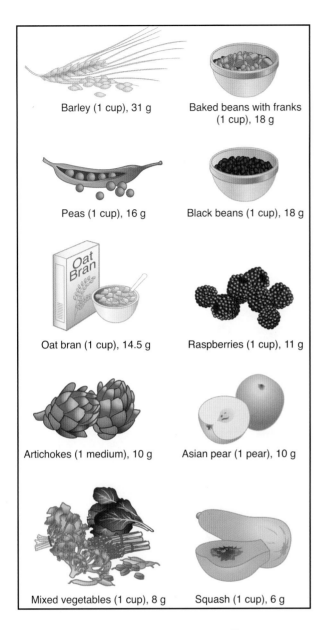

Barley (1 cup), 31 g

Baked beans with franks (1 cup), 18 g

Peas (1 cup), 16 g

Black beans (1 cup), 18 g

Oat bran (1 cup), 14.5 g

Raspberries (1 cup), 11 g

Artichokes (1 medium), 10 g

Asian pear (1 pear), 10 g

Mixed vegetables (1 cup), 8 g

Squash (1 cup), 6 g

Foods rich in fiber. *(Illustration by Electronic Illustrators Group. © 2013 Cengage Learning)*

with special needs or limited access to healthy food. Community dietitians may also make home visits to the elderly or others who cannot travel to provide them with information or advice about grocery shopping and food preparation.

• Food service dietitians. Food service dietitians provide meal plans and oversee food preparation for large organizations or institutions, such as restaurants, schools, prisons, and company cafeterias. They may also be responsible for training and supervising other food workers, including cooks, delivery staff, and dietary assistants.

• Research dietitians. Research dietitians work in universities, pharmaceutical companies, hospitals, government agencies and elsewhere to conduct clinical studies on the effects of diet on health or on specific nutrients. Research dietitians in universities typically have teaching as well as research responsibilities, while those in government agencies may study the effects of public policy on people's food choices and nutritional status.

• Consultant dietitians. Consultant dietitians are dietitians who work in private practice or as independent contractors with healthcare facilities, fitness clubs, sports teams, or other food- or nutrition-related businesses or organizations.

Dietitians in the United States must complete a rigorous program of supervised practical experience as well as classroom instruction. To qualify for the credential of Registered Dietitian (RD), a person must first complete a bachelor's degree in dietetics or an undergraduate degree in a scientific field followed by a master's degree in dietetics. The academic coursework is followed by an internship consisting of at least 1,200 hours in supervised field work placements that include rotations in clinical, community, food service, public health organizations, and other work sites. The candidate must then pass a national registration examination to become a registered dietitian. To maintain the credential, RDs must earn 75 hours of continuing education credit every five years. About half of all RDs in the United States hold advanced degrees as of 2012.

Demographics

Throughout much of the world, families struggle to obtain adequate nutrition. In the United States and other developed countries, nutrition is more often a matter of choice. According to the **Centers for Disease Control and Prevention (CDC)**, American society has become "obesogenic," with increased consumption of non-nutritional foods. Only 25% of Americans consume at least five daily servings of fruits and vegetables—the cornerstones of good nutrition. Americans are also eating more restaurant and fast food than in the past, along with larger portions and other changes in meal patterns and frequency.

Pediatric

The nutritional status and health of American children and adolescents has declined in recent years. As of 2012, 17% of American schoolchildren are overweight or obese. Specific findings include:

• The most recent (2005) Healthy Eating Index from the U.S. Department of Agriculture (USDA) has found that among children aged two through nine, 60–80% have diets in need of improvement and 4–8% have poor

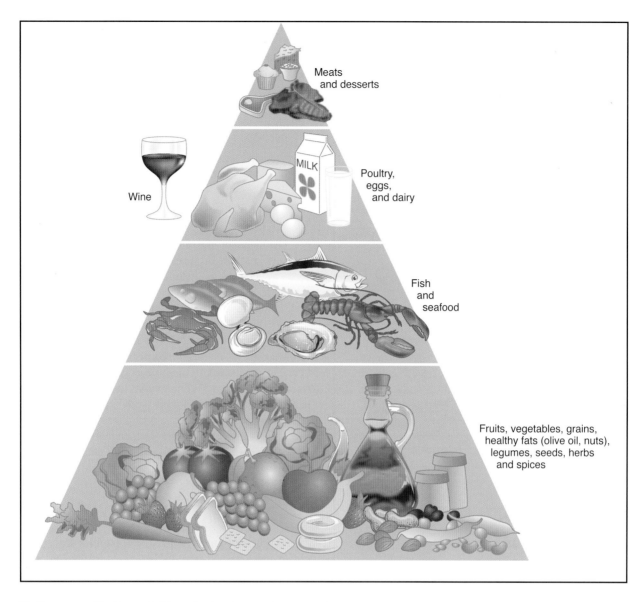

Mediterranean Diet Pyramid *(Illustration by Electronic Illustrators Group. © 2013 Cengage Learning)*

diets, with 63% eating too little fruit and 78% eating too few vegetables.

• Only 21% of high-school students report eating five or more daily servings of fruits and vegetables (other than fried potatoes and chips).

• Whole grains account for only 14% of the total daily grain consumption of children and adolescents.

• Only 39% of children aged two through 17 meet dietary recommendations for fiber (fruits, vegetables, dried beans and peas, and whole grains).

• More than 60% of children and teens eat too much saturated fat.

• Almost two-thirds of teens eat more than the recommended amount of total fat.

• Most teens eat too much processed, prepared, and junk foods.

• Among adolescent girls, 85% do not consume adequate calcium. Milk consumption by teenage girls has decreased 36% in recent decades, while soft-drink consumption has almost doubled among girls and almost tripled among adolescent boys.

• Eating disorders are the third most common chronic illness in adolescent girls, affecting as many as 5%.

Geriatric

According to a report by the Merck Institute of Aging and Health and the **CDC**, two-thirds of older Americans fail to practice good nutrition. Almost 90% of Americans over the age of 65 have one or more

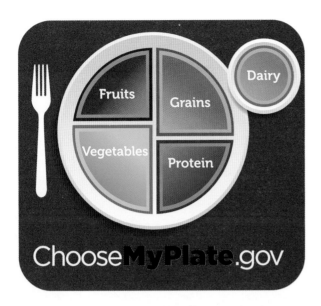

Recommended allotments of food groups for a healthy diet.
(United States Deparment of Agriculture (USDA))

degenerative disorders that may have been prevented by better nutrition.

Pregnant or breastfeeding

Breast milk is ideal nutrition for most infants. Breastfeeding has increased significantly in the United States in recent decades, from 60% in 1993–1994 to 77% in 2005–2006. Breastfeeding rates by black Americans increased from 36% in 1993–1994 to 65% in 2005–2006. Breastfeeding rates are significantly higher among mothers with higher incomes and those aged 30 and over.

Purpose

Nutrition is essential to life. It is required for growth and development from infancy through young adulthood and throughout life to provide energy and maintain bodily tissues and functions. Good nutrition promotes health and helps prevent **obesity** and disease. Nutrition is especially important during pregnancy and childhood to prevent growth retardation. The adequacy of nutrition in childhood and adolescent nutrition can have major ramifications on health in later life.

Benefits

In addition to its essential role in growth and development, maintenance of bodily functions, and energy supply, good nutrition helps prevent weight gain with calories that are high in nutrients other than sugars and fats. Good nutrition also helps prevent or lower the risk of various disorders, including:

- dental caries
- iron-deficiency anemia
- osteoporosis
- hypertension
- heart disease
- type 2 diabetes and gestational diabetes
- some types of cancer

Precautions

In general:

- Fresh foods are usually more nutritious than packaged and processed foods.
- Fast and processed foods contain excess fat and sodium and high amounts of sugar, as well as artificial preservatives and other additives.
- Fast and processed foods are deficient in fiber and such essential vitamins and minerals as vitamin A, riboflavin, folic acid, vitamin E, calcium, magnesium, and potassium.
- It is more difficult to gauge nutrient and calorie content when eating out and buying packaged foods.
- Vegetarians need to choose carefully from the basic foods groups to achieve recommended nutrient intakes, especially of protein, vitamins, and iron.
- Iron-deficiency anemia is very common in women. The recommended iron intake is 15–18 mg daily for females. Good sources of iron include dark-green leafy vegetables, legumes, iron-fortified breads and cereals, and red meat.
- Many adults do not obtain enough calcium from their diets, which can lead to osteoporosis in later life. Women aged 19–50 should consume 1,000 mg of calcium daily. Women over 50 require 1,200 mg. Good sources of calcium include dark-green leafy vegetables, calcium-fortified orange juice, bread, cereal, fish, and low-fat dairy products.
- Although nutritional supplementation is sometimes necessary, if possible, nutrients should come from food. Excessive use of vitamin and mineral supplements can lead to serious health problems.
- Diets should not be radically altered except under medical supervision.

Pediatric

Childhood nutrition requires adequate essential nutrients, fiber, and calories to maintain proper growth, maximize cognitive development, and promote health, while preventing excess weight gain. Poor nutrition in adolescence can cause growth and developmental problems and long-term complications including obesity,

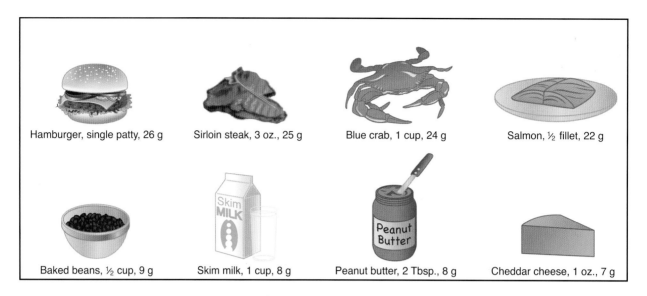

Hamburger, single patty, 26 g

Sirloin steak, 3 oz., 25 g

Blue crab, 1 cup, 24 g

Salmon, ½ fillet, 22 g

Baked beans, ½ cup, 9 g

Skim milk, 1 cup, 8 g

Peanut butter, 2 Tbsp., 8 g

Cheddar cheese, 1 oz., 7 g

Foods containing good amounts of protein. *(Illustration by Electronic Illustrators Group. © 2013 Cengage Learning)*

heart disease, and osteoporosis. Children's diets should include a variety of foods with high nutrient-to-calorie ratios. In addition:

- At age two, 25–33% of grains should be whole-grain, gradually increasing to 50% by age five.
- The average adolescent protein requirement is about 300 mg per 0.4 in (1 cm) of height.
- Physically active adolescents require more fluids and more carbohydrates from fruit and whole grains.
- Requirements for vitamins and minerals increase during adolescence. Teenagers require 1,300 mg of calcium daily. Boys require 10-12 mg of iron and 15 mg of zinc daily. Girls require 15 mg of iron and 12 mg of zinc.
- Vegan and macrobiotic diets for adolescents may require nutritional supplements.

Geriatric

Various factors can interfere with sound nutrition in the elderly:

- medical conditions and/or medications, including medication side effects
- reduced capacity to absorb and utilize nutrients
- oral/dental problems or difficulty chewing or swallowing
- gastrointestinal disturbances
- loss of appetite
- loss of the ability to taste and smell foods
- changes in taste preferences
- loss of manual dexterity
- social isolation, loneliness, or depression

- economic limitations
- lack of cooking skills or desire to cook
- inadequate knowledge of nutrition
- dementia or other problems with cognitive function

The rate of metabolism can decline by as much as 30% over a lifetime and lean muscle mass can decrease by as much as 25% in the elderly, accompanied by an increase in body fat. Therefore, older adults need foods with high nutrient-to-calorie ratios. Although caloric requirements vary greatly, it has been recommended that, after age 50, men reduce their daily intake by 600 calories and women by 300 calories. Because seniors eat less and take in fewer calories, they also consume fewer vitamins and minerals, even though the body's need for some micronutrients may actually increase with age. This is especially true for vitamin D and calcium. A single daily multivitamin/mineral supplement can address nutritional gaps.

Other nutritional recommendations for seniors include:

- adequate protein for immune system health and maintenance and repair of body tissues
- dietary fiber from fruits, vegetables, beans, nuts, seeds, brown rice, and whole grains
- only small amounts of fats, oils, and sweets
- no more than 1,500 mg of sodium daily from all food sources (two-thirds of a teaspoon of table salt)
- adequate fluids—the elderly can easily become dehydrated
- vitamin B_{12} from fortified foods or supplements

KEY TERMS

Antioxidants—A class of biochemicals that have been found to protect cells from free-radical damage.

Calorie—A unit of food energy.

Carbohydrate—A class of nutrients that includes sugars, starches, celluloses, and gums, which are a major source of calories from foods.

Cholesterol—A fat-soluble steroid alcohol (sterol) found in animal fats and oils, and produced in the body from saturated fats. Cholesterol is required to produce vitamin D and various hormones and for the formation of cell membranes. High cholesterol levels contribute to the development of atherosclerosis.

Dietitian—A healthcare professional with specialized training in food and nutrition who advises people on healthful eating, conducts research on nutrition, provides nutritional therapy in healthcare settings, or consults with patients and their families to develop individual diet plans.

Enzymes—Chemical catalysts that help initiate biochemical processes.

Essential fatty acids—Sources of fat in the diet, including omega-3 and omega-6 fatty acids.

Fat—Molecules composed of fatty acids and glycerol; the slowest utilized source of energy, but the most energy-efficient form of food. Each gram of fat supplies about nine calories, more than twice that supplied by the same amount of protein or carbohydrate.

Monounsaturated fat—Fats that contain one double or triple carbon bond per molecule; examples include canola oil and olive oil.

Parenteral nutrition—Feeding a patient intravenously, thus bypassing normal eating and digestive processes.

Polyunsaturated fat—Fats that contain two or more double or triple carbon bonds per molecule; examples include fish, safflower, sunflower, corn, and soybean oils.

Protein—Chains of amino acids that are essential constituents of all living cells and include structural components, enzymes, hormones, and antibodies.

Saturated fat—Fat molecules that contain only single carbon bonds; examples include whole milk, cream, palm and coconut oils, and solid fats such as cheese, butter, and meat.

Trans fat—Fat that is produced by hydrogenation during food processing; trans fats increase bad cholesterol and decrease good cholesterol.

• potassium from leafy green vegetables, tomatoes, bananas, and root vegetables such as potatoes to counter the effects of salt on blood pressure

Pregnant or breastfeeding women

Women have special nutritional needs during menstruation, pregnancy, lactation, and menopause. Pregnant and breastfeeding women have increased requirements for calories and for most nutrients. Pregnant and breastfeeding teenagers have even higher nutritional requirements than other pregnant women. Pregnant women should consume iron-rich plant foods and vitamin-C-rich foods that aid in the absorption of iron. Folic acid, a B vitamin, is particularly important during pregnancy, since it helps protect against brain and spinal cord **birth defects**. All women of childbearing age should consume 400 micrograms (μg) of folic acid daily and 600 μg during pregnancy. Pregnancy and breastfeeding deplete maternal calcium. Pregnant and lactating adult women should consume 1,000 mg of calcium daily. Pregnant and lactating teenagers require 1,300 mg.

Hormonal changes during pregnancy can trigger gestational diabetes, characterized by high levels of sugar in the blood. Changes in diet and exercise are often sufficient to keep blood sugar levels within the normal range. Women who experience gestational diabetes are more likely to develop type 2 diabetes later in life.

Other conditions and allergies

Many people with **allergies** or medical conditions require special diets, such as a low-fat, low-cholesterol diet for heart disease, a low-sodium diet for high blood pressure, or a low-calorie diet for weight reduction. Chronic illnesses, such as diabetes, as well as substance abuse, also create special nutritional requirements.

Nutritional supplements

Nutritional supplements are not regulated by the FDA in the same way that prescription and over-the-counter drugs are. Instead, nutritional supplements are regulated in the same way as food. This means that makers of nutritional supplements do not have to prove

QUESTIONS TO ASK YOUR DOCTOR

- What is your opinion of the new MyPlate food guide icon?
- Have you ever worked with or referred patients to a registered dietitian?
- What nutritional supplements, if any, would you recommend for adults in good health? For children? For teenagers? For older adults?

the effectiveness of their products before putting them on the market. Nutritional supplements that make claims about the benefits of their product are required to carry a label stating that "This statement has not been evaluated by the Food and Drug Administration. This product is not intended to diagnose, treat, cure, or prevent any disease."

Consumers can make wise choices for nutritional supplementation by consulting a physician, pharmacist, nutritionist, or other health professionals. Nutritional supplements are best added into the diet slowly, starting with small dosages and working up to the manufacturers' recommended amounts over time. Also, some supplements, such as herbal medications that may stimulate processes in the body, are best taken intermittently, allowing the body occasional rest periods without the supplement. To avoid unfavorable interactions, nutritional supplements are best used moderately and individually, rather than taking handfuls of capsules and tablets for various needs and conditions at the same time. Finally, consumers should be wary of excessive or grandiose health claims made by manufacturers of nutritional supplements and rely on scientific information to validate these claims.

Resources

BOOKS

Duyff, Roberta Larson. *American Dietetic Association['s] Complete Food and Nutrition Guide*, 4th ed. Hoboken, NJ: John Wiley and Sons, 2012.

Hark, Lisa, Kathleen Ashton, and Darwin Deen, eds. *The Nurse Practitioner's Guide to Nutrition*, 2nd ed. Ames, IA: John Wiley and Sons, 2012.

Insel, Paul M., R. Elaine Turner, and Don Ross. *Discovering Nutrition.* 3rd ed. Sudbury, MA: Jones & Bartlett, 2010.

Smolin, Lori A., and Mary B. Grosvenor. *Basic Nutrition*, 2nd ed. New York: Chelsea House, 2011.

Webb, Geoffrey P. *Dietary Supplements and Functional Foods*, 2nd ed. Ames, IA: Wiley-Blackwell, 2011.

PERIODICALS

Britten, P., et al. "Impact of Typical Rather than Nutrient-Dense Food Choices in the US Department of Agriculture Food Patterns." *Journal of the Academy of Nutrition and Dietetics* 112 (October 2012): 1560–1569.

Clemens, R., et al. "Filling America's Fiber Intake Gap: Summary of a Roundtable to Probe Realistic Solutions with a Focus on Grain-based Foods." *Journal of Nutrition* 142 (July 2012): 1390S–1401S.

Glanz, K., et al. "Effect of a Nutrient Rich Foods Consumer Education Program: Results from the Nutrition Advice Study." *Journal of the Academy of Nutrition and Dietetics* 112 (January 2012): 56–63.

Manger, W.M., et al. "Obesity Prevention in Young School-children: Results of a Pilot Study." *Journal of School Health* 82 (October 2012): 462–468.

Post, R., et al. "Putting MyPlate to Work for Nutrition Educators." *Journal of Nutrition Education and Behavior* 44 (March-April 2012): 98–99.

Slavin, J.L., and B. Lloyd. "Health Benefits of Fruits and Vegetables." *Advances in Nutrition* 3 (July 1, 2012): 506–516.

Tobias, D.K., et al. "Prepregnancy Adherence to Dietary Patterns and Lower Risk of Gestational Diabetes Mellitus." *American Journal of Clinical Nutrition* 96 (August 2012): 289–295.

Troesch, B., et al. "100 Years of Vitamins: Adequate Intake in the Elderly Is Still a Matter of Concern." *Journal of Nutrition* 142 (June 2012): 979–980.

WEBSITES

"Choose My Plate." U.S. Department of Agriculture (USDA). http://www.choosemyplate.gov/ (accessed October 16, 2012).

Dietary Guidelines for Americans, 2010. Center for Nutrition Policy and Promotion, U.S. Department of Agriculture. http://www.cnpp.usda.gov/DGAs2010-PolicyDocument. htm (accessed October 15, 2012).

"Dietary Recommendations for Healthy Children." http://www. heart.org/HEARTORG/GettingHealthy/Dietary-Recommendations-for-Healthy-Children_UCM_ 303886_Article.jsp (accessed October 16, 2012).

"Eat Right Nutrition Tips." Academy of Nutrition and Dietetics. http://www.eatright.org/nutritiontipsheets/#. UH4xslE8H3U (accessed October 16, 2012).

"Nutrition." Centers for Disease Control and Prevention (CDC). http://www.cdc.gov/nutrition/index.html (accessed October 15, 2012).

"Your Guide to Lowering Your Blood Pressure with DASH." National Heart, Lung, and Blood Institute (NHLBI). http:// www.nhlbi.nih.gov/health/public/heart/hbp/dash/new_ dash.pdf (accessed October 16, 2012).

ORGANIZATIONS

Academy of Nutrition and Dietetics [formerly the American Dietetic Association], 120 South Riverside Plaza, Suite 2000, Chicago, IL United States 60606-6995, (312) 899-0040, (800) 877-1600, http://www.eatright.org/

Center for Nutrition Policy and Promotion (CNPP), U.S. Department of Agriculture (USDA), 3101 Park Center Drive, 10th Floor, Alexandria, VA United States 22302-1594, (703) 305-7600, Fax: (703) 305-3300, http://www.cnpp.usda.gov/

Centers for Disease Control and Prevention (CDC), 1600 Clifton Road, Atlanta, GA United States 30333, (800) CDC-INFO (232-4636), http://www.cdc.gov/cdc-info/requestform.html, http://www.cdc.gov/

Food and Drug Administration (FDA), 10903 New Hampshire Ave., Silver Spring, MD United States 20993-0002, (866) INFO-FDA (463-6332), http://www.fda.gov/default.htm

National Heart, Lung, and Blood Institute (NHLBI), P.O. Box 30105, Bethesda, MD United States 20824-0105, (301) 592-8573, Fax: (240) 629-3246, nhlbiinfo@nhlbi.nih.gov, http://www.nhlbi.nih.gov/.

Margaret Alic, PhD
Douglas Dupler
Rebecca J. Frey, PhD

O

Obesity

Definition

Obesity is an abnormal accumulation of body fat—usually 20% or more over an individual's ideal body weight. A person is considered overweight if one's body mass index (BMI) is between 25 and 29.9, and a person is considered obese if the BMI is over 30. Obesity can severely interfere with one's daily functions, and it is associated with increased risk of illness, disability, and even death.

The branch of medicine that deals with the study and treatment of obesity is known as bariatrics. As obesity has become a major health problem in the United States, bariatrics has become a separate medical and surgical specialty.

Demographics

Obesity is a serious public health problem that affects both sexes and all ethnic, racial, age, and socioeconomic groups in the United States and around the world. According to the U.S. **Centers for Disease Control and Prevention (CDC)**, about 31% of adult men and 35% of adult women (a total of about 100 million people) in the United States are obese, as well as 17% of children (aged 2–19). Obesity is the most common nutritional disorder among American children and teens.

The prevalence of obesity varies with age and ethnicity. According to the **CDC**, non-Hispanic blacks have the highest rate of obesity in the United States, with a rate of 44.1%, followed by Mexican Americans (39.3%), Hispanics (37.9%), and non-Hispanic whites (32.6%). The greatest rates of obesity were found in the South and Midwest. With respect to socioeconomic status, non-Hispanic black men and Mexican American men with higher incomes were more likely to be obese than those with lower incomes. With respect to females,

all women with higher incomes were less likely to be obese than lower-income women. Education backgrounds did not seem to affect obesity levels. Among children, African American and Hispanic children are considerably more likely to be overweight than Caucasian Americans.

The **World Health Organization (WHO)** recognizes obesity as a global problem. **WHO** estimated in 2011 that 1.5 billion people worldwide were overweight, of which 500 million were obese. The number of overweight children in Africa and Asia is increasing most rapidly, while in the same countries other children are dying of complications of under- or malnutrition.

Description

Obesity is excessive body weight that develops over time as people consume more calories than they expend in energy. As excess calories accumulate in the body, people first become overweight, then obese. The ability of the human body to store energy can mean the difference between life and death in times of **famine**. However, this protective mechanism becomes a potential problem when food is readily available in unlimited quantities. This is evident in the increasing prevalence of obesity in modern society, particularly in the developed world. As obesity rates have increased, bariatrics—the branch of medicine that studies and treats obesity—has become a separate medical and surgical specialty in developed countries.

The human body is composed of bone, muscle, specialized organ tissues, and fat. Together these comprise the total body mass, measured in pounds (lb) or kilograms (kg). Fat, or adipose tissue, is a combination of essential and storage fats. Essential fat is an energy source for the normal physiologic function of cells and organs. It is tucked in and around internal organs, and is an important building block for all cells of the body. Storage fat is a reserve supply of energy. It accumulates in the chest and abdomen and, in much greater volume,

Height and weight goals

Men

Height	Small frame	Medium frame	Large frame
5'2"	128–134 lbs.	131–141 lbs.	138–150 lbs.
5'3"	130–136	133–143	140–153
5'4"	132–138	135–145	142–153
5'5"	134–140	137–148	144–160
5'6"	136–142	139–151	146–164
5'7"	138–145	142–154	149–168
5'8"	140–148	145–157	152–172
5'9"	142–151	148–160	155–176
5'10"	144–154	151–163	158–180
5'11"	146–157	154–166	161–184
6'0"	149–160	157–170	164–188
6'1"	152–164	160–174	168–192
6'2"	155–168	164–178	172–197
6'3"	158–172	167–182	176–202
6'4"	162–176	171–187	181–207

Women

Height	Small frame	Medium frame	Large frame
4'10"	102–111 lbs.	109–121 lbs.	118–131 lbs.
4'11"	103–113	111–123	120–134
5'0"	104–115	113–126	112–137
5'1"	106–118	115–129	125–140
5'2"	108–121	118–132	128–143
5'3"	111–124	121–135	131–147
5'4"	114–127	124–141	137–151
5'5"	117–130	127–141	137–155
5'6"	120–133	130–144	140–159
5'7"	123–136	133–147	143–163
5'8"	126–139	136–150	146–167
5'9"	129–142	139–153	149–170
5'10"	132–145	142–156	152–176
5'11"	135–148	145–159	155–176
6'0"	138–151	148–162	158–179

SOURCE: Doctors On-Line, Inc. "Height and Weight Goals as Determined by the Metropolitan Life Insurance Company."

(Table by PreMediaGlobal. Reproduced by permission of Gale, a part of Cengage Learning.)

under the skin. When the amount of energy consumed as food exceeds the amount of energy expended in the maintenance of life processes and **physical activity**, storage fat accumulates in excessive amounts.

In the past, obesity was defined as body weight that was at least 20% above one's ideal weight. Ideal weight was defined as the weight at which individuals of the same height, gender, and age had the lowest rate of death. Mild obesity was defined as 20–40% over ideal weight, moderate obesity as 40–100% over ideal, and gross or morbid obesity 100% over ideal weight.

Current guidelines use the body mass index (BMI) to define obesity. The BMI utilizes height and weight to compare the ratio of body fat to total body mass.

To calculate BMI using metric units, weight in kilograms is divided by height in meters squared. To calculate BMI in English units, weight in pounds is divided by height in inches squared and then multiplied by 703. This calculated BMI is compared to the statistical distribution of BMIs for adults aged 20–29 to determine whether an individual is underweight, average, overweight, or obese. The 20–29-year age group was chosen as the standard because it represents fully developed adults at the point in their lives when they have the least amount of body fat. Ideally, body fat is about 15% of total body mass for adult males and about 20–25% for adult females. A simple BMI calculator is available at http://www.nhlbisupport.com/bmi. However, BMI does not distinguish between fat and muscle.

Adult BMIs are age- and gender-independent. All adults aged 20 and older are evaluated on the same BMI scale as follows:

• underweight: BMI below 18.5
• normal weight: BMI 18.5–24.9
• overweight: BMI 25.0–29.9
• obese: BMI 30 and above

Ranges are slightly different for Asian populations. Research has shown that the risk of developing type 2 diabetes and **heart disease** tends to be associated with lower BMIs in Asian populations than in European populations (on which the BMIs are based). Ranges vary, but generally the cap for normal weight is set at 22.9, and a BMI of 23 or higher is considered overweight.

The BMI for children and teens is calculated in the same way as for adults, but the results are interpreted differently. A child's BMI is compared to those of other children of the same age and gender and assigned to a percentile. For example, a girl in the 75th percentile for her age group weighs more than 74 of every 100 girls her age and less than 25 of every 100 girls her age. The percentiles indicate the following:

• underweight: below the 5th percentile
• healthy weight: 5th percentile to below the 85th percentile
• at risk of overweight: 85th percentile to below the 95th percentile
• overweight: 95th percentile and above

The CDC does not use the term "obese" for children and teens because the proportion of body fat fluctuates during growth and development and is slightly higher than in mature adults.

Obesity places stress on the body's organs and puts people at higher risk for many serious and potentially life-threatening health problems:

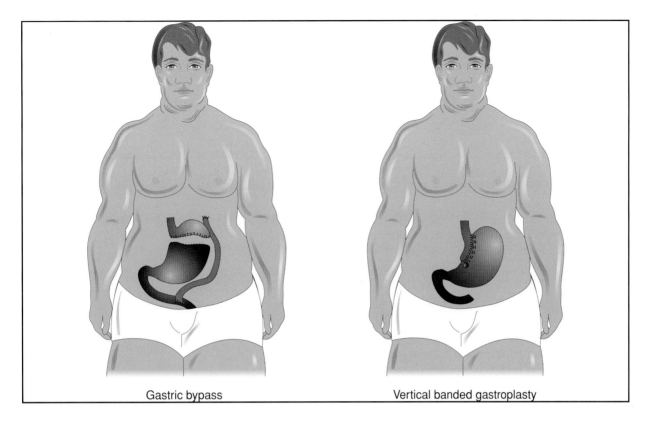

Gastric bypass   Vertical banded gastroplasty

The purpose of obesity surgery is to reduce the size of the stomach and slow the stomach emptying process by narrowing the entrance into the intestine. With this surgery, the volume of food the stomach can hold is reduced from approximately 4 cups to approximately one-half cup. There are two types of procedures used for obesity surgery: gastric bypass surgery and vertical banded gastroplasty, as shown in the illustration above. *(Illustration by Electronic Illustrators Group. Reproduced by permission of Gale, a part of Cengage Learning.)*

- fatigue

- joint problems

- poor physical fitness

- digestive disorders

- dizzy spells

- rashes

- hypertension (high blood pressure)

- menstrual disorders

- complications during childbirth and surgery

- type 2 diabetes mellitus (non-insulin dependent)

- heart disease

- unexplained heart attack

- gallstones

- breathing problems

- hyperlipidemia (high level of fats in the blood)

- infertility

- colon, prostate, endometrial, and breast cancers

- premature aging

Obese individuals have a shorter **life expectancy** than people of normal weight. Many diseases, especially degenerative diseases of the joints, heart, and blood vessels, tend to be more severe in obese individuals, increasing the need for some surgical procedures. Increasing prevalence of type 2 diabetes in the United States and the appearance of type 2 diabetes in children, previously a rarity, are directly related to an increased prevalence of obesity.

Although acute complications of obesity are rare in children, **childhood obesity** is a risk factor for insulin resistance and type 2 diabetes, hypertension, hyperlipidemia, liver and renal disease, and reproductive dysfunction. Childhood obesity increases the risk of deformed bones in the legs and feet. It also can result in emotional disorders, such as depression caused by social isolation and negative comments by peers. Moreover childhood obesity increases the risk of adult obesity and cardiovascular disease.

In 2011, the cost of obesity to the American economy was estimated at more than $100 billion, excluding dollars spent on commercial weight-loss

Body mass index (BMI) calculation and meaning

Body mass index is determined by a person's weight and height:

Pounds/inches		Kilograms/meters	BMI	Weight status
$\dfrac{\text{weight (lb)} \times 703}{[\text{height (in)}]^2}$	(or)	$\dfrac{\text{weight (kg)}}{[\text{height (m)}]^2}$	Below 18.5 18.5–24.9 25.0–29.9 30.0 and above	Underweight Normal Overweight Obese

(Table by PreMediaGlobal. Reproduced by permission of Gale, a part of Cengage Learning.)

programs. The increasing prevalence of obesity and diabetes in children and young adults heralds increased healthcare costs in the future. The social costs of obesity, including decreased productivity, discrimination, depression, and low self-esteem, are less easily measured.

In 1995, the Institute of Medicine of the U.S. National Academies published a report describing obesity as a "complex, multifactorial disease of appetite regulation and energy metabolism." The report cited the following outcomes from even relatively modest weight loss:

• lower blood pressure (and lower risk of heart attack and stroke)

• reduction of abnormally high levels of blood glucose

• lower blood levels of cholesterol and triglycerides (and lower risk of cardiovascular disease)

• lower incidence of sleep apnea

• lower risk for osteoarthritis in weight-bearing joints

• lower incidence of depression

• improved self-esteem

Risk factors

Obesity tends to run in families. Children of obese parents are about 13 times more likely than other children to be obese. Additional obese family members, including siblings and grandparents, greatly increases the likelihood of childhood obesity. The tendency toward a body type with an unusually high number of fat cells—termed *endomorphic*—appears to be inherited. Other genetic factors influence appetite and the metabolic rate at which food is transformed into energy. However, family eating habits are major contributors to the development of obesity. Although the majority of adopted children have patterns of weight gain that more closely resemble those of their birth parents than those of their adoptive parents, normal-weight children adopted into obese families are more likely than other children to become obese. Longitudinal studies of juvenile-onset obesity have demonstrated parental and peer encouragement of

overeating and even deliberate overfeeding of obese children.

Low socioeconomic status is a risk factor for adult-onset obesity. A diet of high-fat, high-sugar refined food and a sedentary lifestyle are also risk factors.

Causes and symptoms

Obesity is caused by the consumption of more calories than the body uses for energy to drive physiological functions. The excess calories are stored as adipose tissue. Although inheritance may play a role, a genetic predisposition toward weight gain alone does not cause obesity. Hormonal and genetic disorders account for less than 10% of obesity in children. Eating habits, physical activity, and environmental, behavioral, social, and cultural factors all contribute to the development of obesity.

Nevertheless, sometimes obesity does have a purely physiological cause, as in the following:

• Cushing's syndrome, a disorder involving the excessive release of the hormone cortisol

• hypothyroidism caused by an underactive thyroid gland, resulting in low levels of the hormone thyroxin and the slow metabolism of food, causing excess unburned calories to be stored as fat

• neurological disturbances, such as damage to the hypothalamus, a structure located deep within the brain that helps regulate appetite

• certain drugs, such as steroids, antipsychotic medications, and antidepressants

Some researchers have suggested that low levels of the neurotransmitter serotonin increase cravings for carbohydrates. In addition, a combination of genetics and early nutritional habits may result in a higher "set point" for body weight that causes obese individuals to feel hunger more often than others. Recent obesity research has focused on two peptide hormones, leptin and ghrelin. Leptin, produced by fat cells, affects hunger and eating behavior; insensitivity to leptin may contribute to obesity. Ghrelin is secreted by cells in the lining of the stomach and is important in appetite regulation and maintaining the body's energy balance.

However, most obesity is caused by simple overeating. During past decades, American eating habits have changed significantly, with many people consuming larger meals and more high-calorie processed foods. School and workplace cafeterias often have a poor selection of nutritional food offerings. Food is sold in many venues besides restaurants and supermarkets. Furthermore, it is estimated that in a given six-month period, 2–5% of Americans binge eat. It has been estimated that approximately 15% of the mildly obese participating in weight-loss programs have binge eating disorder and that the percentage is much higher among the morbidly obese. Current evidence indicates that weight gain depends primarily on total calories consumed, rather than the amount from carbohydrates versus fats, and that low-fat diets are no more effective for weight reduction than low-calorie diets.

Sedentary lifestyles, which are particularly prevalent among affluent socioeconomic groups, also contribute to obesity. Rather than physical labor on farms and in factories, many people are now employed at sedentary jobs in post-industrial service industries. Energy-saving machines and devices—cars, remote control devices, household electric appliances, and power tools—have become standard equipment. One study found that the average Western European adult walks about 8,000–9,000 steps daily. In contrast, among the Amish of Pennsylvania who do not use cars or electricity, men accumulate 18,425 steps daily and have no obesity. Amish women walk 14,196 steps daily and have an obesity rate of only 9%.

Psychological factors, such as depression and low self-esteem, can contribute to overeating and obesity. People may eat compulsively to overcome fear or social maladjustment, express defiance, or avoid intimate relationships.

Some babies are born obese. This can be caused by excessive insulin production in the fetuses of diabetic mothers, excessive trans-placental nutrients in the case of obese mothers, or excessive weight gain during pregnancy.

Some babies become obese because they are overfed. Families may value a plump baby, or caregivers may use a bottle to quiet an infant or to demonstrate their own competence as caregivers. Because obese one-year-olds may be physically delayed in crawling and walking, they become less active toddlers, burning fewer calories. By the age of 10, obese boys and girls are taller than their peers by as much as 4 inches (10 cm). Their skeletal maturation, called bone-age, is also accelerated, so they stop growing earlier. Sexual maturation is advanced. It is not uncommon for obese girls to experience early onset of menstruation, sometimes even before the age of 10. Parental separation and divorce or other psychological stresses may stimulate compensatory overeating in children. Obese teenagers and, increasingly, obese preteens may combine periods of binge eating and caloric deprivation, leading to bulimia or anorexia nervosa.

In developed countries, people generally experience increased BMI with age. The proportion of intra-abdominal fat, which correlates with disease and death, increases progressively with age. There is also a progressive decline in daily total energy expenditure, associated with decreased physical activity and lower metabolic activity, especially in those with chronic disabilities and diseases.

The major symptoms of obesity are excessive weight and large amounts of fatty tissue. Common secondary symptoms include shortness of breath and lower back **pain** from carrying excessive body weight. Obesity can also give rise to secondary conditions including:

• arthritis and other orthopedic problems
• hernias
• heartburn
• adult-onset asthma
• gum disease
• high cholesterol levels
• gallstones
• high blood pressure
• menstrual irregularities or cessation of menstruation (amenorhhea)
• decreased fertility and pregnancy complications
• incapacitating shortness of breath
• sleep apnea and sleeping disorders
• skin disorders from the bacterial breakdown of sweat and cellular material in thick folds of skin or from increased friction between folds
• emotional and social difficulties

Diagnosis

Examination

Obesity is usually diagnosed by observation of excessive storage fat and by calculating BMI from weight and height. Physicians also observe how the excess weight is carried by comparing waist and hip measurements: "apple-shaped" patients—who store most of their weight around the waist and abdomen—are at greater risk for **cancer**, heart disease, **stroke**, and diabetes than "pear-shaped" patients whose extra pounds settle primarily in their hips and thighs.

KEY TERMS

Adipose tissue—Fat tissue.

Anemia—Red blood cell deficiency.

Appetite suppressant—A drug that reduces appetite.

Bariatrics—The branch of medicine that deals with the prevention and treatment of obesity and related disorders.

Binge-eating disorder—A condition characterized by uncontrolled eating.

Body Mass Index (BMI)—A measure of body fat: the ratio of weight in kilograms to the square of height in meters.

Calorie—A unit of food energy.

Carbohydrate—Sugars, starches, celluloses, and gums that are a major source of calories from foods.

Catecholamines—Hormones and neurotransmitters including dopamine, epinephrine, and norepinephrine.

Eating disorder—A condition characterized by an abnormal attitude towards food, altered appetite control, and unhealthy eating habits that affect health and the ability to function normally.

Epidemic—Affecting many individuals in a community or population and spreading rapidly.

Fat—Molecules composed of fatty acids and glycerol; the slowest utilized source of energy, but the most energy-efficient form of food. Each gram of fat supplies about nine calories, more than twice that supplied by the same amount of proteins or carbohydrates.

Gastroplasty—A surgical procedure used to reduce digestive capacity by shortening the small intestine or shrinking the side of the stomach.

Ghrelin—A peptide hormone secreted primarily by the stomach that has been implicated in the control of food intake and fat storage.

Hyperlipidemia—Abnormally high levels of lipids in the blood.

Hyperplastic obesity—Excessive weight gain in childhood, characterized by an increase in the number of fat cells.

Hypertension—Abnormally high arterial blood pressure, which if left untreated can lead to heart disease and stroke.

Hypertrophic obesity—Excessive weight gain in adulthood, characterized by expansion of pre-existing fat cells.

Ideal weight—Weight corresponding to the lowest death rate for individuals of a specific height, gender, and age.

Leptin—A peptide hormone produced by fat cells that acts on the hypothalamus to suppress appetite and burn stored fat.

Metabolic activity—The sum of the chemical processes in the body that are necessary to maintain life.

Metabolic bone disease—Weakening of bones due to a deficiency of certain minerals, especially calcium.

Normal weight—A BMI of less than 25.0.

Obesity—An abnormal accumulation of body fat, usually 20% or more above ideal body weight or a BMI of 30.0 or above.

Off-label use—Drugs in the United States are approved by the Food and Drug Administration (FDA) for specific uses, periods of time, or dosages based on the results of clinical trials. However, it is legal for physicians to administer these drugs for other "off-label" or non-approved uses. It is not legal for pharmaceutical companies to advertise drugs for off-label uses.

Osteoporosis—A disease characterized by low bone mass and structural deterioration of bone tissue, leading to bone fragility.

Overweight—A BMI between 25.0 and 30.0.

Serotonin—A neurotransmitter located primarily in the brain, blood serum, and stomach membrane.

Procedures

BMIs and other measurements do not necessarily accurately reflect body composition and muscle mass. A heavily muscled football player may weigh far more than a sedentary man of similar height, but have significantly less body fat. Chronic dieters, who have lost significant muscle mass during periods of caloric deprivation, may look slim and weigh little but have elevated body fat. Therefore direct measurements of body fat are obtained using calipers to measure skin-fold thickness at the back of the upper arm and other sites, which distinguishes between muscle and adipose tissue.

The most accurate means of estimating body fat is hydrostatic weighing—calculating the volume of water displaced by the body. The patient exhales as completely as possible and is immersed in water and the relative displacement is measured. Women whose body fat exceeds 30–32% of total body mass by this method and men whose body fat exceeds 25–27%, are generally considered obese. Since this method is unpleasant and impractical, it is usually used only in scientific studies.

Treatment

Traditional

Treatment of obesity aims at reducing weight to a BMI within the normal range (below 25.0). The best way to achieve weight loss is to reduce dietary caloric intake and increase physical activity. However obesity will return unless the weight loss includes life-long behavioral changes. "Yo-yo" dieting, in which weight is repeatedly lost and regained, has been shown to increase the likelihood of fatal health problems even more than no weight loss at all.

Behavioral treatment for obesity is goal-directed and process-oriented and relies heavily on self-monitoring, with emphasis on:

• Food intake. This may involve keeping a food diary and learning the nutritional value, caloric content, and fat content of foods. It may involve changing shopping habits, such as only shopping on a certain day and buying only what is on the grocery list, timing meals and planning frequent small meals to prevent hunger pangs, and eating slowly to allow for satiation.

• Response to food. This may involve understanding psychological issues underlying eating habits. For example, some people binge eat when under stress, whereas others use food as a reward. By recognizing psychological triggers, alternate coping mechanisms that do not focus on food, can be developed.

• Time management. Integrating exercise into everyday life is a key to achieving and maintaining weight loss. Starting slowly and building endurance helps to keep patients from becoming discouraged. Varying routines and trying new activities helps to keep interest high.

• Stimulus control. This may involve removing environmental cues for inappropriate eating.

• Contingency management. A system of positive and negative reinforcements may help with behavioral modification.

Most mildly obese individuals can make these lifestyle changes independently with medical supervision. Others may utilize a commercial weight-loss program, such as Weight Watchers. The effectiveness of these programs is difficult to assess, since they vary widely, dropout rates are high, and few employ medical professionals. However, programs that emphasize realistic goals, gradual progress, sensible eating, and exercise can be very helpful and are recommended by many physicians. Programs that promise instant weight loss or utilize severely restricted diets are not effective and, in some cases, can be dangerous.

Moderately obese individuals require medically supervised behavior modification and weight loss. A realistic goal is a 10% weight loss over a six-month period. Most doctors use a balanced, low-calorie diet of 1200–1500 calories a day. However sometimes certain patients may be put on a medically supervised very-low 400–700-calorie liquid protein diet, with supplementation of **vitamins** and minerals, for as long as three months. This therapy should not be confused with commercial liquid-protein diets or weight-loss shakes and drinks. Very-low-calorie diets must be designed for specific patients who are monitored carefully and are used for only short periods. Physicians will also refer patients to professional therapists or psychiatrists for help in changing eating behaviors. Without changing eating habits and exercise patterns, the lost weight will be regained quickly.

For morbidly obese individuals, dietary changes and behavior modification may be accompanied by bariatric surgery. Gastroplasty involves inserting staples to decrease the size of the stomach. Gastric banding is an inflatable band inserted around the upper stomach to create a small pouch and narrow passage into the remainder of the stomach. Bariatric surgery has become less risky in recent years due to innovations in equipment and surgical techniques. However, it is still performed only on patients for whom supervised diet and exercise strategies have failed, who are at least 100 lb (45 kg) overweight or twice their ideal body weight, and whose obesity seriously threatens their health. Risks and possible complications include infections, hernias, and blood clots. Overall, 10–20% of patients who undergo weight-loss surgery require additional operations to correct complications, more than 33% develop gallstones, and 30% develop nutritional deficiencies, such as anemia, osteoporosis, or metabolic bone disease.

Other bariatric surgical procedures—including liposuction, a purely cosmetic procedure in which a suction device removes fat from beneath the skin, and jaw wiring, which can damage gums and teeth and cause painful muscle spasms—have no place in obesity treatment.

Weight loss is recommended for obese children over age seven and for obese children over age two who have medical complications. Weight maintenance is an appropriate goal for children over the age of two who have no medical complications. Most treatment approaches to childhood obesity involve a combination of caloric restriction, physical exercise, and behavioral therapy. Bariatric surgery is considered as a last resort only for adolescents who are fully grown.

Drugs

The short-term use of prescription medications may assist some individuals in managing their condition, but it is never the sole treatment for obesity, nor are drugs ever considered as a cure for obesity. Diet drugs are designed to help medically at-risk obese patients "jump-start" their weight-loss effort and lose 10% or more of their starting body weight, in combination with a diet and exercise regimen. Prescription weight-loss drugs are approved by the U.S. Food and Drug Administration (FDA) only for patients with a BMI of 30 or above, or a BMI of 27 or above and an obesity-related condition, such as high blood pressure, type 2 diabetes, or dyslipidemia (abnormal amounts of fats in the blood). The weight is usually regained as soon as the drugs are discontinued, unless eating and exercise habits have changed.

Most appetite-suppressants are based on amphetamine. They increase levels of serotonin or catecholamine, brain chemicals that control feelings of fullness. Serotonin also regulates mood and may be linked to mood-related eating behaviors. Prescription weight-loss medications include:

• benzphetamine hydrochloride (Didrex)

• diethylpropion (Tenuate, Tenuate Dospan)

• mazindol (Mazanor, Sanorex)

• phendimetrazine (Bontril, Melfiat)

• phentermine (Adipex-P, Ionamin)

• lorcaserin hydrochloride (Belviq)

• phentermine and topiramate (Qsymia)

While most of the immediate side effects of appetite suppressants are harmless, their long-term effects may be unknown. Dexfenfluramine hydrochloride (Redux), fenfluramine (Pondimin), and the fenfluramine-phentermine combination (Fen-Phen) were taken off the market after they were shown to cause potentially fatal cardiac effects. Siburtramine (Meridia) was known to significantly elevate blood pressure and was taken off the market in 2010. Phenylpropanolamine, a component of many nonprescription weight-loss and cold and cough medications (Acutrim, Dex-A-Diet, Dexatrim, Phenldrine, Phenoxine, PPA, Propagest, Rhindecon, Unitrol) was removed from shelves because of an increased risk of stroke. Appetite suppressants can be habit-forming and have the potential for abuse. Appetite suppressants should not be used by patients taking monoamine oxidase inhibitors (MAOIs) and are not recommended for children.

Side effects of prescription and over-the-counter weight-loss products may include:

• constipation

• dry mouth

• headache

• irritability

• nausea

• nervousness

• sweating

Unlike appetite suppressants, orlistat is a lipase inhibitor that reduces the breakdown and absorption of dietary fat in the intestines. Both its prescription (Xenical) and nonprescription (Alli) forms are approved by the FDA. Orilstat is intended to be used with a calorie-controlled diet and exercise program. Side effects may include abdominal cramping, gas, fecal urgency, oily stools, frequent bowel movements, and diarrhea.

Other drugs are sometimes prescribed off-label for treating obesity. For example, fluoxetine (Prozac) is an antidepressant that sometimes aids in temporary weight loss. Side effects of this medication include diarrhea, fatigue, insomnia, nausea, and thirst.

Alternative

Functional food diets are newer, as yet unproven, approaches to weight loss:

• carbohydrates with a low glycemic index, which may help suppress appetite

• green tea extract, which may increase the body's energy expenditure

• chromium, which may encourage the burning of stored fat rather than lean muscle tissue

Various herbs and supplements are promoted for weight loss:

• Diuretic herbs, which increase urine production, can result in short-term weight loss, but do not help with lasting weight control. Increased urine output increases thirst to replace lost fluids and patients who use diuretics for an extended period of time eventually start retaining water anyway.

• In moderate doses, psyllium, a mucilaginous herb available in bulk-forming laxatives like Metamucil, absorbs fluid and provides a feeling of fullness.

• Red peppers and mustard may help encourage weight loss by accelerating the body's metabolic rate. They also cause thirst, so patients crave water instead of food.

• Walnuts can be a natural source of serotonin for providing a feeling of satiation.

• Dandelion (Taraxacum officinale) can increase metabolism and counter a desire for sugary foods.

• The amino acid 5-hydroxytryptophan (5-HTP), which is extracted from the seeds of Griffonia simplicifolia, is thought to increase serotonin levels in the brain. Patients should consult with their healthcare provider before taking 5-HTP, as it may interact with other medications and can have potentially serious side effects.

Acupressure and acupuncture can suppress food cravings. Visualization and meditation can create and reinforce a positive self-image that can enhance a patient's determination to lose weight. By improving physical strength, mental concentration, and emotional serenity, yoga can provide the same benefits. Patients who play soft slow music during meals often find that they eat less food, but enjoy it more.

Home remedies

Eating a reasonable balance of protein, carbohydrates, and high-quality fats are important for weight loss. Support and self-help groups—such as Overeaters Anonymous and TOPS (Taking Off Pounds Sensibly)—that promote nutritious, balanced diets can help patients maintain proper eating regimens. Many diet support groups also exist on the internet.

Fad dieting can have harmful health effects. Weight should be lost gradually and steadily by decreasing calories while maintaining an adequate nutrient intake and level of physical activity. A daily caloric intake of no less than 1,200 calories for women and no less than 1,500 for men enables most people to lose weight safely. A loss of about 1–2 lb (1 kg) per week is recommended. Diets of less than 1,200 calories a day should never be attempted unless prescribed and monitored by a physician.

At least 60–90 minutes of daily moderate-intensity physical activity is usually recommended to maintain weight loss. Obese people who have led sedentary lives may need monitoring to avoid injury as they begin to increase their physical activity. Exercise should be increased gradually, perhaps starting by climbing stairs instead of taking elevators, followed by walking, biking, or swimming at a slow pace. Eventually 15-minute walks can be built up to brisk, 45–60-minute walks.

The American Academy of Family Physicians offers advice for families with children who need to maintain or lose weight:

- Weight-loss interventions should begin as soon as possible in children over two years of age.
- The family must be ready for change; if not, the program is likely to fail.
- The physician should educate the family as to the medical complications of obesity.
- All family members and caregivers should be involved in the treatment program.
- The physician should encourage the child and family, not criticize them.
- The treatment program should institute permanent changes in eating habits and other behaviors.
- The program should help the family to make small gradual changes.
- The program should include learning ways to monitor eating and exercise.
- Goals should be realistic; even a 5% weight loss, if maintained, can reduce risks to health.

Prognosis

The primary factor in achieving and maintaining weight loss is a life-long commitment to sensible eating habits and regular exercise. As many as 85% of dieters who do not exercise on a regular basis regain their lost weight within two years and 90% regain it within five years. Short-term diet programs and repeatedly losing and regaining weight encourage the storage of fat and may increase the risk of heart disease.

However, prudent dieting and exercise are not quick cures for obesity. With decreased caloric intake, the body breaks down muscle for carbohydrates. Much of the early weight loss on a very low-calorie diet represents loss of muscle tissue rather than fat. Similarly, fat is not easily accessed as fuel for exercise.

The chronically or habitually obese tend to come from families with a larger number of risk factors for obesity and have a much more difficult time losing weight than the newly obese. Likewise, previously obese people have a high probability of reverting to obesity.

When obesity develops in childhood, the total number of fat cells increases (hyperplastic obesity), whereas in adulthood the total amount of fat in each cell increases (hypertrophic obesity). Patients who were obese as children may have up to five times as many fat cells as a patient who became obese as an adult. Decreasing the amount of energy (food) consumed or increasing the amount of energy expended reduces the amount of fat in the cells—but does not reduce the number of fat cells already present—and this process is slow, just like the accumulation of excess fat.

Neonatal obesity does not necessarily translate into childhood or adult obesity, but there is an increased probability if the child is born or adopted into a family with multiple obese members. Likewise, excess weight in a child under the age of three does not necessarily predict adult obesity unless one of the parents is obese.

Summer camps specializing in habitually obese children, especially girls, have little long-term success in reducing obesity and a high degree of recidivism for habitual overeating and under-exercising. About 30% of overweight girls eventually develop **eating disorders**.

- Am I obese?
- What factors are contributing to my obesity?
- How can I bring my weight within a normal BMI range?
- Can I get help planning meals?
- How should I increase my exercise level?
- Are any of the advertised obesity diets and products effective or are they dangerous?

According to the Obesity Prevention Center at the University of Minnesota, obesity-control programs that rely on educational messages encouraging greater physical activity and a healthier diet have been only modestly successful. The best outcomes have been with children's programs that have high levels of physical activity.

Prevention

Prevention is far superior to any available treatment for obesity. Obesity can be prevented by eating a healthy diet, being physically active, and making lifestyle changes that help maintain a normal weight. Examples include

- eating smaller portions of food
- taking the time to prepare healthy meals
- avoiding processed foods
- parking farther away from a store
- walking or bicycling instead of driving
- walking the dog instead of just letting it out

Obesity experts suggest that monitoring fat consumption, as well as counting calories, is a key to preventing excess weight gain. The National Cholesterol Education Program of the National Heart, Lung, and Blood Institute maintains that only 30% of calories should be derived from fat and only one-third of those should be saturated fats. High concentrations of saturated fats are found in meat, poultry, and dairy products. Fat replacers or substitutes are now added to many foods. They reduce the amount of fat and usually also reduce the number of calories. It is not clear what effect these will have on the long-term battle against obesity.

However, total caloric intake cannot be ignored, since it is usually the slow accumulation of excess calories, regardless of the source, that results in obesity. A single daily cookie providing 25 excess calories will result in a 5 lb. weight gain by the end of one year. Because most people eat more than they think they do, keeping a detailed and honest food diary is a useful way

to assess eating habits. Eating three balanced, moderate-portion meals a day—with the main meal at mid-day—is a more effective way to prevent obesity than fasting or crash diets that trick the body into believing it is starving. After 12 hours without food, the body has depleted its stores of readily available energy and begins to protect itself for the long term. Metabolic rate starts to slow and muscle tissue is broken down for the raw materials needed for energy maintenance.

The U.S. Department of Agriculture (USDA) food plate, called *MyPlate* to distinguish it from the replaced food pyramid, contains recommendations on diet and exercise based on the *Dietary Guidelines for Americans 2010*, tailored for an individual's BMI. It includes recommendations on physical activity and in five food categories: grains, vegetables, fruits, dairy, and proteins.

It has been suggested that there may be little benefit in encouraging weight loss in older people, especially when there are no obesity-related complications or when promoting changes in lifelong eating habits creates stress. However, studies have shown that weight loss in seniors can lower the incidence of arthritis, diabetes, and other conditions, reduce cardiovascular risk factors, and improve well being. Increased physical activity in the elderly also improves muscle strength and endurance.

The poor prognosis for reversing adult obesity makes childhood prevention imperative. Unhealthy eating patterns and behaviors associated with obesity can be addressed by programs in **nutrition**, exercise, and stress management involving the entire family.

Resources

BOOKS

Adolfsson, Birgitta, and Marilynn S. Arnold. *Behavioral Approaches to Treating Obesity*. Alexandria, VA: American Diabetes Association, 2006.

Gard, Michael. *The End of the Obesity Epidemic*. London: Routledge, 2011.

Hardy, George T., ed. *Encyclopedia of Nutrition Research*. Hauppauge, NY: Nova Science Publishers, 2011.

Hassink, Sandra Gibson. *Guide to Pediatric Weight Management and Obesity*. Philadelphia: Lippincott Williams and Wilkins, 2007.

Thornley, Simon. *Sickly Sweet: Sugar, Refined Carbohydrate, Addiction and Global Obesity*. Hauppauge, NY: Nova Science Publishers, 2011.

PERIODICALS

World Health Organization (WHO) expert consultation. "Appropriate Body-Mass Index for Asian Populations and its Implications for Policy and Intervention Strategies." *Lancet* 363, no. 9403 (2004): 157–63. http://dx.doi.org/10.1016/S0140-6736(03)15268-3 (accessed August 30, 2012).

Yates, Erika A., Alison K. Macpherson, and Jennifer L. Kuk. "Secular Trends in the Diagnosis and Treatment of Obesity Among US Adults in the Primary Care Setting." *Obesity* 20, no. 9 (2012): 1909–14. http://dx.doi.org/10.1038/oby.2011.271 (accessed August 30, 2012).

WEBSITES

Centers for Disease Control and Prevention. "Adult Obesity Facts." http://www.cdc.gov/obesity/data/adult.html (accessed August 24, 2012).

Centers for Disease Control and Prevention. "Body Percentile Calculator for Child and Teen." http://apps.nccd.cdc.gov/dnpabmi/Calculator.aspx (accessed August 13, 2012).

Centers for Disease Control and Prevention. "Overweight and Obesity." http://www.cdc.gov/obesity/index.html (accessed August 13, 2012).

National Heart, Lung, and Blood Institute. "Assessing Your Weight and Health Risk." National Institutes of Health. http://www.nhlbi.nih.gov/health/public/heart/obesity/lose_wt/risk.htm (accessed August 13, 2012).

MedlinePlus. "Obesity." U.S. National Library of Medicine, National Institutes of Health. http://www.nlm.nih.gov/medlineplus/obesity.html (accessed August 13, 2012).

U.S. Department of Agriculture, National Agricultural Library. "Weight and Obesity." Food and Nutrition Information Center. http://fnic.nal.usda.gov/weight-and-obesity (accessed August 30, 2012).

U.S. Department of Agriculture and U.S. Department of Health and Human Services. *Dietary Guidelines for Americans, 2010.* 7th ed. Washington, DC: U.S. Government Printing Office, December 2010. http://health.gov/dietaryguidelines (accessed February 22, 2012).

Weight-Control Information Network. "Overweight and Obesity Statistics. National Institute of Diabetes and Digestive and Kidney Disorders." http://win.niddk.nih.gov/statistics/index.htm (accessed August 24, 2012).

ORGANIZATIONS

Academy of Nutrition and Dietetics, 120 South Riverside Plz., Ste. 2000, Chicago, IL 60606-6995, (312) 899-0040, (800) 877-1600, amacmunn@eatright.org, http://www.eatright.org

American Society for Metabolic and Bariatric Surgery, 100 SW 75th Street, Ste. 201, Gainesville, FL 32607, (352) 331-4900, Fax: (352) 331-4975, info@asmbs.org, http://www.asbs.org

Obesity Prevention Center, University of Minnesota, 1300 S Second St., Ste. 300, Minneapolis, MN 55454, (612) 625-6200, umopc@epi.umn.edu, http://www.ahc.umn.edu/opc/home.html

Overeaters Anonymous, PO Box 44020, Rio Rancho, NM 87174, (505) 891-2664, Fax: (505) 891-4320, http://www.oa.org.

The Obesity Society, 8757 Georgia Ave., Ste. 1320, Silver Spring, MD 20910, (301) 563-6526, Fax: (301) 563-6595, http://www.obesity.orghttp://www.obesity.org/resources-for/consumer.htm

Weight-Control Information Network (WIN), 1 WIN Way, Bethesda, MD 20892-3665, (202) 828-1025, (877) 946-4627, Fax: (202) 828-1028, win@http://win.niddk.nih.gov, http://win.niddk.nih.gov.

Rosalyn Carson-DeWitt, MD
Tish Davidson, AM
William Atkins

Occupational health

Definition

The National Institute of Environmental Health Sciences defines occupational health as "the identification and control of the risks arising from physical, chemical, and other workplace hazards in order to establish and maintain a safe and healthy working environment."

Purpose

Pursuit of occupational safety and health consists of a number of elements, including first recognizing the threats that may be present within any given occupation, followed by plans and actions to eliminate or reduce those hazards from the everyday life of workers in the occupation. Occupational health also involves educating workers and nonworkers about possible hazards and ways that they can avoid these risks in everyday life. It may also may involve the treatment of accidents that occur on the job, as well as recovery and rehabilitation of workers who have been hurt at work.

Description

Among the hazards encountered in workplaces are dangerous machinery, electrical hazards, chemical substances and solvents, heavy metals, noxious gases, and noise. These hazards can cause a wide variety of injuries, such as bruises, sprains, strains, cuts, and broken bones; repetitive motion injuries, such as carpal tunnel syndrome; vision problems that may be as serious as loss of eyesight; hearing problems that may extend to include permanent deafness; acute and chronic illnesses resulting from exposure to disease-causing agents and toxins; **birth defects**; **burns** and illness caused by exposure to **radiation**; and external and internal bodily damage resulting from direct contact with harmful substances. Some of the specific effects of occupational accidents include **asthma** and other types of **allergies**; bloodborne infectious diseases (such as HIV/AIDS and **hepatitis**); many forms of **cancer**; respiratory disorders; skin diseases; emotional **stress**; and traumatic incident stress (TIS).

Procedures for protecting workers against work–related injuries and disease are now highly developed and widely available. Some examples of those procedures include the following:

- Adult Blood Lead Epidemiology and Surveillance (ABLES) is a program for monitoring the lead concentration of workers exposed to metal.

- Chest radiography is available to check on the respiratory health of workers who are regularly exposed to possible carcinogenic substances and other hazards, such as silica and asbestos.

- Chemical databases are extensive and detailed lists of all chemicals to which workers might be exposed, the hazards they pose, and the levels at which they are likely to begin causing damage to one's health.

- Goggles, face shields, safety glasses, full–face respirators, and other equipment are now available for protecting workers against a variety of eye injuries, such as liquid chemicals, metal slivers, pieces of wood or plastic, or blunt impact from larger objects.

- Methane monitors can be used to measure the concentration of this flammable and explosive gas in mines.

- Various types of respirators are available to remove harmful materials from the air a worker breathes or to supply fresh, clean air to workers.

- Regular spirometry testing can be used to measure the health of workers who are exposed to substances that have the potential for compromising their respiratory function.

A number of federal, state, and local agencies oversee the health and safety environment in workplaces. The two largest of these on a federal level are the Occupational Safety and Health Administration (OSHA) and the National Institute for Occupational Safety and Health (NIOSH). OSHA is a division of the U.S. Department of Labor that was established in 1970 to assure safe and healthy working conditions for all Americans by establishing and enforcing standards for good health and safety and to provide education, training, and assistance for workers and their employers. Since its founding, OSHA has issued hundreds of specific standards that deal with virtually every imaginable risk or hazard that workers may face on the job. A summary of those standards is available on the OSHA home page at http://www.osha.gov/pls/oshaweb/owasrch.search_form?p_doc_type=STANDARDS&p_toc_level=1&p_keyvalue=1910. NIOSH was established simultaneously with OSHA in 1970 to serve as the research arm for occupational health within the U.S. government. It is a division of the **Centers for Disease Control and Prevention** that not only conducts and supports original research, but also, based on that research, makes recommendations for new procedures and standards dealing with occupational health and safety. The NIOSH website is an invaluable resource for information on a wide range of occupational risks and hazards ranging from specific chemicals, such as ammonia and antimony, to large-scale issues such as commercial fishing hazards and mining risks, to somewhat more mundane topics such as body art, bicycle saddles, and **reproductive health**.

Federal law permits individual states to develop and implement their own occupational safety and health programs, as long as they provide a level of protection to workers that is at least as great as that provided by federal regulations. As of 2012, 21 states and Puerto Rico had such plans. In addition, four states and the U.S. Virgin Islands had federally approved plans that apply to public workers, but not to private employees.

Professional publications

Both OSHA and NIOSH have extensive lists of publications, usually available for free, that cover almost every imaginable aspect of occupational safety and health. The OSHA list, for example, currently has publications on aerial lifts, amputations, asbestos, blood-borne pathogens, **carbon monoxide poisoning**, catheters, chipper machines, combustible dust, **distracted driving**, protection against falls in a variety of occuptions, grain handling, hand **hygiene**, hydrogen sulfide, ladder safety, and many other subjects.

Resources

BOOKS

Gatchel, Robert, and Izabela Z. Schultz. *Handbook of Occupational Health and Wellness*. New York: Springer Verlag, 2012.

Reese, Charles D. *Accident/Incident Prevention Techniques*, 2nd ed. Boca Raton, FL: Taylor & Francis, 2012.

Vickerstaff, Sarah, Chris Phillipson, and Ross Wilkie, eds. *Work, Health and Wellbeing: The Challenges of Managing Health at Work*. Bristol, UK: Policy Press, 2011.

PERIODICALS

Ikonen, Annukka, et al. "Work-Related Primary Care in Occupational Health Physician's Practice." *Journal of Occupational Rehabilitation* 22. 1. (2012): 88–96

Rand, Robert W., Stephen E. Ambrose, and Carmen M. E. Krogh. "Occupational Health and Industrial Wind Turbines: A Case Study." *Bulletin of Science, Technology & Society* 31. 5. (2011): 359–62

Thompson, M. C., and J. E. Wachs. "Occupational Health Nursing in the United States." *Workplace Health and Safety* 60. 3. (2012): 127–33

WEBSITES

Occupational Health. Medline Plus. http://www.nlm.nih.gov/medlineplus/occupationalhealth.html (accessed October 11, 2012).

Occupational Health. World Health Organization. http://www.who.int/topics/occupational_health/en/ (accessed October 11, 2012).

ORGANIZATIONS

National Institute for Occupational Safety & Health, 395 E St., S.W., Washington, DC 20201, (202) 245-0625, http://www.cdc.gov/niosh/contact/officers.html, http://www.cdc.gov/niosh/.

U.S. Department of Labor. Occupational Safety & Health Administration, 200 Constitution Ave., Washington, DC 20210, (800) 321-OSHA (6742), http://www.osha.gov/ecor_form.html, www.osha.gov.

David E. Newton, EdD

Onchocerciasis

Definition

Onchocerciasis, or river blindness, is an infection that is caused by a parasitic worm (*Oncherocerca volvulus*) that is spread through the bite of black flies. The common name of the disease comes from the tendency of the worm to infect the eye.

Demographics

The **World Health Organization (WHO)** estimates that 37 million people around the world are infected and more than 90 million live in areas that put them at risk. The disease is found in 30 African nations, and 99 percent of victims live in Africa. However, onchocerciasis occurs in Yemen, Mexico, Guatemala, Ecuador, Columbia, Venezuela, and Brazil. Common to these areas are blackflies of the genus *Simulium*. Because of the life cycle of the parasite, casual visitors to these areas are not at risk of developing the infection, but those who visit these areas for extended periods of time (more than three months), such as Peace Corps volunteers and missionaries, may be at risk.

Causes and symptoms

Causes

Onchocerciasis is caused by a parasitic worm. The worm needs two hosts to complete its life cycle: a human being and a blackfly. If a blackfly bites a person who is infected, it can pick up microscopic worm larvae, or microfilariae, from their location in the skin. Once inside the fly, the larvae develop over the next two weeks into a form that is infectious to humans, first entering the midgut of the fly and then its thoracic muscles, then migrating through the body to the head. Ultimately, they reach the proboscis, where they are injected into the skin of another person when the fly next bites. The larvae then remain encased in nodules under the skin as they slowly develop into adult worms. The nodules contain both male and female worms. Males can reach a length of 42 mm while females can measure 33 to 50 cm in length. Encased in their nodules, the worms can live for 15 years; for nine of those years, females are capable of producing microfilariae, which can survive for two years. The microfilariae are usually found in the skin and lymphatic ducts of connective tissue. They are occasionally found in sputum, blood, and urine.

Symptoms

Symptoms result from dead or dying larvae. Larvae that die in the eye cause lesions on the cornea. When these lesions are first formed, they can be reversed. If untreated, they lead to permanent clouding of the cornea that causes blindness. Decreased vision or blindness can also result from inflammation of the optic nerve.

The presence of the larvae does not always trigger a response from the immune system that leads to symptoms. However, individuals who do have symptoms may have vision changes or itchy skin, and the nodules may be felt under the skin. Inflammation can cause long-term damage to the skin and result in thinning as well as a discoloration called "leopard skin."

Diagnosis

Onchocerciasis can be diagnosed in several ways. If nodules are present, one can be removed and examined for the presence of adult worms. A skin shaving can be taken to determine the presence of larvae. Six samples are taken and placed in solutions (such as saline) and observed to see if larvae emerge from the samples. If larvae are not observed, a polymerase chain reaction is often performed as a diagnostic tool. Antibody tests can be used, but these tests cannot distinguish between current and past infections.

Treatment

The recommended treatment for onchocerciasis is ivermectin. The drug must be taken every six months for the life span of the adult worms or for as long as signs of infection are present.

Parasite—an organism that must live on or in another organism in order to survive

Doxycycline eliminates adult worms by killing the bacteria the worms depend on to survive. However, doxycycline can cause severe side effects if another filarial parasite called Loa loa is also present. Before doxycycline is used, The presence of Loa loa should be determined.

Prevention

The best **prevention** methods involve avoiding or preventing blackfly bites. Wearing long sleeves and long pants, as well as wearing clothes that have been treated with permethrin, are recommended. Using an insect repellant containing DEET is also effective.

Efforts and solutions

Efforts to reduce the incidence of onchocerciasis have been spearheaded by the **WHO**. They include spraying of blackfly breeding areas, and the widespread administration of ivermectin, which has been donated by Merck and Co. As a result of these efforts, millions of people who would have suffered skin problems and blindness have been spared. In the Americas, Columbia (in 2007) and Ecuador (in 2008) were the first nations to announce that disease transmission had been halted through these efforts. Mexico and Guatemala made similar announcements in 2011.

Resources

PERIODICALS

Vieia, Juan C,, et al. "Impact of long-term treatment of onchocerciasis with ivermectin in Equador: potential for elimination of infect." *BMC Medicine* 2007 5:9

WEBSITES

Carter Center. "River Blindness Program," accessed September 1, 2012, http://www.cartercenter.org/health/river_blindness/index.html
Centers for Disease Control and Prevention. "Parasites: Onchocerciasis (also known as River Blindness)" accessed September 1, 2012, http://www.cdc.gov/parasites/onchocerciasis/
World Health Organization, "Onchocerciasis," accessed September 1, 2012, http://www.who.int/topics/onchocerciasis

ORGANIZATIONS

Centers for Disease Control and Prevention, 1600 Clifton Road, Atlanta, GA USA 30333, (800) 232-4636, cdcinfo@cdc.gov, www.cdc.gov
World Health Organization, Avenue Appia 20, 1211 Geneva 27, Switzerland 30333, 41 22 (791) 21 11, Fax: 41 22 (791) 21 11, www.who.int.

Fran Hodgkins

Oral health *see* **Dental health**

Organ donation and transplantation

Definition

Organ transplantation involves the giving of a healthy body part from either a living or dead individual to another person.

Purpose

The purpose of organ transplantation is to improve and prolong the life of an ill or impaired individual.

Demographics

In the United States, the number of people who need donated organs outweighs the number of people who donate an organ. At the end of July 2012, according to the U.S. Department of Health and Human Services's Organ Procurement and Transplantation Network (OPTN), about 124,600 people were awaiting donor organs. Of those, about 99,200 needed a kidney donation, and about 16,800 needed a liver donation. Of the 124,600 who were waiting for an organ donation, about 84,000 had been waiting for at least a year, and more than 37,000 of those had been waiting for at least three years.

Most transplanted organs come from deceased donors. The OPTN reported that more than 57 percent of the 14,145 organs that were transplanted in 2011 came from deceased donors.

A special need exists for donors from minority ethnic groups. For example, African Americans have a higher need for organ transplantation than the population overall due to increased incidence of certain medical conditions, such as kidney disease, as well as high blood pressure (hypertension), which can lead to kidney failure. Individuals of Hispanic, Asian, and Pacific Islander descent are also more likely to have kidney disease, and American Indians are more likely to have diabetes. Although matches are possible between people of different ethnic or racial groups, the likelihood of an appropriate genetic match (to prevent organ rejection) is

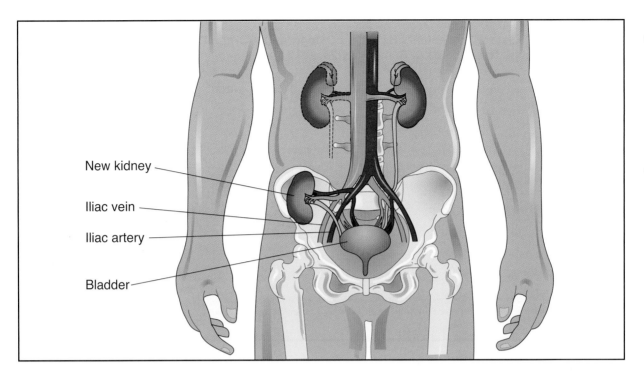

Kidney transplantation involves the surgical attachment of a functioning kidney, or graft, from a donor to a patient with end-stage renal disease (ESRD). During the procedure, the surgeon makes an incision in the patient's flank and implants the new kidney above the pelvic bone and below the non-functioning kidney by suturing the kidney artery and vein to the patient's iliac artery and vein. The ureter of the new kidney is then attached directly to the bladder of the patient. *(Illustration by Electronic Illustrators Group. © 2013 Cengage Learning)*

much higher within those groups. Although the percentage of donors from each minority ethnic group is similar to the percentage of donors from the overall population, the increased transplant demand makes additional donors from these groups important.

Internationally, the rate of organ donation varies with religious and cultural norms and the level of sophistication of medical care. Many countries, such as the United States, are opt-in donation countries. This means that an individual must positively state his or her desire to donate body parts after death. A few countries have an opt-out donor system, where individuals must state before death that they *do not* want to donate organs when they die.

Description

Organ transplantation involves the matching of a person willing to give a healthy body part to an ill person who needs it. There are two types: living donation and cadaver donation (donation after death). In the United States and in many other countries, the costs of organ donation and transplantation may be covered by health insurance. Individual insurance policies vary, and coverage differs, so donors and

transplant recipients should ask their insurance companies detailed questions before the procedure to understand any financial obligations they may incur. In the United States, both citizens and non-citizens can donate and receive body parts, but it is illegal to buy an organ or to receive money for one.

In the United States, individuals who are seeking an organ transplant place their names on the OPTN/United Network for Organ Sharing (UNOS) waiting list, which is a computer database containing patient information. To sign up, each patient must have a doctor referral, must select and then contact one of the 200-plus transplant hospitals across the United States, and must schedule a consultation to determine whether he or she is a good candidate for a transplant. UNOS maintains a centralized computer network, called UNet[SM], that connects all the transplant centers and organ-donation organizations, and matches donated organs to waiting patients.

Several factors can affect the length of time a patient must wait to receive a transplant. These include:

- medical urgency—how long the patient can survive without a transplant

- blood type of the patient and the donor

U.S. Waiting List for Transplants Based on Data from the Organ Procurement and Transplantation Network as of September 29, 2012

All Ages	All Organs	Kidney	Liver	Pancreas	Kidney / Pancreas	Heart	Lung	Heart / Lung	Intestine
	115,837	93,860	16,075	1,233	2,150	3,324	1,638	51	261
< 1 Year	99	5	48	0	0	37	3	1	7
1-5 Years	496	166	164	34	2	95	10	2	108
6-10 Years	346	147	97	11	0	76	9	2	35
11-17 Years	823	512	178	6	2	89	38	3	21
18-34 Years	10,673	9,201	728	175	426	329	184	10	22
35-49 Years	28,596	24,627	2,275	611	1,227	649	231	17	32
50-64 Years	52,633	40,425	9,907	383	484	1,498	846	13	32
65 +	22,179	18,783	2,679	13	9	551	317	3	4

Source: Organ Procurement and Transplantation Network administered by the United Network for Organ Sharing under contract with the U.S. Department of Health and Human Services. Available at http://optn.transplant.hrsa.gov/data/

(Illustration by Electronic Illustrators Group. © 2013 Cengage Learning)

- size and type of organ
- height and weight of transplant candidate, which may limit the pool of potential donor organs
- time on the waiting list
- the distance between the donor's hospital and the potential donor organ, because some organs must be transplanted within a short timeframe
- specific criteria that the transplant center may mandate

Living donation

Donation of a body part by a living person is the less common type of organ donation. Usually, the person who donates is biologically related to the recipient (for example, a parent, sibling, or cousin). Related individuals are more likely to have the same blood type and similar immune-system markers. This helps prevent organ rejection by the recipient's body. Sometimes a relative is willing to donate an organ but is not an adequate match for the recipient. In that case, UNOS may be able to arrange a paired organ exchange with another donor-recipient pair. Living donor transplants are slightly more successful (rejected less frequently) than after-death donations.

To be a living donor, the individual cannot have certain diseases such as **cancer**, HIV infection, **hepatitis**, or major organ disease. Depending on the type of cancer, however, some cancer survivors can become organ donors, especially if a long cancer-free interval has passed. Minors must have parental permission to donate, and all donors undergo extensive medical testing before the donation occurs.

The types of body parts that can be donated by a living person include.

- kidney (most common)
- liver (second most common)
- lung
- intestine
- pancreas
- bone marrow

Donation after death

Individuals who want to donate body parts after death should indicate this desire on their driver's license and in a living will or medical directive, as well as making their wishes known to relatives. Donation after death does not disfigure the body, and a regular funeral can be held. No age limit exists for a donation after death. Individuals can specify in advance which organs they want or do not want to donate. Agreeing to donate after death does not compromise the quality of medical care the individual receives before death.

Organs and tissues that can be transplanted after death include:

- kidneys
- liver

- lungs
- heart
- pancreas
- intestines
- cornea
- skin
- bone
- cartilage
- tendons
- ligaments
- veins
- heart valves
- middle ear

Benefits

The benefit to the recipient is an extended and improved life. On the donor side, many living donors and the families of deceased donors find satisfaction in knowing that their donation has given the gift of life to another person.

Precautions

Living donors undergo extensive medical testing in order to ensure that they are healthy enough to make a donation and that the donated material is compatible with the recipient, as organ and tissue rejection is the most common cause of transplant failure.

Preparation

Living donors receive counseling and must sign a statement of informed consent. Minors must have parental consent to be living donors. Living donors receive a standard pre-operative work-up as well as extensive crossmatching with the recipient to ensure tissue compatibility.

Individuals who wish to donate after death should make this known on their driver's license and in a living will or medical directive, as well as informing their families and their doctors.

Aftercare

The length of the hospital stay and specific aftercare for living donors depends on the organ donated.

Risks

For living donors, the risks are the same as with any operation, mainly infection at the surgical site, uncontrolled bleeding, and adverse reaction to anesthesia. People can live healthy, active lives after donating a kidney, lung, or part of a liver or pancreas. The risk remains, however, that damage by disease or injury to the remaining organ may result in medical problems.

Research and general acceptance

The medical community accepts ethical organ donation as a positive, life-saving procedure. Most religions support organ donation, but when in doubt, individuals should consult their religious leaders.

Efforts and Solutions

One major issue with organ donation is the mismatch between the number of donor organs available and the number of organs needed by patients. Worldwide, roughly 100,000 individuals undergo organ transplantation every year, but many patients remain on waiting lists often as their health deteriorates. This disparity sets up a demand for organs that is sometimes satisfied through the black market. In these cases, which most frequently occur in nations with large, poor populations, buyers arrange the purchase of organs from donors who are in dire financial straits, and unethical doctors then perform transplant operations for affluent transplant patients who are willing to pay for the service. The donors typically receive little for the organs they sell.

A 2011 paper published in *The Lancet* by Francis Delmonico of Harvard University and others, called for governments to "systematically address the needs of their countries according to a legal framework" to help quell this black market activity. The authors asserted that each country or region should strive to provide a sufficient number of organs from within its own population to meet the needs of its citizens, and that the design of those donation programs should be guided by **World Health Organization (WHO)** ethics principles. Specifically, the authors called for each government to develop a framework of legislation with regulatory oversight policy; a supported program to integrate the donation of organs from deceased individuals into the national health system; an ethical practice of live donation that ensures donor safety, donation, and transplantation practices in line with worldwide ethics standards; and a program of preventive medicine that will help decrease the number of needed organ transplants.

Resources

BOOKS

Klein Andrew, Clive Lewis, and Joren Madsen. *Organ Transplantation: A Clinical Guide.* Cambridge, UK: Cambridge University Press, 2011.

Hricik, Donald (ed). *Primer on Transplantation.* 3rd ed. Oxford, UK: Wiley Blackwell, 2011.

PERIODICAL

Delmonico, Francis L., Beatriz Dom'nguez-Gil, Rafael Matesanz, and Luc Noel. "A call for government accountability to achieve national self-sufficiency in organ donation and transplantation." *The Lancet* 378, no. 9800 (2011): 1414–8.

WEBSITES

Becoming a Donor. OrganDonor.gov, U.S. Department of Health and Human Services. http://organdonor.gov/becomingdonor/index.html (accessed August 8, 2012).

"Can I Donate My Organs if I've Had Cancer?" American Cancer Society. http://www.cancer.org/Treatment/SurvivorshipDuringandAfterTreatment/can-i-donate-my-organs (accessed August 8, 2012).

"Living Donation." United Network for Organ Sharing. http://www.unos.org/donation/index.php?topic=living_donation (accessed August 8, 2012).

"OPTN: Organ Procurement and Transplantation Network." U.S. Department of Health and Human Services's Organ Procurement and Transplantation Network http://optn.transplant.hrsa.gov/ (accessed August 8, 2012).

"Organ Donation." MedlinePlus. http://www.nlm.nih.gov/medlineplus/organdonation.html (accessed August 8, 2012).

"Transplantation." World Health Organization. http://www.who.int/topics/transplantation/en/ (accessed August 8, 2012).

Transplant Living. Transplant Living, United Network for Organ Sharing. http://www.transplantliving.org/(accessed August 8, 2012).

"Why Donate?" OrganDonor.gov, U.S. Department of Health and Human Services http://organdonor.gov/whydonate/index.html (accessed August 8, 2012).

ORGANIZATIONS

Donate Life America, 701 E. Bird St., 16th Floor, Richmond, VA 23219, (804) 377-3580, http://www.donatelife.net

National Living Donor Assistance Center, 2461 S. Clark Street, Suite 640, Arlington, VA 22202, (703) 414-1600, NLDCA@livingdonorassistance.org, http://www.livingdonorassistance.org

United Network for Organ Sharing, P.O. Box 2484, Richmond, VA 23218, (804) 782-4800, http://www.unos.org.

Tish Davidson, AM
Leslie Mertz, Ph.D.

P

Pain

Definition

Pain is an unpleasant feeling that is conveyed to the brain by sensory neurons. The discomfort signals actual or potential injury to the body. However, pain is more than a sensation, or the physical awareness of pain; it also includes perception, the subjective interpretation of the discomfort. Perception gives information on the pain's location and intensity and something about its nature. The various conscious and unconscious responses to both sensation and perception, including the emotional response, add further definition to the overall concept of pain.

Purpose

Pain serves to alert a person to potential or actual damage to the body. The definition of damage is quite broad: pain can arise from injury as well as disease. After a pain message has been received and interpreted, further pain can be counterproductive. Pain can have a negative impact on a person's quality of life and impede recovery from illness or injury, thus contributing to escalating health care costs. Unrelieved pain can become a syndrome in its own right and cause a downward spiral in a person's health and emotional outlook. Managing pain properly facilitates recovery, prevents additional health complications, and improves an individual's quality of life.

The experiencing of pain is a completely unique occurrence for each person, a complex combination of several factors other than the pain itself. It is influenced by:

- Ethnic and cultural values. In some cultures, tolerating pain is related to showing strength and endurance. In others, pain is considered punishment for misdeeds.
- Age. Many people have been taught that grownups never cry. On the other hand, in some cultures, the elderly are allowed to complain freely about pain and discomfort.
- Anxiety and stress. This factor is related to being in a strange or unfamiliar place, such as a hospital, and the fear of the unknown consequences of the pain and the condition causing it, which can all combine to make pain feel more severe. For patients being treated for pain, knowing the duration of activity of an analgesic leads to anxiety about the return of pain when the drug wears off. This anxiety can make the pain more severe. In addition, patients who interpret their pain as meaning that their disease is recurring or getting worse often experience pain as more severe.
- Fatigue and depression. It is known that pain in itself can actually cause emotional depression. Fatigue from lack of sleep or the illness itself also contributes to depressed feelings.

Description

Pain arises from any number of situations. Injury is a major cause, but pain may also arise from an illness. It may accompany a psychological condition, such as depression, or may even occur in the absence of a recognizable trigger.

Acute pain

Acute pain often results from tissue damage, such as a skin burn or broken bone. Acute pain can also be associated with headaches or muscle cramps. This type of pain usually goes away as the injury heals, or the cause of the pain (stimulus) is removed.

To understand acute pain, it is necessary to understand the nerves that support it. Nerve cells, or neurons, perform many functions in the body. Although their general purpose, providing an interface between the brain and the body, remains constant, their capabilities vary widely. Certain types of neurons are capable of transmitting a pain signal to the brain.

As a group, these pain-sensing neurons are called nociceptors, and virtually every surface and organ of the body is wired with them. The central part of these cells is located in the spine, and they send threadlike projections to every part of the body. Nociceptors are classified according to the stimulus that prompts them to transmit a pain signal. Thermoreceptive nociceptors are stimulated by temperatures that are potentially tissue damaging. Mechanoreceptive nociceptors respond to a pressure stimulus that may cause injury. Polymodal nociceptors are the most sensitive nociceptors and can respond to temperature and pressure. Polymodal nociceptors also respond to chemicals released by cells in the area from which the pain originates.

Nerve cell endings, or receptors, are at the front end of pain sensation. A stimulus at this part of the nociceptor unleashes a cascade of neurotransmitters (chemicals that transmit information within the nervous system) in the spine. Each neurotransmitter has a purpose. For example, substance P relays the pain message to nerves leading to the spinal cord and brain. These neurotransmitters may also stimulate nerves leading back to the site of the injury. This response prompts cells in the injured area to release chemicals that not only trigger an immune response but also influence the intensity and duration of the pain.

Chronic and abnormal pain

Chronic pain refers to pain that persists after an injury heals, **cancer** pain, pain related to a persistent or degenerative disease, and long-term pain from an unidentifiable cause. It is estimated that one in three people in the United States will experience chronic pain at some point in their lives. Of these people, approximately 50 million are either partially or completely disabled.

Chronic pain may be caused by the body's response to acute pain. In the presence of continued stimulation of nociceptors, changes occur within the nervous system. Changes at the molecular level are dramatic and may include alterations in genetic transcription of neurotransmitters and receptors. These changes may also occur in the absence of an identifiable cause; one of the frustrating aspects of chronic pain is that the stimulus may be unknown. For example, the stimulus cannot be identified in as many as 85% of individuals suffering lower back pain.

Scientists have long recognized a relationship between depression and chronic pain. In 2004, a survey of California adults diagnosed with major depressive disorder revealed that more than half of them also suffered from chronic pain.

Other types of abnormal pain include allodynia, hyperalgesia, and phantom limb pain. These types of pain often arise from some damage to the nervous system (neuropathic). Allodynia refers to a feeling of pain in response to a normally harmless stimulus. For example, some individuals who have suffered nerve damage as a result of viral infection experience unbearable pain from just the light weight of their clothing. Hyperalgesia is somewhat related to allodynia in that the response to a painful stimulus is extreme. In this case, a mild pain stimulus, such as a pin prick, causes a maximum pain response. Phantom limb pain occurs after a limb is amputated; although an individual may be missing the limb, the nervous system continues to perceive pain originating from the area.

Causes and symptoms

Pain is the most common symptom of injury and disease, and descriptions can range in intensity from a mere ache to unbearable agony. Nociceptors can send the brain information that indicates the location, nature, and intensity of the pain. For example, stepping on a nail sends an information-packed message to the brain: the foot has experienced a puncture wound that hurts a lot.

Pain perception also varies, depending on the location of the pain. The kinds of stimuli that cause a pain response on the skin include pricking, cutting, crushing, burning, and freezing. These same stimuli would not generate much of a response in the intestine. Intestinal pain arises from stimuli such as swelling, inflammation, and distension.

Diagnosis

Pain is considered in view of other symptoms and individual experiences. An observable injury, such as a broken bone, may be a clear indicator of the type of pain a person is suffering. Determining the specific cause of internal pain is more difficult. Other symptoms, such as fever or nausea, help narrow down the possibilities. In some cases, such as lower back pain, a specific cause might not be identifiable. Diagnosis of the disease causing a specific pain is further complicated by the fact that pain can be referred to (felt at) a skin site that does not seem to be connected to the site of the pain's origin. For example, pain arising from fluid accumulating at the base of the lung may be referred to the shoulder.

Since pain is a subjective experience, it may be very difficult to communicate its exact quality and intensity to other people. There are no diagnostic tests that can determine the quality or intensity of an individual's pain. Therefore, a medical examination will include many questions about where the pain is located, its intensity, and its nature. Questions are also directed at what kinds of things increase or relieve the pain, how long it has lasted, and whether there are any variations in it. An individual may be asked to use a pain scale to describe the pain. One such scale assigns a number to the pain intensity; for example, 0 may indicate no pain, and 10 may indicate the worst pain the person has ever experienced. Scales are modified for infants and children to accommodate their level of comprehension.

Treatment

Pharmacological options

There are many drugs aimed at preventing or treating pain. Nonopioid analgesics, narcotic analgesics, anticonvulsant drugs, and tricyclic antidepressants work by blocking the production, release, or uptake of neurotransmitters. Drugs from different classes may be combined to treat certain types of pain.

Nonopioid analgesics include common over-the-counter medications such as aspirin, acetaminophen (Tylenol), and ibuprofen (Advil). These are most often used for minor pain, but there are some prescription-strength medications in this class.

Narcotic analgesics are only available with a doctor's prescription and are used for more severe pain, such as cancer pain. These drugs include codeine, morphine, and methadone. **Addiction** to these painkillers is not as common as once thought. Many people who genuinely need these drugs for pain control typically do not become addicted. However, narcotic use is usually limited to patients thought to have a short life span (such as people with terminal cancer) or patients whose pain is only expected to last for a short time (such as people recovering from surgery). In 2004, the Drug Enforcement Administration (DEA) issued new guidelines to help physicians prescribe narcotics appropriately without fear of being arrested for prescribing the drugs beyond the scope of their medical practice. The DEA is trying to work with physicians to ensure that those who need drugs receive them, but to ensure that opioids are not abused.

Anticonvulsants, as well as antidepressant drugs, were initially developed to treat seizures and depression, respectively. However, it was discovered that these drugs also have pain-killing applications. Furthermore, since in cases of chronic or extreme pain, it is not unusual for an individual to suffer some degree of depression; antidepressants may serve a dual role. Commonly prescribed anticonvulsants for pain include phenytoin, carbamazepine, and clonazepam. Tricyclic antidepressants include doxepin, amitriptyline, and imipramine.

Intractable (unrelenting) pain may be treated by injections directly into or near the nerve that is transmitting the pain signal. These root blocks may also be useful in determining the site of pain generation. As the underlying mechanisms of abnormal pain are uncovered, other pain medications are being developed.

Nonpharmacological options

Pain treatment options that do not use drugs are often used as adjuncts to, rather than replacements for, drug therapy. One of the benefits of nondrug therapies is that an individual can take a more active role in pain management. Such relaxation techniques as yoga and meditation are used to focus the brain elsewhere than on the pain, decrease muscle tension, and reduce **stress**. Tension and stress can also be reduced through biofeedback, in which an individual consciously attempts to modify skin temperature, muscle tension, blood pressure, and heart rate.

Hypnosis is another nonpharmacological option for pain relief. Although doctors do not yet fully understand how hypnosis works, it is used successfully in some patients to manage pain related to childbirth, oral surgery, burn treatment, and other procedures that require the patient to remain conscious.

Participating in normal activities and exercising can also help control pain levels. Through physical therapy, an individual learns beneficial exercises for reducing stress, strengthening muscles, and staying fit. Regular exercise has been linked to production of endorphins, the body's natural painkillers.

Acupuncture involves the insertion of small needles into the skin at key points. Acupressure uses these same key points but involves applying pressure rather than inserting needles. Both of these methods may work by prompting the body to release endorphins. Applying heat or being massaged are very relaxing and help reduce stress. Transcutaneous electrical nerve stimulation (TENS) applies a small electric current to certain parts of nerves, potentially interrupting pain signals and inducing release of endorphins. To be effective, use of TENS should be medically supervised.

Two effective pain management treatments that have been used for generations are heat and cold. Both are used to treat acute and chronic pain. Ice is generally used to treat inflammation, especially acute injuries to knees and other joints. Treatment usually lasts three to five days. Often it is used as part of the RICE regimen: rest, ice, compression, and elevation. Heat therapy is generally used for increasing tensile strength, increasing blood flow to the injured area, and helping muscles and tendons to relax. Sometimes ice is used in the early stages of an acute injury, and then heat for the remainder of treatment. In recent years, scientists have identified heat and cold receptors in the body. This has allowed the development of medications, including patches, creams, and gels, that directly target these receptors, increasing the effectiveness of heat and cold treatments.

Invasive procedures

There are three types of invasive procedures that may be used to manage or treat pain: anatomic, augmentative, and ablative. These procedures involve surgery, and certain guidelines should be followed before carrying out a procedure with permanent effects. First, the cause of the pain must be clearly identified. Next, surgery should be done only if noninvasive procedures are ineffective. Third, any psychological issues should be addressed. Finally, there should be a reasonable expectation of success.

Anatomic procedures involve correcting the injury or removing the cause of pain. Relatively common anatomic procedures are decompression surgeries, such as repairing a herniated disk in the lower back or relieving the nerve compression related to carpal tunnel syndrome. Another anatomic procedure is neurolysis, also called a nerve block, which involves destroying a portion of a peripheral nerve.

Augmentative procedures include electrical stimulation or direct application of drugs to the nerves that are transmitting the pain signals. Electrical stimulation works on the same principle as TENS. In this procedure, instead of applying the current across the skin, electrodes are implanted to stimulate peripheral nerves or nerves in the spinal cord. Augmentative procedures also include implanted drug-delivery systems. In these systems, catheters are implanted in the spine to allow direct delivery of drugs to the central nervous system (CNS).

Ablative procedures are characterized by severing a nerve and disconnecting it from the CNS. However, this method might not address potential alterations within the spinal cord. These changes perpetuate pain messages and do not cease, even when the connection between the sensory nerve and the CNS is severed. With growing understanding of neuropathic pain and development of less invasive procedures, ablative procedures are used less frequently. However, they do have applications in select cases of peripheral neuropathy, cancer pain, and other disorders.

Preparation

Dealing with pain is often a long-term process that involves the use of some combination of the treatments described previously. That process is often referred to as a pain management program. The first step in any pain management program usually involves a thorough evaluation of the patient's pain, including a psychosocial

KEY TERMS

Acute pain—Pain in response to injury or another stimulus that resolves when the injury heals or the stimulus is removed.

Chronic pain—Pain that lasts beyond the term of an injury or painful stimulus. The term can also refer to cancer pain, pain from a chronic or degenerative disease, and pain from an unidentified cause.

Neuron—A nerve cell.

Neurotransmitters—Chemicals within the nervous system that transmit information from or between nerve cells.

Nociceptor—A neuron that is capable of sensing pain.

Referred pain—Pain felt at a site different from the location of the injured or diseased part of the body. Referred pain is due to the fact that nerve signals from several areas of the body may "feed" the same nerve pathway leading to the spinal cord and brain.

Stimulus—A factor capable of eliciting a response in a nerve.

as well as a physical assessment. Pain scales or questionnaires can be administered by a member of the healthcare team, although there is no single questionnaire that is universally accepted. Some questionnaires are verbal, while others use pictures or drawings to help the patient describe the pain. Some questionnaires are filled out by the patient, while others may be given to relatives or friends to complete. It is often necessary to ask other family members to complete a pain questionnaire if the patient is cognitively impaired.

In spite of their limitations, questionnaires and self-report forms do allow healthcare workers to better understand the pain being suffered by the patient. Evaluation also includes physical examinations and diagnostic tests to determine the underlying physical causes of the pain. Some evaluations require assessments from several viewpoints, including neurology, psychiatry and psychology, and physical therapy. If the pain is caused by a medical procedure, management consists of anticipating the type and intensity of associated pain and managing it pre-emptively.

Nurses or physicians often take what is called a pain history. This history will help to provide important information that can help healthcare providers to better manage the patient's pain. A typical pain history includes the following questions:

- Where is the pain located?
- On a scale of 1 to 10, with 1 indicating the least pain, how would the person rate the pain being experienced?
- What does the pain feel like?
- When did (or does) the pain start?
- How long has the person had it?
- Is the person sometimes free of pain?
- Is the pain constant, or is it episodic?
- Does the person know of anything that triggers the pain or makes it worse?
- Does the person have other symptoms (e.g., nausea, dizziness, blurred vision) during or after the pain?
- What pain medications or other measures has the person found to help in easing the pain?
- How does the pain affect the person's ability to carry on normal activities?
- What does it mean to the person that he or she is experiencing pain?

Aftercare

The progress of a pain management program should be continually assessed by healthcare providers. Certain signs and symptoms can be taken as an indication that a patient continues to experience pain. Those signs and symptoms include:

- rise in pulse and blood pressure
- more rapid breathing
- perspiring profusely, clammy skin
- taut muscles
- more tense appearance, fast speech, very alert
- unusually pale skin
- dilated pupils of the eye

Signs of chronic pain include:

- lower pulse and blood pressure
- changeable breathing pattern
- warm, dry skin
- nausea and vomiting
- slow or monotone speech
- inability or difficulty in getting out of bed and performing activities of daily living (ADLs)
- constricted pupils of the eye

When these signs are absent, and the patient appears to be comfortable, healthcare providers can consider their interventions to have been successful. It is also important to document interventions used, and which ones were successful.

Prognosis

Successful pain treatment is highly dependent on successful resolution of the pain's cause. Acute pain will stop when an injury heals or when an underlying problem is treated successfully. Chronic pain and abnormal pain are more difficult to treat, and it may take longer to find a successful resolution. Some pain is intractable and will require extreme measures for relief.

Prevention

Pain is generally preventable only to the degree that the cause of the pain is preventable. For example, improved surgical procedures, such as those done through a thin tube called a laparascope, minimize post-operative pain. Anesthesia techniques for surgeries also continuously improve. Some diseases and injuries are often unavoidable. However, pain from some surgeries and other medical procedures and continuing pain are preventable through drug treatments and alternative therapies.

Resources

BOOKS

Bailey, Allison, and Carolyn Bernstein. *Pain in Women: A Clinical Guide*. New York: Springer, 2013.

Brummet, Chad M., and Steven P. Cohen. *Managing Pain: Essentials of Diagnosis and Treatment*. Oxford: Oxford University Press, 2013.

Cervero, Fernando. *Understanding Pain: Exploring the Perception of Pain*. Cambridge, MA: MIT Press, 2012.

Incayawar, Mario, and Knox H. Todd. *Culture, Brain, and Analgesia: Understanding and Managing Pain in Diverse Populations*. New York: Oxford University Press, 2013.

PERIODICALS

Landa, Alla, et al. "Beyond the Unexplainable Pain." *The Journal of Nervous and Mental Disease* 200, 5. (2012): 413–22.

Pergolizzi, Joseph, et al. "The Chronic Pain Conundrum: Should We CHANGE from Relying on Past History to Assessing Prognostic Factors?" *Current Medical Research & Opinion* 28, 2. (2012): 249–56.

Swenson, C.J. "Ethical Issues in Pain Management." *Seminars in Oncology Nursing* 18, Part 2. (2012): 135–42.

Topcu, S.Y., and U.Y. Findik. "Effect of Relaxation Exercises on Controlling Postoperative Pain." *Pain Management Nursing* 13, 1. (2012): 11–17.

WEBSITES

"Chronic Pain." MedicineNet. http://www.medicinenet.com/chronic_pain/article.htm. Accessed on October 31, 2012.

"Pain Management." Everyday Health. http://www.everyday
health.com/pain-management/index.aspx. Accessed on
October 31, 2012.

"Pain Management Health Center." WebMD. http://www
.webmd.com/pain-management/guide/default.htm.
Accessed on October 31, 2012.

"Understanding Pain." Partners against Pain. http://www.
partnersagainstpain.com/understanding-pain/management
.aspx. Accessed on October 31, 2012.

ORGANIZATIONS

American Chronic Pain Association, P.O. Box 850, Rocklin,
CA 95677, Fax: (916) 632–3208, (800) 533–3231,
APA@pacbell.net, http://www.theacpa.org

American Pain Society, 4700 W. Lake Ave., Glenview, IL
60025, (847) 375–4715, Fax: (866) 574–2654, info@
ampainsoc.org, http://www.ampainsoc.org/

Canadian Pain Society, 1143 Wentworth St. West, Suite 202,
Oshawa, Canada ON L1J 8P7, (905) 404–9545, Fax: (905)
404–3727, http://www.canadianpainsociety.ca/en/contact
.html, http://www.canadianpainsociety.ca.

Julia Barrett
Ken R. Wells

Pan American Health Organization (PAHO)

Definition

The Pan American Health Organization (PAHO) is
an international organization working to improve health
and living conditions in 47 countries of the Western
Hemisphere. It serves as the Regional Office of the
Americas of the **World Health Organization (WHO)**
and is part of the Inter-American System, a group of
organizations representing health, finance, development,
and defense in the Western Hemisphere.

Purpose

According to the PAHO constitution, the purpose of
the organization is "to promote and coordinate efforts of
the countries of the Western Hemisphere to combat
disease, lengthen life, and promote the physical and
mental health of the people."

Description

The origin of the PAHO dates to January 1902,
when representatives from 11 Western Hemisphere
nations met in Washington, D.C., for the first International Sanitary Conference. At that conference, a decision

was made to create the International Sanitary Bureau, the
predecessor of the modern Pan American Health
Organization. The mission of the new organization was
to deal with the spread of infectious diseases that were
moving freely throughout the nations of North, South,
and Central America in the early years of the twentieth
century. Biennial meetings were held regularly thereafter,
and at the fifth such conference in 1923, the organization
changed its name to the Pan American Sanitary Bureau
(PASB). In 1949, **WHO** and the Pan American Sanitary
Organization, parent group of PASB, agreed that the
latter would become the official regional office of WHO.
Finally, at the 15th Pan American Sanitary Conference in
San Juan, Puerto Rico, the organization voted to adopt its
modern name.

PAHO consists of four primary bodies: the Pan
American Sanitary Conference, which now meets every
four years and establishes overall policies for the
organization; the Directing Council, which meets annually and approves the organization's program agenda and
budget; the Executive Committee, which deals with
detailed issues related to the organization's operation;
and the Pan American Sanitary Bureau, which carries out
the programs and directives of the three governing
bodies. PAHO has regional offices in 28 nations and
specialized centers in ten countries that deal with issues
such as bioethics (Chile), **epidemiology** (Trinidad), food
and **nutrition** (Jamaica), human ecology and health
(Mexico), and sanitary engineering and environmental
sciences (Peru).

PAHO activities are carried out through a half dozen
major programs, each of which is subdivided into a
number of more specific topics. The major programs are:
family and **community health**; gender, diversity, and
human rights; health surveillance and disease **prevention**
and control; health systems based on primary care; and
sustainable development and **environmental health**. As
an example of the way in which each major topic is
further delineated, the section dealing with health
surveillance and disease prevention and control is further
divided into topics such as chronic diseases, communicable diseases, health information and analysis, international health regulations and epidemic diseases, and
veterinary public health. A topic of special concern to
PAHO is emergency and disaster preparedness. The
association has collected, analyzed, and interpreted
massive amounts of data on past earthquakes, floods,
hurricanes, landslides, and other natural and manmade
disasters, and has produced many publications designed
to aid countries affected by such disasters in the
future. The agency's web page on this topic (http://
www.saludydesastres.info/index.php?lang=en) provides
information on disaster risk reduction in the health sector,
disaster preparedness, health responses in emergencies

and disasters, rehabilitation and reconstruction, and alliances and international assistance. PAHO is also the site of WHO's Regional Health Observatory for the Americas, a center for the collection of health data and statistics intended to provide an objective basis for the determination of future health and safety policies and programs.

Professional publications

PAHO publishes and distributes a large number of books, booklets, pamphlets, brochures, reports, statistical analyses, and other print and electronic publications, some of which are free to the general public. The organization's catalog is available online at http://publications.paho.org/spCall.php?spModule=Story&c_ID=2&catID=13. Its primary regular publication is the monthly journal *Revista Panamericana de Salud Publica/Pan American Journal of Public Health*, a peer–reviewed publication that carries reports of original research. Examples of other books and reports available from PAHO include: *Atlas of Diabetes Education in Latin America and the Caribbean, Domestic Violence: Women's Way Out, Management of Dead Bodies after Disasters: A Field Manual for First Responders, Obesity and Poverty: a New Public Health Challenge*, and *Unhappy Hours: Alcohol and Partner Aggression in the Americas*.

Resources

BOOKS

Cuesto, Marcos. *The Value of Health: A History of the Pan American Health Organization*. Washington, DC: Pan American Health Organization, 2007.

Howard–Jones, Norman. *The Pan-American Health Organization: Origins and Evolution*. Geneva: World Health Organization, 1981.

PERIODICALS

Alleyne, George A. "The Pan American Health Organization's First 100 Years: Reflections of the Director." *American Journal of Public Health* 92. 12. (2002): 1890–4.

Auer, A., and J. E. G. Espinel. "The Pan American Health Organization and International Health: A History of Training, Conceptualization, and Collective Development." *Revista Panamericana de Salud Publica/Pan American Journal of Public Health* 30. 2. (2011): 122–32.

WEBSITES

Guide to the Archives of International Organizations. UNESCO. http://www.unesco.org/archives/sio/Eng/presentation_print.php?idOrg=1028 (accessed October 11, 2012).

The History of the Pan American Health Organization. Global Health Network. http://www.pitt.edu/~super4/lecture/lec0291/index.htm (accessed October 11, 2012).

ORGANIZATIONS

Regional Office for the Americas of the World Health Organization, 525 Twenty Third St., N.W., Washington, DC 20038, (202) 974-3000, Fax: (202) 974-3663, http://new.paho.org/hq/index.php?lang=en.

David E. Newton, EdD

Pandemic

Definition

A pandemic is an epidemic of an **infectious disease** that has spread across large portions of several continents or even worldwide. The English word comes from two Greek words that mean "all" and "people." A noncontagious disease or condition that affects large numbers of people around the world on a steady basis (such as **cancer**, diabetes, or depression) is not a pandemic; the disorder must be an infectious disease to be defined as one.

In the twenty-first century, pandemics are officially identified as such by the **World Health Organization (WHO)**. **WHO** bases its definition of a pandemic on the location of a new epidemic and the stages of its spread, not on the number of people who have the disease or its virulence. The stages defined by WHO are described more fully below.

Description

Pandemics may be caused by either bacteria or viruses. While many of the pandemics from ancient times through the nineteenth century were caused by bacteria (**cholera**, **plague**, **typhus**), the pandemics (including possible future pandemics) of greatest concern in the modern world are caused by viruses (**influenza**, HIV infection, viral hemorrhagic fevers).

Historic pandemics

PLAGUE. Plague is a potentially fatal disease caused by a bacterium, *Yersinia pestis* (formerly called *Pasteurella pestis*). The bacterium enters the human body through the bite of an infected flea carried by rodents or other animal vectors, or (in the case of pneumonic plague) by droplet infection. There are three forms of the disease that may occur during a pandemic: bubonic plague, characterized by buboes, painful swellings in infected lymph nodes, a sudden onset of fever, headache, chills, and weakness; septicemic plague, characterized by fever, chills, extreme weakness, abdominal **pain**, shock,

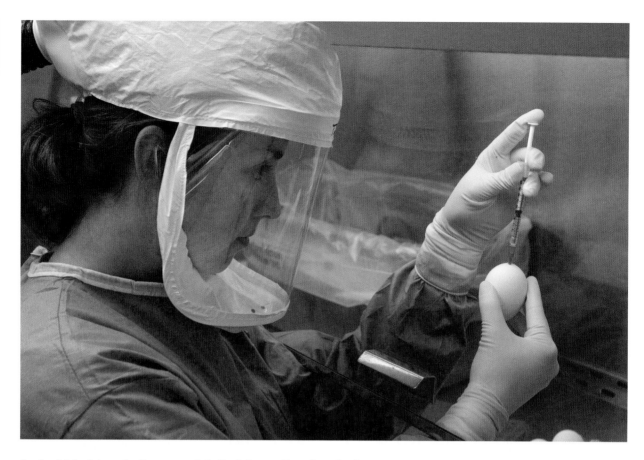

A microbiologist conducting research in the Influenza Branch at the Centers for Disease Control and Prevention.
(CDC/Alexander J. da Silva, PhD/Melanie Moser)

and possibly bleeding into the skin and other organs; and pneumonic plague, characterized by a high fever, headache, weakness, and a rapidly developing **pneumonia** with shortness of breath, chest pain, cough, and sometimes coughing up bloody or watery mucus. Untreated pneumonic plague is invariably fatal.

There were three major pandemics of plague, beginning in the late Roman (Byzantine) Empire and extending into the nineteenth century. The first pandemic, from A.D. 541 to approximately 700, began in Egypt and spread westward; it may have cut the **population** of Europe in half. The second pandemic, which includes the Black Death, extended from 1345 through the 1860s, originated in China and remained in Europe through the end of the seventeenth century. The Black Death of the fourteenth century caused the largest death toll from a bacterial disease in human history. The third pandemic, from the 1860s to the 1960s, began in China and eventually reached India and the United States. It did, however, lead to identification of the plague bacterium and modern methods of effective treatment. As of 2012, plague is an uncommon disease,

limited to isolated cases in the developed world and sporadic localized outbreaks elsewhere.

CHOLERA. Cholera is an infection of the digestive tract caused by the bacterium *Vibrio cholerae* and characterized by severe diarrhea and vomiting. It is transmitted by food or **drinking water** contaminated by fecal matter from infected persons or by eating contaminated shellfish. It is rarely spread by direct contact with an infected person. Untreated persons may die from dehydration and electrolyte imbalance. With proper treatment, cholera has a mortality rate below 1%.

Cholera did not produce pandemics before the nineteenth century, when there were six of them, from 1816 to 1826 (India, China, Indonesia); 1829 to 1851 (Russia, England, Canada, United States); 1852 to 1860 (Russia, China, Japan, Indonesia, Philippines); 1863 to 1875 (Europe and Africa); 1881 to 1896 (Russia, Spain, Japan, Persia); and 1899 to 1923 (Russia, Philippines, Middle East). There was a seventh pandemic in the twentieth century that lasted from 1962 to 1988, which affected Indonesia, Bangladesh, India, and the Soviet Union.

The cholera pandemics are significant in the history of public health for two reasons. First, they were in part the result of increasingly common international travel made possible by steamships and railroads; these means of transportation facilitated the spread of disease from one country or continent to another. Second, the modern field of **epidemiology** grew out of the English physician John Snow's (1813–1858) successful attempt to trace the source of a cholera outbreak in London in 1854. Although the **germ theory** of disease had not yet been proposed, Snow correctly deduced that the source of the outbreak was a public **water** pump whose water was polluted by untreated sewage.

TYPHUS. Typhus is a disease produced by bacteria belonging to the genus *Rickettsia* and characterized by severe headache, a sustained high fever, cough, rash, severe muscle pain, chills, low blood pressure, stupor, heightened sensitivity to light, and delirium. It is transmitted to humans by the bite of the human body louse. Epidemic typhus frequently accompanies wars and **famine**. It is sometimes known as camp fever, jailhouse fever, and ship fever because it spreads rapidly in prisons, military camps, and overcrowded housing. The earliest known epidemic that can be clearly identified as typhus occurred in Italy in 1083; other notable outbreaks followed the Thirty Years War (1618–1648), the Napoleonic Wars (1803–1815), and World War I (1914–1918). During World War II (1939–1945), thousands of prisoners in Nazi concentration camps died of typhus.

Modern methods of **sanitation** and personal cleanliness, the discovery of **antibiotics** and a typhus vaccine, and the use of DDT to kill body lice ended epidemic typhus as a major threat in the developed countries, although occasional outbreaks still occur in the Middle East and parts of Africa.

SMALLPOX. **Smallpox** is a viral disease that killed as many as 400,000 Europeans each year between 1750 and 1800; it is estimated that between 300 million and 500 million people worldwide died of smallpox during the twentieth century alone. The disease was unknown in the Americas prior to the arrival of the Spanish conquistadors in 1520, and it devastated many Native American tribes, who had no resistance to it. Smallpox had a similar effect on the aboriginal population of Australia after Europeans arrived in 1789.

Following Edward Jenner's (1749–1823) discovery of **vaccination** in 1796, various European governments as well as the United States began to institute mandatory vaccination programs, which limited the spread of the disease. Smallpox was eliminated in the United States by 1897 and in northern Europe by 1900. In 1979 WHO officially declared smallpox to have been eradicated around the world.

Pandemics since 1900

INFLUENZA. Influenza is a viral disease that spreads to humans from animals—most often chickens, ducks, other birds, and pigs. Humans can be infected by airborne droplets from infected animals, droppings from infected birds, or direct contact with the nasal secretions, saliva, blood, or feces of infected humans. The symptoms of flu include fever, sore throat, muscle pains, severe headache, coughing, and weakness; in severe cases, the patient develops pneumonia, which is potentially fatal.

Influenza pandemics emerge at irregular intervals; they differ from annual flu epidemics in that they are caused by a new strain of the influenza virus developing in susceptible animal species. The new strain spreads from its animal reservoir to humans and rapidly becomes a pandemic among humans because people lack resistance to the new strain of the virus. There have been five influenza pandemics since 1900. The first pandemic was the so-called Spanish flu, which emerged at the end of World War I in 1918 and killed an estimated 50 million to 100 million people worldwide. The high death toll is attributed to the large proportion of the population that was affected (50% in most countries) and the extreme severity of the symptoms. The second pandemic, the Asian flu of 1957 to 1958, was an avian (bird-related) flu that began in China and spread westward. It caused an estimated 69,000 deaths in the United States and about 4 million deaths worldwide.

The third pandemic, the Hong Kong flu of 1968–1969, caused about 34,000 deaths in the United States and one million deaths worldwide. The fourth pandemic, the Russian flu of 1977, primarily affected people born after 1950, as older adults were partially immune to this new strain. The fifth pandemic, the so-called swine flu of 2009, was caused by a mutation of the virus responsible for the 1918 pandemic. This pandemic began in Mexico in the spring of 2009 and was declared a pandemic by WHO in June 2009. The pandemic was declared over in August 2010. Estimates differ regarding the mortality of this pandemic; 294,500 is the figure most commonly given, the majority of the deaths occurring in Africa and southeastern Asia.

HIV/AIDS. HIV infection is caused by a lentivirus that disrupts the human immune system. Since the disease was first identified in the early 1980s (it may have crossed the species barrier from nonhuman primates like chimpanzees to humans as early as 1910), it has caused as many as 30 million deaths worldwide as of 2012. **AIDS** was first recognized as a pandemic in 1990. At present 68% of AIDS cases worldwide and 66% of all deaths from AIDS are in sub-Saharan Africa (22.9 million and 1.2 million respectively). About 1.2 million people in the United States are presently infected by the virus, with about 17,500 deaths each year.

HIV infection can be transmitted by sexual contact, contaminated syringes, transfusion of contaminated blood, and from mother to child during pregnancy and delivery. While the disease can be treated with a variety of antiretroviral drugs, there is no cure as of 2012, and the disease is considered likely to spread among **vulnerable populations** for the foreseeable future.

POTENTIAL PANDEMICS. Some researchers are concerned about the possibility that one or more viral hemorrhagic fevers (VHFs)—Ebola virus, Marburg virus, Lassa fever virus, and Bolivian hemorrhagic fever—might emerge in pandemic forms at some point in the future. These diseases are caused by five different families of RNA viruses, some of which have been traced to several species of African bats and rodents. All types of VHF are characterized by fever and bleeding disorders; all can progress to high fever, shock, and death. Some observers maintain, however, that large-scale outbreaks of these diseases are unlikely because transmission requires close contact with an infected patient or their body fluids, and the person becomes severely ill so rapidly that there is little time to spread the infection to others. Quarantine followed by decontamination of the patient's environment appears to be effective in limiting the spread of VHFs.

One factor that may contribute to future pandemics of diseases caused by bacteria is the growing development of bacterial resistance to antimicrobial drugs. So-called superbugs (multidrug-resistant **tuberculosis**, gonorrhea, and **staphylococcal infections**) are already widespread in such densely populated countries as China and India, and could easily spread elsewhere.

Origins and staging

With the partial exception of cholera, pandemic diseases originate in animal reservoirs and then spread to humans; they are thus classified as zoonoses. As noted above, the animal species in question that serve as vectors during pandemics range from birds and farm animals to insects, rodents, chimpanzees, and bats. This animal/human connection is the starting point for the World Health Organization's outline of the stages or phases of a pandemic.

The most recent version of WHO's staging of a pandemic was published in 2009. It assumes that the disease is caused by a virus:

- Stage 1: The virus is circulating in animals only and has not yet caused any illness in humans. An outbreak

of a contagious disease in animals is called an epizootic.

- Stage 2: The animal virus has caused some cases of illness in humans. This event establishes a baseline threat of a pandemic because the virus has mutated sufficiently to jump the species barrier.

- Stage 3: Small clusters of humans within a given community have contracted the virus. At this point the disease may be epidemic within that community but it is not yet a pandemic.

- Stage 4: Human-to-animal and human-to-human contacts are causing outbreaks of disease in many communities, and a larger proportion of the population is contracting the disease. A pandemic is not inevitable at this point, however.

- Stage 5: The disease is being transmitted by human-to-human contact in at least two countries within one WHO region. Most countries are not yet affected in stage 5 but a pandemic is considered imminent. This stage indicates that governments and public health officials must be ready to take action.

- Stage 6: The disease is now a full-scale global pandemic, with a large proportion of the populations in the affected countries falling ill.

Stage 6 is followed by a post-pandemic phase in which the number of cases of reportable illness have dropped to the ordinary levels found in countries with adequate disease surveillance. The time frame for the stages of a pandemic varies from a few months to many years.

Efforts and solutions

Efforts to prevent or control pandemics include the following:

- Adequate sanitation, personal hygiene, and hygienic methods of food preparation and service.

- Education of the general public about disease prevention, ranging from general hygiene (including the importance of frequent hand washing), proper food storage and handling, vaccination, and safe sex, to precautions regarding travel abroad, contact with animals, and contact with infected persons or their body fluids.

- Careful surveillance and monitoring of disease outbreaks, including accurate reporting of confirmed cases.

- International as well as national sharing of information and coordination of measures to control the spread of diseases likely to develop into pandemics.

- Quarantining persons or animals diagnosed with a contagious illness. The earliest quarantine in colonial

KEY TERMS

Endemic—Referring to an infectious disease that is constantly present in a particular country or region, though generally under control.

Epidemic—An outbreak of a contagious disease that involves new cases of the disease in a specific human population during a given period substantially exceeding the number expected based on recent experience.

Epizootic—An outbreak of a contagious disease among animals.

Quarantine—The practice of isolating sick persons or animals, or restricting travel or passage in order to prevent the spread of a contagious disease. The English word comes from the Italian word for forty, the number of days customary for quarantining ships visiting Italian ports during the medieval plague epidemics.

Surveillance—In epidemiology, the monitoring and reporting of cases of contagious disease in order to establish patterns of its spread to prevent or minimize the development of epidemics and pandemics.

Vector—In epidemiology, any person, animal, or microorganism that transmits a disease agent into another organism.

Virulence—The degree of a disease organism's ability to produce illness, as indicated by the mortality rate and/or the organism's ability to invade the host's tissues.

Zoonosis (plural, zoonoses)—Any disease that can be transmitted from animals to people or people to animals.

America took place in 1663, when the city of New York imposed a quarantine law in an attempt to curb the spread of smallpox.

Resources

BOOKS

Bissell, Rick. *Preparedness and Response for Catastrophic Disasters*. Boca Raton, FL: Taylor and Francis, 2013.

Bristow, Nancy K. *American Pandemic: The Lost Worlds of the 1918 Influenza Epidemic*. New York: Oxford University Press, 2012.

Dietz, J. Eric, and David R. Black, eds. *Pandemic Planning*. Boca Raton, FL: CRC Press, 2012.

Holmgren, Albin, and Gerhard Borg, eds. *Handbook of Disease Outbreaks: Prevention, Detection, and Control*. Hauppauge, NY: Nova Science, 2009.

Quammen, David. *Spillover: Animal Infections and the Next Human Pandemic*. New York: W.W. Norton and Co., 2012.

PERIODICALS

Adams, P. "The Influenza Enigma." *Bulletin of the World Health Organization* 90 (April 1, 2012): 250–251.

Badiaga, S., and P. Broqui. "Human Louse-transmitted Infectious Diseases." *Clinical Microbiology and Infection* 18 (April 2012): 332–337.

Bos, K.I., et al. "A Draft Genome of *Yersinia pestis* from Victims of the Black Death." *Nature* 478 (October 12, 2011): 506–510.

Kamradt-Scott, A. "Changing Perceptions: Of Pandemic Influenza and Public Health Responses." *American Journal of Public Health* 102 (January 2012): 90–98.

Morens, D.M., and J.K. Taubenberger. "1918 Influenza, A Puzzle with Many Pieces." *Emerging Infectious Diseases* 18 (February 2012): 332–335.

Newsom, S.W. "Pioneers in Infection Control: John Snow, Henry Whitehead, the Broad Street Pump, and the Beginnings of Geographical Epidemiology." *Journal of Hospital Infection* 64 (November 2006): 210–216.

Raabea, V.N., and M. Borcherta. "Infection Control During Filoviral Hemorrhagic Fever Outbreaks." *Journal of Global Infectious Diseases* 4 (January 2012): 69–74.

Sharp, P.M., and B.H. Hahn. "Origins of HIV and the AIDS Pandemic." *Cold Spring Harbor Perspectives in Medicine* 1 (September 2011): a006841.

WEBSITES

"American Experience: Influenza 1918." Public Broadcasting Service (PBS). This is an hour-long video about the effects of the 1918 influenza pandemic on the United States. http://video.pbs.org/video/1378322117 (accessed October 26, 2012).

"CDC Resources for Pandemic Flu." Centers for Disease Control and Prevention (CDC). http://www.cdc.gov/flu/pandemic-resources/ (accessed October 26, 2012).

"Pandemic Influenza Preparedness and Response: WHO Guidance Document." World Health Organization (WHO). This is the most recent (2009) version of a document originally prepared by WHO in 1999 for dealing with influenza pandemics. http://www.who.int/influenza/resources/documents/pandemic_guidance_04_2009/en/index.html (accessed October 26, 2012).

"What Is a Pandemic?" World Health Organization (WHO). http://www.who.int/csr/disease/swineflu/frequently_asked_questions/pandemic/en/index.html (accessed October 26, 2012).

ORGANIZATIONS

Centers for Disease Control and Prevention (CDC), Bacterial Diseases Branch, Foothills Campus, Fort Collins, CO United States 80521, (800) CDC-INFO (232-4636), cdcinfo@cdc.gov, http://www.cdc.gov/

National Institute of Allergy and Infectious Diseases (NIAID), 6610 Rockledge Drive, MSC 6612, Bethesda, MD United States 20892-6612, (301) 496-5717, (866) 284-4107, Fax:

(301) 402-3573, ocpostoffice@niaid.nih.gov, http://www
.niaid.nih.gov/Pages/default.aspx

World Health Organization (WHO), Avenue Appia 20, Geneva,
Switzerland 1211 Geneva 27, +41 22 791 21 11, Fax:
+41 22 791 31 11, http://www.who.int/en/

Rebecca J. Frey, PhD

Parasites

Defintion

A parasite is an organism that lives on or in the body
of a second organism, known as the host. The parasite
generally obtains all of its **nutrition** and the conditions
needed for reproduction from its host. It typically does
not kill the host in the short-term, although it may result
in the host's death in the long term.

Description

Parasites are generally much smaller than their hosts,
on whom they rely for virtually every aspect of their
survival, including food, **water**, warmth, habitat, and
method of transmission. Parasites often interfere with one
or another essential biological function of the host,
causing disease, disability, and, in some cases, death of
the host. Some parasite-like organisms, called parasi-
toids, are distinguished from parasites because their
survival inevitably results in the death of the host.
Parasites range in size from microscopic protozoa to
visible flatworms and roundworms.

Classification

Parasites can be classified in a variety of ways, one
of which is the portion of the host body they habitat.
Those parasites that remain on the outer surface of a host
body are called ectoparasites, while those that inhabit
spaces within a host body are called endoparasites. An
example of an ectoparasite is the tick, which attaches itself
to the outer surface of the host body and then feeds off
blood from the host. An example of an endoparasite is
the roundworm *Trichinella spiralis*, which lives in the
intestinal tract of the host. The relationship between
parasite and host is often considerably more complex
than suggested by this simple classification scheme.
Some parasites go through a number of stages, for
example, in which they may make use of different hosts
at each stage of their life cycle. Some types of ticks, for
example, go through a sequence of stages in which they
depend on three different types of hosts.

Transmission

Since they are dependent on their hosts for most life
activities, parasites face especially challenging problems of
moving between the environment and the host, or, in some
cases, a variety of hosts. One of the most common modes of
transportation makes use of the host's digestive system.
The parasite may reside in the host gut, for example, where
it lays its eggs, which are then expelled by way of the host
excretory system into the outside environment. Once the
eggs hatch, the parasitic young must then find a way to re-
enter a host body and repeat its life cycle. This path explains
one way that parasitic infections among humans are
transmitted. When people handle food or water that has
been contaminated with urine or feces, they may also come
into contact with the eggs of parasites, which are then
transmitted to the new host when he or she eats or drinks
with unclean hands. Parasites are, therefore, the primary
agents through which foodborne and waterborne diseases
are transmitted through human communities.

Another mode of transmission is through the host
circulatory system. Endoparasites that live in host blood
can travel from one host to another when an intermediary
organism—the vector—bites the host and draws blood
from her or his circulatory system. The parasite is then
transferred to a new host when the vector bites a second
individual. Perhaps the best known and most serious of
all parasitic diseases transmitted through blood is
malaria. Malaria is caused by a parasitic protozoa of
the genus *Plasmodium*, which is transferred from one
individual to a second individual by a bite of the female

Disease	Parasite	Insect (vector)
African trypanosomiasis (sleeping sickness)	Trypanosoma brucei gambiense, Trypanosoma brucei rhodesiense	Tsetse flies
Babesiosis	Babesia species	Ixodes (hard-bodied) ticks
Chagas disease	Trypanosoma cruzi	Triatomine ("kissing") bugs
Leishmaniasis	Leishmania species	Phlebotomine sand flies
Malaria	Plasmodium species	Anopheles mosquitoes
Toxoplasmosis	Toxoplasma gondii	No insect vector

(Table by PreMediaGlobal. © 2013 Cengage Learning)

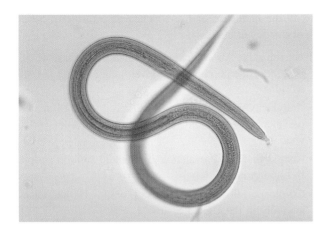

Strongyloides filariform larva. *(CDC/ Dr. Mae Melvin)*

Anopheles mosquito. When the mosquito bites a human, she injects spores of the *Plasmodium* protozoa into the bloodstream of the human. The spores are then carried to the liver, where it reproduces and returns to the bloodstream. In the blood, the mature *Plasmodium* then attacks and destroys red blood cells. When it reproduces within the blood, the new spores thus generated are available for collection by the bit of another mosquito, after which the cycle of infection is repeated.

Human parasitic diseases

Parasitic diseases are among the most devastating health problems encountered in human societies. Although the mode of infection and transmission differs somewhat from disease to disease, most parasitic diseases follow one of the general mechanisms described for foodborne diseases or malaria outlined previously. The U.S. **Centers for Disease Control and Prevention (CDC)** lists close to a hundred parasitic diseases of major concern to humans, including:

• African trypanosomiasis (African Sleeping Sickness)

• American trypanosomiasis (Chagas Disease)

• Ascariasis (intestinal roundworms)

• Cryptosporidiosis

• Dirofilariasis

• Entamoeba histolytica infection (amebiasis)

• Giardiasis

• Lymphatic filariasis (Elephantiasis)

• Leishmaniasis

• Malaria

• Microsporidiosis

• Onchocerciasis (river blindness)

• Pediculosis (head lice infestation)

• Pthiriasis (pubic lice infestation)

• Scabies

• Taeniasis (tapeworm infection)

• Trichuriasis (whipworm infection)

Causes and symptoms

The parasites of greatest concern to human health can be classified into one of three major groups: protozoa, helminths, and ectoparasites.

Protozoa

Protozoa are one-celled organisms that can live freely in nature or as parasites. Some of the protozoa responsible for human diseases are:

• *Entamoeba histolytica* (amebiasis)

• *Cryptosporidium* (cryptosporidiosis)

• *Acanthamoeba* (acanthamoeba keratitis and granulomatous amebic encephalitis)

• *Giardia* (giardiasis)

• *Leishmania* (leishmaniasis)

• *Microsporidia* (microspridiosis)

• *Toxoplasma gondii* (toxoplasmosis)

Parasitic protozoans are transmitted by either of the mechanisms described previously. For example, the primary host for *Toxoplasma gondii* is a member of the family Felidae, including the common house cat. When a cat eats contaminated meat, it eventually sheds oocysts, which are then ingested by other animals, such as birds, rodents, or humans who come into contact with the cat feces. Among humans, that contact comes most commonly when one cleans a cat sandbox and then touches the mouth or face without washing the hands. The **CDC** estimates that toxoplasmosis is the most common cause of foodborne illness in the United States. It estimates that more than 60 million Americans carry the *Toxoplasma gondii* protozoa, although the organism generally produces very mild symptoms, or no symptoms at all.

Helminths

Helminth is the general term given to any type of worm that can infect humans and cause disease. Helminths include a number of worm families, including the platyhelminths (flatworms), nematodes (roundworms), and acanthocephalins (thorny-headed worms). The platyhelminths, in turn, include the cestodes (tapeworms) and trematodes (flukes). Helminths live in the gastrointestinal tract of an animal, where they reproduce by depositing eggs that are then excreted in feces. The eggs normally are deposited in the soil, where they mature and are absorbed into animal bodies in one of two ways primarily. In some cases, for example, a human may ingest foods grown in soil contaminated with parasitic eggs, or a person may handle foods and water without having washed his or her hands after touching contaminated soil. As an example, the nematode *Ascaris lumbricoides* lives in the human gastrointestinal system, from which it excretes its eggs into the soil. When a person comes into contact with that soil and handles food without first having washed her or his hands, the eggs enter the gastrointestinal system of the second person, where they grow and mature. The cycle is then repeated any number of times.

Other helminths enter the body directly through the skin. Eggs that mature in the soil develop into larvae, which are then able to penetrate the skin when someone walks barefoot and sits or lies on contaminated soil. The nematode *Ancylostoma duodenale* uses this mode of transmission. It lives in the small intestine of a human, where it produces its eggs, which are then released during defecation. The eggs mature in the soil and the larvae produced then attach themselves to the skin of a human or other animal with whom they come into contact. They burrow into the body of the new host, are deposited in the small intestine, and they cycle repeats itself.

Ectoparasites

Ectoparasites are organisms that attach themselves to or burrow into the skin and obtain the sustenance they need to stay alive by sucking blood from their host. Some examples of ectoparasites that infect larger animals are leeches, lice, bedbugs, ticks, and mites. Ectoparasites have two quite distinct effects on their hosts. First, they may debilitate the animal directly, by causing dermatitis, skin necrosis, reduced weight gain, anemia, blockage of orifices (such as the ears), and secondary infections. Second, they tend to introduce a variety of infectious diseases into their host by way of pathogens contained within the fluids they exchange with the host. One of the best known ectoparasites in the United States today is the tick *Ixodes scapularis*, which is the vector for bacteria in the genus *Borrelia*, the causative agent for **Lyme disease** and related infectious diseases. Lyme disease is classified as a zoonotic disease because the reservoir for the *Borrelia* bacteria is rodents and deer. When a tick bites an infected rodent or deer and ingests some of its blood, it also absorbs some bacteria. When the tick or one of its progeny then bite a human, it releases some of those bacteria into the bloodstream of the human, where it can cause Lyme disease.

Demographics

Parasitic diseases are among the most common infectious diseases in the world. They tend to be somewhat less common in developed nations with more sophisticated **sanitation** systems. Some recent estimates

as to the incidence and prevalence of parasitic diseases worldwide are as follows:

- Amoebiasis: An estimated prevalence as high as 50 percent of the population in developing countries of the world.
- Ancylostomiasis (hookworm disease): An estimated prevalence of as many as 740 million people worldwide.
- Chagas disease: Prevalence of about 11 million people in Latin America.
- Cryptosporidiosis: Incidence of about 10,000 cases annually in the United States.
- Human African trypanosomiasis (sleeping sickness): Incidence of about 10,000 cases worldwide.
- Leishmaniasis: An estimated worldwide prevalance of about 12 million people with an at risk population of as high as 350 million.
- Malaria: Prevalence of about 216 million cases worldwide.
- Onchocerciasis (river blindness): An estimated prevalence of 17.7 million people in 34 nations worldwide.
- Schistosomiasis: Estimated worldwide prevalence of about 200 million people.
- Toxoplasmosis: An estimated prevalence of 60 million cases in the United States.
- Trichomoniasis: About 3.7 million people in the United States currently infected.

Symptoms

The symptoms of parasitic diseases vary widely, depending to some extent on the specific infection involved. Many parasitic infections are mild, and individuals who are infected with parasites may never be aware that they have been infected. Many parasitic diseases resolve on their own without every having been suspected or detected by the host animal. Other infections have signs and symptoms that are very mild and that can easily be confused with other health and medical conditions, such as low-grade fever, nausea, vomiting, diarrhea, weight loss, abdominal **pain**, disturbed sleep, aching muscles, and general lassitude. In the case of helminthic **infestations**, there may be itchiness or discomfort in the anal or vaginal areas, and worms may actually be visible in stools. Ectoparasites, such as ticks and leeches, are often easily visible to the human eye. The eruptions of the skin caused by burrowing scabies are also easily visible.

Some parasitic diseases cause far more serious health consequences with more obvious and troublesome signs and symptoms. These may include continuous elevated fever, severe gastrointestinal distress, loss of appetite and weight, anemia, sustained and severe diarrhea, profound fatigue, and pneumonia-like symptoms. Some parasitic diseases have very serious, sometimes life-threatening effects with characteristic symptoms. A person with African trypanosomiasis, for example, may develop a characteristic rash at the site of the tsetse fly bite and enlarged lymph nodes. Other symptoms include mental disorientation, a tendency to fall asleep easily (accounting for the common name of the disease: sleeping sickness), vertigo, partial paralysis, and other neurological problems. Death follows within a matter of months or a few years.

Onchocerciasis (river blindness) is also accompanied by a number of characteristics signs and symptoms, the most prominent of which are itchiness, the development of nodules under the skin, and vision changes that ultimately result in complete blindness in some cases. Another characteristic sign is a change in the color and texture of the skin, which result in a so-called "leopard-skin" appearance with a "cigarette-paper" texture.

Diagnosis

Some ectoparasitic diseases can be diagnosed by direct observation, often supplemented by patient history. For example, a diagnosis of Lyme disease may be indicated by signs and symptoms presented by the patient along with a collection of the suspected agent (a tick) itself. Scabies and pediculosis are other examples of diseases that can often be diagnosed simply by visual examination of a patient's body. Many parasitic diseases are never diagnosed because patients are never aware of their presence, and the diseases resolve on their own with no permanent or temporary harm to the host.

Many other parasitic diseases are more difficult to diagnose and require either relatively simple technologies or more sophisticated (and more accurate) tests. First level diagnostic technologies fall into two categories, those that involve parasites present in the gastrointestinal system and those for parasites present in the circulatory system. Tests in the first category involve visual and/or microscopic examination of the feces, in which the investigator looks for eggs produced by the parasite or for direct evidence of the parasite itself. Urinalysis can also be used for the identification of evidence for a few parasitic diseases, such as the eggs produced in **schistosomiasis**. An endoscopy or colonoscopy can also be used to examine the interior of the gastrointestinal system with the objective of obtaining visual evidence of parasites or their eggs directly. Diagnosis can also be based on a variety of blood tests. In some cases, a sample of blood can be examined under the microscope to look for direct evidence of a parasite, while in other cases,

blood samples may have to undergo more sophisticated serological tests for analysis.

One problem with direct tests for parasites is that the organisms may be too few in number or may no longer be present in the body, making detection and diagnosis difficult or impossible. In such cases, a battery of second-level tests is available that are aimed to detecting more subtle evidence of the existence of parasites, such as antibodies the body may have developed in response to the parasite infestation. Such tests include complement fixation, (CFT), immunodiffusion (ID), indirect hemagglutination (IHA), indirect immunofluorescent antibody (IFA), enzyme-linked immunosorbent assay (ELISA), radioimmunoassay (RIA), latex agglutination, capillary agglutination and card agglutination. These tests use one method or another to look for antigens, antibodies, or antigen-antibody complexes formed during a parastic invasion. Finally, x-ray, magnetic resonance imaging (MRI), computerized axial tomography (CAT), or other imaging technologies can be used to look for scarring, lesions, or other evidence of damage to organs caused by parasites.

Prevention

One broad general rule for the **prevention** of parasitic diseases is based on the improvement of hygienic practices. Most parasitic diseases are transmitted when an individual comes into contact with the wastes of another human or an animal that is already infected with a disease. When one does not wash her or his hands, clean one's food, drink or cook only with clean water, keep one's own body clean, or maintain other basic hygienic practices, one is at risk for contracting a parasitic disease. The specific steps one can take to reduce the risk of catching a parasitic disease include

- Observe basic hygienic practices, with special attention to handwashing after using the toilet or whenever one has come into contact with any material or object that may have been contaminated by parasites.

- Make sure that water used for drinking, cooking, bathing, and other household and personal purposes has been purified by one process or another.

- Clean all fruits and vegetables before eating.

- Make sure all cooked foods have been heated to a high enough temperature to kill any parasites that may be present.

- Be aware that domestic pets and farm animals often carry and transmit parasites and wash your hands after handling any such animal.

- Recognize that some kinds of parasites can be transmitted through oral sex and take necessary precautions in engaging in such types of contact.

- Be aware of the possibility of being in contact with fecal matter as, for example, if you work in a garden where natural fertilizer may have been used.
- Research areas of the world to which you may travel where sanitary procedures are not as sophisticated as they may be in most developed countries.
- Do not go barefoot in areas where soilborne parasites may be present.
- Thoroughly clean all clothing, bedding, and other items in areas where parasites are known or suspected to be present as, for example, in travelers lodging where bedbugs have been observed.

Treatment

Treatment of parasitic diseases fall into two general categories: those that depend on drugs and those that make use of herbal and other complementary and alternative methods. The specific choice of a drug for the treatment of a parasitic disease depends on the disease itself. In every case, the objective is to use a specific chemical capable of killing the parasite and/or its eggs to prevent transmission of the disease. Some of the drugs used for this purpose include:

- for use against roundworms: benzimidazoles, Emodepside, Levamisole, Morantel, Pyrantel
- for use against tapeworms: benzimidazoles, Niclosamide, Praziquantel
- for use against blood flukes: antimonials, Metrifonate, Oxamnaquine, Praziquantel
- for use aginst liver flukes: Closantel, Praziquantel
- for use against ectoparasites: Crotamiton, Lindane, Malathion, Permethrin

The list of drugs approved for use against various protozoa is very long, with many drugs developed for use against a specific protozoan. Some examples include:

- for treatment of malaria: Chloroquine, Mefloquine, Primaquine, Quinine
- for treatment of trichomoniasis: Metronidazole, Tinidazole
- for treatment of giardiasis: Meparcine hydrochloride, Metronidazole, Tinidazole
- for treatment of toxoplasmosis: Atovaquone, Azithromycin, Clindamycin, Sulfadiazine
- for treatment of leishmaniasis: Amphotericin, Pentamidine isetionate

Complementary and alternative therapists recommend a variety of techniques and substances for the treatment of parasitic infections. They tend to argue that the use of synthetic chemicals is harmful to the body and should be avoided in preference to the use of natural

---

KEY TERMS

Ectoparasite—A parasite that lives on or just below the exterior surface of an animal.

Endoparasite—A parasite that lives within the body of an animal.

Helminth—A worm that causes disease in an animal.

Incidence—The rate at which a disease occurs over some given period of time, usually a year.

Necrosis—Death of living tissue.

Oocyte—An immature female egg.

Parasitoid—A parasite whose presence on or in an animal ultimately causes the death of that animal.

Protozoa—A single-celled eukaryotic organism.

Prevalence—The total number of cases of a disease present in a region at any given time.

Zoonotic—Having an origin in animals, as in zoonotic diseases that normally occur in nonhuman animals.

---

materials and procedures. Some of the herbs recommended for the treatment of parasitic infections are agrimony, artemesia, barberry, black walnut, cloves, echinacea, garlic, goldenseal, prickly ash, qing hao, quassia, tansy, and wormwood. Such practitioners may also recommend mechanical methods for cleaning out the digestive system (called "colonic cleansing") to physically expel worms and their eggs. Most complementary and alternative procedures and materials have not been tested under controlled laboratory conditions, so their value depends largely on observational reports of their effects.

Prognosis

The prognosis for the majority of parasitic diseases is generally very good. Many people infected with parasites are not aware of their condition, and any disease that develops is likely to resolve on its own with little or no long-lasting effect on the individual. Such is not the case with diseases that are not treated or that by their very nature carry high risks for an individual. Malaria, for example, remains one of the most serious diseases in the world because of its long-term effects on individuals, in spite of the fact that effective methods of prevention and treatment are available. Control of the disease depends not so much on developing new methods of preventing and treating the disease as it does on finding ways of implementing current knowledge and technology in

Vaughan, A. M., and S. H. Kappe. "Malaria Vaccine Development: Persistent Challenges." *Current Opinion in Immunology* 24, 3. (2012): 324–31.

WEBSITES

"Humaworm." https://humaworm.com/welcome.html. Accessed on October 23, 2012.

Ndao, Momar. "Diagnosis of Parasitic Diseases: Old and New Approaches." Interdisciplinary Perspectives on Infectious Diseases. http://www.hindawi.com/journals/ipid/2009/278246/. Accessed on October 23, 2012.

"Parasites." Centers for Disease Control and Prevention. http://www.cdc.gov/parasites/. Accessed on October 23, 2012.

Wilcox, Glenn Lockhart. "Parasite Prevention." http://drglennwilcox.com/pdf/Parasite_Prevention.pdf. Accessed on October 23, 2012.

ORGANIZATIONS

Centers for Disease Control and Prevention (CDC), 1600 Clifton Rd., Atlanta, GA 30333, (800) 232–4636, http://www.cdc.gov/cdc-info/requestform.html, http://www.cdc.gov.

David E. Newton, Ed.D.

regions where it is needed. The prognosis for untreated cases of diseases like human African trypanosomiasis (sleeping sickness) is also poor since the disease develops fairly rapidly and causes death within a few months or few years.

Resources

BOOKS

Boglish, Burton Jerome, Clint Earl Carter, and Thomas N. Oeltmann. *Human Parasitology*, 4th ed. Amsterdam: Elsevier, 2013.

Davis, Charles E. *The International Traveler's Health Book: A Complete Guide to Avoiding Infections*. Baltimore: Johns Hopkins University Press, 2012.

Hughes, David P., Jacques Brodeur, and Frederic Thomas. *Host Manipulation by Parasites*. Oxford: Oxford University Press, 2012.

Karlan, Dean S., and Jacob Appel. *More than Good Intentions: Improving the Ways the World's Poor Borrow, Save, Farm, Learn, and Stay Healthy*. New York: Plume, 2012.

PERIODICALS

Jones, J. L., and J. P. Dubey. "Foodborne Toxoplasmosis." *Clinical Infectious Diseases* 55, 6. (2012): 845–51.

Mali, Sonja, S. Patrick Kachur, and Paul M. Arguin. "Malaria Surveillance—United States, 2010." *MMWR: Morbidity and Mortality Weekly Report* 61, 2. (2012): 1–17.

Muänoz-Saravia, Silvia Gilka, et al. "Chronic Chagas Heart Disease: A Disease on its Way to Becoming a Worldwide Health Problem: Epidemiology, Etiopathology, Treatment, Pathogenesis and Laboratory Medicine." *Heart Failure Reviews* 17, 1. (2012): 45–64.

Parrot fever

Definition

Parrot fever is a rare **infectious disease** that causes **pneumonia** in humans. It is transmitted from pet birds or poultry. The illness is caused by a chlamydia, which is a type of intracellular parasite closely related to bacteria. Parrot fever is also called chlamydiosis, psittacosis, or ornithosis.

Description

Parrot fever, which is referred to as avian psittacosis when it infects birds, is caused by *Chlamydia psittaci*. Pet birds in the parrot family, including parrots, parakeets, macaws, and cockatiels, are the most common carriers of the infection. Other birds that may also spread *Chlamydia psittaci* include pigeons, doves, mynah birds, and turkeys. Birds that are carrying the organism may appear healthy, but can shed it in their feces. The symptoms of avian psittacosis include inactivity, loss of appetite and ruffled feathers, diarrhea, runny eyes and nasal discharge, and green or yellow-green urine. Sick birds can be treated with **antibiotics** by a veterinarian.

Chlamydia psittaci is usually spread from birds to humans through exposure to infected bird feces during cage cleaning or by handling infected birds. In humans, parrot fever ranges in severity from minor flu-like symptoms to severe and life-threatening pneumonia.

Causes and symptoms

Parrot fever is usually transmitted by inhaling dust from dried bird droppings or by handling infected birds. Humans can also spread the disease by person-to-person contact, but that is very rare. The symptoms usually develop within five to 14 days of exposure and include fever, headache, chills, loss of appetite, cough, and tiredness. In the most severe cases of parrot fever, the patient develops pneumonia. People who work in pet shops or who keep pet birds are the most likely individuals to become infected.

Diagnosis

Only 100–200 cases of parrot fever are reported each year in the United States. It is possible, however, that the illness is more common since it is easily confused with other types of **influenza** or pneumonia. Doctors are most likely to consider a diagnosis of parrot fever if the patient has a recent history of exposure to birds. The diagnosis can be confirmed by blood tests for antibodies, usually complement fixation or immunofluorescence tests. The organism is difficult to culture. A chest x-ray may also be used to diagnose the pneumonia caused by *Chlamydia psittaci*.

Treatment

Psittacosis is treated with an antibiotic, usually tetracycline (Achromycin, Sumycin); doxycycline (Doxy, Vibramycin); or erythromycin (Eryc, Ilotycin). Oral medication is typically prescribed for at least 10–14 days. Severely ill patients may be given intravenous antibiotics for the first few days of therapy.

Prognosis

The prognosis for recovery is excellent; with antibiotic treatment, more than 99% of patients with parrot fever will recover. Severe infections, however, may be fatal to the elderly, untreated persons, and persons with weak immune systems.

Prevention

There is no vaccine that is effective against parrot fever. Birds that are imported into the country as pets should be quarantined to ensure that they are not infected before they can be sold. Health authorities recommend that breeders and importers feed imported birds a special blend of feed mixed with antibiotics for 45 days to ensure that any *Chlamydia psittaci* organisms are destroyed. In

KEY TERMS

Avian chlamydiosis—An illness in pet birds and poultry caused by *Chlamydia psittaci*. It is also known as parrot fever in birds.

Chlamydia psittaci—An organism related to bacteria that infects some types of birds and can be transmitted to humans to cause parrot fever.

Chlamydiosis, psittacosis, or ornithosis—Other names for parrot fever in humans.

addition, bird cages and food and water bowls should be cleaned daily.

Resources

BOOKS

Hobson, Jeremy. *Keeping Chickens,* 2nd ed. Cincinnati, OH: David&Charles, 2010.

Sachs Jessica Snyder. *Good Germs, Bad Germs: Health and Survival in a Bacterial World.* New York, NY: Hill and Wang, 2008.

ORGANIZATIONS

Centers for Disease Control and Prevention, 1600 Clifton Rd., Atlanta, GA 30333, (404) 639–3311, (800) 311–3435, http://www.cdc.gov.

Altha Roberts Edgren
Laura Jean Cataldo, RN, Ed.D.

Pasteurization

Definition

Pasteurization is a process by which food is flash heated to a relatively high temperature in order to reduce the number of microorganisms, thereby increasing the product's shelf life and making it healthier for human consumption.

Description

Pasteurization is used to increase the shelf life of many food and beverage products and to make them safer to consume by reducing their microbe content. Milk and dairy products are some of the most frequently pasteurized foods. Other commonly pasteurized products, which are often liquids, include beer, juice, and eggs. Pasteurization removes many of the microorganisms in

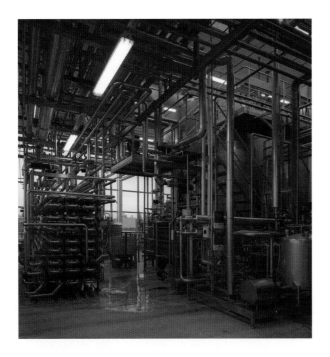

A facility in the dairy industry. *(© iStockphoto.com/ alaincouillaud)*

these food products, but it does not completely sterilize them. Sterilization of these products would produce undesirable textures and flavors in most pasteurized food. Some products, like yogurts, contain bacteria that are helpful to the human digestive tract. Yogurt is made by combining milk and these "good" bacteria. When yogurt is pasteurized after the bacteria cultures have been added, it kills them and renders them useless. For these bacteria cultures to still be viable, the milk must be pasteurized separately, before the addition of the cultures.

The temperatures to which an item is heated and the length of time it is heated depend on the product. Temperatures often range from between 151 and 212 degrees Fahrenheit (66 and 100 degrees Celsius), and exposure times between 0.01 seconds and 30 minutes. Ultra-high-temperature (UHT) processing is accomplished above 268 degrees Fahrenheit (131 degrees Celsius) for approximately two to five seconds. Sometimes lower temperatures may be used when products are heated in bulk in large vats.

Excepting UHT, pasteurized products need to be refrigerated immediately and continuously after processing. UHT leaves products nearly sterile and does not impose the same refrigeration requirements. Normal pasteurization reduces the microbial content of a product but does not prevent the proliferation of slow-growing bacteria or bacteria that produce endospores.

Dairies utilize the Hazard Analysis and Critical Control Program (HACCP) for the points of **sanitation** and contamination monitoring. Contamination of the milk comes after it has left the cow's udder, unless the cow is somehow diseased or infected. Dangerous microorganisms can enter the milk during the milking, handling, and packaging processes.

Origins

The process of pasteurization was developed in the 1860s by French scientist, Louis Pasteur (1822–1895). Pasteur was studying the presence and effects of microorganisms and the potential relationships between these and disease in human beings. He presented evidence that living organisms participated in the process of fermentation and that specific organisms aided specific fermentations. At the request of the French emperor, Napoleon III, Pasteur looked for a way to minimize the spoiling of wine during shipping. Based on his knowledge of microorganisms, Pasteur heated the wine. Despite the ability of Pasteur's new technique to improve the shelf life of wine, many manufacturers felt that it altered the taste of the wine too much to be worth the increased lifespan. Among the organisms pasteurization kills are those that contribute to the aging of a wine. Though the wine industry in general abandoned the process, it was adapted to other food and beverage industries, particularly dairy.

Prior to the Industrial Revolution, milk and other dairy products had been consumed for thousands of years in rural settings, without consequence. After the industrial revolution, however, urban areas began to further develop and expand, as did the consumption of milk and milk products in these areas. By the end of the nineteenth century, the unsanitary conditions of urban areas resulted in many outbreaks of milk-borne disease— like **scarlet fever**, **diphtheria**, typhoid, and diarrhea. Widespread commercial use of the pasteurization process and the implementation of dairy industry regulations helped combat these issues in Europe and the United States in the late nineteenth and early twentieth centuries.

Demographics

The use of pasteurization today varies. In some states the sale of raw milk products is legal; in others it is prohibited. Outside the United States, the laws are highly varied. Many rural populations still consume raw milk and dairy products. Other areas have prohibitions on such products, though enforcement varies.

It is estimated that the process of pasteurization removes between 97–99 percent of bacteria such as **mycobacterium tuberculosis**, **salmonella**, and streptococcus species.

Raw milk from a healthy animal contains approximately 1,000 microorganisms (or fewer) per milliliter.

PASTEUR, LOUIS (1822–1995)

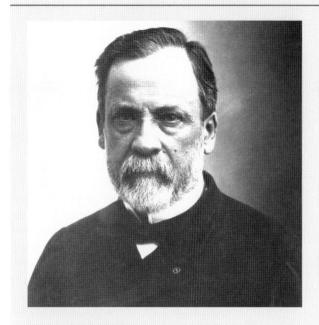

(© Bettmann/CORBIS)

Pasteur the experimenter revolutionized public health by proving bacterial pollution, demonstrating pollution prevention through pasteurization, describing the microbial etiology of infectious diseases, and demonstrating that disease could be prevented through vaccination.

Louis Pasteur was born at Dole, France, into a modest family with a father who operated a tannery. In October 1843 he entered the École Nationale in Paris and worked in the laboratory of Jerome Balard. Pasteur built his first discovery on tartaric and para-tartaric acids: he showed that the two substances are identical but that their atomic positions are reversed. This success led Pasteur to study the optical activity of a whole series of substances.

At the University of Strasbourg, where he was appointed as professor of chemistry in January 1849, Pasteur examined meticulously diverse kinds of molecules. Pasteur deduced that the molecules of life are asymmetrical. Applying this discovery to fermentation, he went on to consider it as a natural biological occurrence, not as an artificial chemical synthesis. To prove that the fermentation was a germ of life he switched from crystals to microbes, from chemistry to microbiology and immunology.

Pasteur had begun his studies on fermentation in 1854 at the University of Lille, where he had been appointed dean of the science faculty two years earlier,

and he soon turned his attention to incomplete distillation. He took a microscope to a beet sugar factory and spent days on end making alcohol. Looking through the eyepiece he watched the growth of the globules that were present as sugar was being turned into alcohol. Pasteur showed that minute organisms acted because they were alive and breathing. In holding his own against some of the greatest biochemical theories of the time, which maintained that fermentus was indispensable because of its capacity to disappear, Pasteur was going to give the germ its due importance in alcohol and lactic fermentation and then in the rotting process. Aerobic germs are necessary to the life cycle since they take in oxygen and expel carbon dioxide, which is absorbed by plants. Building on this, he held that microorganisms, both parasitic and useful ones, must be everywhere-in the water, the air, the ground. This hypothesis from the outset was waged against one of the major philosophical and biological problems of the nineteenth century: the theory of spontaneous generation, which claimed that germs are born directly in mineral matter.

To show that such theory was wrong and that spontaneous generation does not occur, Pasteur first had to develop a new experimental strategy. At the École Normale SupÉrieure, where he had been appointed director of scientific studies in 1857, he invented an external device used to pump air from the school's garden and filter it through a fluff of cotton. Microbes could be detected when the cotton was washed on a watch glass. This debate on spontaneous generation was to turn into an analysis of air and the first epidemiological analyses of the presence of microorganisms in the environment. Pasteur showed that germs vary in relation to place and season depending on climatic conditions and hygiene.

In 1865, upon orders from Napoleon III, Pasteur went to work on wine diseases, using heat as a source of prevention. He adopted Nicolas Appert's procedure for food keeping and recommended a new method for conserving wine: heating between 60°C and 100°C in an air-free environment for one to two hours. The pasteurization method circled the globe.

From 1865 through 1869 he investigated the pebrine disease that had been devastating the production of raw silk. He discovered that silkworms were contaminated when hatched, as the butterfly was already sick because of a minuscule parasite. Pasteur demonstrated that healthy eggs could be seen under a microscope and hatched. His cellular system helped end the disease by 1875.

Pasteurized milk reduces that number so that it falls in a range from between a few cells and a few dozen cells per milliliter.

Effects on public health

The U.S. **Centers for Disease Control and Prevention (CDC)** advise against using raw milk products and cite recent disease outbreaks related to unpasteurized dairy products in 2001, 2003, and 2004. Proponents for raw milk and dairy products, however, argue that pasteurization reduces the nutrient content of these products—destroying hormones, enzymes, and "good" bacteria. There are grassroots movements in both the United States and the United Kingdom that advocate for the availability and primacy of raw milk products. These movements have come largely out of other food movements that favor consuming food in its most natural and unprocessed states.

The 2010 (most recent available) U.S. Dietary Guidelines, created by the U.S. **Department of Health and Human Services** recommend consuming more low-fat and fat-free dairy products. This endorsement of dairy products for the everyday diet of Americans increases the importance of the availability of safe dairy products.

Efforts and solutions

The original pasteurization regulations evolved into the Grade A Pasteurized Milk Ordinance (PMO), which is handled by the U.S. Department of Health and Human Services and the Public Health Service. It is the responsibility of the U.S. Food and Drug Administration (FDA), however, to determine the particulars related to sanitation, milking methods, milk handling, and other standards that constitute the ordinance. Each state is then responsible for enforcing their standards and regulating local production.

Local and state **health departments** report instances of foodborne disease outbreaks to the **CDC** via the Foodborne Disease Outbreak Surveillance System. This process helps generate regional and national statistics as well as detecting trends in outbreaks. Such data can help determine the relative efficacy of pasteurization methods themselves and the regulations enforcing these processes.

Salmonella outbreaks are a serious health concern as they result in illness and often deaths. Roughly 96 percent of salmonella cases are caused by **food contamination**. Some raw or fresh food products—like produce, meat, and eggs—cannot withstand the heat of pasteurization and still maintain their fresh state. Some products, like peanut butter, have shown to be able to support strains of salmonella after pasteurization.

KEY TERMS

Sterilization—Any procedure that kills all micro-organisms in and on a product.

Ultra High Temperature (UHT) Processing—Procedure in food processing where a product is heated, for a short time, to a higher temperature than those used in pasteurization. Result of UHT processing is near sterilization of the food product.

Microorganism—A microscopic organism made up of one cell or a small cluster of cells.

Scientists are working on alternative methods of pasteurization that do not require the temperatures of traditional pasteurization. *Food Research International* reported in March 2012, the testing of an electron beam (e-beam). This e-beam is a form of **ionizing radiation** that accelerates electrons. There is potential for this beam to be incorporated into a device similar to a microwave oven—this would allow food service companies and even individual households to pasteurize fresh foods without the heat of pasteurization.

Resources

BOOKS

"Pasteurization." *The Britannica Guide to Inventions That Changed the Modern World.* Ed. Robert Curley. New York: Britannica Educational Publishing with Rosen Educational Services, 2010.

"Pasteurization." *The Encyclopedia of the Digestive System and Digestive Disorders.* Anil Minocha and Christine Adamex. 2nd ed. New York: Facts on File, 2011.

McIntosh, Philip. "Pasteurization." *Encyclopedia of Micro-biology.* Ann Maczulak. New York: Facts on File, 2012.

McIntosh, Philip. "Pasteurization." *Food: In Context.* Ed. Brenda Wilmoth Lerner and K. Lee Lerner. Vol. 2: Junk Food to Yeast and Leavening Agents. Detroit: Gale, 2011.

PERIODICALS

Jaczynski, Jacek, Kristen E. Matak, and Reza Tahergorabi. "Application of electron beam to inactivate Salmonella in food: Recent developments." *Food Research International* 45.2 (2012): 685+.

Angulo, Frederick J., et al. "Nonpasteurized dairy products, disease outbreaks, and state laws—United States, 1993–2006." *Emerging Infectious Diseases.* 18.3 (2012): 385+.

WEBSITES

U.S. Department of Health and Human Services. "Dietary Guidelines for Americans, 2010." http://health.gov/dietaryguidelines/2010.asp. Accessed September 12, 2012.

Grade "A" Pasteurized Milk Ordinance. U.S. Department of Health and Human Services, Public Health Service, and

Food and Drug Administration, 2009. http://www.fda.gov/downloads/Food/FoodSafety/Product-SpecificInformation/MilkSafety/NationalConferenceonInterstateMilkShipments NCIMSModelDocuments/UCM209789.pdf. Accessed September 12, 2012.

ORGANIZATIONS

U.S. Department of Health and Human Services, 200 Independence Avenue, Washington, D.C. USA 20201, (877) 696-6775, www.hhs.gov.

Andrea Nienstedt, MA

Pertussis *see* **Whooping cough**

Physical activity

Definition

Physical activity can be defined as actions that involve planned, structured, and repetitive bodily movements for the purpose of maintaining or improving physical fitness and overall health. Physical activity includes cardiovascular training, muscle-strength training, and stretching activities for flexibility and to prevent injury. Typical physical activities include walking, running, cycling, swimming, weight training, aerobics, and individual and team sports.

Purpose

Regular physical activity is important for the physical, mental, and emotional health of people of all ages—from young children to the elderly. It promotes:

- weight maintenance or weight loss
- cardiovascular efficiency
- musculoskeletal strength and flexibility
- improved functioning of the metabolic, endocrine, and immune systems
- adequate bone density
- lower cholesterol levels
- recovery from illness, injury, or surgery
- mental and emotional well-being

The beneficial effects of physical activity diminish within two weeks of substantially reducing the activity. Physical fitness is lost completely if physical activity is not resumed within two to eight months.

Demographics

The National Institutes of Health (NIH) has identified inactivity as a major public health problem in the United States, and most North American adults would benefit from increasing their level of physical activity. More than 60% of American adults do not get enough physical activity to provide health benefits, and more than 25% are inactive during their leisure time. Lack of physical activity is a major contributor to the current epidemic of **obesity**, since people who are overweight or obese burn fewer calories than they take in, resulting in weight gain. Sedentary lifestyles and unhealthy eating patterns are responsible for at least 300,000 deaths from chronic disease each year in the United States. Likewise, a recent survey in the United Kingdom found that only one-third of adults meet recommended goals for physical activity.

Insufficient physical activity is more prevalent among women than men and among those with lower levels of economic stability and educational achievement. However, the number of adult Americans who are exercising regularly is on the increase. According the **Centers for Disease Control and Prevention (CDC)**, between 2001 and 2005 the number of women exercising at least 30 minutes per day increased by 8.6% and the number of men increased by 3.5%.

Geriatric

Physical activity generally decreases with age. It is estimated that two-thirds of Americans over age 65 have at least one chronic condition, with 36 million suffering from some form of arthritis. Lack of physical activity is a significant contributor to conditions such as osteoarthritis, lower back **pain**, and osteoporosis. More than 300,000 total joint replacements are performed each year due to osteoarthritis.

Description

Programs of physical activity should include three types of exercise: strengthening (including weight or resistance training), stretching and flexibility exercises, and cardiovascular exercise. Recent studies have indicated that muscle strength and aerobic fitness make independent contributions to health and that more muscle strength correlates with lower death rates, regardless of aerobic fitness. The American College of Sports Medicine recommends two strength-training workouts per week, each consisting of about 10 repetitions of 10 exercises for strengthening all of the major muscle groups. Yoga is often recommended for stretching, bending, and improving overall flexibility.

The physical activities one chooses should be interesting and appealing: studies have found that people are more likely to stick with an exercise program when they enjoy the activity, whether as an individual, with a

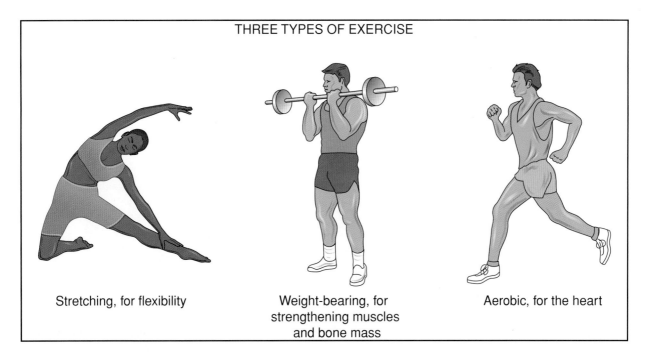

THREE TYPES OF EXERCISE

Stretching, for flexibility

Weight-bearing, for
strengthening muscles
and bone mass

Aerobic, for the heart

Physical activity is utilized to improve health, maintain fitness, and is important as a means of physical rehabilitation.
(Illustration by Electronic Illustrators Group. © 2013 Cengage Learning)

partner, or with a group or team. Convenience is also an important consideration. Physical activities can take place at home, outdoors, or at a health club or fitness center, school, church, or community center. Taking a class, working out with a friend, competing, or setting personal goals can help maintain motivation. Walking for exercise can be combined with various enjoyable activities, such as bird watching, museum visits, window shopping, or exercising the dog. Group physical activities and team sports are good ways to socialize. Varying exercise routines every few weeks can benefit different muscle groups and help prevent boredom. In addition, since the human body adjusts rapidly to most exercises, continuing the same routine for too long can result in decreased benefits.

The most efficient cardiovascular exercises for improving physical fitness include:

• brisk walking (3–4 mph), whether outside, in a mall, or on a treadmill
• jogging
• running
• bicycling, either outside or on a stationary bike
• stair climbing
• elliptical cross-training on exercise machines
• aerobics
• swimming
• water exercise or aerobics
• rowing
• cross-country (Nordic) skiing
• jumping rope—a particularly good form of physical activity for children

Other activities that provide cardiovascular conditioning—but are less endurance-promoting because they usually require frequent starting and stopping—include:

• dancing
• basketball
• soccer
• softball
• badminton
• racquetball
• squash
• tennis
• table tennis
• volleyball
• skating
• golfing, if walking and carrying clubs

Teenagers can get cardiovascular exercise through school sports including:

• baseball
• cross country
• track and field
• cheerleading

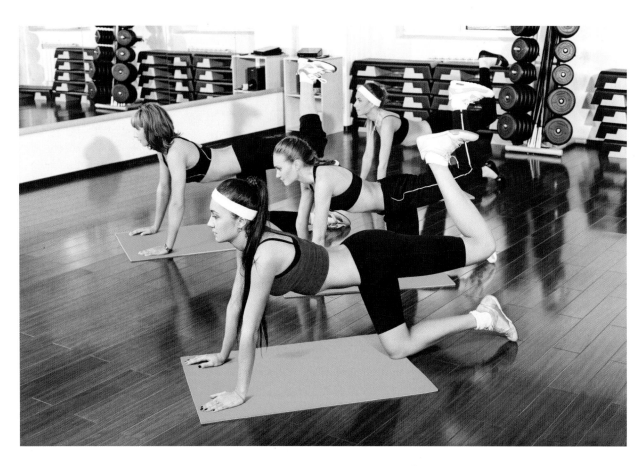

Group of women in an exercise class. *(Kiselev Andrey Valerevich/Shutterstock.com)*

- drill team

- field hockey

- football

- lacrosse

- wrestling

People who are generally sedentary can still get exercise through their occupation, housework, home repair, gardening, using stairs instead of an elevator, and various recreational pursuits. People with health problems can find physical activities that accommodate their injuries or disorders. The American Council on Exercise suggests specific exercises for the elderly and for adults with problems such as **asthma**, chronic pain, bad knees, shoulder injuries, arthritis, and flat feet.

Regularity and intensity are key elements of any physical activity. It has generally been recommended that all adults get at least 30 minutes of moderate-intensity exercise on most days of the week. However, the most recent consensus is to aim for 150 minutes per week, regardless of how it is divided up. The latest evidence suggests that three 10-minute bouts of physical activity are as beneficial as one 30-minute workout. Improving cardiovascular endurance requires at least 20–60 minutes of cardiovascular exercise three to five days per week. The U.S. **Department of Health and Human Services** recommends at least 60 minutes of physical activity for children and teens on most or all days of the week.

Defining "moderate intensity" can be tricky. Until recently, exercise intensity was generally gauged by increased heart rate. However intensity is more accurately measured by metabolic rate, as represented by units of metabolic equivalents or METS, an individual's metabolic rate during physical activity divided by the metabolic rate when sitting still. The latter is defined as 1 kilocalorie per kilogram (kg) of body weight per hour or an oxygen uptake of 3.5 milliliters per kg per minute. Moderate activity is defined as 3–6 METS. Although a precise measurement requires determining oxygen intake in a laboratory, charts of average METS for various activities are available. Examples of METS include:

- walking, 2–8

- running, 8–18

- bicycling, 4–16

- stationary bicycling, 3–12.5

- general health-club exercise, 5.5
- calisthenics, 3–8
- weight lifting, 3–6
- swimming, 6–11
- cross-country skiing, 7–16.5
- downhill skiing, 5–8
- volleyball, 3–8
- dancing, 3–10
- basketball, 4.5–8
- tennis, 5–8
- tai chi, 4
- stretching, hatha yoga, 2.5
- household tasks, 2–9
- mowing with a hand mower, 6

Physical activity geared to a target heart rate is typically about 70% of the maximum heart rate for one's age. Heart rate is calculated by counting the pulse, usually about halfway through a 20–30-minute workout. Fingers are placed firmly but lightly over the inside of the wrist or on the neck just below the angle of the jaw; however, too much pressure on the neck can slow down the heart rate. The palm also can be placed over the heart to count the number of beats. A zero is added to a six-second count, or a 10-second count is multiplied by six to obtain the beats per minute (bpm). Maximum bpm is calculated by subtracting one's age from 220. For example:

- Target heart rate during cardiovascular exercise for a healthy 50-year-old might be 170 multiplied by 70% or 119 bpm.
- A particularly fit 50-year-old might have a target heart rate of 80% of maximum or 136 bpm.
- A 50-year-old with a medical condition may have a target exercising heart rate of only 50% or 85 bpm. A bpm above the target rate indicates a need to slow down, whereas a bpm below the target indicates a need to speed up the pace of physical activity.

There are other methods for measuring the intensity of cardiovascular exercise:

- Classes and DVDs usually include a timed heart-rate check and a chart of target rates by age.
- Electronic exercise pulse monitors are available.
- A simple "talk test" is based on speaking a complete sentence: the pace of physical activity is too high if the sentence cannot be completed, and too low if it is overly easy to speak the sentence.
- Cardiovascular exercise usually involves sweating; therefore, people who no longer sweat during their exercise routine may need to increase the intensity, duration, or frequency of their workouts.

Improved fitness in response to physical activity appears to be genetically determined and to run in families. Some previously sedentary people show less improvement in fitness than would be expected following weeks of a vigorous exercise program, and about 10% show no improvement at all. However, even those who show no improvement in fitness measures still respond to physical activity with lowered blood pressure and cholesterol, improved insulin levels, and less abdominal fat.

Origins

Throughout most of human history, most people were adequately active. Then, early in the twentieth century, the rate of heart attacks in Western countries began to increase dramatically. The first indication that this might be due to lack of physical activity came in a landmark 1953 study of London bus conductors: conductors, who spent their days collecting fares from seated passengers and walking up and down the stairs of double-decker buses, had half the number of heart attacks as seated bus drivers. Since then, countless studies have confirmed the positive effects of physical activity, not just on the heart and circulatory system, but on virtually every system of the body.

Benefits

Physical activity promotes:

- cardiovascular fitness, including improved heart function and increased heart, lung, and muscle endurance
- muscle strength and mass
- flexibility
- weight loss
- lowered blood pressure
- bone density and strength, which reduces the risk of fractures and osteoporosis
- mental health and psychological and emotional well-being from the release of brain hormones called endorphins

Additional benefits of cardiovascular exercise include:

- improved immune system function
- improved utilization and control of blood sugar
- decreased cholesterol and triglycerides
- decreased abdominal fat
- increased energy levels
- less fatigue

- improved appetite
- improved sleep
- reduced stress
- pain reduction

Regular physical activity lowers the risk of a heart attack by 50–80%. Physical activity also has been shown to reduce the risk of:

- stroke
- cancer
- diabetes
- liver and kidney disease
- osteoporosis
- depression
- dementia

Even those who are overweight or obese can become aerobically fit with physical activity. Studies have found that the risk of dying is more closely related to fitness than to weight. In fact, people who are fit but obese have a lower risk of dying than people who are unfit but of normal weight.

More than 30 million Americans undergo surgery each year. Each patient's surgical risk, complications, and outcome depend, at least in part, on their physical fitness: how well their cardiovascular and pulmonary systems withstand the stress of anesthesia; how quickly their bones and muscles recover after surgical procedures; and how well their metabolic and immune systems respond to surgery and the risk of infection.

Precautions

- Everyone should have a physical examination before embarking on a program of physical activity for the first time or after a long period of inactivity.
- Exercise intensity and duration should be increased gradually.
- People who are very weak may need to build strength before they can participate in cardiovascular exercise.
- Warming up before, and stretching after, physical activity are very important.
- People should pace themselves and check their heart rate or otherwise judge their level of exertion.
- If exercising becomes "very hard" or worse, it is important to slow the pace.
- Although some discomfort, such as aches or stiffness, are to be expected during the first few days of a new type of physical activity, if pain is intrusive it is important to stop the activity or get instruction on technique.

- Strenuous cardiovascular exercise should never be halted abruptly without a cool-down, since blood that has concentrated in the working muscles can pool and cause dizziness or lightheadedness.
- Cardiovascular exercise requires a healthy diet with plenty of vegetables.
- It is best to wait up to two hours after a full meal before exercising, and about an hour after exercising before having a meal, although a small healthy snack before exercising can boost energy levels.
- It is important to drink enough fluid to replace water that is lost as sweat; however, coffee, tea, colas, chocolate, or alcohol can cause the body to lose fluid.
- Simple types of physical exercise in the home, such as a balance board, can reduce the risk of recurrent sprained ankles.
- Taking a few days off from cardiovascular exercise every month can help rejuvenate the body.

Geriatric

Both maximum heart rate and cardiac output are lower in older adults, in part due to a decrease in the beta-adrenergic response. Older adults should have a stress test before embarking on a cardiovascular exercise program. A good result on a stress test is a bpm that is 80% of the age-adjusted maximum, with 90% considered excellent.

Other conditions

Various medical conditions can affect physical activity. For example, people with back problems should avoid activities that require twisting or vigorous forward movements, such as aerobic dancing or rowing. People with spinal disk disease should avoid high-impact activities.

Preparation

Physical activity should begin with a light or very light warm-up of five to ten minutes that may include gentle stretching to loosen muscles and joints and help prevent injury. The warm-up may involve slowly beginning the conditioning activity—warming up for a brisk walk or jog by walking slowly or strolling, or warming up to ride a stationary bike by pedaling slowly with no resistance. Warming up increases blood flow to the muscles, increases muscle temperature, and prepares them to work harder.

Aftercare

Cardiovascular exercise should be followed by a light or very light five- or 10-minute cool-down to allow the heart and circulation to gradually return to a resting

Aerobic exercise—Any exercise that increases the body's oxygen consumption and improves the functioning of the cardiovascular and respiratory systems.

Cholesterol—A fat-soluble steroid alcohol (sterol) found in animal fats and oils and produced in the body from saturated fats. High cholesterol levels contribute to the development of cardiovascular disease.

Endorphins—A class of peptides in the brain that are produced during exercise and bind to opiate receptors, resulting in pleasant feelings and pain relief.

Exercise—Any type of physical activity requiring physical effort, generally carried out for the purpose of maintaining or improving health and fitness.

Metabolic equivalent of task; MET—The energy cost of a physical activity, measured as a multiple of the resting metabolic rate, which is defined as 3.5 milliliters of oxygen consumed per kilogram (kg) of body weight per minute, equivalent to 1 kilocalorie per kg per hour.

Obesity—Excessive weight due to accumulation of fat, usually defined as a body mass index (BMI) of 30 or above or body weight greater than 30% above normal on standard height-weight tables.

Physical activity—Any activity that involves moving the body and burning calories.

Physical fitness—A combination of muscle strength, cardiovascular health, and flexibility that is usually attributed to regular exercise and good nutrition.

Sedentary—Inactivity and lack of exercise; a lifestyle that is a major risk factor for becoming overweight or obese and developing chronic diseases.

Stress test—An electrocardiogram recorded before, during, and after a period of increasingly strenuous cardiovascular exercise, usually on a treadmill or stationary bicycle.

Target heart rate—The heart rate, in beats per minute (bpm), that should be maintained during cardiovascular exercise by an individual of a given age.

Triglycerides—Neutral fats; lipids formed from glycerol and fatty acids that circulate in the blood as lipoprotein. Elevated triglyceride levels contribute to the development of cardiovascular disease.

state. The cool-down can include the same activity as the conditioning phase at a slower pace—slower walking or pedaling with reduced resistance on a stationary bike.

Most doctors encourage patients to become active as soon as possible following surgery. Aftercare is individualized, and there may be limitations on physical activity; however, the goal is to return the patient to normal daily activities and exercise routines. Patients should ask for explicit guidelines concerning exercise.

Risks

Physical activity poses a risk of injury, particularly if exercises are inappropriate or improperly performed. Too much physical activity can be as harmful as too little; overuse of certain muscles and joints can lead to problems such as tennis elbow or shin splints. High-intensity physical activity, such as high-impact aerobics and jogging, are not recommended as frequently as in the past. Running, in particular, is hard on the knees and ankle joints, and there is a risk of sprained ankles and injuries from falls. About one-half of all regular runners and players of team sports suffer some type of musculoskeletal injury each year.

Inadequate rest increases the risk of **stroke** and circulatory problems. Injury or illness from overtraining is sometimes indicated by a high resting heart rate, sleeping difficulties, or exhaustion. The risk of a heart attack can rise as much as 100-fold for a completely unfit individual who undertakes vigorous exercise, such as jogging or shoveling snow. In contrast, a person who runs five times per week merely doubles their risk of heart attack during vigorous exercise. The risk of heart attack subsides about one-half hour after exercising and pales in comparison to the lifetime benefits of regular exercise.

Pregnant or breastfeeding

Some types of physical activity are inappropriate for pregnant women. Pregnant women are generally advised not to exercise for two consecutive days.

Resources

BOOKS

Bouchard, Claude, Steven N. Blair, and William Haskell, eds. *Physical Activity and Health*, 2nd ed. Champaign, IL: Human Kinetics, 2012.

Dishman, Rod, Gregory Heath, and I-Min Lee. *Physical Activity Epidemiology*, 2nd ed. Champaign, IL: Human Kinetics, 2012.

Kotecki, Jerome E. *Physical Activity and Health: An Interactive Approach*, 3rd ed. Sudbury, MA: Jones & Bartlett Learning, 2010.

Ransdell, Lynda, et al. *Developing Effective Physical Activity Programs*. Champaign, IL: Human Kinetics, 2009.

PERIODICALS

Rasberry, C.N., et al. "The Association between School-based Physical Activity, including Physical Education, and Academic Performance: A Systematic Review of the Literature." *Preventive Medicine* 52, Suppl. 1. (2011): S10–20.

Rock, C.L., et al. "Nutrition and Physical Activity Guidelines for Cancer Survivors." *CA: A Cancer Journal for Clinicians* 62, 4. (2012): 243–74.

Singh, L., et al. "Physical Activity and Performance at School: A Systematic Review of the Literature including a Methodological Quality Assessment." *Archives of Pediatrics and Adolescent Medicine* 166, 1. (2012): 49–55.

Wen, C.P., et al. "Minimum Amount of Physical Activity for Reduced Mortality and Extended Life Expectancy: A Prospective Cohort Study." *Lancet* 378, 9798. (2011): 1244–53.

WEBSITES

"Global Recommendations on Physical Activity for Health." World Health Organization. http://www.who.int/dietphysicalactivity/factsheet_recommendations/en/index.html. Accessed on October 18, 2012.

"National Guidelines for Physical Activity." National Association for Sport and Physical Education. http://www.aahperd.org/naspe/standards/nationalGuidelines/PAguidelines.cfm. Accessed on October 18, 2012.

"Physical Activity." Centers for Disease Control and Prevention. http://www.cdc.gov/physicalactivity/everyone/guidelines/index.html. Accessed on October 18, 2012.

"Physical Activity Guidelines." U.S. Department of Health and Human Services. http://www.health.gov/paguidelines/. Accessed on October 18, 2012.

ORGANIZATIONS

American College of Sports Medicine, PO Box 1440, Indianapolis, IN 46202-1440, (317) 637-9200, Fax: (317) 634-7817, http://www.acsm.org

American Council on Exercise, 4851 Paramount Drive, San Diego, CA 92123, (858) 279-8227, (888) 825-3636, Fax: (858) 576-6564, support@acefitness.org, http://www.acefitness.org

American Heart Association, 7272 Greenville Avenue, Dallas, TX 75231, (800) 242-8721, http://www.americanheart.org

National Institute of Arthritis and Musculoskeletal and Skin Diseases, Information Clearinghouse, 1 AMS Circle, Bethesda, MD 20892-3675, (301) 495-4484, (877) 22-NIAMS (226-4267), Fax: (301) 718-6366, NIAMSinfo@mail.nih.gov, http://www.niams.nih.gov

U.S. Centers for Disease Control and Prevention, 1600 Clifton Road, Atlanta, GA 30333, (800) CDC-INFO (232-4636), cdcinfo@cdc.gov, http://www.cdc.gov.

Margaret Alic, PhD

Plague

Definition

Plague is a contagious febrile disease caused by the bacterium *Yersinia pestis* (formerly called *Pasteurella pestis*). The bacterium is named for Alexandre Yersin (1863–1943), a Swiss/French bacteriologist who identified it during an outbreak of plague in Hong Kong in 1894.

The English word *plague* is derived from the Latin *plaga*, which means "wound" or "blow." As of 2012, the term *plague* is applied primarily to bubonic plague; however, historians of medicine often use the word to refer to major pandemics in general, including some whose infectious agent is debated or unknown.

Description

Plague is a disease that has profoundly affected human history; it is still considered potentially dangerous, particularly in underdeveloped parts of the world. Until 2007, plague was one of only three diseases that were directly reportable to the **World Health Organization (WHO)**, the others being **cholera** and **yellow fever**. Plague is classified as a **zoonosis** because it is transmitted to humans by contact with animals. Plague affects animals—particularly rodents and such animals as squirrels, rabbits, and chipmunks—more severely than humans; humans are only the incidental host of the plague bacterium. The continued existence of the plague bacterium depends solely on its transmission between fleas and rodents; human infection does not play a part in its persistence.

The most problematic animal vectors of plague are rodents and the fleas carried in their fur. The regions of the world most susceptible to plague in the modern era are those with tropical or subtropical climates, specifically those that lie between 55 degrees north of the Equator and 40 degrees south. The major exception is Australia.

There are three basic forms of plague in humans:

• Bubonic plague: Bubonic plague is the form most often associated with the Black Death and other major outbreaks of plague in Western Europe. Bubonic plague results when a flea infected with *Y. pestis* bites a human and regurgitates a mass of bacteria in its blood into the wound. The plague bacteria can reproduce inside skin cells and eventually enter the lymphatic system, which will carry them to a lymph node. Inside the node, *Y. pestis* can multiply rapidly, secreting several toxins and causing inflammation and hemorrhage. The lymph node will swell, producing the characteristic bubo that gives this form of plague its name.

• Septicemic plague: This form of plague develops when the plague bacteria enter the bloodstream from the lymphatic system. They secrete an endotoxin called coagulase that causes disseminated intravascular coagulation (DIC), a potentially fatal condition in which small clots form throughout the body's blood vessels, destroying the body's ability to control bleeding elsewhere. People with septicemic plague develop bleeding into the skin and other organs, and will typically vomit or cough up blood. This form of plague is almost always fatal without treatment.

• Pneumonic plague: Pneumonic plague is transmitted person-to-person via respiratory droplets. The plague bacteria infect the lungs, resulting in headaches, coughing, sneezing, and coughing up or vomiting blood. Although the usual incubation period for pneumonic plague is 2 to 4 days, it can develop in as little as a few hours. Untreated pneumonic plague is invariably fatal.

Origins

Plague has caused high mortality among humans and other animals for millennia. As of 2012, epidemiologists believe that the modern form of *Y. pestis* is descended from a bacterium that lives in the gut known as *Yersinia pseudotuberculosis*, and that it has generated variant strains across the course of recorded human history through the evolutionary mechanism known as selective pressure. Some historians of medicine speculated that the Black Death was caused by a virus rather than *Y. pestis*; however, recent DNA studies of medieval plague victims across Europe have shown that they died from earlier strains of *Y. pestis* that are now extinct. The present biovars (strains) of *Y. pestis* are known as Orientalis and Medievalis.

Historians of medicine usually describe three pandemics (worldwide or continent-wide outbreaks) of plague:

• First pandemic, A.D. 541 to approximately 700: This pandemic includes the so-called Plague of Justinian (Byzantine emperor, 482–565) in 541–542, followed by further outbreaks in 588 and 700. It is estimated that

Europe lost 50% of its population between 541 and 700.

• Second pandemic, 1345 to the 1860s: this pandemic includes the Black Death, which entered Europe from China in 1347; the Great Plague of London in 1665; and the Great Plague of Vienna in 1679. According to one historian, plague was present somewhere in Europe in every single year from 1347 to 1671. The Black Death of the fourteenth century caused the largest death toll in history from a nonviral disease.

• Third pandemic, 1860s to the 1960s: this pandemic began in China and spread to India and the west coast of the United States; it eventually affected all continents around the world. The third pandemic did, however, lead to the scientific identification of the plague bacterium and modern methods of effective treatment. The last outbreak of plague in the United States occurred in Los Angeles in 1924.

Demographics

Plague in the modern world is largely limited to underdeveloped countries with humid tropical or subtropical climates. According to **WHO**, there are about 5,000 cases of plague reported each year, almost all of them (95%) in Africa. The last major outbreak of plague occurred in Surat, India, in 1994, and caused 52 deaths. About 300,000 people fled the area, fearing infection. It is thought that the Surat epidemic was triggered by unusually heavy rainfall that caused flooding and a large number of drowned animals that were not properly disposed of.

Plague first entered the United States in 1900 via infected rats on ships from Asian port cities that docked in ports on the west coast. Following the Los Angeles outbreak in 1924, infected urban rodents then transmitted the plague bacterium to rodents in rural areas across the western states. Most cases of plague since 1970 have occurred as scattered instances in the desert Southwest, particularly northern New Mexico, northern Arizona, and southern Colorado. Another cluster of cases has occurred in California, southern Oregon, and far western Nevada. There are on average 10 to 15 cases of plague in humans reported to the **CDC** each year in the United States.

Apart from rodents, cats are the animal most likely to become infected because they are particularly susceptible to plague, and can be infected by eating diseased rodents. Several cases of human plague in recent years involved veterinarians who became infected by treating sick cats. One warning sign of plague in the desert Southwest is an epizootic, or outbreak of plague among the local animals. Such epizootics are most common in cool summers that follow unusually wet winters. Native Americans are at greater risk of contracting plague than members of other races or ethnic groups in the United States. Men and women are equally likely to become infected by the plague bacterium.

Causes and symptoms

Causes

As noted, plague is caused by a bacterium, *Y. pestis*, that lives in the gut of infected fleas. The bacterium multiplies and forms a mass that extends into the flea's esophagus. When the flea bites an animal or human host, the mass of bacteria is injected into the host's bloodstream and lymphatic system. The most common paths of transmission in the modern world, either from animals to humans or from one human to another, are:

- Being bitten by fleas. Flea bites may lead to bubonic or septicemic plague.
- Exposure to a person with pneumonic plague.
- Handling infected laboratory animals or dead animal carcasses. Contact with contaminated animal tissue may lead to either bubonic or septicemic plague.
- Droplet infection. This type of transmission has not been documented in the United States since 1924, but still occurs with some frequency in developing countries.
- Scratches or bites from an infected cat.

Symptoms

The symptoms of plague vary somewhat depending on the type of plague:

- Bubonic plague: Patients with bubonic plague develop a sudden onset of fever, headache, chills, and weakness along with one or more swollen, sore, and painful buboes. The bacteria multiply in the lymph node closest to where the bacteria entered the human body.
- Septicemic plague: Septicemic plague may occur either as the first form of plague in a patient or develop from untreated bubonic plague It is characterized by fever, chills, extreme weakness, abdominal pain, shock, and possibly bleeding into the skin and other organs. The patient's skin and other tissues may turn black and die; the fingers, toes, and the nose are the parts of the body most commonly affected by tissue necrosis. Diarrhea may be a prominent symptom of septicemic plague, particularly in the elderly.
- Pneumonic plague: This form of plague may develop either from inhaling infected droplets from another person, or from untreated bubonic or septicemic plague spreading to the lungs. It is the only form of plague that can be transmitted directly from person to person. The patient with pneumonic plague has a high fever, headache, weakness, and a rapidly developing pneumonia with shortness of breath, chest pain, cough, and sometimes coughing up bloody or watery mucus. The pneumonia may cause respiratory failure and shock.

Diagnosis

Diagnosis begins with a careful patient history, particularly a known flea bite or recent travel to an area where plague is endemic. The patient's occupation may provide an additional clue, particularly if he or she works with animals or engages in hunting and trapping in rural areas.

The presence of a bubo combined with a visible flea bite will lead the doctor to suspect bubonic plague. Septicemic and pneumonic plague may not have any unique symptoms at first; however, the doctor can make a diagnosis of plague by taking a tissue sample from a bubo or a sample of the patient's blood and submitting them to a laboratory for analysis. In the United States, the sample must be sent either to a reference laboratory or directly to the CDC. The plague bacterium has a characteristic "safety pin" appearance when it is stained on a blood smear.

Confirmed cases of plague must be reported to the local health department, the CDC, and WHO.

Prevention

There have been different vaccines for plague in use in humans since 1897, when a Russian physician working in Paris developed a plague vaccine for use in India. As of 2012, however, there is no longer a plague vaccine licensed for use in the United States, according to the CDC. However, the CDC states that several new vaccines are in development.

The CDC recommends the following measures to lower the risk of contracting plague:

- Clear away brush, rock piles, junk, and other objects near the house where rodents could shelter and reproduce. Also remove pet food or food set out for wild animals, and make the house and any outbuildings on the property rodent-proof.
- Wear gloves when handling or skinning potentially infected animals to prevent contact between the skin and the plague organisms.
- Use flea repellents when hiking, camping, or working outdoors. Products containing DEET can be used on clothing as well as skin; products containing permethrin are for clothing only.
- Cats and dogs should be treated with flea control products, particularly if they are allowed outside.

KEY TERMS

Bubo—A swollen lymph node resulting from an infection. Buboes are characteristic of bubonic plague but may also occur in syphilis, tuberculosis, or gonorrhea. The English word is derived from the Greek word for groin, which is the most common location for buboes to appear.

DEET—A slightly yellow oily substance that can be applied to skin or clothing to protect against flea bites, tick bites, and the bites of other insects that can spread disease. The full chemical name of DEET is N,N-Diethyl-meta-toluamide.

Disseminated intravascular coagulation (DIC)—An abnormal activation of blood clotting mechanisms that occurs in response to various diseases, including plague. Small blood clots form inside the blood vessels, disrupting normal clotting elsewhere in the body and leading to abnormal bleeding in the skin, digestive tract, and other organs.

Endemic—Referring to an infectious disease that is constantly present in a particular country or region, though generally under control.

Epizootic—An outbreak of a contagious disease among animals.

Febrile—Characterized or caused by fever.

Necrosis—A form of cell injury that results in the death of living tissue. Tissue necrosis is a common symptom of septicemic plague.

Pandemic—An epidemic of infectious disease that spreads over several continents or worldwide.

Reportable disease—Any disease that is required by law to be reported to government authorities or to such organizations as the CDC or WHO. Reportable diseases are also called notifiable diseases.

Selective pressure—Influence exerted by an antibiotic or other factor on natural selection to promote the survival of one group of organisms over another.

Septicemia—The presence of disease organisms and their toxins in the bloodstream.

Vector—In epidemiology, any person, animal, or microorganism that transmits a disease agent into another organism.

Zoonosis (plural, zoonoses)—Any disease that can be transmitted from animals to people or people to animals.

Animals allowed to roam freely are more likely to come in contact with plague-infected animals or fleas and could bring the infected fleas into the home.

• Do not allow a cat or dog that has been allowed to roam freely in a plague-endemic area to sleep in a human bed inside the house.

Treatment

Plague is treatable with **antibiotics**, most commonly streptomycin, gentamicin, or doxycycline. The Food and Drug Administration (FDA) has also approved levoflox-acin for prophylactic (preventive) treatment as well as diagnosed cases of plague. Trimethoprim-sulfamethoxazole has been used on occasion to treat bubonic plague; however, it is not considered first-line therapy. Patients are typically given a ten-day course of medication; those with advanced forms of plague are given such supportive measures as intravenous fluids and ventilator support.

As of 2012, studies of *Y. pestis* samples taken from Asia, Africa, and North and South America indicate that the bacterium has *not* developed resistance to the eight antimicrobials most often used to treat it.

In spite of the fact that plague can be treated, healthcare and laboratory personnel must always be warned of a possible diagnosis of plague in a specific patient. All body fluid specimens must be handled with gloves and mask to prevent the infected fluids from forming aerosol droplets and spreading the disease further.

Prognosis

The prognosis depends on the type of plague and the speed of diagnosis and treatment. Patients who are diagnosed and treated early have the best chance of full recovery. Bubonic plague has a mortality rate of 10 to 20% when treated, 50% when untreated. Septicemic plague has a mortality rate of 20 to 25%. Pneumonic plague has a mortality rate of 50% when treated, 100% when untreated.

Effects on public health

The effects of plague on public health are most noticeable in underdeveloped countries and in the western United States. Because plague cannot be completely eradicated due to its animal reservoirs, ongoing surveillance, careful reporting of diagnosed cases, and education of the public about the need to control local rodent populations are still necessary. Another task for researchers is further work on one or more vaccines effective against plague.

The other major consideration for public health workers is the possibility that *Y. pestis* could be used as an agent of bioterrorism. The Japanese were the first to weaponize plague by breeding large numbers of infected fleas during World War II and injecting Chinese and Allied prisoners of war with *Y. pestis*. During the Cold War, both the Soviet Union and the United States experimented with weaponizing pneumonic plague by various methods that included freeze drying, vacuum drying, developing drug-resistant strains of *Y. pestis*, and genetic engineering. Aerosolized pneumonic plague remains the most significant threat; however, there have been no post-World War II incidents of bioterrorism involving plague as of 2012.

Resources

BOOKS

Holmgren, Albin, and Gerhard Borg, eds. *Handbook of Disease Outbreaks: Prevention, Detection, and Control.* Hauppauge, NY: Nova Science, 2009.

Little, Lester K., ed. *Plague and the End of Antiquity: The Pandemic of 541–750.* New York: Cambridge University Press, 2007.

Sherman, Irwin W. *Twelve Diseases That Changed Our World.* Washington, DC: ASM Press, 2007.

PERIODICALS

Anderson, P.D., and G. Bokor. "Bioterrorism: Pathogens as Weapons." *Journal of Pharmacy Practice* 25 (October 2012): 521–529.

Bevins, S.N., et al. "*Yersinia pestis*: Examining Wildlife Plague Surveillance in China and the USA." *Integrative Zoology* 7 (March 2012): 99–109.

Centers for Disease Control and Prevention (CDC). "Fatal Laboratory-acquired Infection with an Attenuated *Yersinia pestis* Strain—Chicago, Illinois, 2009." *Morbidity and Mortality Weekly Report* 60 (February 25, 2011): 201–205.

Haench, S., et al. "Distinct Clones of *Yersinia pestis* Caused the Black Death." *PLoS Pathogens* 6 (October 7, 2010): e1001134.

Hotez, P.J. "The Four Horsemen of the Apocalypse: Tropical Medicine in the Fight against Plague, Death, Famine, and War." *American Journal of Tropical Medicine and Hygiene* 87 (July 2012): 3–10.

Rosenzweig, J.A., and A.K. Chopra. "The Future of Plague Vaccines: Hopes Raised by a Surrogate, Live-attenuated Recombinant Vaccine Candidate." *Expert Review of Vaccines* 11 (June 2012): 659–661.

Steneroden, K.K., et al. "Zoonotic Disease Awareness in Animal Shelter Workers and Volunteers and the Effect of Training." *Zoonoses and Public Health* 58 (November 2011): 449–453.

Urich, S.K., et al. "Lack of Antimicrobial Resistance in *Yersinia pestis* Isolates from 17 Countries in the Americas, Africa, and Asia." *Antimicrobial Agents and Chemotherapy* 56 (January 2012): 555–558.

WEBSITES

"The Black Death." History Channel. This is a 26-minute video from the History Channel's series "History's Turning Points." http://www.youtube.com/watch?v=4y_qVG8xnjY (accessed October 24, 2012).

"Plague." Centers for Disease Control and Prevention (CDC). http://www.cdc.gov/plague/ (accessed October 23, 2012).

"Plague." Mayo Clinic. http://www.mayoclinic.com/health/plague/DS00493 (accessed October 24, 2012).

"Plague." Medscape. http://emedicine.medscape.com/article/235627-overview (accessed October 23, 2012).

ORGANIZATIONS

Centers for Disease Control and Prevention (CDC), Bacterial Diseases Branch, Foothills Campus, Fort Collins, CO United States 80521, (800) CDC-INFO (232-4636), cdcinfo@cdc.gov, http://www.cdc.gov/

Food and Drug Administration (FDA), 10903 New Hampshire Ave., Silver Spring, MD United States 20993-0002, (866) INFO-FDA (463-6332), http://www.fda.gov/default.htm

National Institute of Allergy and Infectious Diseases (NIAID), 6610 Rockledge Drive, MSC 6612, Bethesda, MD United States 20892-6612, (301) 496-5717, (866) 284-4107, Fax: (301) 402-3573, ocpostoffice@niaid.nih.gov, http://www.niaid.nih.gov/Pages/default.aspx

World Health Organization (WHO), Avenue Appia 20, Geneva, Switzerland 1211 Geneva 27, +41 22 791 21 11, Fax: +41 22 791 31 11, http://www.who.int/en/

Rebecca J. Frey, PhD

| Pneumonia

Definition

Pneumonia is an infection of the lung that can be caused by nearly any class of organism known to cause human infections. These include bacteria, amoebae, viruses, fungi, and **parasites**. Pneumonia may also result from non-infectious causes, such as inhalation of food, liquids, gases, or dust. Pneumonia often develops as a complication of a pre-existing condition or infection or when a patient's immune system is weakened by a condition such as a simple viral respiratory tract infection

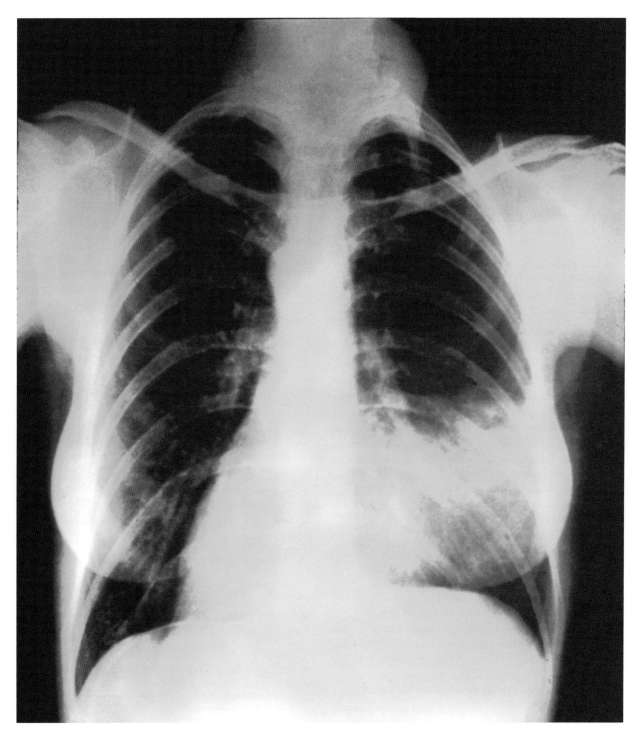

X-Ray showing pneumonia in the right lung. *(© SPL/Photo Researchers, Inc. Reproduced by permission.)*

or by **influenza**. Pneumonia and influenza together are ranked as the eighth leading cause of death in the United States, with pneumonia accounting for most of those deaths. In the elderly, pneumonia is the fourth leading cause of death and the leading infectious cause of death. In 2011, 53,692 people in the United States died of pneumonia and influenza.

When a person has pneumonia, the air sacs in the lungs become filled with pus and other liquids, and oxygen transfer from the lungs to the blood stream is inhibited. Without sufficient oxygen, body cells cannot function properly. Lobar pneumonia affects a section (lobe) of a lung while bronchial pneumonia affects patches throughout both lungs.

Description

Anatomy of the lung

To better understand pneumonia, it is important to understand the basic anatomic features of the respiratory system. The human respiratory system begins at the nose and mouth, where air is breathed in (inspired) and out (expired). The air tube extending from the nose is called the nasopharynx. The tube carrying air breathed in through the mouth is called the oropharynx. The nasopharynx and the oropharynx merge into the larynx. The oropharynx also carries swallowed substances, including food, **water**, and salivary secretion, which must pass into the esophagus and then the stomach. The larynx is protected by a trap door called the epiglottis. The epiglottis prevents substances that have been swallowed, as well as substances that have been regurgitated (thrown up), from heading down into the larynx and toward the lungs.

A useful method of picturing the respiratory system is to imagine an upside-down tree. The larynx flows into the trachea, which is the tree trunk, and thus the broadest part of the respiratory tree. The trachea divides into two tree limbs, the right and left bronchi. Each one of these branches off into multiple smaller bronchi, which course through the tissue of the lung. Each bronchus divides into tubes of smaller and smaller diameter, finally ending in the terminal bronchioles. The air sacs of the lung, in which oxygen-carbon dioxide exchange actually takes place, are clustered at the ends of the bronchioles like the leaves of a tree. They are called alveoli.

The tissue of the lung which serves only a supportive role for the bronchi, bronchioles, and alveoli is called the lung stroma (or lung parenchyma).

Function of the respiratory system

The main function of the respiratory system is to provide oxygen, the most important energy source for the body's cells. Inspired air (the air we breathe in) contains the oxygen, and travels down the respiratory tree to the alveoli. The oxygen moves out of the alveoli and is sent into circulation throughout the body as part of the red blood cells. The oxygen in the inspired air is exchanged within the alveoli for the waste product of human metabolism, carbon dioxide. The air we breathe out contains the gas called carbon dioxide. This gas leaves the alveoli during expiration. To restate this exchange of gases simply, we breathe in oxygen, we breathe out carbon dioxide.

Respiratory system defenses

The healthy human lung is sterile. There are no normally resident bacteria or viruses (unlike the upper respiratory system and parts of the gastrointestinal system, where bacteria dwell even in a healthy state). There are multiple safeguards along the path of the respiratory system. These are designed to keep invading organisms from leading to infection.

The first line of defense includes the hair in the nostrils, which serves as a filter for large particles. The epiglottis is a trap door of sorts, designed to prevent food and other swallowed substances from entering the larynx and then trachea. Sneezing and coughing, both provoked by the presence of irritants within the respiratory system, help to clear such irritants from the respiratory tract.

Mucus, produced through the respiratory system, also serves to trap dust and infectious organisms. Tiny hair like projections (cilia) from cells lining the respiratory tract beat constantly. They move debris trapped by mucus upwards and out of the respiratory tract. This mechanism of protection is referred to as the mucociliary escalator.

Cells lining the respiratory tract produce several types of immune substances which protect against various organisms. Other cells (called macrophages) along the respiratory tract actually ingest and kill invading organisms.

The organisms that cause pneumonia, then, are usually carefully kept from entering the lungs by virtue of these host defenses. However, when an individual encounters a large number of organisms at once, the usual defenses may be overwhelmed, and infection may occur. This can happen either by inhaling contaminated air droplets, or by aspiration of organisms inhabiting the upper airways.

Conditions predisposing to pneumonia

In addition to exposure to sufficient quantities of causative organisms, certain conditions may make an individual more likely to become ill with pneumonia. Various conditions are listed below.

Cigarette smoke, inhaled directly by a smoker or second-hand by a innocent bystander, interferes significantly with ciliary function, as well as inhibiting macrophage function, thus predisposing in individual to pneumonia.

Stroke, seizures, alcohol, and various drugs interfere with the function of the epiglottis. This leads to a leaky seal on the trap door, with possible contamination by swallowed substances and/or regurgitated stomach contents. Alcohol and drugs also interfere with the normal cough reflex. This further decreases the chance of clearing unwanted debris from the respiratory tract.

Viruses may interfere with ciliary function, allowing themselves or other microorganism invaders (such as bacteria) access to the lower respiratory tract. One of the most important viruses is HIV (human immunodeficiency virus), the causative virus in **AIDS** (acquired immunodeficiency syndrome). In recent years this virus has resulted in a huge increase in the incidence of pneumonia. Because AIDS results in a general decreased effectiveness of many aspects of the host's immune system, a patient with AIDS is susceptible to all kinds of pneumonia. This includes some previously rare parasitic types which would be unable to cause illness in an individual possessing a normal immune system.

Pneumonia is sometimes a pulmonary condition affecting **cancer** patients, and may indicate that the cancer is progressing or that the patient has developed a new problem. Both cancer and the therapies used to treat it can injure the lungs or weaken the immune system in ways that make cancer patients especially susceptible to the bacteria, fungi, viruses, and other organisms that cause pneumonia. Tumors and infections can block the patient's airway or limit the lungs' ability to rid themselves of fluid and other accumulated secretions that make breathing difficult. **Radiation** treatment for breast cancer increases the risk of pneumonia in some patients by weakening lung tissue. Other factors that increase a cancer patient's risk of developing pneumonia include:

• radiation therapy

• chemotherapy

• surgery

• depressed white blood cell count (neutropenia)

• antibiotics

• steroids

• malnutrition

• limited mobility

• splenectomy-immune system deficits

Various chronic conditions predispose a person to infection with pneumonia. These include **asthma**, cystic fibrosis, and neuromuscular diseases which may interfere with the seal of the epiglottis. Esophageal disorders may result in stomach contents passing upwards into the esophagus. This increases the risk of aspiration into the lungs of those stomach contents with their resident bacteria. Diabetes, sickle cell anemia, lymphoma, leukemia, and emphysema also predispose a person to pneumonia.

Pneumonia is also one of the most frequent infectious complications of all types of surgery. Many drugs used during and after surgery may increase the risk of aspiration, impair the cough reflex, and cause a patient to under fill their lungs with air. **Pain** after surgery also discourages a patient from breathing deeply enough, and from coughing effectively.

Certain other conditions can increase the risk of pneumonia. These include the following:

• abnormal anatomical structure, particularly of the chest or lungs

• advanced age and associated immune system weakness

• esophageal disorders that may result in stomach contents passing upwards

• genetic factors and associated changes in DNA

• malnutrition

Pneumonia in children

Pneumonia can develop gradually in children after exposure to the causative organism, or it can develop quickly after another illness, reducing the lungs' ability to receive and distribute oxygen. It can be mild and easily cured with **antibiotics** and rest, or it can be severe and require hospitalization. The onset, duration, and severity of pneumonia depend upon the type of infective organism invading the body and the response of the child's immune system in fighting the infection. Respiratory distress represents 20% of all admissions of children to hospitals, and pneumonia is the underlying cause of most of these admissions.

Bacterial pneumonia develops after the child inhales or aspirates pathogens. Viral pneumonia stems primarily from inhaling infected droplets from the upper airway into the lungs. In neonates, pneumonia may result from colonization of the infant's nasopharynx by organisms that were in the birth canal at the time of delivery.

Pneumonia in the elderly

Pneumonia is one of the common and significant diseases of the elderly, especially those over the age of 70. In general, the elderly are more susceptible to pneumonia than younger people. The elderly are also more likely to be hospitalized for pneumonia and need mechanical ventilation, resulting in a longer hospital stay than younger persons. In addition, many elderly people contract pneumonia while staying in a hospital for other conditions, because their immune systems are often compromised due to the condition that initially required treatment.

The elderly have a less effective mucociliary escalator, as well as changes in their immune system. This causes this age group to be more at risk for the development of pneumonia.

The intensity of symptoms and clinical manifestations of pneumonia are often less in the elderly than in younger patients, thus complicating diagnosis of the disease. The elderly may lose lung capacity as they age, making it harder for them to cough productively. They are also often used to feeling ill so may not recognize new symptoms of illness. Elderly people with pneumonia commonly exhibit acute confusion or delirium and deterioration of base metabolic functions.

Incidence

In the United States, pneumonia is the sixth most common disease leading to death; two million Americans develop pneumonia each year, and 40,000–70,000 die from it. Pneumonia is also the most common fatal infection acquired by already hospitalized patients. In developing countries, pneumonia ties with diarrhea as the most common cause of death. According to the **Centers for Disease Control and Prevention (CDC)**, the number of deaths from pneumonia in the United States has declined slightly since 2001, however, even in nonfatal cases, pneumonia is a significant economic burden on the health care system. One study estimates that people in the American workforce who develop pneumonia cost employers five times as much in health care as the average worker.

The epidemic of HIV, has resulted in a huge increase in the incidence of pneumonia. Because AIDS results in immune system suppression, individuals with AIDS are highly susceptible to all kinds of pneumonia, including some previously rare parasitic types that would not cause illness in someone with a normal immune system.

Demographics

Every year in the United States, two million people of all ages develop pneumonia, including 4% of all the children in the country. It is the sixth most common disease leading to death and the fourth leading cause of death in the elderly; 40,000 to 70,000 people die from pneumonia each year. The incidence of pneumonia in children younger than one year of age is 35 to 40 per 1,000; 30 to 35 per 1,000 children ages two to four; and 15 per 1,000 children between ages five and nine. Fewer than 10 children in 1,000 over age nine are reported to develop pneumonia.

One sixth of the six million pneumonia cases that develop each year occur primarily in persons aged 65 years and older. Over 90% of all deaths from pneumonia occur in the older population. The incidence of development of pneumonia in the elderly is 20 to 40 illnesses per 1,000 persons for pneumonia acquired in community settings, while the incidence rises to 100 to 250 per 1000 persons in cases acquired in long-term care facilities. An estimated 2.1% of elderly residents in long-term care facilities at any one time have pneumonia. About one billion dollars per year are spent on medical therapy to treat bacterial pneumonia in the elderly.

Causes

The list of organisms which can cause pneumonia is very large, and includes nearly every class of infecting organism: viruses, bacteria, bacteria-like organisms, fungi, and parasites. Some organisms are more frequently encountered by specific age groups. In addition, some characteristics of an individual may place him or her at greater risk for infection by particular types of organisms:

- Viruses cause the majority of pneumonias in young children (especially respiratory syncytial virus, parainfluenza and influenza viruses, and adenovirus).

- Adults are more frequently infected with bacteria (such as *Streptococcus pneumoniae*, *Haemophilus influenzae*, and *Staphylococcus aureus*).

- Pneumonia in older children and young adults is often caused by the bacteria-like *Mycoplasma pneumoniae* (often referred to as "walking" pneumonia).

- *Pneumocystis carinii pneumonia* (PCP) is an important cause of pneumonia in patients with immune problems (such as patients being treated for cancer with chemotherapy, or patients with AIDS). Classically considered a parasite, it appears to be more related to fungi.

- People who have reason to come into contact with bird droppings, such as poultry workers, are at risk for pneumonia caused by the organism *Chlamydia psittaci*.

- A very large, serious outbreak of pneumonia occurred in 1976, when individuals attending an American Legion convention were infected by a previously unknown organism. The outbreak caused 29 deaths among American Legion members who were staying at a Philadelphia hotel. Subsequently named *Legionella pneumophila*, it causes what is now called "Legionnaire's disease." The Legionella bacteria can live in water and can spread through air conditioning systems in hotels and hospitals. Susceptibility to the disease increases with increasing age.

Other bacteria that cause pneumonia, especially in institutional settings, include *Klebsiella*, *Pseudomonas aeruginosa*, *Enterobacter* species, *Proteus* species, *Escherichia coli*, and other gram negative bacteria. Strains of anaerobic bacteria can be aspirated into the lungs by the elderly due to conditions associated with **aging** (such as sedative use or neurological conditions) and cause pneumonia. *Haemophilus influenzae* is a bacterium that causes pneumonia more frequently in patients with chronic bronchitis.

Pneumonia caused by *Mycoplasma pneumoniae* is a common cause of pneumonia that is usually not a significant threat to the health of the elderly, as it usually affects people younger than 40. Persons at highest risk for mycoplasma pneumonia are those living or working in crowded areas such as schools and homeless shelters, although many people who contract mycoplasma pneumonia have no identifiable risk factor. Symptoms typical of pneumonia are usually mild and appear over a period of one to three weeks. They may become more severe in some people.

PCP is caused by a fungus, *Pneumocystis jiroveci*. PCP develops in persons with weakened immune systems from causes such as cancer, chronic use of corticosteroids or other medications that affect the immune system, HIV/AIDS, or solid organ and/or bone marrow transplants. Symptoms of PCP include a mild and dry cough, fever, rapid breathing, and shortness of breath, especially upon exercise or activity. PCP was a rare disease before the AIDS disease developed. This type of pneumonia may also be referred to as pneumocystis pneumonia.

Chemical pneumonia is an unusual type of lung irritation. Although pneumonia usually is caused by a bacterium or virus, in chemical pneumonia, inflammation of lung tissue can be caused by many types of chemicals, including liquids, gases, and small particles, such as dust or fumes. Only a small percentage of pneumonias are caused by chemicals. Some chemicals harm only the lungs; however, some toxic chemicals may affect other organs in addition to the lungs and can result in serious organ damage or death. Aspiration pneumonia is another form of chemical pneumonia, where oral secretions or stomach contents are aspirated into the lungs. Inflammation develops from the toxic effects of stomach acid and enzymes on lung tissue. Symptoms of chemical pneumonia may include:

- burning of the nose, eyes, lips, mouth, and throat
- dry cough
- wet cough producing clear, yellow, or green mucus
- cough producing blood or frothy pink matter
- nausea or abdominal pain
- chest pain
- shortness of breath
- painful breathing or pleuritis (an inflammation of the outside covering of the lungs)
- headache
- flu symptoms
- weakness or a general ill feeling
- delirium or disorientation

Half of all pneumonia cases are caused by viruses, including the influenza virus, parainfluenza virus, adenovirus, rhinovirus, **herpes** simplex virus, respiratory synctial virus, hantavirus, and **cytomegalovirus**. Many of these pneumonia infections are mild and may last only a short time. However pneumonia caused by the influenza virus may be severe and occasionally fatal. The symptoms of influenza pneumonia are similar to those of influenza, including fever, dry cough, headache, muscle pain, and weakness. However, within 12 to 36 hours, breathlessness develops, and the coughing increases, with a small amount of mucus produced. Patients have a high fever and may develop blueness of the lips. Eighty percent of deaths in recent influenza epidemics occurred in persons aged 65 and older, mostly due to development of complications such as sepsis or acute respiratory distress syndrome. Viral pneumonia can be further complicated by development of bacterial pneumonia.

Symptoms

Pneumonia is suspected in any patient who has fever, cough, chest pain, shortness of breath, and increased respirations (number of breaths per minute). Fever with a shaking chill is even more suspicious. Many patients cough up clumps of sputum, commonly known as spit. These secretions are produced in the alveoli during an infection or other inflammatory condition. They may appear streaked with pus or blood. Severe pneumonia results in the signs of oxygen deprivation. This includes blue appearance of the nail beds or lips (cyanosis).

The invading organism causes symptoms, in part, by provoking an overly-strong immune response in the lungs. In other words, the immune system, which should help fight off infections, kicks into such high gear that it damages the lung tissue and makes it more susceptible to infection. The small blood vessels in the lungs (capillaries) become leaky, and protein-rich fluid seeps into the alveoli. This results in less functional area for oxygen-carbon dioxide exchange. The patient becomes relatively oxygen deprived, while retaining potentially damaging carbon dioxide. The patient breathes faster and faster in an effort to bring in more oxygen and blow off more carbon dioxide.

Mucus production is increased, and the leaky capillaries may tinge the mucus with blood. Mucus plugs actually further decrease the efficiency of gas exchange in the lung. The alveoli fill further with fluid and debris from the large number of white blood cells being produced to fight the infection.

Consolidation, a feature of bacterial pneumonias, occurs when the alveoli, which are normally hollow air spaces within the lung, instead, become solid due to quantities of fluid and debris.

Viral pneumonias and mycoplasma pneumonias do not result in consolidation. These types of pneumonia primarily infect the walls of the alveoli and the stroma of the lung.

Severe acute respiratory syndrome (SARS)

Severe acute respiratory syndrome, or **SARS**, is a contagious and potentially fatal disease that first appeared in the form of a multi-country outbreak in early February 2003. Later that month, the **CDC** began to work with the **World Health Organization (WHO)** to investigate the cause(s) of SARS and to develop guidelines for **infection control**. SARS has been described as an "atypical pneumonia of unknown etiology;" by the end of March 2003, the disease agent was identified as a previously unknown coronavirus.

The early symptoms of SARS include a high fever with chills, headache, muscle cramps, and weakness. This early phase is followed by respiratory symptoms, usually a dry cough and painful or difficult breathing. Some patients require mechanical ventilation. The mortality rate of SARS is thought to be about 3%.

Diagnosis

For the most part, diagnosis is based on the patient's report of symptoms, combined with examination of the chest. Listening with a stethoscope will reveal abnormal sounds, and tapping on the patient's back (which should yield a resonant sound due to air filling the alveoli) may instead yield a dull thump if the alveoli are filled with fluid and debris.

Laboratory diagnosis can be made of some bacterial pneumonias by obtaining a sputum specimen and staining the sputum with special chemicals and looking at it under a microscope. Identification of the specific type of bacteria may require culturing the sputum (using the sputum sample to grow greater numbers of the bacteria in a lab dish).

X-ray examination of the chest may reveal certain abnormal changes associated with pneumonia. Localized shadows obscuring areas of the lung may indicate a bacterial pneumonia, while streaky or patchy appearing changes in the x-ray picture may indicate viral or mycoplasma pneumonia. These changes on x-ray, however, are known to lag in time behind the patient's actual symptoms.

The doctor may do a bronchoscopy (visualizing inside the airway via a scope), or may remove a small piece of lung tissue (transbronchial biopsy) for microscopic examination and cultures. If the patient's condition continues to worsen, the doctor may remove additional lung tissue via thoracic needle biopsy or open lung biopsy, for microscopic analysis and cultures.

Treatment

Prior to the discovery of penicillin antibiotics, bacterial pneumonia was almost always fatal. Today, antibiotics, especially given early in the course of the disease, are very effective against bacterial causes of pneumonia. Erythromycin and tetracycline improve recovery time for symptoms of mycoplasma pneumonia. They do not, however, eradicate the organisms. Amantadine and acyclovir may be helpful against certain viral pneumonias.

A newer antibiotic named linezolid (Zyvox) is being used to treat penicillin-resistant organisms that cause pneumonia. Linezolid is the first of a new line of antibiotics known as oxazolidinones. Another new drug known as ertapenem (Invanz) is reported to be effective in treating bacterial pneumonia.

Patients may also be given fluids and possibly drug therapy to thin mucus secretions (mucolytic agents) or medication to open the airways of the lung (brochodilators). Cough suppressants may be given as well as pain medication and fever-reducing medication. Hospitalized patients often receive oxygen, respiratory therapy, and intravenous antibiotics and fluids.

Pneumonia in cancer patients must be treated promptly in order to speed recovery and prevent complications that could arise if the inflammation were allowed to linger. Treatment always includes bed rest and coughing to expel phlegm and other fluids from the lungs (productive cough). To determine which course of treatment would be most appropriate, a doctor considers when symptoms first appeared, what pattern the illness has followed, and whether cancer or its treatments have diminished the patient's infection-fighting ability (immune response).

Public health response

Most forms of pneumonia are not reportable diseases, and so are reported to public health agencies only through informal procedures, such as calls from primary healthcare workers. Knowing about the existence of such cases in a community can be of importance to public health agencies because they allow public health workers to follow up on possible sources of the disease and its spread among members of the community. When cases of pneumonia are identified within a community, public health workers collect basic information about the disease characteristics, patients' symptoms,

KEY TERMS

Acute respiratory distress syndrome—A serious reaction to various forms of injuries to the lung, which is characterized by inflammation of the lung, leading to impaired gas exchange and release of inflammatory mediators causing inflammation and low blood oxygen and frequently resulting in multiple organ failure. This condition is life threatening and often lethal, usually requiring mechanical ventilation and admission to an intensive care unit.

Alveoli—The little air sacs clustered at the ends of the bronchioles, in which oxygen-carbon dioxide exchange takes place.

Aspiration—A situation in which solids or liquids which should be swallowed into the stomach are instead breathed into the respiratory system.

Bronchoscopy—The examination of the bronchi (the main airways of the lungs) using a flexible tube (bronchoscope). Bronchoscopy helps to evaluate and diagnose lung problems, assess blockages, obtain samples of tissue and/or fluid, and/or to help remove a foreign body.

CD4 count—A measure of the strength of the immune system. HIV continually kills CD4 cells. Over time, the body can not replace these lost CD4 cells and their number declines. AS this happens, the body becomes more susceptible to infections. A normal CD4 count is 1,000. The body starts to get more frequent common infections at around a count

of 400. At around a CD4 count of 200, the body becomes susceptible to many unusual infections. It is best to start medications for HIV before the CD4 count drops below 200 to prevent these infections from developing.

Cilia—Hair-like projections from certain types of cells.

Consolidation—A condition in which lung tissue becomes firm and solid rather than elastic and air-filled because it has accumulated fluids and tissue debris.

Coronavirus—One of a family of RNA-containing viruses known to cause severe respiratory illnesses. In March 2003, a previously unknown coronavirus was identified as the causative agent of severe acute respiratory syndrome, or SARS.

Cyanosis—A bluish tinge to the skin that can occur when the blood oxygen level drops too low.

Sepsis—Presence of various pus-forming and other pathogenic organisms, or their toxins, in the blood or tissues.

Sputum—Material produced within the alveoli in response to an infectious or inflammatory process.

Stroma—A term used to describe the supportive tissue surrounding a particular structure. An example is that tissue which surrounds and supports the actually functional lung tissue.

and other relevant information that can be used to decide on the most reasonable treatment to be recommended. That information can also be used to provide information about an pneumonia outbreak to health professionals and to the general public. This type of educational program about pneumonia would normally include possible sources of the disease, methods of transmission, treatment options, and methods of **prevention**.

Prognosis

Prognosis varies according to the type of organism causing the infection. Recovery following pneumonia with *Mycoplasma pneumoniae* is nearly 100%. *Staphylococcus pneumoniae* has a death rate of 30–40%. Similarly, infections with a number of gram negative bacteria (such as those in the gastrointestinal tract which can cause infection following aspiration) have a death rate of 25–50%. *Streptococcus pneumoniae*, (also referred to as pneumococcal pneumonia), the most common organism causing pneumonia, produces a death

rate of about 5%. More complications occur in the very young or very old individuals who have multiple areas of the lung infected simultaneously. Individuals with other chronic illnesses (including cirrhosis of the liver, congestive heart failure, individuals without a functioning spleen, and individuals who have other diseases that result in a weakened immune system, experience complications. Patients with immune disorders, various types of cancer, transplant patients, and AIDS patients also experience complications.

The chances of an early recovery (within two to three weeks) from pneumonia are enhanced if the pneumonia is detected early, if the patient has a strong immune system, if the infection has not spread throughout the body, and if the patient is not suffering from other diseases.

Prevention

Measures that can be taken to prevent pneumonia include frequent washing of hands, elimination of the use of tobacco (which damages the ability of the lungs to withstand infections), and wearing of masks in dusty or moldy areas. Since pneumonia often follows common respiratory infections such as the cold or flu, an important preventive measure is to be alert to any symptoms of respiratory illness that last for more than a few days. The practice of deep breathing for patients recovering in the hospital from various diseases or surgeries is recommended to help prevent them from developing pneumonia.

Because many bacterial pneumonias occur in patients who are first infected with the influenza virus (the flu), yearly **vaccination** against influenza can decrease the risk of pneumonia for certain patients. This is particularly true of the elderly and people with chronic diseases (such as asthma, cystic fibrosis, other lung or heart diseases, sickle cell disease, diabetes, kidney disease, and forms of cancer).

A specific vaccine against *Streptococcus pneumoniae* is very protective, and should also be administered to patients with chronic illnesses.

Patients who have decreased immune resistance are at higher risk for infection with *Pneumocystis carinii*. They are frequently put on a regular drug regimen of trimethoprim sulfa and/or inhaled pentamidine to avoid pneumocystis pneumonia.

The flu vaccine helps prevent pneumonia caused by influenza viruses. This vaccine must be given yearly to protect against new viral strains.

Additional preventive therapy may be necessary for:

• AIDS patients with CD4 counts below 200

• people on chronic high-doses of corticosteroids

• people who have had previous episodes of PCP

Health care team roles

In most cases, a diagnosis of pneumonia is made in a physician's office, a general medical clinic, or emergency room by a primary care practitioner. Children and adolescents with pneumonia are most likely to be diagnosed by their primary care physician or pediatrician.

When patients are hospitalized for pneumonia, good nursing assessment and observation are primary requirements. These include monitoring vital signs, including oxygen saturation (the amount of oxygen circulating in the blood), encouraging the patient to move, breathe deeply, cough, and get out of bed with assistance (if indicated) to facilitate good lung expansion. The nurse should also provide education to the patient about the importance of coughing, breathing deeply, and taking in adequate fluid.

When at home, patients should be encouraged to drink fluids to loosen secretions and bring up phlegm. Both patients and care givers should be made aware of potential drug interactions with other medications that the patient may be taking (for example, warfarin and antibiotics). Regular communication between the physician and the care giver is essential.

Resources
BOOKS

Fein, Alan, and Ronald Grossman. *Diagnosis and Management of Pneumonia ad Other Respiratory Infections.* West Islip, NY: Professional Communications, Inc., 2006.

Icon Group International. *Pneumonia: Webster's Timeline History, 1998 - 2005.* San Diego, CA: ICON Group International, Inc., 2009.

Mays, Thomas Jefferson. *Pulmonary Consumption, Pneumonia, and Allied Diseases of the Lungs.* New York, NY: General Books LLC, 2009.

Niederman, Michael S., ed. *Severe Pneumonia (Lung Biology in Health and Disease).* London, United Kingdom: Informa Healthcare, 2005.

Petty, Thomas, and James S. Seebass, eds. *Pulmonary Disorders of the Elderly: Diagnosis, Prevention, and Treatment.* Philadelphia, PA: American College of Physicians, 2007.

PERIODICALS

Gulland, A. "Simple Measures Could Prevent More than Two Million Child Deaths from Pneumonia and Diarrhoea." *BMJ* 344, e4025. (2012): 344.

Saltzman, R. W., et al. "Clinical Conditions Associated with PCP in Children." *Pediatric Pulmonolgy* 47, 5. (2012): 510-6.

Von Baum, H., et al. "How Deadly Is Seasonal Influenza-associated pneumonia? The German Competence Network for Community-Acquired Pneumonia." *European Respiratory Journal* 37, 5. (2011): 1151–57.

WEBSITES

Pneumonia. American Lung Association. http://www.lung.org/lung-disease/pneumonia/ (accessed August 23, 2012).

Pneumonia. Mayo Clinic. http://www.mayoclinic.com/health/pneumonia/DS00135 (accessed August 23, 2012).

Pneumonia–Topic Overview. WebMD. http://www.webmd.com/lung/tc/pneumonia-topic-overview (accessed August 23, 2012).

ORGANIZATIONS

American Lung Association, 1301 Pennsylvania Ave. NW, Washington, D.C. 20004. (202) 785 3355; Fax: (202) 452 1805. http://www.lungusa.org.

Centers for Disease Control and Prevention. 1600 Clifton Rd., NE, Atlanta, GA 30333. (800) CDC-INFO (800 232-4636) or (404) 639-3534. cdcinfo@cdc.gov, www.cdc.gov.

National Heart Lung and Blood Institute. P.O. Box 30105, Bethesda, MD 20824-0105. 301-592-8573. nhlbiinfo@nhlbi.nih.gov, http://www.nhlbi.nih.gov.

World Health Organization, Communicable Diseases, 20 Avenue Appia, 1211, Geneva 27, Switzerland. +41 22 791 4140. http://www.who.int/gtb.

Rosalyn Carson-DeWitt, MD
Rebecca J. Frey, Ph.D.
Laura Jean Cataldo, RN, Ed.D.

Poisoning

Definition

Poisoning occurs when any substance interferes with normal body functions (that is, disturbs an organism by chemical reaction or other activity on the molecular level) after it is swallowed, inhaled, injected, or absorbed in a sufficient quantity. The substance that does the poisoning is called a poison. The branch of medicine that deals with the detection and treatment of poisons is known as "toxicology." In actuality, any substance can be poisonous if too much is taken. For example, water taken in extremely large amounts—called "water intoxification"—can cause death in humans. However, water is generally not considered a poison. Poisons normally are considered within the following groups: carbon monoxide in appliances, household products (such as furniture polish), indoor/outdoor plants, heavy metals such as lead, overdoses of illegal drugs, pesticides, and prescription or over-the counter medicines that are taken in extreme doses.

Description

Poisons are common in the home and workplace, yet there are basically two major types. One group consists of products that were never meant to be ingested or inhaled, such as shampoo, paint thinner, pesticides, houseplant leaves, and carbon monoxide. The other group contains products that can be ingested in small quantities but are harmful if taken in large amounts, such as pharmaceuticals, medicinal herbs, and alcohol. Other types of poisons include the bacterial toxins that cause food poisoning, such as *Escherichia coli*; heavy metals, such as the lead found in the paint on older houses; and the venom found in the bites and stings of some animals and insects. The staff at a poison control center and emergency room doctors have the most experience diagnosing and treating poisoning cases.

Demographics

Poisonings are a common occurrence and can be intentional or unintentional. About 10 million cases of poisoning occur in the United States each year. As of 2012, the U.S. **Centers for Disease Control and Prevention (CDC)** state every day, on average, 87 Americans die because of unintentional poisoning, and another 2,277 are treated in emergency departments (EDs). The **CDC** also reports that deaths from unintentional poisoning increased by 160% from 1999 to 2009. At the end of that period, unintentional poisoning was the second leading cause of unintentional injury death (second only to motor vehicle fatalities). That same year, the most common cause of unintentional poisoning deaths was drugs, with opioid **pain** medications, cocaine, and heroin being the most common ones used. Between 2004 and 2005, around 71,000 children, less than 18 years of age, were seen in EDs each year because of medication poisonings. Over 80% of these visits were involved an unsupervised child. Curiosity, inability to read warning labels, a desire to imitate adults, and inadequate supervision lead to childhood poisonings.

The elderly are the second most likely group to be poisoned. Mental confusion, poor eyesight, and the use of multiple drugs are the leading reasons that this group has a high rate of accidental poisoning. A substantial number of poisonings also occur as **suicide** attempts or drug overdoses.

Costs to society

In 2005, according to the CDC, poisonings led to $33.4 billion in medical and productivity costs within the United States.

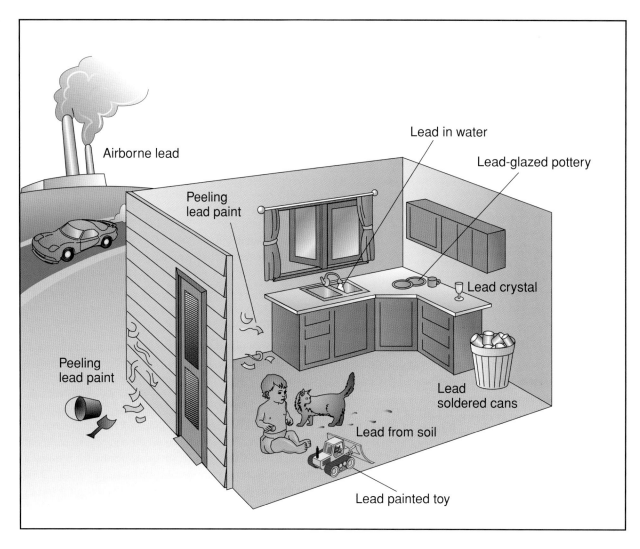

Continuous exposure to lead can damage nearly every system in the human body and is particularly harmful to the developing brain of fetuses and young children. Common sources of lead exposure include lead-based paint, dust and soil, drinking water, food from cans, and eating utensils, such as plates and drinking glasses, that are lead-based. *(Illustration by Electronic Illustrators Group. Reproduced by permission of Gale, a part of Cengage Learning.)*

Causes and symptoms

The causes of poisons are wide in numbers, and the symptoms vary widely as well.

Causes

The effects of poisons are as varied as the poisons themselves. However, the medical community understands the exact mechanisms of only a few. Some poisons interfere with metabolism. Others destroy the liver or kidneys. Some examples include the consumption of heavy metals and the overdosing of some pain relief medications, including acetaminophen (Tylenol) and nonsteroidal anti–inflammatory drugs (Advil, Ibuprofen). A poison may severely depress the central nervous system, leading to coma and eventual respiratory and circulatory failure. Potential poisons in this category include anesthetics (e.g., ether and chloroform), opiates (e.g., morphine and codeine), and barbiturates. Some poisons directly affect the respiratory and circulatory systems. Carbon monoxide causes death by binding with hemoglobin that normally transports oxygen throughout the body. Certain corrosive vapors trigger the body to flood the lungs with fluids, effectively drowning the person. Cyanide interferes with respiration at the cellular level. Another group of poisons interferes with the electrochemical impulses that travel between neurons in the nervous system. Yet another group, including cocaine, ergot, strychnine, and some snake venoms, causes potentially fatal seizures.

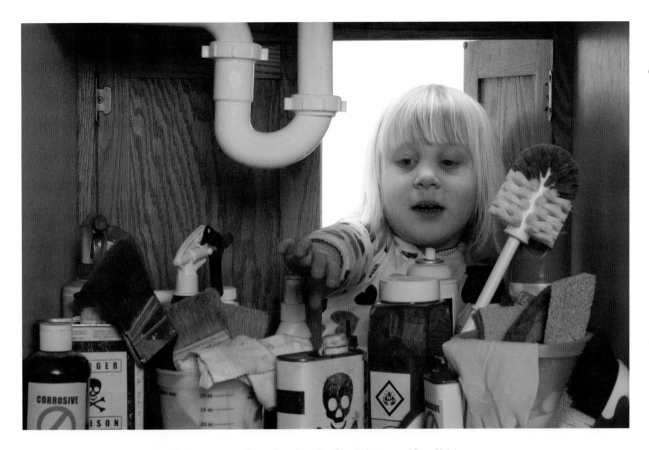

A child depicted in a household danger zone for poisoning. *(© iStockphoto.com/GaryAlvis)*

Symptoms

Severity of symptoms can range from headache and nausea to convulsions and death. The type of poison; the amount and time of exposure; and the age, size, and health of the victim are all factors that determine the severity of symptoms and the chances for recovery.

Symptoms of plant poisoning range from irritation of the skin or mucous membranes of the mouth and throat to nausea, vomiting, convulsions, irregular heartbeat, and even death. It is often difficult to tell whether a person has eaten a poisonous plant because there are no tell-tale empty containers and no unusual lesions or odors around the mouth.

Many cases of plant poisoning involve plants that contain hallucinogens, such as peyote cactus buttons, certain types of mushrooms, and marijuana. A recent case of plant poisoning in France concerned *Datura*, or moonflower, a plant that has become popular with young people trying to imitate Native American puberty rites.

Other cases of plant poisoning result from the use of herbal dietary supplements that have been contaminated by toxic substances. The Food and Drug Administration (FDA) has the authority to monitor herbal products on the market and issue warnings about accidental poisoning or other adverse effects associated with these products. For example, in 2011, the U.S. confectionery company Candy Dynamics voluntarily recalled its gum called "Toxic Waste Short Circuits" bubblegum because the FDA found it contained unsafe levels of lead, along with other heavy metals.

Household chemicals

Many products used daily in the home are poisonous if swallowed. These products often contain strong acids or strong bases (alkalis). Toxic household cleaning products include:

- ammonia
- bleach
- dishwashing liquids
- drain openers
- floor waxes and furniture polishes
- laundry detergents, spot cleaners, and fabric softeners
- mildew removers
- oven cleaners
- toilet bowl cleaners

Personal care products found in the home can also be poisonous. These include:

- deodorant
- hairspray
- hair straighteners
- nail polish and polish remover
- perfume
- shampoo

Signs that a person has swallowed one of these substances include evidence of an empty container nearby, nausea or vomiting, and **burns** on the lips and skin around the mouth if the substance was a strong acid or alkali. The chemicals in some of these products may leave a distinctive odor on the breath.

Pharmaceuticals

Both over-the-counter and prescription medicines can help the body heal if taken as directed. However, when taken in large quantities or with other drugs where there may be an adverse interaction, they can act as poisons. Drug overdoses, both accidental and intentional, are the leading cause of poisoning in adults. Medicinal herbs should be treated like pharmaceuticals. They should be taken only in designated quantities and under the supervision of a knowledgeable person. Herbs that have healing qualities when taken in small doses can be toxic in larger doses or can interact with prescription medications in unpredictable ways.

Drug overdoses cause a range of symptoms, including excitability, sleepiness, confusion, unconsciousness, rapid heartbeat, convulsions, nausea, and changes in blood pressure. The best initial evidence of a drug overdose is the presence of an empty container near the victim.

Other causes of poisonings

People can be poisoned by fumes they inhale. Carbon monoxide is the most common form of inhaled poison. Other toxic substances that can be inhaled include:

- farm and garden insecticides and herbicides
- gasoline fumes
- insect repellent
- paint thinner fumes

Diagnosis

Initially, poisoning is suspected if the victim shows changes in behavior and signs or symptoms previously described. Hallucinations or other psychiatric symptoms may indicate poisoning by a hallucinogenic plant. Evidence of an empty container or information from the victim is helpful in determining exactly what substance has caused the poisoning. Some acids and alkalis leave burns on the mouth. Petroleum products, such as lighter fluid or kerosene, leave a distinctive odor on the breath. The vomit may be tested to determine the exact composition of the poison. Once hospitalized, the patient may be given blood and urine tests to determine his or her metabolic condition.

Prevention

Most accidental poisonings are preventable. The number of deaths of children from poisoning has declined since the 1960s but the U.S. National Center for Health Statistics stated that 972 American children died in 2007 from poisonings. The CDC states in 2012 that the lowest mortality rates for poisonings were among children less than 15 years old because they do not abuse drugs as frequently as do older people. This decline has occurred mainly because of better packaging of toxic materials and better public education.

Actions to prevent poisonings include:

- removing plants that are poisonous
- keeping medicines and household chemicals locked and in a place inaccessible to children
- keeping medications in child-resistant containers
- never referring to medicine as "candy"
- keeping cleaners and other poisons in their original containers
- disposing of outdated prescription medicines
- not purchasing over-the-counter medications with damaged protective seals or packaging
- avoiding the use of herbal preparations not made by a reputable manufacturer

Treatment

Treatment for poisoning depends on the poison swallowed or inhaled. Contacting the poison control center or hospital emergency room is the first step in getting proper treatment. The poison control center's telephone number is often listed with emergency numbers on the inside cover of the telephone book, or it can be reached by dialing the operator. The poison control center will ask for specific information about the victim and the poison, then give appropriate first aid instructions. If the patient is to be taken to a hospital, a sample of vomit and the poison container should be taken along, if they are available.

Most cases of plant poisoning are treated by inducing vomiting, if the patient is fully conscious. Vomiting can be induced by taking syrup of ipecac, an over-the-counter emetic (an agent that induces vomiting) available at any pharmacy.

For acid, alkali, or petroleum product poisonings, the patient should not vomit. Acids and alkalis can burn the esophagus if they are vomited, and petroleum products can be inhaled into the lungs during vomiting, resulting in **pneumonia**.

Once under medical care, doctors have the option of treating the patient with a specific remedy to counteract the poison (antidote) or with activated charcoal to absorb the substance inside the patient's digestive system. In some instances, pumping the stomach may be required. This technique, which is known as "gastric lavage," involves introducing 20–30 milliliters (mL) of tap water or 9% saline solution into the patient's digestive tract and removing the stomach contents with a siphon or syringe. The process is repeated until the washings are free of poison. Medical personnel will also provide supportive care as needed, such as intravenous fluids or mechanical ventilation.

If the doctor suspects that the poisoning was not accidental, he or she is required to notify law enforcement authorities. Most cases of malicious poisoning concern family members or acquaintances of the victim, but the number of intentional random poisonings of the public has increased in recent years. In 2009, according to the U.S. Substance Abuse and Mental Health Services Administration (SAMHSA), 14,270 emergency room visits were reported for intentional drug poisoning. Intentional poisonings often occur inside bars or nightclubs. An illicit drug is placed into a person's alcoholic drink by someone aiming to sexually assault or rob that person. One such illicit drug used in this scenario is the so-called date rape drug, which is the general name for one of two prescription sleep-aid drugs—gamma-hydroxybutyric acid (GHB) or benzodiazepines (Rohypnol or "roofies") used in combination with alcohol.

Prognosis

The outcome of poisoning varies from complete recovery to death and depends on the type and amount of the poison, the health of the victim, and the speed with which medical care is obtained.

Precautions

Nancy Harvey Steorts, the author of *Safety and You* and the former chair of the U.S. Consumer Product Safety Commission, makes the following statement, "It can happen so fast! A poison can get into your system

and you can get deathly ill or even die. You can be a little child, or a grown adult. Poisoning can happen to anyone." Steorts also offers the following precautions to prevent food poisonings:

- Thoroughly wash all fruits and vegetables before eating them.
- Thoroughly wash off the tops of any canned soft drinks or foods before opening them.
- Make sure the kitchen is clean, and that all counters are disinfected, and utensils are thoroughly washed before using them.
- Thoroughly cook all meats, poultry, and fish before eating them, as a potentially toxic substance could be on such items.
- Always use a meat thermometer.

Risks

The U.S. **Department of Health and Human Services** (HHS) reported that, in 2008, 2.5 million people called a poison center because someone had been exposed to a poison. Children under the age of six years accounted for half of all human poison exposures reported to poison centers. However, adults are also at risk. That year, more than three-quarters of all poisoning deaths reported to poison centers occurred among people ages 20 to 59 years.

The HHS also stated that different types of poisonings are more frequent, depending on age. For example, older adults are more prone to being poisoned from taking prescription medications. On the other hand, children are more likely to be poisoned through painkillers, cosmetics, personal care or cleaning products,

QUESTIONS TO ASK YOUR DOCTOR

- How long will it take me to recover from food poisoning?
- How do I reduce my risk, and my children's risk, of lead poisoning?
- Where can I learn more about poisons and poisoning?
- What are my treatment options with respect to my particular form of poisoning?
- What are the risks associated with treatment?
- Will I recover completely from being poisoned?

pest killers, and plants. Preteens through older adults are commonly poisoned through alcohol, herbal products, over-the-counter medicines, prescription drugs, and spoiled food.

Aftercare

If two days after being treated for food poisoning, one is not feeling better, and symptoms have not markedly improved, make an appointment to see a family doctor or primary healthcare provider.

Resources

BOOKS

Beers, Mark H. *The Merck Manual of Diagnosis and Therapy.* Rahway: Merck, 2006.

Shannon, Michael W., et al. *Haddad and Winchester's Clinical Management of Poisoning and Drug Overdose.* Philadelphia: Saunders/Elsevier, 2007.

WEBSITES

Baker, David E. *Homeowner Chemical Safety.* National Ag Safety Database, University of Missouri-Columbia. (April 2002). http://nasdonline.org/document/1088/d000874/ homeowner-chemical-safety.html (accessed August 13, 2012).

Candy Dynamics Recalls Toxic Waste® Short Circuits™ Bubble Gum. Canadian Food Inspection Agency. (March 28, 2011). http://www.inspection.gc.ca/english/corpaffr/recarapp/ 2011/20110328e.shtml (accessed August 14, 2012).

Cunha, John P. *Poisoning.* eMedicineHealth.com. http:// www.emedicinehealth.com/poisoning/article_em.htm (accessed August 14, 2012).

Emergency Manual. American Academy of Emergency Physicians. http://www.emergencycareforyou.org/Emergency Manual/Default.aspx (accessed August 13, 2012).

FDA Poisonous Plant Database. Food and Drug Administration. (May 2008). http://www.accessdata.fda.gov/scripts/ plantox/index.cfm. (accessed August 13, 2012).

Intentional Poisonings in Clubs, Bars May Be on the Rise. CBS News. (November 10, 2011). http://www.cbsnews.com/ 8301-500368_162-57322016/intentional-poisonings-in-clubs-bars-may-be-on-the-rise/ (accessed August 14, 2012).

Poisoning. Medline Plus. (June 12, 2012). http://www.nlm.nih .gov/medlineplus/poisoning.html (accessed August 14, 2012).

Steorts. Nancy Harvey. *Poison Precautions.* ParentsTalk.com. http://www.parentstalk.com/expertsadvice/ea_fs_0008. html (accessed August 14, 2012).

Unintentional Poisoning Data & Statistics. Centers for Disease Control and Prevention. (June 29, 2012). http://www .cdc.gov/homeandrecreationalsafety/poisoning/data.html (accessed August 14, 2012).

ORGANIZATIONS

American Association of Poison Control Centers, (800) 222-1222, http://www.aapcc.org

American Medical Association, 515 N. State St., Chicago, IL U.S.A. 60654, (800) 621-8335, http://www.ama-assn.org/

Food and Drug Administration, 10903 New Hampshire Ave., Silver Spring, MD U.S.A. 20993, (888) INFO-FDA (463-6332), http://www.fda.gov/

National Toxicology Program (National Institute of Environmental Health Sciences), PO Box 12233, Research Triangle Park, NC U.S.A. 27709, 1 (541-3419), http://ntp .niehs.nih.gov/

Tish Davidson, A.M.
Rebecca J. Frey, PhD
Karl Finley
William A. Atkins, B.B., B.S., M.B.A.

Polio

Definition

Poliomyelitis, or polio, is an **infectious disease** caused by a virus that normally lives in the human digestive tract. About 90% of persons infected by the virus have no symptoms at all. In the other 10%, the polio virus causes an infection with symptoms ranging from a mild flu-like illness to paralysis of the lower limbs or death from paralysis of the muscles that control breathing.

Description

The term poliomyelitis comes from the Greek words *polio*, meaning gray, and *myelon*, referring to the spinal cord. The term is accurate, as an important consequence of the disease is the involvement of the spinal cord.

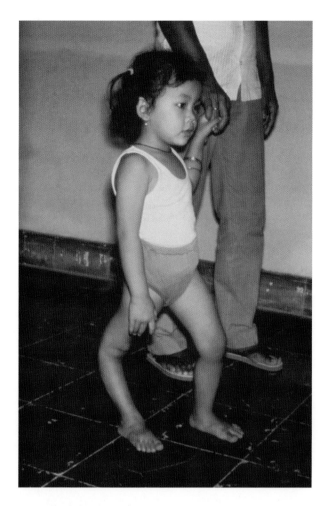

A young girl with a deformity in her right lower extremity due to Polio. *(© CDC)*

of paralysis, which is the most severe manifestation of the infection.

When the poliovirus reaches the central nervous system, inflammation and destruction of the spinal cord motor cells (anterior horn cells) occurs, which prevents them from sending out impulses to muscles. Loss of impulse transmission causes the muscles to become limp or soft and they cannot contract. This condition is referred to as flaccid paralysis. The extent of the paralysis depends on where the virus strikes and the number of cells that it destroys. Usually, some of the limb muscles are paralyzed; the abdominal muscles or muscles of the back may be paralyzed, affecting the person's posture. The neck muscles may become too weak for the head to be lifted. Paralysis of the face muscles may cause the mouth to twist or the eyelids to droop. According to **WHO**, one of every 200 infections leads to paralysis. Of those, between 5% and 10% die because their breathing muscles become paralyzed.

Risk factors

Humans are the only natural host of polioviruses; these viruses are not transmitted by animals. Some people are more likely than others to develop the paralytic form of the disease if they do become infected. These include:

- young children
- elderly adults
- people who engage in hard physical labor or strenuous exercise
- people who have recently had a tonsillectomy or dental surgery
- pregnant women
- people who travel frequently to areas where polio is still endemic
- people with an immune system weakened by HIV/AIDS or certain types of cancer treatment

Demographics

According to the **Centers for Disease Control and Prevention (CDC)**, the incidence rate has been less than 0.01 cases per 100,000 people in the United States since 1965.

Worldwide, polio has come close to being eradicated. In 1988, polio was endemic in 125 countries. By mid-2012, it was endemic in only 3—Afghanistan, Pakistan, and Nigeria. However, in June 2012, the Taliban, a fundamentalist insurgent group in Afghanistan and Pakistan, forced stoppage of the polio **vaccination** program in Pakistan for fear that doctors with the program were working as spies for the United States. As

Polio was widespread in the developed countries of Europe and North America in the first part of the twentieth century. The epidemics not only became more severe, but also affected adolescents and adults rather than mostly children. The older average age of patients was also marked by increased severity of symptoms. Since the introduction of effective vaccines, paralytic polio is almost unknown in the United States except for a few cases among recent immigrants and travelers who have contracted the disease outside the United States; the last case of wild polio occurred in the United States in 1979. In 1988, the **World Health Organization (WHO)** began the Global Polio Eradication Initiative with the goal of wiping out endemic polio by 2006.

There are three known types of polioviruses (called 1, 2, and 3), each causing a different strain of the disease. All are members of the viral family of enteroviruses, which are viruses that infect the gastrointestinal tract. Type 1 is the cause of epidemics and about 85% of cases

DR. JONAS E. SALK (1914–1995)

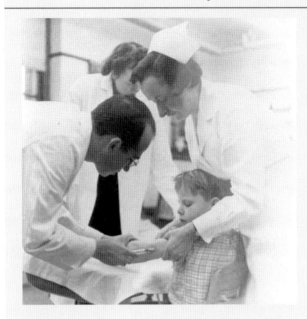

(Library of Congress)

Jonas Salk was born in New York, New York, on October 28, 1914. He received his medical degree from New York University in 1939. In 1942, Salk began working for a former teacher, Thomas Francis, Jr., to produce influenza vaccines, a project that continued until 1949.

That year, as a research professor, Salk began a three-year project sponsored by the National Foundation for Infantile Paralysis, also known as the March of Dimes. Caused by the poliomyelitis virus, polio was also known as infantile paralysis. Periodic outbreaks of the disease, which attacks the nervous system, caused death or a lifetime of paralysis, especially in children. It was a difficult disease to study because sufficient viruses could not be obtained. Unlike bacteria, which can be grown in cultures, viruses need living tissue on which to grow. Once a method for preparing viruses was discovered and improved, sufficient viruses became available for research.

Salk first set out to confirm that there were three virus types responsible for polio and then began to experiment with ways to kill the virus and yet retain its ability to produce an immune response. By 1952, he had produced a dead virus vaccine that worked against the three virus types. He began testing. First the vaccine was tested on monkeys, then on children who had recovered from the disease, and finally on Salk's own family and children, none of whom had ever had the disease. Following large-scale trials in 1954, the vaccine was finally released for public use in 1955. The Salk vaccine was not the first vaccine against polio, but it was the first to be found safe and effective. By 1961, there was a 96 percent reduction in polio cases in the United States.

of this writing, the polio vaccination program in the Afghanistan-Pakistan border region had not resumed. A similar boycott of the polio vaccination program occurred in Nigeria in 2003 when rumors were spread that the vaccine contained anti-fertility drugs to prevent Muslim men from fathering children. Although the vaccination program resumed 12 months later, the disease had returned to large areas of Nigeria and as of 2012 had not yet been eradicated.

Causes and symptoms

Polio is caused by a virus that enters the mouth through food or **water** that has been contaminated by fecal matter. It is an extremely contagious illness; anyone living with a recently infected person is likely to become infected too. Although people carrying the poliovirus are most contagious for 7–10 days before and after symptoms (if any) appear, they can spread the virus for weeks in their bowel movements.

Once inside the body, the polio virus takes between 6 and 20 days to incubate. It finds its way to the tissues

lining the throat and the intestinal tract, where it multiplies rapidly. After about a week in the intestines, the virus travels to the tonsils and the lymph nodes, where it multiplies further and then enters the bloodstream. It can remain within the blood and lymphatic system for as long as 17 weeks. In a minority of cases, the virus enters the central nervous system from the blood and lymph. It then multiplies in and destroys the nerve cells (motor neurons) in the brain and spinal cord that control the movements of the muscles. The location and severity of the paralytic polio that results when the motor neurons are damaged varies with the part of the central nervous system that is affected.

Minor forms of acute polio infection

Between 4 and 8% of acute polio infections are characterized by influenza-like symptoms. This type of infection is called abortive poliomyelitis. People with this form of polio infection experience sore throat and fever, nausea, vomiting, abdominal **pain**, constipation, or diarrhea. Abortive polio is difficult to distinguish from influenza or other viral infections. Patients recover completely in about a week.

About 10% of people infected with poliovirus develop severe headache and pain and stiffness of the neck and back. These symptoms are due to an inflammation of the meninges (tissues that cover the spinal cord and brain). This syndrome is called nonparalytic or aseptic **meningitis**. The term "aseptic" is used to differentiate this type of meningitis from those caused by bacteria. Patients with nonparalytic meningitis may experience a brief period of general illness followed by stiffness in the neck, back, or legs. They may also experience other abnormal sensations for a period of 2–10 days. As with abortive polio, patients with nonparalytic meningitis recover completely.

Paralytic polio

Between 1 and 2% of people infected with poliovirus develop the most severe form, paralytic polio. Some of these individuals may have 2–3 symptom-free days between the minor illness and the major illness, but often the symptoms appear without any previous minor illness. Symptoms again include headache and back and neck pain. The major symptoms, however, are due to invasion of the motor nerves, which are responsible for movement of the muscles.

Paralytic polio is usually divided into three types, depending on whether the paralysis affects the arms and legs (spinal polio; accounts for 79% of cases of paralytic polio); breathing, speaking, and swallowing (bulbar polio; 2% of cases); or the limbs as well as breathing and other functions (bulbospinal polio; 19% of cases). Bulbar polio is particularly likely to lead to death if the patient is not placed on a respirator because the virus affects the brain stem—the part of the brain that controls heartbeat as well as breathing and other vital functions.

The maximum state of paralysis in paralytic polio is usually reached within a few days of the onset of symptoms. The remaining unaffected nerves then begin the process of attempting to grow branches to compensate for the destroyed nerves. Often, the nerve cells are not completely destroyed. By the end of a month, the nerve impulses start to return to the apparently paralyzed muscle and by the end of six months, recovery is almost complete. In cases where the nerve cells are completely destroyed, however, paralysis is permanent.

Diagnosis

The diagnosis of polio is based on a combination of the patient's history and the type and location of symptoms—particularly such symptoms as a stiff neck, difficulty breathing, or abnormal reflexes. Fever and

---

KEY TERMS

Aseptic—Sterile; containing no microorganisms, especially no bacteria.

Asymptomatic—Having no symptoms of a disease even though the person may be infected by the organism that causes the disease.

Brainstem—The stalk of the brain that connects the two cerebral hemispheres to the spinal cord.

Endemic—A term applied to a disease that maintains itself in a particular area without reinforcement from outside sources of infection.

Flaccid—Weak, soft, or floppy.

Gastrointestinal—Pertaining to the stomach and intestines.

Lymph/lymphatic—One of the three body fluids that is transparent and a slightly yellow liquid that is collected from the capillary walls into the tissues and circulates back to the blood supply.

Meningitis—Inflammation of the membranes that cover the brain and spinal cord.

Motor neuron—A type of cell in the central nervous system that controls the movement of muscles either directly or indirectly.

Neurologic—Pertaining to the nervous system.

Paralysis—The inability to voluntarily move.

---

asymmetric flaccid paralysis without sensory loss in a child or young adult almost always indicate poliomyelitis. Nonparalytic poliomyelitis cannot be distinguished clinically from aseptic meningitis due to other agents. Virus isolated from a throat swab and/or feces or blood tests that demonstrate the rise in a specific antibody are required to confirm the diagnosis.

Examination

TESTS. To confirm the diagnosis, samples of the patient's stool, spinal fluid, or throat mucus may be collected and sent to a laboratory for analysis to see whether the sample contains the virus itself. A blood sample early in the infection may also be analyzed for evidence of antibodies to the poliovirus.

PROCEDURES. A lumbar puncture is the procedure performed in order to obtain a sample of the patient's spinal fluid. A long, thin needle is inserted into the lower back between the vertebrae to withdraw spinal fluid. This test can be used to reveal an increased number of white blood cells and no bacteria (aseptic meningitis).

Treatment

Traditional

There is no drug that can cure polio as of 2012. **Antibiotics** are ineffective against any viral infection, including polio. Patients with abortive polio or nonparalytic meningitis do not usually need treatment other than resting at home.

Patients with paralytic polio may be placed on a respirator to help them breathe, particularly if they are diagnosed with bulbar polio. Other treatments include painkillers and hot packs for muscle aches, physical therapy to restore muscle strength, and occupational or speech therapy as needed. Physical therapy is the most important part of management of paralytic polio during recovery. Braces or special shoes may be recommended for some patients. A few patients may undergo surgery to restore limb function.

Prognosis

The overall prognosis for recovery from an acute attack of paralytic polio is generally good. Mortality is about 5–10%, mostly in elderly and very young patients; however, the death rate can reach 20–60% in cases of bulbar involvement. Half the patients with spinal polio recover fully; 25% have mild disabilities; and the remaining 25% are left with severe disabilities. Most patients recover from breathing problems, and only a small percentage of patients need long-term treatment on a respirator. Patients with muscle paralysis typically recover about 60% of their strength in the first 3–4 months of treatment.

About a quarter of patients who have recovered from paralytic polio develop a disorder called post-polio syndrome (PPS) between 10 and 40 years after the initial infection. PPS is not a re-infection although its cause is not completely understood. PPS is marked by:

• muscular weakness

• fatigue

• being easily exhausted after even small amounts of activity

• joint pain

• sleep disorders

• difficulty breathing or swallowing

• inability to tolerate cold temperatures

PPS is treated with rest and such supportive measures as powered wheelchairs, pain relievers, and medications to help the patient sleep. Patients are also encouraged to simplify their work habits and take frequent rest breaks.

Public health role and response

The **World Health Organization** has sponsored the initiative to eradicate polio. They work in conjunction with public health agencies and non-governmental organizations around the world, with their effort concentrated in countries where polio is still present. Because humans are the only host to the polio virus, it is possible that the virus can, like the **smallpox** virus, be completely eliminated by properly supported and coordinated vaccination efforts.

Prevention

Polio can easily be prevented by administration of either the Salk vaccine, which contains an inactivated poliovirus, or the Sabin oral vaccine, which contains a weakened live virus. The Salk vaccine (also called the inactivated polio vaccine or IPV) is given as a series of four shots administered at 2 months, 4 months, between 6 and 18 months and a booster given between 4 and 6 years. This **immunization** contains no live virus, just the components of the virus that provoke the recipient's immune system to react as if the recipient were actually infected with the poliovirus without causing polio symptoms. The recipient thus becomes immune to infection with the poliovirus in the future. The United States switched exclusively to using IPV rather than oral polio vaccine in 1999. It is the only polio vaccine that can safely be given to people with weakened immune systems.

The Sabin vaccine (also called the oral polio vaccine or OPV) is given to infants and adults by mouth in several doses. OPV contains the live, but weakened, poliovirus, which make the recipient immune to future infections with poliovirus. OPV is less expensive to administer than IPV. It requires no injections, thus no sterile needles, and is easily administered to both children and adults. For these reason, it is often used in the developing world. It is not routinely given to people with weakened immune systems because it contains a live virus and can very rarely cause polio.

Resources

BOOKS

Closser, Svea. *Chasing Polio in Pakistan: Why the World's Largest Public Health Initiative May Fail.* Nashville, TN: Vanderbilt University Press, 2010.

Hecht, Alan. *Polio.* New York: Chelsea House, 2009.

Krasner, Robert I. *Twentieth-century Microbe Hunters: Their Lives, Accomplishments, and Legacies.* Sudbury, MA: Jones and Bartlett Publishers, 2008.

Presley, Gary. *Seven Wheelchairs: A Life beyond Polio.* Iowa City: University of Iowa Press, 2008.

WEBSITES

Polio and Post-Polio Syndrome. MedlinePlus March 6, 2012 [accessed June 25, 2012]. http://www.nlm.nih.gov/medlineplus/polioandpostpoliosyndrome.html

Polio Vaccination. Centers for Disease Control and Prevention. January 3, 2012 [accessed June 25, 2012]. http://www.cdc.gov/vaccines/vpd-vac/polio/default.htm

Weiler, Christine. Acute Poliomyelitis. Medscape.com January 18, 2012 [accessed June 25, 2012]. http://emedicine.medscape.com/article/306440-overview

World Health Organization (WHO). Poliomyelitis 2012 [accessed June 25, 2012]. http://www.who.int/topics/poliomyelitis/en

ORGANIZATIONS

American Physical Therapy Association, 1111 North Fairfax Street, Alexandria, VA 22314-1488, (703) 684-APTA (2782). TDD: (703) 683-6748, (800) 999-APTA (2782, Fax: (703) 683-6748, http://www.apta.org

March of Dimes Foundation, 1275 Mamaroneck Avenue, White Plains, NY 10605, (914)997-4488, askus@marchofdimes.com, http://www.marchofdimes.com

National Institute of Allergy and Infectious Diseases Office of Communications and Government Relations, 6610 Rockledge Drive, MSC 6612, Bethesda, MD 20892-6612, (301) 496-5717, (866) 284-4107 or TDD: (800)877-8339 (for hearing impaired), Fax: (301) 402-3573, http://www3.niaid.nih.gov

United States Centers for Disease Control and Prevention (CDC), 1600 Clifton Road, Atlanta, GA 30333, (404) 639-3534, 800-CDC-INFO (800-232-4636). TTY: (888) 232-6348, inquiry@cdc.gov, http://www.cdc.gov

World Health Organization, Avenue Appia 20, 1211 Geneva 27, Switzerland, +22 41 791 21 11, Fax: +22 41 791 31 11, info@who.int, http://www.who.int.

Linda K. Bennington, CNS
Rebecca J. Frey, PhD
Tish Davidson, AM

Pollution *see* **Air pollution**

▌Population

Definition

Population is a term to denote all of the organisms of the of the same species that occupy some specific area. It is a measurement used on local, state, national, and international levels to determine or measure such important information as governmental representation, appropriation of government funds and benefits, distribution of wealth and other resources, and severity of threats like crime and disease. For instance, electoral votes available in the United States are determined by population counts within a given state, and the spread of disease is usually measured by the number of cases compared against a measure of the population.

Description

Humans in their earliest form first appeared nearly one million years ago. During the first 990,000 years of human existence, the human population grew at a relatively slow rate—15 people per million, annually. In the last 300 years, this rate has climbed drastically. Generally, the three largest changes in human growth rates are attributed to the Agricultural Revolution, the Industrial Revolution, and the more recent Green Revolution.

The Agricultural Revolution happened around 5,000 B.C., when humans ceased to be primarily hunter-gatherers and began to domesticate plants and animals. For thousands of years after that, the human growth rate is estimated at somewhere around 0.03% per year, reaching approximately 300 million people around the year 0. This ongoing growth was naturally countered in the Middle Ages—as humans began to form more populated and condensed urban environments, disease spread more rapidly and to greater effect. Diseases like the bubonic **plague** managed to kill immense quantities of people—roughly 25% of population of Europe in approximately 50 years.

The Industrial Revolution began in the mid-seventeenth century. From this time through approximately the following 300 years, the human population grew from approximately 500 million to over six billion; the population growth rate climbed from a mere 0.1% annually to 1.8% annually.

The Green Revolution is generally placed somewhere in the 1960s. This revolution has consisted of the advances of modernity that have improved quality of life and reduced death rates globally. These advances include the creation and widespread use of vaccines and **antibiotics** after World War II, increased crop

World population growth from 1950–2020

Year	Population	Average annual growth rate (%)	Average annual population change
1950	2,555,982,611	1.47	37,768,237
1951	2,593,750,848	1.61	42,042,862
1952	2,635,793,710	1.70	45,320,983
1953	2,681,114,693	1.77	47,842,880
1954	2,728,957,573	1.86	51,339,043
1955	2,780,296,616	1.88	52,854,158
1956	2,833,150,774	1.95	55,718,773
1957	2,888,869,547	1.93	56,393,986
1958	2,945,263,533	1.76	52,218,932
1959	2,997,482,465	1.39	41,951,479
1960	3,039,433,944	1.33	40,629,803
1961	3,080,063,747	1.80	56,018,983
1962	3,136,082,730	2.19	69,405,494
1963	3,205,488,224	2.19	71,002,977
1964	3,276,491,201	2.08	68,918,678
1965	3,345,409,879	2.07	70,135,995
1966	3,415,545,874	2.02	69,649,013
1967	3,485,194,887	2.04	71,751,266
1968	3,556,946,153	2.07	74,532,014
1969	3,631,478,167	2.05	75,123,281
1970	3,706,601,448	2.07	77,395,382
1971	3,783,996,830	2.01	76,793,114
1972	3,860,789,944	1.96	76,389,273
1973	3,937,179,217	1.91	75,725,073
1974	4,012,904,290	1.81	73,483,375
1975	4,086,387,665	1.75	72,049,425
1976	4,158,437,090	1.72	72,331,131
1977	4,230,768,221	1.69	72,268,962
1978	4,303,037,183	1.73	75,188,498
1979	4,378,225,681	1.71	75,638,139
1980	4,453,863,820	1.69	76,035,404
1981	4,529,899,224	1.75	80,163,373
1982	4,610,062,597	1.73	80,244,759
1983	4,690,307,356	1.68	79,323,181
1984	4,769,630,537	1.68	80,594,461
1985	4,850,224,998	1.68	82,355,074
1986	4,932,580,072	1.72	85,713,224
1987	5,018,293,296	1.71	86,343,509
1988	5,104,636,805	1.67	86,061,173
1989	5,190,697,978	1.66	87,027,432
1990	5,277,725,410	1.56	82,903,255
1991	5,360,628,665	1.54	83,112,161
1992	5,443,740,826	1.50	82,013,172
1993	5,525,753,998	1.45	80,584,690
1994	5,606,338,688	1.43	80,672,638
1995	5,687,011,326	1.39	79,424,294
1996	5,766,435,620	1.39	80,435,809
1997	5,846,871,429	1.34	78,899,442
1998	5,925,770,871	1.31	78,001,123
1999	6,003,771,994	1.28	77,230,943
2000	6,081,002,937	1.25	76,753,814
2001	6,157,756,751	1.24	76,520,745
2002	6,234,277,496	1.22	76,271,568
2003	6,310,549,064	1.20	75,993,822
2004	6,386,542,886	1.18	75,638,540
2005	6,462,181,426	1.16	75,478,997
2006	6,537,660,423	1.15	75,561,947
2007	6,613,222,370	1.14	75,666,070
2008	6,688,888,440	1.13	75,761,868
2009	6,764,650,308	1.11	75,772,948
2010	6,840,423,256	1.10	75,755,042
2011	6,916,178,298	1.09	75,622,621
2012	6,991,800,919	1.07	75,164,045
2013	7,066,964,964	1.05	74,468,973
2014	7,141,433,937	1.03	73,604,414
2015	7,215,038,351	1.00	72,747,545

[continued]

(Table by PreMediaGlobal. © 2013 Cengage Learning)

World Population Growth from 1950–2020

Year	Population	Average annual growth rate (%)	Average annual population change
2016	7,287,785,896	0.98	71,952,940
2017	7,359,738,836	0.96	71,088,531
2018	7,430,827,367	0.94	70,179,131
2019	7,501,006,498	0.92	69,208,946
2020	7,570,215,444	0.90	68,403,637

SOURCE: U.S. Bureau of the Census

(Table by PreMediaGlobal. © 2013 Cengage Learning)

production, and general improvements in areas like medical care, medicine, and **sanitation**. The current human population is over 6 billion.

Since the Agricultural Revolution, humans have tended increasingly to gravitate toward more organized, urban environments. As the human growth rate increases, so does the percentage of humans living in cities. As the human population has grown, historically, humans have adapted and improved in efficiency in order to continue to support and feed the rapidly growing numbers.

Historically, overpopulations have been attributed to the end of complete civilizations, including the various Mesopotamian peoples in the third millennium B.C. and the Mayans in the ninth century. In both cases, it is believed that overuse of the land due to rapid population growths led to a situation in which the ecological environments could no longer support the populations dependent on them, and the human populations did not survive.

Effects on public health

As the human population grows, there are consequences to the rapid expansion. Human growth has significant impact on ecological factors—from the emission of fossil fuels to the percentage of occupied land and available natural resources. Growth in human populations also leads to increased rates of migration as local areas become overpopulated, as well as changes in social complexities, largely as a result of migration. Migration and social diversification are not necessarily problematic, as long as the social and governmental infrastructures are able to adapt to the sometimes rapid changes.

Efforts and solutions

The rapid growth of the human population and the current human population have been used to assert the need for drastic medical or economic measures to curb the current growth rate. There is disagreement, however, about whether lack of development in countries is caused by overpopulation or whether lack of development is itself the cause of overpopulation. There is even debate over whether overpopulation is an accurate representation of the current human population. Neo-Malthusians have asserted that overpopulation causes **poverty** and that contraception would end poverty. Some Marxists have argued that a more equal distribution of wealth would be enough to satisfy the needs of all people, even in less-developed countries (LDCs), while representatives from LDCs at a United Nations (UN) conference in the 1970s argued that development would be the most effective contraceptive.

There have been movements to reduce or halt population growth, but these movements often come with questionable costs. Probably the most popular population-reduction policy has been China's "one child" policy, which made having one child per family the law. This policy, combined with a cultural preference for males, has led to a drastic population imbalance in which girls and women have become scarce in China. Other movements, often by international aid groups, to increase the availability of contraception to women around the world have proven problematic because they can lead to violation of **human rights** when women are either unable to make decisions about whether to employ contraception and the method of contraception used. Human rights violations also become an issue when there is not sufficient medical care to administer or respond to the complications of contraception.

Now, in the twenty-first century, many affluent countries report no net population growth, and fertility rates in LDC are declining. Many governments and aid organizations are now shifting their focuses toward other issues, including **aging** populations, effects of migratory patterns, irreplaceably low fertility rates in some European countries, and global access to adequate food, **water**, and health care.

Resources

BOOKS

Brunson, Jan. "Overpopulation." *Encyclopedia of Women in Today's World.* Ed. Mary Zeiss Stange, Carol K. Oyster, and Jane E. Sloan. Vol. 3. Thousand Oaks, CA: Sage Reference, 2011. 1058-1060.

Christian, David. "Population Growth." *Bershire Encyclopedia of World History.* Ed. William H. McNeill, et al. 2nd ed. Vol. 5. Great Barrington, MA: Berkshire Publishing, 2010. 2018-2022.

Jackson, William A. "Overpopulation." *Encyclopedia of Global Studies.* Ed. Helmut K. Anheier, Mark Juergensmeyer, and Victor Faessel. Vol. 3. Thousand Oaks, CA: Sage Reference, 2012. 1285-1286.

"Population Growth." *Encyclopedia of Global Warming.* Ed. Steven I. Dutch. Vol. 3. Pasadena, CA: Salem Press, 2010. 854–857.

WEBSITES

World Health Organization. "Urban Population Growth."http://www.who.int/gho/urban_health/situation_trends/urban_population_growth/en/index.htmlAccessed November 14, 2012.

ORGANIZATIONS

World Health Organization, Avenue Appia 20, 12 Geneva 27, Switzerland, 41 22 791-2111, Fax: 41 22 791-3111, www.who.int.

Andrea Nienstedt, MA

Post–partum depression *see* **Reproductive health**

Post-traumatic stress disorder

Definition

Post-traumatic stress disorder (PTSD) is a complex anxiety disorder that may occur when an individual experiences or witnesses an event perceived as a threat and in which he or she experiences fear, terror, or helplessness. PTSD is sometimes summarized as "a normal reaction to abnormal events." It was first defined as a distinctive disorder in 1980. Originally diagnosed in veterans of the Vietnam War, it is now recognized in civilian survivors of trauma, such as rape or other criminal assaults; **natural disasters**; plane crashes, train collisions, or industrial explosions; acts of terrorism; **child abuse**; or war.

Demographics

PTSD can develop in almost anyone in any age group exposed to a sufficiently terrifying event or chain of events. The **National Institute of Mental Health** (NIMH) estimated in 2007 that about 7.7 million adults in the United States have PTSD. One study found that 3.7% of a sample of teenage boys and 6.3% of adolescent girls had PTSD. It is estimated that people's risk of developing PTSD over the course of their life is between 8 and 10%. Women are at greater risk of PTSD following **sexual assault** or domestic **violence**, whereas men are at greater risk of developing PTSD following military combat. On average, 30% of soldiers who have been in a war zone develop PTSD. Recent statistics on PTSD in U.S. military personnel returning from Iraq demonstrated that, using more inclusive parameters, between 20.7% and 30.5% of troops suffered from PTSD; using stricter parameters, PTSD was present in 5.6–11.3% of troops.

Traumatic experiences are surprisingly common in the general North American **population**. More than 10% of the men and 6% of the women in one survey reported experiencing four or more types of trauma in their lives. The most frequently mentioned traumas are:

• witnessing someone being badly hurt or killed
• being involved in a fire, flood, earthquake, severe hurricane, or other natural disaster
• being involved in a life-threatening accident (workplace explosion or transportation accident)
• being in military combat

PTSD is more likely to develop in response to an intentional human act of violence or cruelty, such as a rape or mugging, than as a reaction to an impersonal catastrophe like a flood or hurricane. It is not surprising that the traumatic events most frequently mentioned by men diagnosed with PTSD are rape, combat exposure, childhood neglect, and childhood physical abuse. For women diagnosed with PTSD, the most common traumas are rape, sexual molestation, physical attack, being threatened with a weapon, and childhood physical abuse.

PTSD can also develop in therapists, rescue workers, or witnesses of a frightening event as well as in those who were directly involved. This process is called "vicarious traumatization."

Description

The experience of PTSD has sometimes been described as like being in a horror film that keeps replaying and cannot be shut off. It is common for people with PTSD to feel intense fear and helplessness and to relive the frightening event in nightmares or in their waking hours. Sometimes the memory is triggered by a sound, smell, or image that reminds the sufferer of the traumatic event. These re-experiences of the event are called "flashbacks." Persons with PTSD are also likely to be jumpy and easily startled or to go numb emotionally and lose interest in activities they used to enjoy. They may have problems with memory and with getting enough sleep. In some cases, they may feel disconnected from the real world or have moments in which their own bodies seem unreal; these symptoms are indications of dissociation, a process in which the mind splits off certain memories or thoughts from conscious awareness. Many people with PTSD turn to alcohol or drugs in order to escape the flashbacks and other symptoms of the disorder, even if only for a few minutes.

Risk factors

Factors that influence the likelihood of a person's developing PTSD include:

- The nature, intensity, and duration of the traumatic experience. For example, someone who just barely escaped from the World Trade Center before the towers collapsed is at greater risk of PTSD than someone who saw the collapse from a distance or on television.

- The person's previous history. People who were abused as children, who were separated from their parents at an early age, or who have a previous history of anxiety or depression are at increased risk of PTSD.

- Genetic factors. Vulnerability to PTSD is known to run in families.

- The availability of social support after the event. People who have no family or friends are more likely to develop PTSD than those who do.

HIGH-RISK POPULATIONS. Some subpopulations in the United States are at greater risk of developing PTSD. The lifetime prevalence of PTSD among persons living in depressed urban areas or on Native American reservations is estimated at 23%. For victims of violent crimes, the estimated rate is 58%.

PTSD also appears to be more common in seniors than in younger people. Thirteen percent of the senior population reports they are affected by PTSD, in comparison to 7–10% of the entire population. Reports of elder abuse crimes have gone up by 200% since 1986. The incidence of PTSD is also known to be higher among Holocaust survivors, war veterans, and **cancer** or heart surgery survivors, which accounts for a significant portion of older Americans. Of those seniors who are military veterans, there is an increasing number who are isolated and/or in poor health as a result of PTSD.

Children are also susceptible to PTSD, and their risk is increased exponentially as their exposure to the event increases. Children experiencing abuse, the death of a parent, or those located in a community suffering a traumatic event can develop PTSD. Two years after the Oklahoma City bombing of 1995, 16% of children within a 100-mile radius of Oklahoma City with no direct exposure to the bombing had increased symptoms of PTSD. Weak parental response to the event, having a parent suffering from PTSD symptoms, and intensified exposure to the event via the media all increase the possibility of a child's developing PTSD symptoms. In addition, a developmentally inappropriate sexual experience for a child may be considered a traumatic event, even though it may not have actually involved violence or physical injury. Proposed changes to the fifth edition of the *Diagnostic and Statistical Manual of Mental Disorders* (*DSM-5*, 2013) include post-traumatic stress disorder in preschool children among its new diagnoses.

MILITARY VETERANS. Studies conducted between 2004 and 2006 with veteran participants from the wars in Iraq and in Afghanistan found a strong correlation between duration of combat exposure and PTSD. Veterans of combat in Iraq reported a higher rate of PTSD than those deployed to Afghanistan because of longer exposure to warfare.

Information about PTSD in veterans of the Vietnam era is derived from the National Vietnam Veterans Readjustment Survey (NVVRS), conducted between 1986 and 1988. The estimated lifetime prevalence of PTSD among American veterans of this war is 30.9% for men and 26.9% for women. An additional 22.5% of the men and 21.2% of the women have been diagnosed with partial PTSD at some point in their lives. The lifetime prevalence of PTSD among veterans of World War II and the Korean War is estimated at 20%.

CROSS-CULTURAL ISSUES. Further research needs to be done on the effects of ethnicity and culture on post-traumatic symptoms. As of the early 2010s, most PTSD research had been done by Western clinicians working with patients from a similar background. Researchers do not yet know whether persons from non-Western societies have the same psychological reactions to specific traumas or whether they develop the same symptom patterns.

PROTECTIVE OR RESILIENCE FACTORS. As important as the question of *who* gets PTSD is also the question of who does *not* get PTSD. Why do some people who are exposed to traumatic events succumb to the long-lasting after-effects of PTSD, whereas others seem to endure the trauma and successfully move on? Researchers have identified the following resilience factors, which seem to decrease the likelihood that traumatic exposure will lead to PTSD:

- actively seeking support from friends, family, or others following a traumatic incident
- engaging with a formal support group
- maintaining a positive view of personal actions during the course of, or in response to, the traumatic incident
- implementing a coping strategy
- feeling as if a lesson has been learned from the traumatic event
- not becoming paralyzed with terror; being able to respond and react effectively despite fear

Causes and symptoms

The causes of PTSD are not completely understood. One major question that has not yet been answered is: Why do some people involved in a major disaster develop PTSD, while other survivors of the same event do not? For example, a survey conducted in November 2001 of 988 adults living close to the World Trade Center found that only 7% had been diagnosed with PTSD following the events of September 11; the other 93% were anxious and upset, but they did not develop PTSD. Research into this question is ongoing.

Causes

When PTSD was first suggested as a diagnostic category for *DSM-III* in 1980, it was controversial precisely because of the central role of outside stressors as causes of the disorder. Psychiatry has generally emphasized the internal abnormalities of individuals as the source of mental disorders; prior to the 1970s, war

veterans, rape victims, and other trauma survivors were often blamed for their symptoms and regarded as cowards, moral weaklings, or masochists. The high rate of psychiatric casualties among Vietnam veterans, however, led to studies conducted by the Department of Veterans Affairs. These studies helped to establish PTSD as a legitimate diagnostic entity with a complex set of causes.

BIOCHEMICAL/PHYSIOLOGICAL CAUSES. Present neurobiological research indicates that traumatic events cause lasting changes in the human nervous system, including abnormal levels of secretion of stress hormones. In addition, in PTSD patients, researchers have found changes in the amygdala and the hippocampus—the parts of the brain that form links between fear and memory. Experiments with ketamine, a drug that inactivates one of the neurotransmitters in the central nervous system, suggest that trauma works in a similar way to damage associative pathways in the brain. Positron emission tomography (PET) scans of PTSD patients suggest that trauma affects the parts of the brain that govern speech and language.

SOCIOCULTURAL CAUSES. Studies of specific populations of PTSD patients (e.g., combat veterans, survivors of rape or genocide, former political hostages or prisoners) have shed light on the social and cultural causes of PTSD. In general, societies that are highly authoritarian, glorify violence, or sexualize violence have high rates of PTSD even among civilians.

OCCUPATIONAL FACTORS. Persons whose work exposes them to traumatic events or who treat trauma survivors may develop secondary PTSD (also known as compassion fatigue or burnout). These occupations include specialists in emergency medicine, police officers, firefighters, search-and-rescue personnel, psychotherapists, and disaster investigators. The degree of risk for PTSD is related to three factors: the amount and intensity of exposure to the suffering of trauma victims, the worker's degree of empathy and sensitivity, and unresolved issues from the worker's personal history.

PERSONAL VARIABLES. Although the most important causal factor in PTSD is the traumatic event itself, individuals differ in the intensity of their cognitive and emotional responses to trauma; some persons appear to be more vulnerable than others. In some cases, this greater vulnerability is related to temperament or natural disposition, with shy or introverted people being at greater risk. In other cases, the person's vulnerability results from chronic illness, a physical disability, or previous traumatization—particularly abuse in childhood. Studies done by the U.S. Department of Veterans Affairs have found some evidence that race and ethnicity may also be factors, with veterans who belong to ethnic minority groups at higher risk of experiencing PTSD after combat.

Symptoms

DSM-IV-TR specifies six diagnostic criteria for PTSD:

• Traumatic stressor: The patient has been exposed to a catastrophic event involving actual or threatened death or injury or a threat to the physical integrity of the self or others. During exposure to the trauma, the person's emotional response was marked by intense fear, feelings of helplessness, or horror. In general, stressors caused intentionally by human beings (genocide, rape, torture, abuse) are experienced as more traumatic than accidents, natural disasters, or "acts of God."

• Intrusive symptoms: Patients experience flashbacks, traumatic daydreams, or nightmares, in which they relive the trauma as if it were recurring in the present. Intrusive symptoms result from an abnormal process of memory formation. Traumatic memories have two distinctive characteristics: they can be triggered by stimuli that remind the patient of the traumatic event, or they may have a "frozen" or wordless quality, consisting of images and sensations rather than verbal descriptions.

• Avoidant symptoms: Patients attempt to reduce the possibility of exposure to anything that might trigger memories of the trauma and to minimize their reactions to such memories. This cluster of symptoms includes feeling disconnected from other people, psychic numbing, and avoidance of places, persons, or things associated with the trauma. Patients with PTSD are at increased risk of substance abuse as a form of self-medication to numb painful memories.

• Hyperarousal: Hyperarousal is a condition in which the nervous system is always on "red alert" for the return of danger. This symptom cluster includes hypervigilance, insomnia, difficulty concentrating, general irritability, and an extreme startle response. Some clinicians think that this abnormally intense startle response may be the most characteristic symptom of PTSD.

• Duration of symptoms: The symptoms must persist for at least one month.

• Significance: Patients suffer from significant social, interpersonal, or work-related problems as a result of the PTSD symptoms. One common social symptom of PTSD is a feeling of disconnection from other people (including loved ones); from the larger society; and from spiritual, religious, or other significant sources of meaning.

KEY TERMS

Benzodiazepines—A class of drugs that have a hypnotic and sedative action, used mainly as tranquilizers to control symptoms of anxiety.

Cognitive-behavioral therapy—A type of psychotherapy used to treat anxiety disorders (including PTSD) that emphasizes behavioral change as well as alteration of negative thought patterns.

Cortisol—A hormone produced by the adrenal glands near the kidneys in response to stress.

Dissociation—The splitting off of certain mental processes from conscious awareness. Many PTSD patients have dissociative symptoms.

Flashback—A temporary reliving of a traumatic event.

Hyperarousal—A state of increased emotional tension and anxiety, often including jitteriness and being easily startled.

Hypervigilance—A condition of abnormally intense watchfulness or wariness. Hypervigilance is one of the most common symptoms of PTSD.

Prevalence—The percentage of a population that is affected by a specific disease at a given time.

Selective serotonin reuptake inhibitors (SSRIs)—A class of antidepressants that works by blocking the reabsorption of serotonin in the brain, raising the levels of serotonin.

Trauma—A severe injury or shock to a person's body or mind.

Diagnosis

The diagnosis of PTSD is based on the patient's history, including the timing of the traumatic event and the duration of the patient's symptoms.

Examination

Consultation with a mental health professional for diagnosis and a plan of treatment is always advised. Many of the responses to trauma, such as shock, terror, irritability, blame, guilt, grief, sadness, emotional numbing, and feelings of helplessness, are natural reactions. For most people, resilience is an overriding factor, and trauma effects diminish within six to sixteen months. It is when these responses continue or become debilitating that PTSD is often diagnosed.

As outlined in *DSM-IV,* the exposure to a traumatic stressor means that an individual experienced, witnessed, or was confronted by an event or events involving death or threat of death, serious injury or the threat of bodily harm to oneself or others. The individual's response must involve intense fear, helplessness, or horror. A two-pronged approach to evaluation is considered the best way to make a valid diagnosis because it can gauge under-reporting or over-reporting of symptoms. The two primary forms are structured interviews and self-report questionnaires. Spouses, partners, and other family members may also be interviewed. Because the evaluation may involve subtle reminders of the trauma in order to gauge a patient's reactions, individuals should ask for a full description of the evaluation process beforehand. Asking what results can be expected from the evaluation is also advised.

A number of structured interview forms have been devised to facilitate the diagnosis of post-traumatic stress disorder:

• Clinician Administered PTSD Scale (CAPS), developed by the National Center for PTSD

• Structured Clinical Interview for DSM (SCID)

• Anxiety Disorders Interview Schedule-Revised (ADIS)

• PTSD-Interview

• Structured Interview for PTSD (SI-PTSD)

• PTSD Symptom Scale Interview (PSS-I)

Self-reporting checklists provide scores to represent the level of stress experienced. Some of the most commonly used checklists are:

• The PTSD Checklist (PCL), which has one list for civilians and one for military personnel and veterans

• Impact of Event Scale-Revised (IES-R)

• Keane PTSD Scale of the MMPI-2

• Mississippi Scale for Combat Related PTSD and the Mississippi Scale for Civilians

• Posttraumatic Diagnostic Scale (PDS)

• Penn Inventory for Post-Traumatic Stress

• Los Angeles Symptom Checklist (LASC)

Tests

There are no laboratory or imaging tests that can detect PTSD, although a doctor may order imaging studies of the brain to rule out head injuries or other physical causes of the patient's symptoms.

Treatment

Various treatments are used for post-traumatic stress disorder.

Traditional

Treatment for PTSD usually involves a combination of medications and psychotherapy. If patients have started to abuse alcohol or drugs, they must be treated for the substance abuse before being treated for PTSD. If they are diagnosed with coexisting depression, treatment should focus on the PTSD because its course, biology, and treatment response are different from those associated with major depression. Patients with the disorder are usually treated as outpatients; they are not hospitalized unless they are threatening to commit **suicide** or harm other people.

Mainstream forms of psychotherapy used to treat patients who have already developed PTSD include:

• Cognitive-behavioral therapy. There are two treatment approaches to PTSD included under this heading: exposure therapy, which seeks to desensitize the patient to reminders of the trauma; and anxiety management training, which teaches the patient strategies for reducing anxiety. These strategies may include relaxation training, biofeedback, social skills training, distraction techniques, or cognitive restructuring.

• Psychodynamic psychotherapy. This approach helps the patient recover a sense of self and learn new coping strategies and ways to deal with intense emotions related to the trauma. Typically, it consists of three phases: establishing a sense of safety for the patient; exploring the trauma itself in depth; and helping the patient re-establish connections with family, friends, the wider society, and other sources of meaning.

• Discussion groups or peer-counseling groups. These groups are usually formed for survivors of specific traumas, such as combat, rape or incest, and natural or transportation disasters. They help patients to recognize that other survivors of the shared experience have had the same emotions and reacted to the trauma in similar ways. They appear to be especially beneficial for patients with guilt issues about their behavior during the trauma (e.g., submitting to rape to save one's life, or surviving the event when others did not).

• Family therapy. This form of treatment is recommended for PTSD patients whose family life has been affected by the PTSD symptoms.

Drugs

In general, medications are used most often in patients with severe PTSD to treat the intrusive symptoms of the disorder as well as feelings of anxiety and depression. These drugs are usually given as one part of a treatment plan that includes psychotherapy or group therapy. As of 2012, no single medication was considered a primary cure for PTSD. The selective serotonin reuptake inhibitors (SSRIs) appear to help the core symptoms when given in higher doses for five to eight weeks, while the tricyclic antidepressants (TCAs) or the monoamine oxidase inhibitors (MAOIs) are most useful in treating anxiety and depression.

Sleep problems can be lessened with brief treatment with an antianxiety drug, such as a benzodiazepine like alprazolam (Xanax), but long-term usage can lead to disturbing side effects, including increased anger, drug tolerance, dependency, and abuse. Benzodiazepines are also not given to PTSD patients diagnosed with coexisting drug or alcohol abuse.

Alternative

Relaxation training, which is sometimes called anxiety management training, includes breathing exercises and similar techniques intended to help the patient prevent hyperventilation and relieve the muscle tension associated with the fight-or-flight reaction of anxiety. Yoga, aikido, tai chi, and dance therapy help patients work with the physical as well as the emotional tensions that either promote anxiety or are created by the anxiety.

Other alternative or complementary therapies are based on physiological and/or energetic understanding of how the trauma is imprinted in the body. These therapies affect a release of stored emotions and resolution of them by working with the body rather than merely talking through the experience. One example of such a therapy is somatic experiencing (SE), developed by Peter Levine. SE is a short-term, biological, body-oriented approach to PTSD or other trauma. It heals by emphasizing physiological and emotional responses, without re-traumatizing the person, without placing the person on medication, and without the long hours of conventional therapy.

When used in conjunction with therapies that address the underlying cause of PTSD, relaxation therapies such as hydrotherapy, massage therapy, and aromatherapy are useful to some patients in easing PTSD symptoms. Essential oils of lavender, chamomile, neroli, sweet marjoram, and ylang-ylang are commonly recommended by aromatherapists for stress relief and anxiety reduction.

Some patients benefit from spiritual or religious counseling. Because traumatic experiences often affect patients' spiritual views and beliefs, counseling with a trusted religious or spiritual advisor may be part of a treatment plan. A growing number of pastoral counselors in the major Christian and Jewish bodies in North America hold advanced credentials in trauma therapy. Native Americans are often helped to recover from PTSD by participating in traditional tribal rituals for cleansing memories of war and other traumatic events. These rituals may include sweat lodges, prayers and chants, or consultation with a shaman or tribal healer.

Several controversial methods of treatment for PTSD have been introduced since the mid-1980s. Some have been developed by mainstream medical researchers, while others are derived from various forms of **alternative medicine**. These methods are controversial because they do not offer any scientifically validated explanations for their effectiveness. They include:

- Eye Movement Desensitization and Reprocessing (EMDR). This is a technique in which the patient re-imagines the trauma while focusing visually on movements of the therapist's finger. It is claimed that the movements of the patient's eyes reprogram the brain and allow emotional healing.

- Tapas Acupressure Technique (TAT). TAT was developed in 1993 by licensed acupuncturist Tapas Fleming. It is derived from traditional Chinese medicine (TCM), and its practitioners maintain that a large number of acupuncture meridians enter the brain at certain points on the face, especially around the eyes. Pressure on these points is thought to release traumatic stress.

- Thought Field Therapy. This therapy combines the acupuncture meridians of TCM with analysis of the patient's voice over the telephone. The therapist then provides an individualized treatment for the patient.

- Traumatic Incident Reduction. This is a technique in which the patient treats the trauma like a videotape and "runs through" it repeatedly with the therapist until all negative emotions have been discharged.

- Emotional Freedom Techniques (EFT). EFT is similar to TAT in that it uses the body's acupuncture meridians, but it emphasizes the body's entire "energy field" rather than just the face.

- Counting Technique. Developed by a physician, this treatment consists of a preparation phase, a counting phase in which the therapist counts from 1 to 100 while the patient re-imagines the trauma, and a review phase. Like Traumatic Incident Reduction, it is intended to reduce the patient's hyperarousal.

Healthcare team roles

It is essential for all treatment team members to know their roles and execute them properly throughout the treatment and recovery phases of this disorder. Depending on whether outpatient or inpatient treatment is being provided, the team leaders may include psychiatrists, psychologists, nursing staff, behavior specialists, physical therapists, and other medical or behavioral staff. In some cases, it may be appropriate to include the patient's religious or spiritual advisor as a member of the team.

QUESTIONS TO ASK YOUR DOCTOR

- What are my chances of recovering completely from PTSD? How long do you think it might take?
- What medications would you recommend and why?
- What should I do when I have a flashback?
- Can you help me explain my symptoms to my family and friends?

Prognosis

The prognosis of PTSD is difficult to determine because patients' personalities and the experiences they undergo vary widely. A majority of patients get better, including some who do not receive treatment. One study reported that the average length of PTSD symptoms in patients who seek treatment is 32 months, compared to 64 months in patients who are not treated.

Factors that improve a patient's chances for full recovery include prompt treatment, early and ongoing support from family and friends, a high level of functioning before the frightening event, and an absence of alcohol or substance abuse. About 30% of people with PTSD never recover completely, however.

Efforts and solutions

PTSD is impossible to prevent completely because natural disasters and human acts of violence will continue to occur. In addition, it is not possible to tell beforehand how any given individual will react to a specific type of trauma. Prompt treatment after a traumatic event may lower the survivor's risk of developing severe symptoms.

As a result of the U.S. presence in Afghanistan and the Iraq war, military members are experiencing prolonged exposure to combat and increases in PTSD. As of May 2012, the U.S. military was making a concerted and organized effort to redefine PTSD and its diagnostic criteria for members of the military. Members of the military do not necessarily respond with feelings of fear or helplessness the way that a member of the general population might, because they are trained to compartmentalize emotion in order to complete their duties. The military is hoping to expand recognition and treatment of PTSD in soldiers and veterans who—though they may appear to be moving on and dealing with trauma—may still need treatment for PTSD. By changing the way PTSD is viewed in relation to military members, the U.S. military aims to help remove the stigma attached to PTSD, with the hope that more military members will feel comfortable seeking treatment. Elaine Miller-Karas, director of the Trauma Resource Institute, told National Public Radio (NPR) that "Many of our young men and women coming back don't want to go to a mental health therapist. But they will go someplace and learn skills for wellness to increase their resiliency." The military is hoping that by reducing the stigma of PTSD and increasing the availability and use of alternative therapies, more soldiers and veterans in need of care for PTSD will feel comfortable enough to seek it out.

Resources

BOOKS

American Psychiatric Association. *Diagnostic and Statistical Manual of Mental Disorders*. 4th ed., text rev. Washington, DC: American Psychiatric Publishing, 2000.

Antony, Martin M., and Murray B. Stein, eds. *Oxford Handbook of Anxiety and Related Disorders*. New York: Oxford University Press, 2009.

Bradley, W., et al. *Neurology in Clinical Practice,* 5th ed. Philadelphia: Butterworth-Heinemann, 2008.

Brohl, Kathryn. *Working with Traumatized Children: A Handbook for Healing,* rev. ed. Arlington, VA: CWLA Press, 2007.

Grey, Nick, ed. *A Casebook of Cognitive Therapy for Traumatic Stress Reactions.* New York: Routledge, 2009.

Slone, Laurie B., and Matthew J. Friedman. *After the War Zone: A Practical Guide for Returning Troops and Their Families.* Cambridge, MA: Da Capo Lifelong, 2008.

PERIODICALS

Cohen, J.A., and M.S. Scheeringa. "Post-traumatic Stress Disorder Diagnosis in Children: Challenges and Promises." *Dialogues in Clinical Neuroscience* 11 (2009): 91–99.

Evans, S., et al. "Disability and Posttraumatic Stress Disorder in Disaster Relief Workers Responding to September 11, 2001, World Trade Center Disaster." *Journal of Clinical Psychology* 65 (April 22, 2009): 684–94.

Hamblen, J.L., et al. "Cognitive Behavioral Therapy for Postdisaster Distress: A Community-Based Treatment Program for Survivors of Hurricane Katrina." *Administration and Policy in Mental Health* 36 (May 2009): 206–14.

Smith, T.C., et al. "PTSD Prevalence, Associated Exposures, and Functional Health Outcomes in a Large, Population-Based Military Cohort." *Public Health Reports* 124 (January-February 2009): 90–102.

WEBSITES

Abramson, Larry. "Military Looks to Redefine PTSD, Without Stigma" http://www.npr.org/2012/05/14/152680944/

military-looks-to-redefine-ptsd-without-stigma Accessed August 20, 2012.

"Helping Children Cope with Violence and Disasters: What Parents Can Do." National Institute of Mental Health. http://www.nimh.nih.gov/health/publications/helping-children-and-adolescents-cope-with-violence-and-disasters-what-parents-can-do/index.shtml (accessed September 16, 2011).

Hope for Recovery: Understanding PTSD [video]. National Center for PTSD. http://www.ncptsd.va.gov/ncmain/ncdocs/videos/emv_hoperecovery_gpv.html (accessed September 16, 2011).

"Post-Traumatic Stress Disorder." National Alliance on Mental Illness. http://www.nami.org/Template.cfm?Section=By_Illness&Template=/TaggedPage/TaggedPageDisplay.cfm&TPLID=54&ContentID=23045 (accessed September 16, 2011).

"What Is PTSD?" National Center for PTSD Fact Sheet http://www.ncptsd.va.gov/ncmain/ncdocs/fact_shts/fs_what_is_ptsd.html (accessed September 16, 2011).

ORGANIZATIONS

American Academy of Experts in Traumatic Stress, 203 Deer Rd., Ronkonkoma, NY 11779, (631) 543-2217, Fax: (631) 543-6977, info@aaets.org, http://www.aaets.org

American Psychiatric Association, 1000 Wilson Blvd., Ste. 1825, Arlington, VA 22209-3901, (703) 907-7300, apa@psych.org, http://www.psych.org

Anxiety Disorders Association of America, 8730 Georgia Ave., Silver Spring, MD 20910, (240) 485-1001, Fax: (240) 485-1035, http://www.adaa.org

National Alliance on Mental Illness, 2107 Wilson Blvd., Ste. 300, Arlington, VA 22201-3042, Fax: (703) 524-9094, (800) 950-6264, http://www.nami.org

National Center for PTSD, U.S. Department of Veterans Affairs, 810 Vermont Ave. NW, Washington, DC 20420, (802) 296-6300, ncptsd@va.gov, http://www.ncptsd.va.gov

National Institute of Mental Health, 6001 Executive Blvd., Rm. 8184, MSC 9663, Bethesda, MD 20892-9663, (301) 433-4513; TTY: (301) 443-8431, Fax: (301) 443-4279, (866) 615-6464; TTY: (866) 415-8051, nimhinfo@nih.gov, http://www.nimh.nih.gov

Rebecca J. Frey, PhD
Andrea Nienstedt, MA

Poverty

Definition

Despite its social stigmas and social associations, poverty is a fluid idea with different meanings in different places. Poverty generally represents earning or living off of less money than adequate, as deemed by a particular country or region.

Description

There are different degrees of poverty—extreme poverty, in much of the world, equates to living on less than $1 per day. As of 2012, the poverty line for the United States is $11,170 per year for one person, which equals just under $31 per day. The poverty threshold in the U.S. increases by $3,960 annually per additional person in the household.

Multiple factors usually go into assessing poverty guidelines, including the cost of living in the area. Cost of living represents the change over time in the cost of maintaining a specific standard of living. It fluctuates between any two areas and any two time periods—for instance, the cost of living in major cities is often greater than in rural areas. Complex economic systems—like inflation and supply and demand—interact to produce cost-of-living changes.

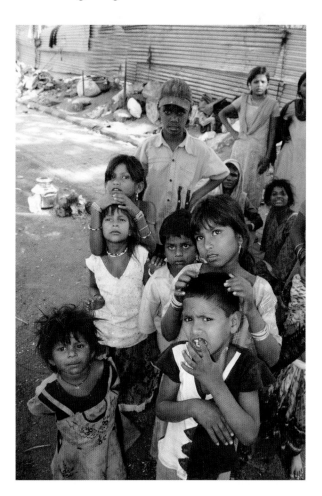

Poor street children in India. (© *iStockphoto.com/Nikhil Gangavane*)

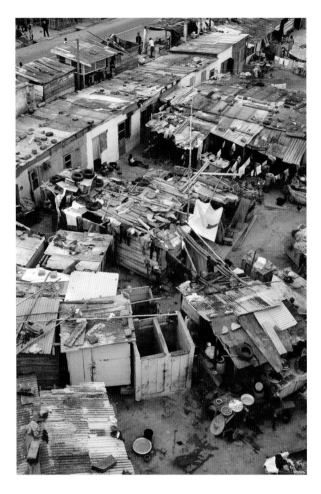

A poor community with fishing houses in Ghana. (© trevor kittelty/Shutterstock.com)

People living in poverty are living, or attempting to sustain themselves, without adequate funds. Lack of adequate financial resources means inadequate levels of healthy food and **water**, medical care, shelter, clothing, education, and other basic necessities. These basic inadequacies lead to malnutrition, disease, exposure to the elements, and greatly increased death rates.

There are a number of factors that contribute to poverty including climate change and subsequent **natural disasters**, geopolitical conflict and instability, and economic instability.

During his administration, after the assassination of President John F. Kennedy, President Lyndon Johnson declared a "war on poverty." During his presidency, the national poverty rate fell from 22% to 13%. After Johnson's presidency, Americans began to reply more on the federal government to ensure adequate standards of living including housing, health care, education, employment, and income. Since the United States began to experience a recession in 2008, national poverty levels

have begun to increase, with children being the most affected.

In recent years, poverty has become an increasingly important global issue. Both India and China have made great progress in reducing the number of their citizens living in poverty—India has diversified its industries to become a hub for pharmaceuticals and telecommunications. In just over 20 years, China has drastically reduced its poverty rate (down to 27% from 85%); however, even with such a drastic reduction, approximately 130 million Chinese people still live in poverty.

Inadequate access to clean water and **sanitation** greatly contribute to malnutrition and the spread of disease globally. According to Water.org—a nonprofit organization dedicated to increasing global access to clean water and sanitation—approximately 3.4 million people die every year from water-related diseases, and 99% of those deaths occur in the developing world. Additionally, 780 million people do not have access to clean water. When a population is unable to have its basic needs met—like access to clean water, sanitation, food, basic medical care—it is far less likely to be able to succeed and contribute to their communities socially and economically.

In its efforts to reduce, and hopefully end, global poverty, the United Nations (UN) has stressed the interconnected nature of many of the major issues facing the global community—including poverty, education, and gender equality. Of the eight developmental goals listed in the UN's Millennium Delcaration, the UN Population Fund asserts that gender equality is a key to achieving the other goals, including ending global poverty. Unequal opportunities for women—particularly in terms of economics and education—stunt the ability of local and national economies to thrive, because such a large portion of their populations is effectively removed from active participation.

Recent movements like microloans seek to eliminate poverty not through charity, but by providing access to resources in order for those in poverty to create new economic opportunities for themselves and their communities. In 2006, the Nobel Peace Prize was

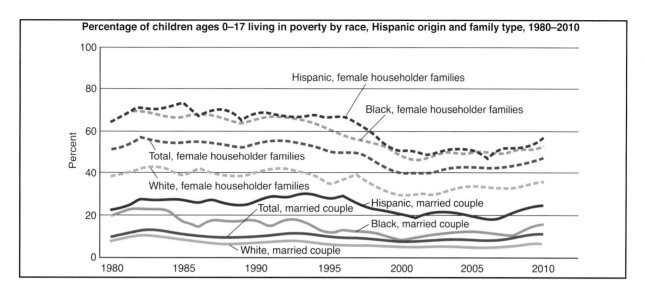

Percentage of children ages 0–17 living in poverty by race, Hispanic origin and family type, 1980–2010

Hispanic, female householder families

Black, female householder families

Total, female householder families

White, female householder families

Total, married couple

Hispanic, married couple

Black, married couple

White, married couple

(Illustration by Electronic Illustrators Group. © 2013 Cengage Learning)

awarded to the Grameen Bank of Bangladesh, and its founder, Muhammad Yunus, who developed the concept of microloans, or microcredit. Yunus's concept, which has since become a common international practice, seeks to provide small loans to women in developing countries to help them build a business. The businesses formed vary in size and specialty, from agriculture to retail to food service. After the woman has established her business, she repays the money, and with her new income, she is providing influxes of new money into her local economy. Statistically, women tend to spend their money on the care of their families, so by increasing their economic status, these women are able to provide better food, shelter, and education for their families, and often breaking the cycle of poverty.

An increasing number of organizations are seeking to change Western attitudes toward developing and impoverished countries. Like Grameen Bank, and often utilizing microloans, many organizations attempt to approach issues like global poverty and gender equality as problems that can only be solved by those experiencing the situation, with slight assistance—not necessarily hand outs—from others. Pulitzer-Prize-winning New York Times journalists, and husband and wife, Nicholas Kristof and Sheryl WuDunn started a movement—including a book, documentary, and nonprofit initiative—called *Half the Sky*, based on their experiences working with impoverished women around the world. Like Yunis, Kristof and WuDunn, through awareness, donations, and microfinance, are making efforts to reduce or eliminate global poverty by improving attitudes toward women and increasing their economic opportunities worldwide.

Demographics

According to the **World Health Organization (WHO)**, approximately 1.2 billion people around the world live in extreme poverty (under $1 per day).

According to the most recent data from the National Poverty Center at the University of Michigan, 15.1% of all Americans were living in poverty. That is the highest national poverty rate since 1993.

Contrary to previous trends, children now have a higher poverty rate (22%) in the U.S. than the elderly (9%).

Effects on public health

Environmental experts anticipate that increased climate changes in the coming years will lead to increased levels of poverty and difficulty in accessing basic resources like food and water. Additionally, the needs of the impoverished put extra stress on governmental and economic systems. In countries like the U.S. with a national welfare-type system, there must be sufficient revenue to cover the benefits being provided to poor citizens, but these systems increase the likelihood of basic nutritional and medical needs being met. In countries without such infrastructures, malnourishment and the spread of chronic and often deadly diseases is more likely, making the danger of poverty an ever bigger concern.

Efforts and solutions

In 2000, 189 countries signed the Millennium Declaration, initiated by the United Nations, which

Recent poverty statistics for the United States

- The official poverty rate in 2010 was 15.1 percent—up from 14.3 percent in 2009. This was the third consecutive annual increase in the poverty rate. Since 2007, the poverty rate has increased by 2.6 percentage points, from 12.5 percent to 15.1 percent.
- In 2010, 46.2 million people were in poverty, up from 43.6 million in 2009—the fourth consecutive annual increase in the number of people in poverty.
- Between 2009 and 2010, the poverty rate increased for non-Hispanic Whites (from 9.4 percent to 9.9 percent), for Blacks (from 25.8 percent to 27.4 percent), and for Hispanics (from 25.3 percent to 26.6 percent). For Asians, the 2010 poverty rate (12.1 percent) was not statistically different from the 2009 poverty rate.
- The poverty rate in 2010 (15.1 percent) was the highest poverty rate since 1993 but was 7.3 percentage points lower than the poverty rate in 1959, the first year for which poverty estimates are available.
- The number of people in poverty in 2010 (46.2 million) is the largest number in the 52 years for which poverty estimates have been published.
- Between 2009 and 2010, the poverty rate increased for children under age 18 (from 20.7 percent to 22.0 percent) and people aged 18 to 64 (from 12.9 percent to 13.7 percent), but was not statistically different for people aged 65 and older (9.0 percent).

SOURCE: Current Population Survey (CPS), 2011 Annual Social and Economic Supplement (ASEC), the source of official poverty estimates. The CPS ASEC is a sample survey of approximately 100,000 households nationwide. These data reflect conditions in calendar year 2010.

(Table by PreMediaGlobal. © 2013 Cengage Learning)

includes both poverty and environmental stability as two of eight connected **Millennium Development Goals** (MDGs). The Millennium Declaration set 2015 as its deadline for ending poverty. This declaration is momentous not only in the number of countries participating, but in a consensus among both poor and wealthy nations that poverty is not only an issue that needs to be addressed, but also one that countries from all socioeconomic levels share a responsibility to end.

Resources

BOOKS

"Fighting Poverty." *Poverty*. Tina Kafka. Detroit: Lucent Books, 2010. 39-59. Hot Topics.

"Poverty." *Encyclopedia of Global Warming*. Ed. Steven I. Dutch. Vol. 3. Pasadena, CA: Salem Press, 2010. 858-860.

"Poverty." *American Incomes: Demographics of Who Has Money*. 8th ed. Ithaca, NY: New Strategist Publications, Inc., 2011. 329. American Money Series.

PERIODICALS

Giridharadas, Anand, and Keith Bradsher. "Microloan Pioneer and His Bank Win Nobel Peace Prize." *The New York Times*.13 October 2006.http://www.nytimes.com/2006/10/13/business/14nobelcnd.html?pagewanted=all&_r=0 Accessed November 14, 2012.

WEBSITES

Half the Sky. http://www.halftheskymovement.org. Accessed November 14, 2012.

National Poverty Center, University of Michigan. "Poverty in the United States." http://www.npc.umich.edu/poverty/. Accessed November 14, 2012.

U.S. Department of Health and Human Services. "2012 HHS Poverty Guidelines." http://aspe.hhs.gov/poverty/12poverty.shtml. Accessed November 14, 2012.

Water.org. "Water Facts." http://water.org/water-crisis/water-facts/water/. Accessed November 14, 2012.

World Health Organization. "Poverty and Health." http://www.who.int/hdp/poverty/en/. Accessed November 14, 2012.

ORGANIZATIONS

U.S. Department of Health & Human Services, 200 Independence Avenue, S.W., Washington, DC USA 20201, (877) 696-6775, www.hhs.gov

World Health Organization, Avenue Appia 20, 12 Geneva 27, Switzerland, 41 22 (791) 2111, Fax: 41 22 (791) 3111, www.who.int

Andrea Nienstedt, MA

Pregnancy *see* **Reproductive health**

▌Prevention

Definition

In public health, prevention refers to all those actions used to prevent the occurrence of disease and injury. Authorities recognize at least three levels of prevention. Universal prevention involves actions appropriate for use with the general public or a whole population, such as providing immunizations against common infectious diseases. Selective prevention involves preventive actions for subgroups of individuals at risk for specific health risks, such as providing informational programs for people at risk for sickle-cell anemia. Targeted prevention involves preventive actions for high-risk individuals who have not yet been diagnosed for a disease, but who show minimal signs or symptoms for the disease. Some authorities also recognize various levels of prevention. In such cases, primary prevention refers to actions taken before any physical evidence of a disease is available. Secondary prevention occurs when the first signs or symptoms of the disease develop. And tertiary prevention is used when the disease or injury has developed; it aims to reduce further deterioration as a result of the disease or injury.

Purpose

The purpose of preventive actions is to reduce or eliminate the risk of disease or injury or to limit the deleterious effects of a disease or injury.

Description

The general principle underlying public health preventive programs is that it is almost always more efficacious and economically beneficial to prevent disease and injury from occurring than it is to treat the results of such conditions. In light of that principle, virtually all public health agencies at all levels have developed and implemented some type of preventive program as a fundamental part of their missions. The U.S. **Department of Health and Human Services** (HHS) has developed a strategy for the development of prevention programs in virtually any area. That strategy begins with a definition of the problem and the collection of data and information about its prevalence. From this information, public health officials can then begin to identify possible causes of the problem which, in turn, can lead to the development of methods for dealing with those causes. Those methods are then tested in the field to determine their effectiveness in eliminating or reducing the cause of the disease or injury, and those that prove to be effective can become the core of the preventive program. The program is then put into practice with members of the community for whom it is appropriate and continuously evaluated for its effectiveness in the field.

This type of preventive program can be used for a wide variety of disease, injuries, and conditions, such as the prevention of:

- infectious diseases, such as measles, mumps, polio, and hepatitis
- chronic diseases, such as diabetes, cancer, and cardio-vascular disease
- drug abuse and addiction
- accidents
- tobacco and alcohol abuse
- obesity and other nutritional issues
- lack of physical activity
- suicide and other related psychological disorders
- childhood and adolescent disease disorders
- sexual disorders
- oral health

The specific elements of every prevention program vary from topic to topic, although most share certain common elements. An example of a prevention program is the San Francisco (California) Department of Health (SFDH) Childhood Lead Prevention Program. The purpose of that program is to reduce the number of children who develop lead-related health issues as a result of exposure to the element in their own homes or communities. The primary elements of that program are as follows:

- provision for collection of reports on all environmental sources of lead in the Bay Area
- follow-up on all such reports, which includes detailed studies of the area and collection and analysis of all data collected at the contaminated site
- collection of information and data about specific cases of lead poisoning among families in the Bay Area
- provision of a range of information about lead poisoning and its prevention to parents, contractors, property owners, and other stakeholders for whom lead contamination may be an issue
- provision of case management support for families with children who have been exposed to or are at risk for lead in their environment

The SFDH also publishes a number of newsletters, brochures, and other print materials dealing with lead **poisoning**, including *Information for Parents*; *Information for Contractors*; *Information for Property Holders*; a quarterly newsletter; lead hazard bulletins and requirements with city, state, and federal law information; brochures on related health issues, such as childhood **asthma**.

Health Screenings

Some of the most effective preventive programs involve screening protocols. A screening program is one in which large numbers of individuals are tested for the presence of a disease or for risk factors for a disease or potential injury before any signs or symptoms are present. One of the most common screening programs involves mammographies for women who are known to be at risk for breast **cancer**. A mammography is a procedure in which low-intensity x-rays are used to examine breast tissue. The procedure is able to detect the presence of cancer cells before other signs or symptoms are present. In such a case, patients may be offered therapeutic procedures such as breast-conserving procedures or mastectomies to deal with the potential of advanced breast cancers.

Governmental agencies and professional societies have now developed recommendations for a number of diseases and injuries for which screenings may be appropriate. For example, the U.S. Preventive Services

Task Force (USPSTF) has made the following recommendations:

- Alcohol misuse: Screening for all adults, including pregnant women, along with behavioral counseling, where indicated and appropriate, in a primary care setting; additional recommendations have been made by the American Medical Association (AMA) and the Canadian Task Force on Preventive Health Care (CTFPHC).

- Breast cancer: Screening mammography every 1-2 years for women over the age of 40; additional recommendations from the American Cancer Society (ACS), American College of Preventive Medicine (ACPM), National Institutes of Health (NIH), AMA, and CTFPHC.

- Cervical cancer: Screening for women who have been sexually active; additional recommendations from the AMA, ACPM, and CTFPHC.

- Chlamydial infection: Screening for all women aged 25 and younger, and all women who are at risk for chlamydial infection; screening for all asymptomatic pregnant women under the age of 26; additional recommendations by the Centers for Disease Control and Prevention (CDC), ACPM, and CTFPHC.

- Colorectal cancer: Screening for men and women over the age of 50; additional recommendations by the American Gastroenterological Society, ACS, and CTFPHC.

- Depression: All adults in healthcare systems where adequate facilities for such screenings are available; additional recommendations by the CTFPHC.

- Diabetes mellitus, type 2: Adults with hypertension or hyperlipidemia; additional recommendations by the American Diabetes Association and CTFPHC.

- Hepatitis B: Pregnant women during their first prenatal visit; additional recommendations by the Advisory Committee on Immunization Practices (ADIP).

- Human immunodeficiency virus: Screening for known at-risk men and women; additional recommendations by the Joint National Committee (JNC) and the CTFPHC.

- High blood pressure and lipid disorders: Routine screening for men over the age of 35 and women over the age of 45; routine screening for younger men and women with known risk factors for coronary heart disease; additional recommendations by the AMA and CTFPHC.

- Obesity: Routine screening for all adult men and women; additional recommendations by the CTFPHC, ACPM, American Diabetes Association, and NIH.

- Osteoporosis: Routine screening for women over the age of 65; additional recommendations by the National Osteoporosis Foundation and the CTFPHC.

- Tobacco use: Routine screening for all tobacco users and all pregnant women; additional recommendations by CTFPHC and U.S. Public Health Service.

- Visual impairment: Routine screening for all elderly persons; additional recommendations by American Academy of Ophthalmology (AAO).

Additional screening recommendations have been made for dental and periodontal disease by the American Dental Association; for glaucoma by the AAO; hearing impairment by the Speech-Language-Hearing Association and the CTFPHC; **hepatitis** C by the **CDC**; oral cancer by the ACS, CTFPHC, National Cancer Institute (NCI), National Institute of Dental Research, and the ADA; prostate cancer by the ACS, AMA, American Urologic Association, ACPM, and CTFPHC; and skin cancer by CTFPHC, ACS, ACPM, NCI.

Costs to Society

Reducing the financial cost of disease and injury is one of the major objectives of prevention programs. Many studies have been conducted to determine the estimated cost to society of diseases such as diabetes, **obesity**, and HIV/AIDS, behavioral problems such as drug abuse and unintended pregnancies; and injuries, such as those caused by firearms. Some of the findings of those studies include the following:

- The estimated cost of health care associated with tobacco use in the United States in 2008 was $96 billion.

- Employers in the United States lose an estimated $6.4 billion annually because of absence of work resulting from obesity-related causes, and obsese males pay an additional $1,152 annually for obesity-related hospitalizations and drug costs; for women, that additional cost amounts to $3,613 per year.

- The annual cost to U.S. employers for drug-abuse-related problems (including alcohol) in 2012 was $276 billion.

- As of 2008, accidents involving consumer products in the home were estimated to affect more than 180,000 Americans annually at a cost of about $3.3 billion.

- Total dental care costs in the United States in 2006 were estimated at $17.9 billion.

Efforts and solutions

As noted previously, virtually all public health agencies at all levels of government now recognize prevention programs as an essential part of their missions. Perhaps the most comprehensive and detailed effort to emphasize the role of prevention in public health in recent times was contained in the 2010 Patient

Protection and Affordable Care Act, signed by President Barack Obama on March 23, 2010. One provision of that act created the National Prevention Council (NPC) with the charge of developing a National Prevention Strategy. The NPC consists of heads of 17 federal agencies, departments, and offices with responsibilities for health prevention activities. In June 2011, the NPC released its first version of the National Prevention Strategy. That strategy consists of two primary elements, four Strategic Directions and seven Strategic Priorities. The overall goal of these Directions and Priorities is to "increase the number of Americans who are healthy at every stage of life."

The four Strategic Directions listed in the National Prevention Strategy are:

• Healthy and safe community environments, which means the creation and maintenance of communities that develop prevention programs that promote wellness and the recognition of such communities when and where they exist.

• Clinical and community preventive services, which requires that preventive healthcare programs are available in all communities and that such communities are intergrated with each other and mutually reinforcing.

• Empowered people, which implies that communities will develop specific mechanisms by which individual health prevention decisions are supported and enforced.

• Elimination of health disparities, which calls for communities to eliminate differences in access to all forms of health care among all races, ethnic groups, and other classifications of individuals.

The seven Strategic Priorities that have been selected for the current National Prevention Strategy and the recommended actions for achieving these objectives include:

• Tobacco-free Living: support for tobacco-free control policies; support for the 2009 Family Smoking Control and Prevention Act; expand tobacco use cessation programs; develop and implement educational programs to encourage people to live tobacco-free lives.

• Preventing Drug Abuse and Excessive Alcohol Use: support tobacco control policies and programs at local, state, tribal, and terretorial levels; create environments that empower young people not to drink or not to start drinking; identify drug abuse and alcohol use problems early and provide intervention programs for those involved in such activities; reduce inappropriate access to and use of prescription drugs.

• Healthy Eating: increase access to nutritious, affordable foods in all communities; implement existing

nutritional standards and policies; improve the nutritional quality of food supplies; help people understand and make healthy food and beverage choices; support policies and programs that promote breastfeeding.

• Active Living: encouragement design of community facilities that supports all types of physical activity; promote and strengthen school programs that involve physical activity; facilitate access to safe, accessible, affordable places for physical activity; support policies and programs for physical activity in the workplace; provide physical activity counseling and referrals.

• Injury and Violence Free Living: develop and implement policies and programs for transportation safety; promote community designs that promote safety and prevents injuries; promote policies and practices that reduce the risk of falls among the elderly; improve policies and programs that reduce the number of workplace injuries; strengthen policies and programs designed to prevent violence; develop programs that help individuals to make choices that lead to safer, more injury-free lives.

• Reproductive and Sexual Health: increase the use of preconception and prenatal care; provide support for sexual health care for pregnant and parenting women; provide sexual health education, especially for adolescents; enchance early detection programs for certain sexual infections, such as hepatitis and HIV.

• Mental and Emotional Well-Being: promote early childhood development that includes positive parenting and violence-free homes; facilitate the connection across all elements of the community throughout the lifespan; provide families and individuals with the

QUESTIONS TO ASK YOUR DOCTOR

- Are there any medical conditions for which my children should be screened? If so, what are they?

- What household safety issues do you think should be of special concern to our family, and what preventive steps can we take against those issues?

- What safety precautions do you recommend for use when our one-year-old child travels in a car?

- Can you explain the reason that preventive services are so focused on the use of tobacco products?

- At what point, if any, should members of our family begin considering taking action against obesity problems? What steps would be included in such preventive actions?

- How, if at all, do health preventive recommendations differ for women and for men?

support needed to promote mental health; promote policies and programs for the early identification and treatment of mental health disorders.

Resources

BOOKS

Compton, Michael T., ed. *Clinical Manual of Prevention in Mental Health*. New York: American Psyciatric Publishing 2009.

Kumanyika, Shiriki, and Ross Brownson, eds. *Handbook of Obesity Prevention: A Resource for Health Professionals*. New York: Springer, 2010.

Maffetone, Philip. *The Big Book of Health and Fitness: A Practical Guide to Diet, Exercise, Healthy Aging, Illness Prevention, and Sexual Well-Being*. New York: Skyhorse Publishing, 2012.

Rethman, Jill, and Trisha O'hehir. *Prevention Strategies For Oral Health: A Lifetime of Healthy Smiles*. New York: Blackwell Publishing, 2013.

PERIODICALS

Braithwaite, D., et al. "Cancer Prevention for Global Health: A Report from the ASPO International Cancer Prevention Interest Group." *Cancer Epidemiology, Biomarkers, and Prevention* 21, 9. (2012): 1606–10.

Catalano, R. F., et al. "Worldwide Application of Prevention Science in Adolescent Health." *Lancet* 379, 9826. (2012): 1653–64.

García-Huidobro D, K. Puschel, and G. Soto. "Family Functioning Style and Health: Opportunities for Health Prevention in Primary Care." *British Journal of General Practice* 62, 596. (2012): e198–203.

Hawk, C, H. Ndetan, and M. W. Evans, Jr. "Potential Role of Complementary and Alternative Health Care Providers in Chronic Disease Prevention and Health Promotion: An Analysis of National Health Interview Survey Data." *Preventive Medicine* 54, 1. (2011): 18–22.

WEBSITES

"The Guide to Community Preventive Services." Community Preventive Services Task Force. http://www.thecommunity guide.org/index.html. Accessed on October 2, 2012.

"Health, Prevention, and Wellness Program." Administration on Aging. http://www.aoa.gov/AoARoot/AoA_Programs/ HCLTC/Evidence_Based/index.aspx. Accessed on October 2, 2012.

"National Prevention Strategy." National Prevention Council. http://www.healthcare.gov/prevention/nphpphc/strategy/ report.pdf. Accessed on October 2, 2012.

"Prevention for a Healthier America." Trust for America's Health. http://healthyamericans.org/reports/prevention08/. Accessed on October 2, 2012.

ORGANIZATIONS

Office of Disease Prevention and Health Promotion, U.S. Department of Health and Human Services, 1101 Wootton Pkwy., Suite LL100, Rockville, MD USA 20852, 1 (240) 453–8280, Fax: 1 (240) 453–8282, http://odphp.osophs .dhhs.gov/.

David E. Newton, Ed.D.

Prison health *see* **Correctional health**

Public Health Accreditation Board (PHAB)

Definition

The Public Health Accreditation Board (PHAB) is a national nonprofit organization established to oversee and implement accreditation of public **health departments** and to develop and administer training programs designed toward that end.

Purpose

The purpose of PHAB is to protect and advance the quality of local, state, tribal, and territorial public health departments by testing and certifying departments for certain essential characteristics of an efficient public health entity.

Description

The principles on which PHAB was founded were first outlined in a strategic plan called the Futures Initiative released by the U.S. **Centers for Disease Control and Prevention (CDC)** in 2004. That plan suggested that accreditation of public health departments was a key element in strengthening public health programs throughout the United States. Release of the report set into motion a series of meetings in which the concept of national accreditation programs were discussed in more detail. Those meetings culminated in May 2007 with the formation of the PHAB, which was charged with the task of developing accreditation standards, training programs for the development of needed skills, and a testing and accreditation program for public health programs. The final accreditation process was finally announced in February 2009, and 30 health departments took part in the beta testing of the program in 2009 and 2010. The testing phase of the program was completed in the spring of 2011 and the final standards and testing program were released to the general public in July of that year. Accreditation opportunities for public health departments then became available in September 2011.

The PHAB accreditation process consists of seven steps:

- Pre–application, during which a health department informs PHAB of its intention to apply for accreditation and begins to collect relevant materials for the process.

- Application, which involves submitting the actual application and application fee, and health department employees complete the training phase of the process.

- Document selection and submission, at which point an agency collects all documents needed to demonstrate that it meets PHAB standards.

- Site visit, which allows three to four PHAB inspectors to visit the applying facility to confirm the accuracy of submitted data and carry out discussions about the agency's activities.

- Decision, which may be either "approved" (for five years) or "not approved." Agencies that are not approved may appeal this decision to a special board of the PHAB. A formal appeals process is outlined in the PHAB Guide to National Public Health Department Accreditation Version 1.0.

- Reports, which are required annually of agencies that are approved.

- Reaccreditation, a process through which every approved agency must pass at the end of five years, often with the requirement of additional training sessions and the submission of more recent documents.

As of late 2012, no public health department had yet received approval as a result of completing this series of seven steps.

The PHAB website provides detailed information on the process needed to achieve accreditation. In addition to an online orientation program, the organization also provides in-person training that deals with topics such as selection of documents needed for accreditation, how to upload documents, how to prepare for an official site visit, and how to prepare the required annual report to the PHAB. Instruction is also provided for individuals who are interested in becoming inspectors for the PHAB site visitations of applicants.

Professional publications

PHAB provides a limited number of documents related to its work, the most important of which is the *Final Recommendations for a Voluntary National Accreditation Program for State and Local Health Departments*, on which the philosophy and work of the agency is based. A special issue of the *Journal of Public Health Management & Practice* (January/February 2010) is available from PHAB and provides a number of articles on various aspects of the program. An irregular electronic newsletter is also available at no cost to professionals and the general public.

Resources

PERIODICALS

Riley, William J., et al. "Public Health Department Accreditation." *American Journal of Preventive Medicine* 42. 3. (2012): 263–71.

Riley, William J., Kaye Bender, and Elizabeth Lownik. "Public Health Department Accreditation Implementation: Transforming Public Health Department Performance." *American Journal of Public Health* 102. 2. (2012): 237–42.

WEBSITES

Public Health Accreditation: Q&A with Kaye Bender. Public Health Newswire. http://www.publichealthnewswire.org/?p=2573 (accessed October 11, 2012).

Public Health Accreditation Board. Centers for Disease Control and Prevention. http://www.cdc.gov/stltpublichealth/partnerships/phab.html (accessed October 11, 2012).

ORGANIZATIONS

Public Health Accreditation Board (PAHB), 1600 Duke St., Suite 440, Alexandria, VA 22314, (703) 778-4549, Fax: (703) 778-4556, info@phaboard.org, http://www.phaboard.org/.

David E. Newton, EdD

Public health administration

Definition

Public health administration is the aspect of the field of public health that concentrates on management of personnel and programs. Administration is needed on a day-to-day basis to ensure that organizations operate efficiently and successfully, as programs require supervision and guidance. The field of administration is concerned with theories and techniques derived from a variety of fields, including statistics, behavioral psychology, policy analysis, communications, budgeting, and other aspects of organizational management.

Description

The work of a public health administrator is at the same time similar to and different from that of persons engaged in administration in other fields. The administrative elements are similar; they include supervising employees, coordinating programs, preparing budgets, monitoring programs, and evaluating results and outcomes. Aspects that are specific to the field of public health include health and disease **prevention** programs. Public health administrators conduct educational campaigns and try to maintain the health of the people they serve. Other health professionals have similar aims of maintaining health but often focus on restorative or curative measures rather than preventive programs.

There are 10 core public health functions with which an administrator must be familiar. There is a specialized body of public health law. Data are constantly being generated. These data must be sorted, classified, stored, and interpreted. There are highly sophisticated computer systems and databases to keep track of diseases, vital events, waste materials, insects, pollutants, and a host of other aspects of public health. Data that are collected must be organized, analyzed, and presented to such constituencies as members of the public, governmental agencies, and other health care professionals. The overall health of the public being served must be periodically assessed. Intervention programs must be designed, implemented, and evaluated. Other forms of research are also conducted.

The day-to-day activities of a public health administrator include human resources management, finance, performance measurement and improvement, communications, and marketing, which maintains relations with members of the media and local government. A public health administrator must build relationships with such various constituencies as consumer groups, healthcare providers, and legislators. Leadership is an important aspect of public health administration.

Work settings

The most common work setting for a public health administrator is an office within a local health department or public health agency. There are approximately 3,300 local boards of health in the United States. Their sizes vary from a single municipality to an entire state. Many consist of one or more counties. Each employs a staff of professionals that provide specialized services. Each provider has a supervisor; larger organizations have more than one layer of supervision. In addition, there are public and private organizations that provide public health services, including nonprofit organizations like the American Red Cross and the American **Cancer** Society. Governments also employ public health administrators. The number of persons who provide some administrative services within the realm of public health is thus extensive.

Undergraduate education and postgraduate training

Basic preparation for a career in public health administration usually begins with a college degree but does not end at the undergraduate level. It is possible to learn administration from experience on the job but the time required is increasing each year. As of 2012, a master's degree is the functional minimum level of education for admission into the field of public health administration; the different types of master's degrees are described in the next section. The actual field of study at the college level can vary; however, an undergraduate degree in management, public health, nursing, **community health**, applied health, allied health or a related discipline is useful preparation for graduate work in public health administration. An optimal undergraduate curriculum should include course work in the following subject areas: management, accounting, finance, economics, biology, **environmental health** or science, marketing, business, health law, and budgeting.

Initial training following completion of the master's degree begins with job orientation. This is relatively similar for most entry-level positions in the field. During orientation, the structure and reporting relationships of an organization are described. Basic laws and other legal requirements are outlined. Job duties of a particular position are explained. Organizational regulations and requirements are reviewed.

A high level of interpersonal and communications skills is vital to public health administrators, as much of their time is spent writing reports and explaining their decisions to other healthcare professionals and the wider community. With healthcare budgets shrinking as of 2012, many administrators must also be skilled in writing grant proposals as well as budgeting increasingly scarce funding resources. In addition, public health administrators must acquire competence in cross-cultural communication, as many public health programs at the local level are intended to reach minorities and other underserved populations.

Ongoing training occurs at two levels. The first is specific to a particular working agency or environment. It consists of office and organizational updates, program changes, and information pertaining to other local issues. The second is specific to the field of public health. These updates typically occur at professional conferences and through articles in the secondary literature of public health. They consist of changes in programs that have been proposed or imposed by federal or other funding agencies. They also include new findings related to theories or practice that have been developed by researchers. Changes in reporting procedures fall within this category.

Advanced education and training

There are 49 schools of public health accredited by the Council on Education for Public Health (CEPH) in the United States as of 2012 that offer master's degrees in the field. Master's-level training in public health administration is obtained by completing a formal graduate degree program. The most commonly earned graduate credential is a Master of Public Health (MPH) degree. This degree provides a broad-based curriculum for anyone in the field of public health and is appropriate for persons just entering the field as well as those with experience. Other master's degrees are also useful. These include Master of Business Administration (MBA), Master of Health Services Administration (MHSA), Master of Public Administration (MPA), Master of Hospital Administration (MHA), and Master of Management (MM) degrees. The core requirements of the different degree programs are similar and typically include course work in statistics, economics, management, finance, marketing, issues, law, and human resource administration. Elective courses help to tailor a graduate curriculum to the specific needs of each student.

There are some differences among the degree courses described. These are typically related to the focus afforded by the training. For example, a MPH degree is specifically concentrated on public health. An MBA provides more general training. While both degrees are useful, the MPH is focused on health. In an analogous manner, MHSA coursework focuses on issues related to managing health service providers and organizations. MPA focuses on administration in a public or not for profit environment. The MHA is geared for hospital

KEY TERMS

Credential—A document that serves as proof of a person's competence in a specific field. Academic degrees, diplomas, certificates given on completion of an examination, and identification badges are all examples of credentials.

Epidemiology—The study of patterns and distribution of disease in large groups of people.

Vital event—An occurrence for which a certificate is typically issued. Examples of vital events include births, deaths, marriages, and adoptions.

administrators, while the MM is very general. MPH degree curriculum includes courses in **epidemiology** and environmental health. The others typically substitute additional courses in economics, accounting, or labor relations.

Some workers in public health administration require continuing education units to maintain a license or certification. Examples of such workers include nurses, social workers, health officers, sanitarians, and physicians. The rules for many of these professionals are not set by federal or national agencies, but rather may be specific to the state that has issued the credential. Professionals earning continuing education credits may include courses and seminars that cover aspects of public health administration. In this way, they acquire new and updated knowledge. The Association of Schools of Public Health (ASPH) offers both a basic Certified in Public Health (CPH) credential and Certified in Public Health Continuing Education (CPHCE) credits for professionals in public health. The CPH credential, which was first offered in 2008, requires passing an examination; maintaining the credential requires recertification every two years. The cost of the CPH examination as of 2012 is about $400.

All persons seeking to enter the field of public health administration will require professional training and preparation. This requirement will translate into opportunities for teachers of this subject. With demand for trained persons increasing, the demand for teachers is also likely to increase.

Future outlook

The outlook for persons seeking employment in public health administration is ambiguous as of 2012. On the one hand, the Bureau of Labor Statistics (BLS) expects jobs in this field to increase at an above-average

749

QUESTIONS TO ASK YOUR DOCTOR

- Would you recommend public health administration as a career choice?
- What is your opinion of the impact of the current crisis in health care on this field?

rate. With recent rapid changes in managed care and the restructuring of healthcare delivery, disease prevention and public health have assumed new importance in the mainstream practice of medicine. New emphases in the field of public health since the early 2000s include environmental health, drug abuse and **addiction** treatment, and women and children's health; startup programs in these areas will require persons with training in public health administration.

In spite of the favorable job outlook, however, entry into the field is increasingly competitive because stiff performance standards have been instituted since the early 2000s. With increased requirements for training and preparation, salaries for public health administrators are likely to increase. As the baby boomer generation ages and retires, the number of agencies and organizations providing services is expected to rise. These demands, too, are likely to drive up salaries for public health administrators. As of 2012, salaries in the field range from $45,000 to $95,000 per year; the salary depends on the applicant's experience and credentials, and the size of the public health department or organization.

The downside of job opportunities in the field, however, is the increasing levels of pressure on public health administrators to accomplish more in less time with fewer support staff as a result of shrinking funding. The economic downturn of 2008 coupled with the ever-increasing cost of health care in general means that public health administrators face numerous financial as well as managerial challenges in meeting their organizations' goals. According to a report published in the spring of 2012, over 23,000 jobs in local **health departments** were lost between 2008 and 2010 because of the recession and subsequent funding cuts. In addition, a June 2012 editorial in the *New England Journal of Medicine* noted that the number of healthcare- and public health-related jobs is not by itself a measure of improved health care: "The key policy goals should be to achieve better health outcomes and increase overall economic productivity, so that we can all live healthier and wealthier lives."

Resources

BOOKS

Levy, Barry S, and Joyce R. Gaufin, eds. *Mastering Public Health: Essential Skills for Effective Practice.* New York: Oxford University Press, 2012.

Novick, Lloyd F., Cynthia B. Morrow, and Glen P. Mays. *Public Health Administration: Principles for Population-based Management,* 2nd ed. Sudbury, MA: Jones and Bartlett, Publishers, 2008.

Rose, Patti Renee. *Cultural Competency for Health Administration and Public Health.* Sudbury, MA: Jones and Bartlett, 2011.

Turnock, Bernard J. *Essentials of Public Health,* 2nd ed. Sudbury, MA: Jones and Bartlett Learning, 2012.

PERIODICALS

Baicker, Katherine, and Amitabh Chandra. "The Health Care Jobs Fallacy." *New England Journal of Medicine* 366 (June 28, 2012): 2433–2435.

Drehobl, P.A., et al. "Public Health Surveillance Workforce of the Future."*Morbidity and Mortality Weekly Report: Surveillance Summaries* 61 (July 27, 2012): Supplement 25–29.

Willard, R., et al. "Impact of the 2008–2010 Recession on Local Health Departments." *Journal of Public Health Management and Practice* 18 (March-April 2012): 106–114.

WEBSITES

"Member Schools." Association of Schools of Public Health. http://www.asph.org/document.cfm?page=200 (accessed October 4, 2012).

"What Is Public Health?" Association of Schools of Public Health. http://www.whatispublichealth.org/what/index .html (accessed October 4, 2012).

ORGANIZATIONS

American Public Health Association (APHA), 800 I Street, NW, Washington, DC United States 20001-3710, (202) 777-APHA, Fax: (202) 777-2534, http://apha.org/

Association of Schools of Public Health (ASPH), 1900 M Street NW, Suite 710, Washington, DC United States 20036, (202) 296-1099, Fax: (202) 296-1252, info@asph.org, http://www.asph.org/

Association of State and Territorial Health Officials (ASTHO), 2231 Crystal Drive, Suite 450, Arlington, VA United States 22202, (202) 371-9090, Fax: (571) 527-3189, http://www.astho.org/

Council on Education for Public Health (CEPH), 1010 Wayne Avenue, Suite 220, Silver Spring, MD United States 20910, (202) 789-1060, Fax: (202) 789-1895, http://www .ceph.org/

National Association of County and City Health Officials (NACCHO), 1100 17th Street, NW, Seventh Floor, Washington, DC United States 20036, (202) 783-5550, Fax: (202) 783-1583, info@naccho.org, http://naccho.org/

National Association of Local Boards of Health (NALBOH), 1840 East Gypsy Lane Road, Bowling Green, OH United States 43402, (419) 353-7714, Fax: (419) 352-6278, http://www.nalboh.org/.

L. Fleming Fallon, Jr., MD, PhD, Dr.PH.
Rebecca J. Frey, PhD

Public health engineers

Definition

Public health engineering is a specialized field of environmental engineering which deals with the **prevention**, control, and remediation of potential hazards to public health.

Purpose

The purpose of public health engineering is to design and construct systems that prevent or control conditions that might contribute to a reduction in the quality of public health, such as designing **water** control and purification systems that prevent the spread of water-borne diseases.

Description

The mid-nineteenth century saw the rise of a relatively new profession known as public health engineering, in which trained professionals attacked a number of environmental problems associated with public health issues. Primary among these challenges was dealing with impure water and sewage systems that contributed to the spread of communicable diseases in a community. Over time, public health engineering became subsumed in a newer and more comprehensive field of study known as environmental engineering, which today deals with any factor that threatens the biological, physical, or human environment. As with other environmental engineering programs, specializing in public health engineering usually requires a bachelor's or master's degree, with a heavy emphasis on courses in biology, chemistry, physics, and mathematics. In some states, a public health engineer is required to be certified by a professional board, such as the Accreditation Board for Engineering and Technology.

Public health engineers are involved in dealing with environmental hazards that pose a threat to human health. They may be required to assess the status of some existing natural or manmade system, such as a lake waterfront, municipal water purification system or sewage system, a public campground, a high school campus, the indoor pollution status of a large building, or a municipal swimming pool. Based on that assessment, they may develop recommendations for improvements or modifications in existing systems to make them more effective in protecting human health and may be asked to design new structures and systems to achieve that objective. They may then be expected to supervise and oversee the actual construction and installation of such a system and to evaluate its functioning at the conclusion of construction. Public health engineers may also be expected to conduct routine tests and inspections of existing systems, such as **chlorination** systems in water plants, **sanitation** practices in local food establishments, and soil composition in public gathering areas. Many public health engineers also have public education responsibilities in which they are expected to improve the general public's understanding of the risks posed by natural and manmade systems and the way in which those systems affect human health for better or worse.

Public health engineers must have a number of basic skills common to all environmental engineers, such as:

• A general understanding and command of the principles of environmental science and environmental engineering procedures and principles.

• An ability to collect, collate, and interpret both qualitative and quantitative data.

• An ability to read and write technical reports dealing with health and environmental issues.

• Communication skills that can be used both with fellow professionals and with the general public.

• An understanding of systems analysis, in which any one element functions as a part of a larger whole.

• Problem solving skills that allow one to define a specific problem and develop a specific solution for that problem.

Professional publications

A number of peer-reviewed professional journals carry papers of interest to public health engineers. These include: *Journal of Environmental Engineering*, published by the Environmental Engineering Division of the American Society of Civil Engineers; *Environmental Engineering*, published by the Society of Environmental Engineers (Great Britain); *Environmental Science & Technology*, published by the American Chemical Society; *Environmental Engineer*; and *Environmental Engineer: Applied Research and Practice*, both published by the American Academy of Environmental Engineers (AAEE). In addition, all of the professional organizations listed here also publish and distribute a very large array of specialized texts on topics of interest to public health engineers. Examples of books available from the AAEE include: *Creative Safety Solutions, Environmental, Safety, and Health Engineering, Handbook of Ecotoxicology, Impact of Hazardous Waste on Human Health, Microbial Food Contamination*, and *Safety, Health and Environmental Protection*.

Resources

BOOKS

Assistant Public Health Engineer. Syosset, NY: National Learning Corp., 2003.

Public Health Engineer: Test Preparation Study Guide: Questions & Answers. Syosset, NY: National Learning Corp., 2009.

PERIODICALS

Ehrenhard, Michael L., Dennis R. Muntslag, and Celeste P. M. Wilderom. "Challenges to the Implementation of Fiscal Sustainability Measures." *Journal of Organizational Change Management* 25. 4. (2012): 612–29.

Gute, David M. "Public Health Engineering: Water as a Focus in Restoring the Connection between Engineering and Public Health." *Journal of Water Resources Planning and Management* 130 Part 6. (2004): 425–28

WEBSITES

Public Health Engineer. MyMajor. http://www.mymajors.com/careers-and-jobs/Public-Health-Engineer (accessed October 11, 2012).

Public Health Engineer I. Onandaga County, New York. http://www.ongov.net/employment/jobs/specs/sp10350.htm (accessed October 11, 2012).

ORGANIZATIONS

American Academy of Environmental Engineers (AAEE), 130 Holiday Ct., Suite 100, Annapolis, MD 21401, (410) 266-3311, Fax: (410) 266-7653, info@aaee.net, www.aaee.net.

David E. Newton, EdD

Public Health Foundation (PHF)

Definition

The Public Health Foundation (PHF) is a nonprofit association chartered in the District of Columbia with the mission of conducting research, providing training, and distributing information about the best practices in public health care. A number of countries other than the United States (notably India and Pakistan) also have national public health foundations, as do a number of states, regional partnerships, and cities in the United States.

Purpose

A key aspect of PHF's work consists of research that can be used by state and local public health agencies to develop better health policies. The organization also provides training programs for public health workers and distributes a wide variety of information about best practices in public health care.

Description

PHF was founded in 1968 to advance the quality of public health care in the United States through research, training, and distribution of information about the best available public health care practices. Today, its work is organized into two major focus areas: performance management/quality improvement and workforce development. The first of these terms refers to a combination of programs designed to improve the effectiveness of a public health agency's programs, empowering its workforce, streamlining its decision-making process, and improving the quality of services provided by a local health agency. PHF offers a number of services in its efforts to achieve this goal, including demonstration programs on topics such as **asthma**, sexually transmitted infections, and performance management improvement; online training sessions; a clearinghouse of tools and resources; personalized guidance from trained coaches and consultants; and specific examples of practical applications in the practice of public health. The second focus area, workforce development, consists of TrainingFinder Real-time Affiliate Integrated Network (TRAIN), a combination of public health-related courses offered through PHF state affiliates. A second element of this focus area is the PHF Online Store, which has available over 300 resources dealing with all aspects of the public health profession for use in training and development of staff personnel.

In addition to these two major focus areas, PHF sponsors a number of specific programs dealing with essential topics in public health, such as accreditation, **community health assessment**, data, infrastructure, management, policy, quality improvement, recruitment and retention, strategic planning, training, and workforce development. An example of the type of programs available from PHF is one called Winnable Battles, a program originally developed by the U.S. **Centers for Disease Control and Prevention (CDC)**. Winnable Battles is a program aimed at public health priorities that have a large-scale impact on public health and known and effective strategies for dealing with them. PHF participates in this effort by providing the research that can be used by local public health agencies to initiate an attack on a Winnable Battle in some specific area. A key tool in the PHF arsenal in this regard is its publication *Guide to Community*

Preventative Services, which summarizes research evidence on a number of important public health issues.

Professional publications

PHF publishes and distributes publications on public health issues in a number of formats, including books, brochures, CD-ROMs and software, DVDs, posters, and videos. These publications cover topics such as adolescent health, asthma and **allergies**, diabetes, **environmental health**, evaluation and planning, hand **hygiene**, immunizations, maternal and child health, **minority health, nutrition**, preparedness, prescription drugs, **school health**, veterinary public health, and winnable battles. The organization does not publish a journal or newsletter of its own.

Resources

BOOKS

Odo, Francine. *Public Health Memory Jogger II*. Salem, NH: GOAL/QPC, 2007.

PERIODICALS

Bialek, R., J. Carden, and G. L. Duffy. "Supporting Public Health Departments' Quality Improvement Initiatives: Lessons Learned from the Public Health Foundation." *Journal of Public Health Management and Practice* 16. 1. (2010): 14–8.

Kanarek, Norma, Ron Bialek, and Yoku Shaw–Taylor. "A New Methodology for Reporting the Status of Community Health Improvement in the United States." *Applied Research in Quality of Life* 1, 2, (2006): 159–168.

WEBSITES

Nevada Public Health Foundation. http://www.nevadapubli-chealthfoundation.org/home.asp (accessed October 12, 2012).

Public Health Foundation Enterprises. http://www.phfe.org/ (accessed October 12, 2012).

ORGANIZATIONS

Public Health Foundation (PHF), 1300 L St., Suite 800, Washington, DC 20005, (202) 218-4400, Fax: (202) 218-4409, info@phf.org, www.phf.org.

David E. Newton, EdD

Public health nurses

Definition

A public health nurse is a person with an educational degree in nursing with special expertise in working with **community health** problems.

Purpose

Public health nurses carry out a number of responsibilities aimed at assessing the current health status of a community, working to improve the health of individuals in the community, and educating men, women, and children about health issues.

Description

Public health nurses differ from other types of nurses in that they tend to work with large groups of individuals at the same time, rather than individual patients as a hospital or private nurse might do. Among the many responsibilities of a public health nurse are the following:

- Conduct surveys, interviews, and other procedures to determine the health trends within a community and the specific health risks the community faces.

- Work with other members of the public health service to develop public health goals and public health policy for the community.

- Advocate on behalf of the community for local, state, federal, and other policies that will benefit the general health status of the community.

- Understand the range of diversity present within a community and incorporate that information into the development and execution of local public health policy and practices.

- Design and implement health education policies and programs that are appropriate to the needs and resources of a community.

- Conduct home visits to assess individual health needs, to educate individuals about healthful practices, and to provide health services where necessary.

- Cooperate and collaborate with other health–related services for groups and individuals.

- Administer and interpret patient tests and screenings that may be conducted on individuals and groups.

- Collect and review data and documents required to meet federal, state, local, and other governmental requirements.

- Conduct routine preventative and diagnostic procedures, such as taking blood pressure and temperature, administering vaccinations, conducting physical examinations and mental health interviews, and administering pregnancy tests.

- Organize and conduct classes on topics of special interest in a community, such as parenting classes, classes on nutrition, prenatal clinics, and courses on substance abuse.

- Visit schools to conduct educational seminars, screening, testing, and other routine health programs.

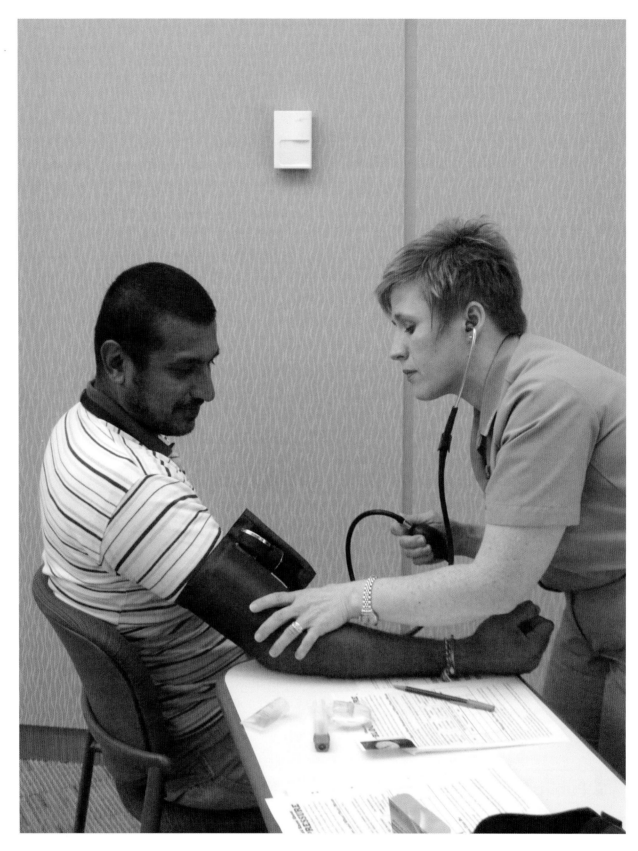

A blood pressure (BP) screening exercise that was being conducted by Centers for Disease Control (CDC) nurses in order to help employees monitor their BP. *(CDC/Nasheka Powell)*

Public health nurses work in a variety of conditions that include public health offices and clinics, schools, youth centers, women's shelters, migrant camps, and individual homes. They may travel and work alone or as members of a team. In addition to possessing basic nursing skills, public health nurses must have superior communication skills and be strong and healthy to carry out the physically stressful tasks associated with their work. A nursing certificate obtained after two years of study is a minimum educational requirement, with many agencies requiring more advanced training such as a bachelor's degree in nursing and, in some cases, licensing as a registered nurse. Special training in community health nursing may also be required.

Professional publications

The professional organization for public health nurses is the Association of Public Health Nurses (APHN), formed in July 2012. APHN grew out of an earlier group, the Association of State & Territorial Directors of Nursing (ASTDN), which had existed as an independent association since 1935. ASTDN consisted only of nurses employed at state **health departments**, and APHN was created to expand that population to include all public health nurses at all levels of employment. One of the important documents produced by the ASTDN was a 2011 report, The Future of Nursing, available online at http://www.phnurse.org/docs/ASTDN_Position_on_The_Future_of_Nursing_Report_2011.pdf. The current APHN contains a number of important archived documents from ASTDN, including reports on health equity, nursing shortages, standards of care, state health department needs, and **emergency preparedness** and response. The APHN also provides a number of webinars on topics of interest to public health nurses, such as **environmental health**, vaccinations, sexual health in adolescents, and **tuberculosis**. The organization does not publish a journal or newsletter.

Resources

BOOKS

Harkness, Gail A., and Rosanna DeMarco. *Community and Public Health Nursing: Evidence for Practice* Philadelphia: Wolters Kluwer Health/Lippincott Williams & Wilkins, 2012.

Maurer, Frances A., and Claudia M. Smith. *Community/Public Health Nursing Practice: Health for Families and Populations*, 5th ed. Philadelphia; London: Saunders, 2012

Stanhope, Marcia, and Jeanette Lancaster. *Public Health Nursing: Population-Centered Health Care in the Community*, 8th ed. St. Louis, MO: Mosby Elsevier, 2012.

PERIODICALS

Coverdale, G. "Ready, Willing and Able? Specialist Community Public Health Nurses's Views of Their Public Health Role." *Journal of Research in Nursing* 17. 1. (2012): 47–63.

Issel, L. M., et al. "Public Health Nursing Job Descriptions: Are They Aligned with Professional Standards?" *Journal of Public Health Management and Practice* 18. 3. (2012): E1–E8.

Peltzer, Jill N., and Cynthia S. Teel. "The Development of a Comprehensive Community Health Center in a Rural Community: A Qualitative Case Study." *Leadership in Health Services* 25. 1. (2012): 52–61.

WEBSITES

Public Health Nurse. Explore Health Careers.org. http://explorehealthcareers.org/en/Career/149/Public_Health_Nurse (accessed October 11, 2012).

Public Health Nurse. The Campaign for Nursing's Future. http://www.discovernursing.com/specialty/public-health-nurse#.UEUoi9b8u5I (accessed October 11, 2012).

Why Choose Public Nursing? You Tube. http://www.youtube.com/watch?v=9PEOYW69Z5c (accessed October 11, 2012).

ORGANIZATIONS

Association of Public Health Nurses (APHN), PO Box 7440, Oklahoma City, OK 73153, (405) 271-9444, X56531, askaphn@phnurse.org, http://www.phnurse.org/.

David E. Newton, EdD

Q fever

Definition

Q fever is an illness caused by a type of bacterium, *Coxiella burnetii*, resulting in a fever and rash.

Description

C. burnetii lives in many different kinds of animals, including cattle, sheep, goats, ticks, cats, rabbits, birds, and dogs. In sheep and cattle the bacteria tends to accumulate in large numbers in the female's uterus (the organ where lambs and calves develop) and udder. Other animals have similar patterns of bacterial accumulation within the females. As a result, *C. burnetii* can cause infection through contaminated milk, or when humans come into contact with the fluids or tissues produced when a cow or sheep gives birth. The bacteria can also survive in dry dust for months; therefore, if the female's fluids contaminate the ground, humans may become infected when they come in contact with the contaminated dust.

Persons most at risk for Q fever include anybody who works with cattle or sheep, or products produced from them. These include farm workers, slaughterhouse workers, workers in meat-packing plants, veterinarians, and wool workers. Since September 2001, however, Q fever has become an additional concern because of its potential as an agent of bioterrorism.

Q fever has been found all over the world, except in some areas of Scandinavia, Antarctica, and New Zealand.

Causes and symptoms

C. burnetii causes infection when a human breathes in tiny droplets, or drinks milk, containing the bacteria. After 3 to 30 days, symptoms of the illness appear.

The usual symptoms of Q fever include fever, chills, heavy sweating, headache, nausea and vomiting, diarrhea, fatigue, and cough. Also, a number of other problems may present themselves, including inflammation of the liver

(**hepatitis**); inflammation of the sac containing the heart (pericarditis); inflammation of the heart muscle itself (myocarditis); inflammation of the coverings of the brain and spinal cord, or of the brain itself (meningoencephalitis); and **pneumonia**.

Chronic Q fever occurs most frequently in patients with other medical problems, including diseased heart valves, weakened immune systems, or kidney disease. Such patients usually have about a year's worth of vague symptoms, including a low fever, enlargement of the spleen and/or liver, and fatigue. Testing almost always reveals that these patients have inflammation of the lining of the heart (endocarditis).

Diagnosis

Q fever is diagnosed by demonstrating that the patient's immune system is making increasing numbers of antibodies (special immune cells) against markers (antigens) that are found on *C. burnetii.*

Treatment

Doxycycline and quinolone **antibiotics** are effective for treatment of Q fever. Treatment usually lasts for two weeks. Rifampin and doxycycline together are given for chronic Q fever. Chronic Q fever requires treatment for at least three years.

Minocycline has been found to be useful in treating post-Q fever fatigue. The dosage is 100 mg per day for three months.

Public Health Response

Q fever is a notifiable disease in the United States and most other developed nations. This designation means that any health or medical facility that learns of a case of Q fever is required to notify the federal and/or state government of this fact. Upon notification, federal and/or state public health workers begin an investigation of that report, determining the type of Q fever involved, the number of patients who have the disease, possible source(s) of the infection, and the pattern by which the disease has been spread within the community. Public health workers then contact other individuals who may have been exposed to the infectious agent or to individuals who have become infected to determine whether they are immune to the disease and, if not, to make arrangements for their **vaccination**. In this process, public health workers typically carry out an aggressive educational program in which they teach individuals how to avoid contracting Q fever, the steps to take in case infection occurs, prognosis, and other information that may be relevant to the outbreak. These elements are also essential factors in long-term educational programs for the general public and for workers who come into contact with animals through whom Q fever may be transmitted.

Prognosis

Death is rare from Q fever. Most people recover completely, although some patients with endocarditis will require surgery to replace their damaged heart valves.

Prevention

Q fever can be prevented by the appropriate handling of potentially infective substances. For example, milk should always be pasteurized, and people who work with animals giving birth should carefully dispose of the tissues and fluids associated with birth.

Industries which process animal materials (meat, wool) should take care to prevent the contamination of dust within the plant.

Vaccines are available for workers at risk for Q fever.

Resources

BOOKS

Toman, Rudolf, et al., eds. *Coxiella Burnetii: Recent Advances and New Perspectives in Research of the Q Fever Bacterium.* Dordrecht; London: Springer, 2012.

PERIODICALS

de Valk, H. "Q Fever: New Insights, Still Many Queries." *Euro Surveillance: European Communicable Disease Bulletin* 17, 3. (2012): 20062.

Kemp, M., et al. "A Program against Bacterial Bioterrorism: Improved Patient Management and Acquisition of New Knowledge on Infectious Diseases." *Biosecurity and Bioterrorism* 10, 2. (2012): 203-207.

Raoult, D. "Chronic Q Fever: Expert Opinion versus Literature Analysis and Consensus." *Journal of Infection* 65, 2. (2012): 102-108.

ORGANIZATIONS

Centers for Disease Control and Prevention, 1600 Clifton Rd., NE, Atlanta, GA 30333, (800) CDC-INFO (800 232-4636) or (404) 639-3534, cdcinfo@cdc.gov, www.cdc.gov.

Rosalyn Carson-DeWitt, MD
Rebecca J. Frey, PhD

Quarantine and isolation

Definition

Quarantine and isolation describes the voluntary or involuntary removal of one or more persons, animals, or

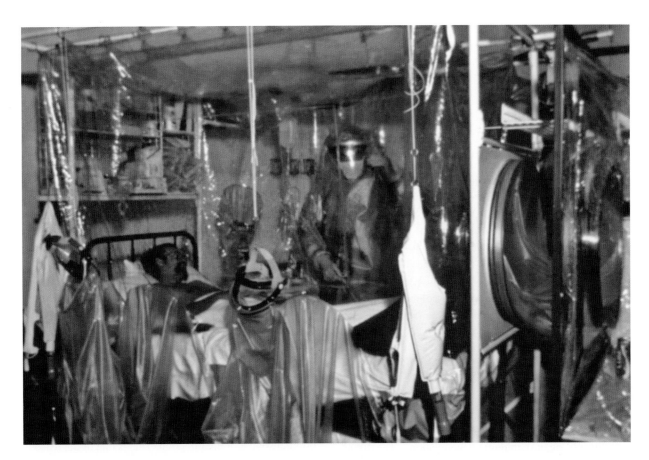

An Ebola patient in an isolation unit. *(CDC/Dr. Lyle Conrad)*

goods from the general population for the purpose of providing special treatment, interrupting the spread of a disease or protecting other elements (persons, animals, or goods).

Description

Though imported freight can be quarantined if suspected of carrying a disease, infestation, or other potentially harmful item, quarantine and isolation usually refer to methods used to treat and prevent the spread of illness and disease. The terms "quarantine" and "isolation" are often used interchangeably. However, the terms are not identical and there are slight differences in their purpose.

Isolation describes the removal of persons to their house or to a medical facility, away from unnecessary contact with others. Isolation is used (usually voluntarily) when a person is known to be sick with a communicable illness. Isolation will usually last as long as the person is infected with the illness.

Quarantine describes the removal of one or more persons to a private location, similar to the process of isolation. Quarantine is used when a person is believed to

have been infected or has had contact with someone infected with a communicable disease. The quarantine will last long enough for any necessary treatments (medication or immunizations) to be administered. Quarantine will be long enough to make sure that the person is not showing symptoms of the disease or illness, and is, therefore, not a threat to the general population.

The time of quarantine for contemporary illnesses varies depending on the incubation period of the illness. A quarantined person stays isolated in order to be monitored for symptoms, for a period from five days, for an illness like **measles**, to forty days, for an illness like **whooping cough**.

Modern quarantine or isolation areas can be established in an individual's home, a hospital, or medical care facility. During a period of quarantine or isolation, patients have little if any contact with other healthy individuals. If patients are quarantined or isolated at home, they will likely need to wear protective clothing and a mask when around family members and will need to avoid sharing any items with other members of the household. Patients that are quarantined or isolated in a hospital or medical facility will be cared for by trained personnel taking the necessary precautions to minimize the chances of the disease spreading to healthcare personnel. In either location, patients will need to avoid having visitors in order to reduce the likelihood of spreading infection.

Origins

The word "quarantine" is derived from the Latin *quaranta* ("forty"), which was the number of days of confinement for foreign ships docking in European ports in the fourteenth century. Quarantine has been used historically to isolate cargo or populations believed to be dangerous or contagious, such as the banishing of those suffering with **leprosy** to leper colonies.

The process of quarantining was used in the Americas, particularly by European colonizers, as they became exposed to insects and diseases. Newer colonists were more susceptible than generations that had been established in the Americas. African slaves and Native Americans were susceptible to diseases brought over by the Europeans, but they did not have the freedom to practice quarantining.

In the nineteenth and twentieth centuries, the process of quarantining in America has been used multiple times prejudicially against immigrant populations. The Immigration Restriction League utilized pseudosciences to justify procedures that limited the diversity of incoming immigrants. The **Centers for Disease Control and Prevention (CDC)** has the authority to monitor travelers coming into the United States for infectious diseases. Occasionally, the **CDC** only needs to quarantine a small number of people as a precautionary measure. Should a quarantine be necessary, the U.S. maintains 20 quarantine stations at ports of entry and border crossings. The "Spanish Flu" **pandemic** of 1918–1919 is the last large-scale quarantine that occurred in the United States.

Risks

Any infectious or communicable disease carries with it many direct and peripheral risks. For instance, in addition to the risks and symptoms associated of the disease, many victims of infectious diseases experience other medical, emotional, and financial hardships. This is especially true in cases of quarantine and isolation—those that have been in quarantine or isolation report feelings of alienation and depression, in addition to worries about financial ramifications and the potential to infect loved ones. In addition, individuals who have been quarantined or isolated have the added stigma of the quarantine or isolation, in addition to any associated with the initial disease.

KEY TERMS

Communicable Disease—an infectious, contagious disease transmitted by bacteria or viral organisms.

Contagious Disease—a highly communicable disease with the ability to spread rapidly from one source to other through contact or proximity.

Infectious Disease—a disease caused by a microorganism; may or may not be communicable. A non-communicable disease would be one spread through food or environmental sources.

Pandemic—an epidemic involving more than one continent or region of the world, without regard to geopolitical boundaries.

Another risk associated with quarantine and isolation is efficacy. Despite the historic reliance on these methods to prevent the spread of disease, they have not proved to be very effective for most diseases. Many diseases are spread through an intermediate contact—the bite of a rat, flea, or mosquito, for instance—so quarantining or isolating individual patients will prevent those persons from causing additional infections, but will not stop the original source of the infection. This is one of the reasons why quarantine and isolation are used far less frequently today than they have been in previous centuries. Mathematical models of responses to a pandemic using quarantine and isolation, however, suggest that this method—if used in a precise way—has the potential to be effective in a large-scale outbreak.

More recent debates on quarantine and isolation have also highlighted the delicate **human rights** balance required in the use of these preventative measures. When deciding whether or not quarantining or isolating a patient is appropriate and the specific measures to take, healthcare professionals have to weigh the risks to society at large with the rights of the individual(s) to refuse the proposed treatment. In the 2000s, both the American Medical Association (AMA) and the **World Health Organization (WHO)** modified their protocols on quarantine and isolation, in order to address these concerns.

Costs to Society

On the small scale with which they are normally used, quarantine and isolation are not major costs to the United States. In the event of a pandemic, the costs for maintaining large-scale quarantine or isolation units would be large; however, if the containment efforts were successful, those costs would be significantly less than the costs of an uncontained disease outbreak.

Efforts and Solutions

In 2005, The American Medical Association (AMA) drafted guidelines—found in "The Use of Quarantine and Isolation as Public Health Interventions"—to establish standardized handling of quarantining situations in an effective and ethical manner. The following year, the **World Health Organization (WHO)** adopted its own, similar guidelines.

In the event of a pandemic, American state and federal authorities have the ability to isolate or quarantine mass groups of people in order to protect public health. A list of diseases, named by Executive Order of the President, dictates the diseases for which quarantine can be imposed. As of the last amendment in 2003, this list includes: **cholera**, **diphtheria**, infectious **tuberculosis**, **plague**, **smallpox**, **yellow fever**, viral hemorrhagic fevers, and **severe acute respiratory syndrome (SARS)**.

Resources

BOOKS

"Infectious Diseases." *Encyclopedia of American Immigration.* Ed. Carl L. Bankston, III. Vol. 2. Pasadena, CA: Salem Press, 2010.

Thivierge, Bethany. "Quarantine." *Infectious Diseases & Conditions.* Ed. H. Bradford Hawley. Vol. 3. Ipswich, MA: Salem Press, 2012.

"Prevention." *Battling and Managing Disease.* Ed. Kara Rogers. New York: Britannica Educational Publishing with Rosen Educational Services, 2011.

Evans, Merrill. "Psychological Effects of Infectious Disease." *Infectious Diseases & Conditions.* Ed. H. Bradford Hawley. Vol. 2. Ipswich, MA: Salem Press, 2012.

"Quarantine and Isolation to Control the Spread of Contagious Diseases." *Contagious Diseases Sourcebook.* Ed. Joyce Brennfleck Shannon. 2nd ed. Detroit: Omnigraphics, 2010.

PERIODICALS

Gumel, Abba B., and Mohammad A. Safi. "Mathematical analysis of a disease transmission model with quarantine, isolation, and an imperfect vaccine." *Computers and Mathematics with Applications* 61.10 (2011).

Gonzalez-Medina, Diego, Quan Le, and Joan Williams. "Infectious diseases and social stigma." *Medical and Health Science Journal* 7 (2011).

WEBSITES

American Medical Association "The Use of Quarantine and Isolation as Public Health Interventions." http://www.ama-assn.org/ama/pub/physician-resources/medical-ethics/code-medical-ethics/opinion225.page Accessed September 26, 2012.

Centers for Disease Control and Prevention "Quarantine and Isolation." http://www.cdc.gov/quarantine/ Accessed September 26, 2012.

ORGANIZATIONS

Centers for Disease Control and Prevention, 1600 Clifton Road, Atlanta, GA USA 30333, (800) 232-4636, cdcinfo@cdc.gov, www.cdc.gov.

Andrea Nienstedt, MA

R

Rabies

Definition

Rabies is an acute viral disease of the central nervous system that affects humans and other mammals but is most common in carnivores. It is sometimes referred to as a **zoonosis**, or disease of animals that can be communicated to humans. Rabies is almost exclusively transmitted through saliva from the bite of an infected animal. Another name for the disease is *hydrophobia*, which literally means "fear of water," a symptom shared by half of all people infected with rabies. Other symptoms include fever; depression; confusion; painful muscle spasms; sensitivity to touch, loud noise, and light; extreme thirst; painful swallowing; excessive salivation; and loss of muscle tone.

Description

Cases of rabies in humans are very infrequent in the United States and Canada, averaging one or two a year (down from over 100 cases annually in 1900), but, according to the **World Health Organization**, about 55,000 people worldwide die of the infection each year; about one person every ten minutes. Of all suspected rabid animal bites, 40% of victims are children under the age of 15. Rabies is most common in developing countries in Africa, Latin America, and Asia, particularly India. Dog bites are the origin of 99% of infections in humans, but other important host animals may include the wolf, mongoose, raccoon, jackal, and bat. A group of researchers in India found that monkeys as well as dogs were frequent vectors of rabies. The team also reported that the male:female ratio of rabies patients in India is 4:1.

Most deaths from rabies in the United States and Canada result from bat bites. In January 2012, a 63-year-old Massachusetts man died of **encephalitis**, which was caused by rabies. The man, who had been bitten by a rabid bat, was the first case of human rabies in Massachusetts since 1935.

On October 18, 2004, a Wisconsin teenager was diagnosed with rabies after suffering from a minor bat bite on September 12, 2004. Miraculously, she was cured of rabies after doctors induced coma and administered four antiviral drugs.

People whose work frequently brings them in contact with animals are considered to be at higher risk than the general population. This would include those in the fields of **veterinary medicine**, animal control, wildlife work, and laboratory work involving live rabies virus. People in these occupations and residents of, or travelers to, areas where rabies is a widespread problem should consider being immunized.

In late 2002, rabies re-emerged as an important public health issue. Dr. Charles E. Rupprecht, director of the **World Health Organization (WHO)** Collaborating Center for Rabies Reference and Research, has listed several factors responsible for the increase in the number of rabies cases worldwide:

• Rapid evolution of the rabies virus. Bats in the United States have developed a particularly infectious form of the virus

• Increased diversity of animal hosts for the disease

• Changes in the environment that are bringing people and domestic pets into closer contact with infected wildlife

• Increased movement of people and animals across international borders. In one case in 2012, a man who had contracted rabies in the Philippines was not diagnosed until he began to feel ill in the United Kingdom

• Lack of advocacy about rabies

Causes and symptoms

Rabies is caused by a rod- or bullet-shaped virus that belongs to the family Rhabdoviridae. The rabies virus is a

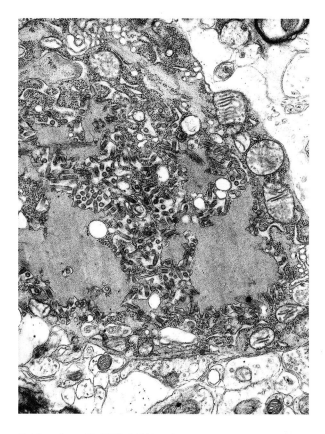

Rabies virus. *(© BSIP SA/Alamy)*

member of a genus of viruses called lyssaviruses, which include several related viruses that infect insects as well as mammals. The rabies virus is usually transmitted via an animal bite, however, cases have also been reported in which the virus penetrated the body through infected saliva, moist tissues such as the eyes or lips, a scratch on the skin, or the transplantation of infected tissues. Inhalation of the virus in the air, as might occur in a highly populated bat cave, is also thought to occur.

From the bite or other area of penetration, the virus multiplies as it spreads along nerves that travel away from the spinal cord and brain (efferent nerves) and into the salivary glands. The incubation period of the rabies virus can be several weeks or months, but rarely much longer, after which time symptoms appear. Initially, the area around the bite may burn and be painful. Early symptoms may also include a sore throat, low-grade fever, headache, loss of appetite, nausea and vomiting, and diarrhea. Painful spasms develop in the muscles that control breathing and swallowing. The individual may begin to drool thick saliva and may have dilated or irregular pupils, increased tears and perspiration, and low blood pressure.

Later, as the disease progresses, the patient becomes agitated and combative and may exhibit increased mental confusion. The affected person usually becomes sensitive to touch, loud noises, and bright lights. The victim also becomes extremely thirsty but is unable to drink because swallowing is painful. Some patients begin to dread water because of the painful spasms that occur. Other severe symptoms during the later stage of the disease include excessive salivation, dehydration, and loss of muscle tone. Death usually occurs three to 20 days after symptoms have developed. Unfortunately, recovery is very rare.

Diagnosis

After the onset of symptoms, blood tests and cerebrospinal fluid (CSF) analysis tests will be conducted. CSF will be collected during a procedure called a lumbar puncture, in which a needle is used to withdraw a sample of CSF from the area around the spinal cord. The CSF tests do not confirm diagnosis but are useful in ruling out other potential causes for the patient's altered mental state.

The two most common diagnostic tests are the fluorescent antibody test and isolation of the rabies virus from an individual's saliva or throat culture. The fluorescent antibody test involves taking a small sample of skin (biopsy) from the back of the neck of the patient. If specific proteins, called "antibodies," that are produced only in response to the rabies virus are present, they will bind with the fluorescent dye and become visible. Another diagnostic procedure involves taking a corneal impression in which a swab or slide is pressed lightly against the cornea of the eye to determine whether viral material is present.

Treatment

Until the results of the most recent successful cure of a late-term rabies case can be repeated successfully and validated by the medical community, the historic treatment options for rabies **prevention** immediately following a bite remain the most viable treatment. Because of the extremely serious nature of a rabies infection, the need for rabies immunizations will be carefully considered for anyone who has been bitten by an animal, based on a personal history and results of diagnostic tests.

If necessary, treatment includes the following:

- The wound is washed thoroughly with medicinal soap and water. Deep puncture wounds should be flushed with a catheter and soapy water. Unless absolutely necessary, a wound should not be sutured.

- Tetanus toxoid and antibiotics will usually be administered.

KEY TERMS

Active immunization—Treatment that provides immunity by challenging an individual's own immune system to produce antibodies against a particular organism, in this case the rabies virus.

Antibody—A specific protein produced by the immune system in response to a specific foreign protein or particle called an "antigen."

Biopsy—The removal of a small sample of tissue for diagnostic purposes.

Efferent nerves—Nerves that convey impulses away from the central nervous system to the periphery.

Enchephalitis—Swelling of the brain and spinal cord, which is often what makes rabies fatal.

Fluorescent antibody test (FA test)—A test in which a fluorescent dye is linked to an antibody for diagnostic purposes.

Lumbar puncture—A procedure that involves withdrawing a small sample of cerebrospinal fluid from the back around the spinal cord.

Lyssavirus—A genus of viruses that includes the rabies virus and related viruses that infect insects as well as mammals.

Passive immunization—Treatment that provides immunity through the transfer of antibodies obtained from an immune individual.

Rhabdovirus—A type of virus named for its rod- or bullet-like shape. The rabies virus belongs to a family of viruses called Rhabdoviridae.

Vector—An animal or insect that carries a disease-producing organism.

Zoonosis—Any disease of animals that can be transmitted to humans. Rabies is an example of a zoonosis.

• Rabies vaccination may or not be given, based on the available information. If the individual was bitten by a domestic animal, and the animal was captured, the animal will be placed under observation in quarantine for ten days. If the animal does not develop rabies within four to seven days, then no immunizations are required. If the animal is suspected of being rabid, it is killed, and the brain is examined for evidence of rabies infection. In cases involving bites from domestic animals where the animal is not available for examination, the decision for vaccination is made based on the prevalence of rabies within the region where the bite

occurred. If the bite was from a wild animal, and the animal was captured, it is generally killed because the incubation period of rabies is unknown in most wild animals.

• If necessary, the patient is vaccinated immediately, generally through the administration of human rabies immune globulin (HRIG) for passive immunization, followed by human diploid cell vaccine (HDCV) or rabies vaccine adsorbed (RVA) for active immunization. Passive immunization is designed to provide the individual with antibodies from an already immunized individual, while active immunization involves stimulating the individual's own immune system to produce antibodies against the rabies virus. Both rabies vaccines are equally effective and carry a lower risk of side effects than some earlier treatments. Unfortunately, in underdeveloped countries, these newer vaccines are usually not available. Antibodies are administered to the patient in a process called "passive immunization." To do this, the HRIG vaccine is administered once, at the beginning of treatment. Half of the dose is given around the bite area, and the rest is administered into the muscle. Inactivated viral material (antigenic) is then given to stimulate the patient's own immune system to produce antibodies against rabies. For active immunization, either the HDCV or RVA vaccine is given in a series of five injections. Immunizations are typically given on days one, three, seven, fourteen, and twenty-eight.

In instances in which rabies has progressed beyond the point where **immunization** would be effective, a radical treatment involving a drug-induced coma and the administration of four different antiviral drugs could be an option. The traditional approach prior to October 2004 was to provide as much relief from **pain** and suffering as possible through medical intervention while waiting to see if survival was possible. The patient would be given medication to prevent seizures, relieve some of the anxiety, and relieve painful muscle spasms. Pain relievers would also be given. In the later stages, aggressive supportive care would be provided to maintain breathing and heart function. Survival via the traditional treatment is rare.

Prognosis

If preventative treatment is sought promptly, rabies need not be fatal. Immunization is almost always effective if started within two days of the bite. Chance of effectiveness declines, however, the longer **vaccination** is put off. It is, however, important to start immunizations, even if it has been weeks or months following a suspected rabid animal bite, because the vaccine can be effective even in these cases. If immunizations do not prove effective or are not received, rabies is usually fatal with a few days of the onset of symptoms.

Public Health Costs

Though there are few cases of rabies in the United States and Canada and even fewer deaths than historically, this decline is not spontaneous. The United States' spending on rabies prevention has increased to approximately $300 million annually. These funds go to things like animal vaccinations, animal-control programs, rabies laboratories, and other medical costs.

Efforts and Solutions

One promising preventive strategy that has been used since the early 2000s is the distribution of wildlife baits containing an oral vaccine against rabies. This strategy has been used in Germany to vaccinate wild foxes, which are frequent carriers of the disease in Europe. In the United States, veterinary researchers at Kansas State University have developed an oral vaccine for fruit bats; early trials of the vaccine have yielded promising results.

Prevention

The following precautions should be observed in environments where humans and animals may likely come into contact.

• Domesticated animals, including household pets, should be vaccinated against rabies. If a pet is bitten by an animal suspected to have rabies, its owner should contact a veterinarian immediately and notify the local animal-control authorities. Domestic pets with current vaccinations should be revaccinated immediately; unvaccinated dogs, cats, or ferrets are usually euthanized (put to sleep). Further information about domestic pets and rabies is available on the American Veterinary Medical Association (AVMA) web site.

• Wild animals should not be touched or petted, no matter how friendly they may appear. It is also important not to touch an animal that appears ill or passive, or whose behavior seems odd, such as failing to show the normal fear of humans. These are all possible signs of rabies. Many animals, such as raccoons and skunks, are nocturnal, and their activity during the day should be regarded as suspicious.

• People should not interfere in fights between animals.

• Because rabies is transmitted through saliva, a person should wear rubber gloves when handling a pet that has had an encounter with a wild animal.

• Garbage or pet food should not be left outside the house or camp site, because it may attract wild or stray animals.

• Windows and doors should be screened. Some victims of rabies have been attacked by infected animals, particularly bats, that entered through unprotected openings.

• State or county health departments should be consulted for information about the prevalence of rabies in an area. Some areas, such as New York City, have been rabies-free, only to have the disease reintroduced at a later time.

• Preventative vaccination against rabies should be considered if one's occupation involves frequent contact with wild animals or non-immunized domestic animals.

• Bites from mice, rats, or squirrels rarely require rabies prevention, because these rodents are typically killed by any encounter with a larger, rabid animal and would, therefore, not be carriers.

• Travelers should ask about the prevalence of the disease in countries they plan to visit.

Resources

BOOKS

Cohen, J. et al. Infectious Diseases. 3rd ed. St. Louis: Mosby, 2010.

Gershon, A.A. et al. Infectious Diseases of Children. 11th ed. St. Louis: Mosby, 2004.

Long, S.S. et al. Principles and Practice of Pediatric Infectious Diseases. 3rd ed. London: Churchill Livingstone, 2009.

Mandell, G.L. et al. Principles and Practice of Infectious Diseases. 7th ed. London: Churchill Livingstone, 2010.

PERIODICALS

Chhabra, M., R.L. Ichhpujani, K.N. Tewari, and S. Lal. "Human Rabies in Delhi." Indian Journal of Pediatrics 71 (March 2004): 217-220.

Fooks, A.R., N. Johnson, S.M. Brookes, et al. "Risk Factors Associated with Travel to Rabies Endemic Countries." Journal of Applied Microbiology 94, Supplement (2003): 31S-36S.

"Human Death Associated with Bat Rabies—California, 2003." Morbidity and Mortality Weekly Report 53 (January 23, 2004): 33-35.

Messenger, S.L., J.S. Smith, L.A. Orciari, et al. "Emerging Pattern of Rabies Deaths and Increased Viral Infectivity." Emerging Infectious Diseases 9 (February 2003): 151-154.

Peters, C., R. Isaza, D.J. Heard, et al. "Vaccination of Egyptian Fruit Bats (Rousettus aegyptiacus) with Monovalent Inactivated Rabies Vaccine." Journal of Zoo and Wildlife Medicine 35 (March 2004): 55-59.

Rosenthal, Elisabeth. "Girl is first to survive rabies without a shot." The New York Times November 25, 2004: A28.

Smith, J., L. McElhinney, G. Parsons, et al. "Case Report: Rapid Ante-Mortem Diagnosis of a Human Case of Rabies Imported Into the UK from the Philippines." Journal of Medical Virology 69 (January 2003): 150-155.

Stringer, C. "Post-Exposure Rabies Vaccination." Nursing Standard 17 (February 5-11, 2003): 41-42.

Thulke, H.H., T. Selhorst, T. Muller, et al. "Assessing Anti-Rabies Baiting—What Happens on the Ground?" BMC Infectious Diseases 4 (March 9, 2004): 9.

Weiss, R.A. "Cross-Species Infections." Current Topics in Microbiology and Immunology 278 (2003): 47-71.

WEBSITES

CDC.Gov http://www.cdc.gov/rabies Accessed July 10, 2012

National Association of State Public Health Veterinarians, Inc. "Compendium of Animal Rabies Prevention and Control, 2011." Morbidity and Mortality Weekly Report Recommendations and Reports (May 31, 2011). http://www.nasphv.org/Documents/RabiesCompendium.pdf Accessed July 10, 2012

Reutershttp://www.reuters.com/article/2012/01/30/us-rabies-massachusetts-idUSTRE80T1W220120130 Accessed July 10, 2012

ORGANIZATIONS

American Veterinary Medical Association (AVMA), 1931 North Meacham Road, Suite 100, Schaumburg, IL 60173-4360, http://www.avma.org

Centers for Disease Control and Prevention, 1600 Clifton Rd., NE, Atlanta, GA 30333, (404) 639-3311, (800) 311-3435, http://www.cdc.gov

Institut Pasteur, 25-28, Rue du Dr. Roux, 75015, Paris, France +33 0 1 45 68 80 00, http://www.pasteur.fr/haut_ext.html.

Janet Byron Anderson
Rebecca J. Frey, Ph.D.
Andrea Nienstedt, MA

Radiation

Definition

Radiation and radioisotopes are extensively used medications to allow physicians and other medical professionals to image internal structures and processes *in vivo* (in the living body) with a minimum of invasion to the patient. Higher doses of radiation are also used as means to kill cancerous cells.

Radiation is actually a term that includes a variety of different physical phenomena. However, in essence, all these phenomena can be divided in two classes: phenomena connected with nuclear radioactive processes are one class, the so-called radioactive radiation (RR); electromagnetic radiation (EMR) may be considered as the second class.

Both classes of radiation are used in diagnoses and treatment of neurological disorders.

Demographics

Devices such as x-ray machines and computed tomography (CT) medical imaging instruments are used commonly in the medical community. Any patient of a physician or other such medical professional in need of such devices for diagnosis and/or treatment would be subjected to various amounts of radiation or radio-isotopes.

Description

There are three kinds of radiation useful to medical personnel: alpha, beta, and gamma radiation. Alpha radiation is a flow of alpha particles that have been emitted by an atomic nucleus; beta radiation is a flow of electrons (or positrons) emitted by radioactive nuclei such as strontium-90; and gamma radiation is electromagnetic radiation of very high frequency (very short wavelength), otherwise called gamma rays.

Radioisotopes for medical use, containing unstable combinations of protons and neutrons, are made by neutron activation. This process involves the capture of a neutron by the nucleus of an atom, resulting in an excess of neutrons (neutron rich). Proton-rich radioisotopes are manufactured in cyclotrons. During radioactive decay, the nucleus of a radioisotope seeks energetic stability by emitting particles (alpha, beta, or positron) and photons (including gamma rays).

Radiation produced by radioisotopes allows accurate imaging of internal organs and structures. Radioactive tracers are formed from the bonding of short-lived radioisotopes with chemical compounds that, when in the body, allow the targeting of specific body regions or physiologic processes. Emitted gamma rays (photons) can be detected by gamma cameras, and computer enhancement of the resulting images allows quick and relatively noninvasive (compared to surgery) assessments of trauma or physiological impairments.

Causes and symptoms

Radiation can damage any and all tissues in the body. The particular manifestation will depend upon the amount of radiation, the time during which it is absorbed, and the susceptibility of the particular type of tissue. However, in small doses, radiation can be helpful in the diagnosis and treatment of medical conditions. Some symptoms may occur when radiation is used on humans.

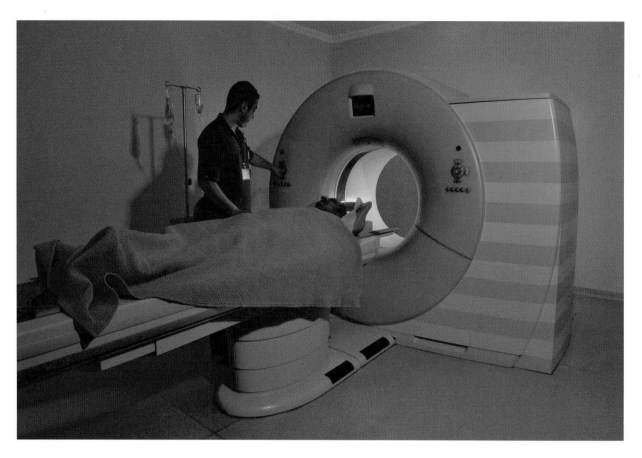

Radiation can come from a Magnetic Resonance Imaging machine. (© Levent Konuk/Shutterstock.com)

These symptoms depend on the amount of dosage used and the region of the body in which the radiation is applied. Commonly felt symptoms include skin reactions (such as redness or itchiness), tiredness, and loss of appetite. Inflammation of the tissues in and around the affected area can also occur. Such tissue inflammation depends on the particular organs affected. For instance, radiation of the colon may cause diarrhea, whereas radiation to the lungs may cause radiation pneumonitis (or inflammation of lung tissue caused by radiation), with symptoms that include difficulty breathing, chest **pain**, and coughing. Other signs of radiation exposure are bruising, skin **burns**, vomiting of blood, hair loss, mouth ulcers, and open sores. Even though undesirable and temporary symptoms often occur, they can be minimized with the use of caution and expertise by medical professionals.

Diagnosis

The use of radiation for the diagnosis of disease or damage to the body can greatly benefit patients, but the benefit must outweigh its risk when recommending such procedures. In almost all cases, the amount of radiation given in such diagnoses is generally low. For instance, a single diagnostic radiology examination of the (lateral) chest provides about 4 millirem (mrem), or 0.04 milli-Sievert (mSv), of radiation to the patient, while an exam to the abdomen gives approximately 53 mrem (0.53 mSv). As a comparison, the amount of natural background radiation that the average American receives each year is approximately 300 mrem (3 mSv). Consequently, the benefits typically outweigh the risks. Research has consistently shown that such low doses of radiation, used for diagnostic radiological examinations, do not cause any serious harm to the human body. However, the increasing use of medical radiation is a growing concern to the medical profession. In fact, a 2010 article in *The Wall Street Journal* stated that "Americans get the most medical radiation in the world—even more than folks in other rich countries—and the average American's dose has grown sixfold over the last couple of decades."

Nuclear radiation

The diagnosis of certain medical conditions is commonly performed with the use of nuclear radiation. Some of these methods include the use of x rays and tomography.

Computed tomography—Abbreviated CT, a medical imaging method that uses tomography along with computer processing to generate three-dimensional images from a series of two-dimensional x-ray images.

Electromagnetic radiation—Abbreviated EMR or EM radiation, a form of energy that contains components of both an electric field and a magnetic field.

Radioactive radiation—Radiation produced from radioactive substances.

Radioisotope—An unstable isotope that emits radiation when it decays or returns to a stable state.

Radiotherapy—The use of x rays or radioactive substances to treat disease.

Rem—Short for roentgen equivalent in man, it is a dose equivalent radiation. One rem is equal to 0.01 Sievert (Sv).

Sievert—Abbreviated Sv, it is a unit of dose equivalent radiation in the International System of Units (SI). One Sv is equal to 100 rem, or 100,000 millirem (mrem).

Tomography—Any of a number of medical imaging procedures that image sections of a body with the use of various types of penetrating waves, such as x rays.

X RAYS. The use of x rays for examining people and animals is called diagnostic radiology. Because the density of tissues is unequal, x rays (a high-frequency and energetic form of electromagnetic radiation) pass through tissues in an unequal manner. The beam passed through the body layer is recorded on special film to produce an image of internal structures. However, conventional x rays produce only a two-dimensional (2D) picture of the body structure under investigation.

TOMOGRAPHY. Tomography (from the Greek *tomos*, meaning "to slice") is a method developed to allow the detailed construction of images of the target object. Initially using the x rays to scan layers of the area in question, with computer assisted tomography, a computer then analyzes data of all layers to construct a three-dimensional (3D) image of the object.

Computed tomography (also known as CT, CT scan) and computerized axial tomography (CAT) scans use x rays to produce images of anatomical structures.

Single proton (or photon) emission computed tomography (SPECT) produces three-dimensional images of an organ or body system. SPECT detects the presence and course of a radioactive substance that is injected, ingested, or inhaled. In neurology, a SPECT scan can allow physicians to examine and observe the cerebral circulation. SPECT produces images of the target region by detecting the presence and location of a radioactive isotope. The photon emissions of the radioactive compound containing the isotope can be detected in a manner that is similar to the detection of x rays in computed tomography (CT). At the end of the SPECT scan, the stored information can be integrated to produce a computer-generated composite image.

Positron emission tomography (PET) scans use isotopes produced in a cyclotron. Positron-emitting radionuclides are injected and allowed to accumulate in the target tissue or organ. As the radionuclide decays, it emits a positron that collides with nearby electrons to result in the emission of two identifiable gamma photons. PET scans use rings of detectors that surround the patient to track the movements and concentrations of radioactive tracers. PET scans have attracted the interest of physicians because of their potential use in research into metabolic changes associated with mental diseases such as schizophrenia and depression. PET scans are used in the diagnosis and characterizations of certain cancers and **heart disease**, as well as clinical studies of the brain. PET uses radio-labeled tracers, including deoxyglucose, which is chemically similar to glucose and is used to assess metabolic rate in tissues and to image tumors, and dopa (3,4-dihydroxyphenylalanine), within the brain.

Another type of CT scan device was first tested in 2007. Using what are called super x rays, the device has the capability of directing a much more concentrated beam of x rays than any older type of technology. The new super x-ray device is called 64-slice CT because it uses 64 detectors to produce the images. It is faster and less expensive at diagnosing heart disease. One day, such advanced technology may eliminate the need for millions of cardiac catheterizations (procedures to unblock clogged arteries) performed annually in the United States. However, a much larger amount of radiation is directed into the patient, which raises much controversy in the medical profession. The risk for **cancer** when such procedures are performed is a major concern of doctors and patients alike.

Electromagnetic radiation

In contrast to imaging produced through the emission and collection of nuclear radiation (e.g., x rays, CT scans), magnetic resonance imaging (MRI) scanners rely on the emission and detection of electromagnetic radiation.

MAGNETIC RESONANCE IMAGING. Electromagnetic radiation consists of oscillations of components of electric and magnetic fields. In the simplest cases, these oscillations occur with definite frequency; the unit of frequency measurement is 1 hertz (Hz), which is one oscillation per second. Arising in some point (under the action of the radiation source), electromagnetic radiation travels with the velocity that is equal to the velocity of the light, and this velocity is equal for all frequencies. Another quantity, wavelength, is often used for the description of electromagnetic radiation. (This quantity is similar to the distance between two neighboring crests of waves spreading on a **water** surface, which appeared after dropping a stone on the surface.) Because the product of the wavelength and frequency must equal the velocity of light, the greater the wave frequency, the less its wavelength.

MRI scanners rely on the principles of atomic nuclear-spin resonance. Using strong magnetic fields and radio waves, MRIs collect and correlate deflections caused by atoms into images. MRIs allow physicians to see internal structures with great detail and also allow earlier and more accurate diagnosis of disorders.

MRI technology was developed from nuclear magnetic resonance (NMR) technology. Groups of nuclei brought into resonance, that is, nuclei absorbing and emitting photons of similar electromagnetic radiation such as radio waves, make subtle yet distinguishable changes when the resonance is forced to change by altering the energy of impacting photons. The speed and extent of the resonance changes permit a nondestructive (because of the use of low-energy photons) determination of anatomical structures.

MRI images do not utilize potentially harmful **ionizing radiation** generated by three-dimensional x-ray CT scans; rather, they rely on the atomic properties (nuclear resonance) of protons in tissues when they are scanned with radio frequency radiation. The protons in the tissues, which resonate at slightly different frequencies, produce a signal that a computer uses to tell one tissue from another. MRI provides detailed three-dimensional soft tissue images.

Treatment

These methods are used successfully for the treatment of medical conditions. Because higher doses of radiation are used, when compared to diagnosis procedures, the risks are much greater. Consequently, physicians seriously consider the risks and benefits of the treatments for the patient.

Radiation therapy (radiotherapy)

When radiation beams are used for the treatment of patients, the procedure is called radiotherapy. As such, radiotherapy requires the use of radioisotopes and higher doses of radiation that are used diagnostically to treat some cancers (including brain cancer) and other medical conditions that require destruction of harmful cells.

Radiation therapy is delivered via external radiation or via internal radiation therapy (the implantation/injection of radioactive substances).

Cancer, tumors, and other rapidly dividing cells are usually sensitive to damage by radiation. The goal of radiation therapy is to deliver the minimally sufficient dosage to kill cancerous cells or to keep them from dividing. Cancer cells divide and grow at rates more rapid than normal cells and so are particularly susceptible to radiation. Accordingly, radioisotope irradiation can restrict or eliminate some cancerous growths. The most common forms of external radiation therapy use gamma rays and x rays. During the second half of the twentieth century, the radioisotope cobalt-60 was the frequently used source of radiation used in such treatments. Subsequent methods of irradiation included the production of x rays from linear accelerators.

Iodine-131 and phosphorus-32 are commonly used in radiotherapy. The use of boron-10 to specifically attack tumor cells is one of several more radical uses of radioisotopes. Boron-10 concentrates in tumor cells and is then subjected to neutron beams that result in highly energetic alpha particles that are lethal to the tumor tissue.

PRECAUTIONS. Radiation therapy is not without risk to healthy tissue and to persons on the healthcare team, and precautions (shielding and limiting exposure) are taken to minimize exposure to other areas of the patient's body and to personnel on the treatment team.

Therapeutic radiologists, radiation oncologists, and a number of technical specialists use radiation and other methods to treat patients who have cancer or other tumors.

Care is taken in the selection of the appropriate radioactive isotope. Ideally, when the radioactive compound is used, it loses its radioactive potency rapidly. (This is expressed as the half-life of a compound.) For example, gamma-emitting compounds used in SPECT scans can have a half-life of just a few hours. This is beneficial for the patients, as it limits the contact time with the potentially damaging radioisotope.

The selection of radioisotopes for medical use is governed by several important considerations involving dosage and half-life. Radioisotopes must be administered in sufficient dosages so that emitted radiation is present in sufficient quantity to be measured. Ideally, the radioisotope has a short enough half-life that, at the delivered dosage, there is insignificant residual radiation following the desired length of exposure.

QUESTIONS TO ASK YOUR DOCTOR

- How does radiation therapy work?
- How much does radiation therapy cost? Will my health insurance cover it?
- What should I expect as side effects of radiation? Are there any long-term effects that I should consider?
- Can you help me assess the benefits compared to the risks?

Prognosis

The use of radiation for therapy widely varies due primarily to the type of cancer being treated, the location of the cancer, the degree that the cancer has spread in the body, and the type of radiation therapy being administered to the patient. In some cases, radiation can cure the cancer, such as in the treatment for skin tumors, laryngeal cancer (of the vocal cords), and early-stage breast cancer (after a lumpectomy has been performed). In other cases, radiation does not cure the cancer but prevents the cancer from spreading and improves the patient's quality of life.

Prevention

New areas of radiation therapy that may prove more effective in treating brain tumors (and other forms of cancers) include three-dimensional conformal radiation therapy (a process where multiple beans are shaped to match the contour of the tumor) and stereotactic radiosurgery (used to irradiate certain brain tumors and obstructions of the cerebral circulation). Gamma knives use focused beams (with the patient often wearing a special helmet to help focus the beams), while cyberknifes use hundreds of precise pinpoint beams emanating from a source of irradiation that moves around the patient's head.

Resources

BOOKS

Adler, Arlene M, and Richard R. Carlton, eds. *Introduction to Radiologic Sciences and Patient Care.* St. Louis: Elsevier Saunders, 2012.

Khalil, Magdy M. *Basic Sciences of Nuclear Medicine.* Berlin: Springer, 2011.

Saha, Gopal B. *Fundamentals of Nuclear Pharmacy.* New York: Springer, 2010.

Yarbro, Connie Henke, Debra Wujcik, and Barbara Holmes Gobel, eds. *Cancer Nursing: Principles and Practice.* Sudbury, MA: Jones and Bartlett, 2011.

WEBSITES

"Medical Radiation Is a Growing Concern." The Wall Street Journal, June 15, 2010. http://online.wsj.com/article/SB10001424052748704324304575306940440759082.html (accessed March 23, 2011).

"Radiation, People, and the Environment." International Atomic Energy Agency. http://www.iaea.org/Publications/Booklets/RadPeopleEnv/index.html (accessed March 21, 2011).

Stabin, Michael G. "Doses from Medical Radiation Sources." Health Physics Society. http://www.hps.org/hpspublications/articles/dosesfrommedicalradiation.html (accessed March 21, 2011).

"What Is Nuclear Medicine?" Society of Nuclear Medicine. http://www.snm.org/index.cfm?PageID=3106&RPID (accessed March 21, 2011).

"'Super X-rays' Spot Heart Ills, Spark Debate." MSNBC. http://www.msnbc.msn.com/id/21642624/ns/health-heart_health/ (accessed March 21, 2011).

ORGANIZATIONS

Environmental Protection Agency, 1200 Pennsylvania Ave. NW, Washington, DC 20460, (202) 272-0167, http://water.epa.gov

National Cancer Institute, 6116 Executive Blvd., Rm. 3036A, Bethesda, MD 20892-8322, (800) 422-6237, cancergovstaff@mail.nih.gov, http://www.cancer.gov..

Alexander Ioffe

Rape *see* **Sexual assault**

Refugee health

Definition

Refugees are persons who have been displaced from their home or native country. Generally understood, the reasons for this unrest can include: oppression or persecution, political unrest, war, drought, **famine**, and **natural disasters**. However, in terms of international and U.S. law, refugees must be fleeing their native country because of "a well-founded fear of persecution on account of race, religion, nationality, membership in a particular social group or political opinion" (8 USC sec. 2201(a)(42)). Status as a refugee denotes someone who is seeking safety across a national border, whereas internally displaced persons (IDPs) are people who, for any of the same reasons, are seeking safety within their native country. Refugees should not be confused with the terms "aliens," "illegal aliens," or "immigrants." Refugee health encompasses the myriad potential health considerations for various refugee populations.

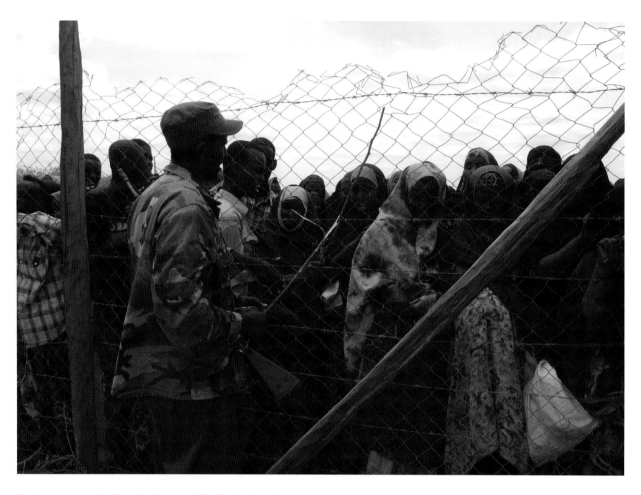

A refugee camp in Somalia. (homeros/Shutterstock.com)

Description

The primary international policy governing the rights and treatment of refugees is the *The 1951 Convention Relating to the Status of Refugees,* which is also the basis for the refugee policies of the United Nations (UN) Refugee Convention. Historically, policies regarding refugees have been centered on war—the League of Nations first addressed Russian refugees after World War I, and the 1951 policies evolved out of concerns over those displaced from Europe after World War II. The UN refugee policies govern the type of relief and the freedoms that host nations are to provide to qualifying persons. However, these terms have proven to be inadequate in definition and subject to selective manipulation.

The UN Refugee Convention policies are specific in the requirements for the situation that produces a qualifying refugee. Though this protection has aided countless lives endangered by persecution, it has proven to be unable to adapt to changes in the nature of persecutions. For instance, because of the wording of these original policies, women fleeing genital mutilation do not qualify for refugee status under the statutes, despite the horrific nature of the **violence** they are fleeing. The UN policies also make no provisions for IDPs or non-states, like the territory of Palestine.

The Refugee Convention has also allowed refugee policy to be subject to political manipulation—which has occurred to some degree in all of the nations that host refugees. For instance, during the Cold War, the United States was incredibly flexible with the definition of refugee provided in the convention, in order to accommodate the few defectors that were able to escape the Eastern Bloc. These defectors were then touted as evidence of Western superiority over communist forces. After the end of the Cold War, the definition of refugee became much stricter and less accommodating. In America and abroad, refugee-hosting governments have adapted and changed their policies based on political pressure or popularity.

There are a number of health concerns regarding refugees, depending on their reasons for fleeing, the countries from which they fled, and their environment after fleeing. Many refugees—especially if fleeing as part of a large exodus—are displaced to small or large state-run communities called refugee camps. These camps are often rudimentary in structure, sometimes consisting of a small city of tents. Refugee camps lack some of the infrastructures of an actual city, including usual **water** and **sanitation**, and there are often overcrowded. These conditions frequently result in a variety of health problems and aid in the spread of illness and disease. Additionally, refugees may already be ill or malnourished upon arrival to such a camp. Though refugee camps are often perceived as temporary operations, many refugees live for prolonged periods of time—even decades—in these camps.

There are additional health concerns for women and children refugees. Whether in a refugee camp or a new country population, many female refugees become victims of rape, and refugees who are also mothers often suffer from overwork. Many women flee to refugee camps as places of safety but are subsequently raped and become pregnant. Women giving birth in refugee camps are often doing so in unsanitary conditions without the aid of a skilled person—these conditions pose significant health risks for both mother and child. Women in refugee camps are often also victims of patriarchal and even abusive gender-power schemas within many refugee camps. The existing power structures often allow women to be intimidated and controlled by male leaders, as well as expected to do the labor within the camp. Additionally, these women face the physical and psychological effects of their original persecution, the trauma of displacement, and subsequent hardships. Refugee mothers are often very resilient in their efforts to provide safety for their children, but they face substantial obstacles in their daily tasks and are often dealing with loss of loved ones, identity, and the shock of often entirely unfamiliar surroundings, food, customs, and even language. As a result of their various traumas, many refugee women and mothers suffer from symptoms of **post-traumatic stress disorder** (PTSD).

Whether within a refugee camp or situated in a more natural domestic setting, refugees fall outside of the traditional infrastructures of health care and are at risk for subsequent health problems. Within refugee camps, resources are often very strained, and refugees may get emergency medical attention at best. Outside of refugee camps, when proper health care is available, refugees face financial, cultural, and linguistic difficulties in obtaining medical treatment. Large cultural gaps also tend to produce different beliefs in appropriate medical treatment and the protocol for seeking out that treatment. Refugees resettled in urban areas are often beset by

poverty, while those resettled in more suburban areas often face isolation and discrimination. Refugee children are also likely to have learning and behavioral problems. Many cultures are reluctant to understand or accept Western medical treatments—for example, many patriarchal cultures would be uncomfortable with female practitioners or female patients seeking treatment unaccompanied, and many cultures are also reluctant to seek or accept mental health treatment.

Another problematic group includes persons displaced by natural disasters or occurrences such as hurricanes, floods, famines, or droughts. According to the internationally accepted definitions, these are not refugees. If these individuals were to stay in their own countries, they would be IDPs, but if they were to be relocated even out of necessity to another country, their status would be more ambiguous. These events can have serious health effects. The initial event—such as a hurricane or flood—poses immediate bodily threat, but after the event, with local infrastructures damaged, there can be additional health risks, including exposure to contaminated water and sewage. Those displaced by weather may be temporarily housed in a shelter similar to a refugee camp where they may be exposed to additional illnesses. These illnesses often make basic resources like clean food, water, and necessary medication scarce. Like traditional refugees, those displaced by significant weather or natural disasters may also experience psychological symptoms like depression or PTSD.

Demographics

Between the 1970s and the 2000s, the United States settled more refugees than all other countries combined. After September 11, 2001, the U.S. has drastically cut back on the number of persons granted refugee status. According to the most recent data available from the United Nations High Commissioner for Refugees (UNHCR), the U.S. is now ranked 10th among countries resettling refugees.

The United Nations High Commissioner for Refugees (UNHCR) estimates that there are 16 million refugees worldwide; 47% of these are women, and another 44% are children.

The top five countries for the resettlement of refugees are: Pakistan, Syria, Iran, Germany, and Jordan.

Costs to Society

The burden of refugee health falls internationally. Without a home, refugees are each—either for a time or indefinitely—dependent on the world at large to maintain their substandard basic provisions. Refugees in refugee camps usually depend entirely on international aid and charity. Settled refugees have the opportunity to become less dependent financially, but they are still dependent on their new countries to accept and orient them. The financial cost of the world's refugee population is too great for any one nation to bear. Additionally, host nations are responsible for the care of the refugees within their borders.

As refugee response efforts become more coordinated and sophisticated, the unique dynamics of the refugee state and experience are better understood. Research and data continue to grow and help the international community better understand the plight and needs of refugee communities—both in refugee camps and settled. Internationally speaking, there is an infrastructure to help refugee populations—managed by branches of the United Nations like the UNHCR, **WHO**, and UNICEF. These programs, however, are always in desperate need of funding, and instances of war, genocide, or unrest around the world increase the need for this funding. In the United States and other countries that resettle refugees, there are minimal and insufficient programs and infrastructures to provide the necessary assistance and orientation for refugees as they attempt to assimilate themselves into a new society. Though the financial costs of maintaining international and domestic refugee programs are immense, so are the loss of life and the medical repercussions for refugee populations that receive inadequate care.

Efforts and Solutions

In 2000, the **World Health Organization (WHO)**, the International Red Cross and Red Crescent Societies, the Disaster Mental Health Institute, and the University of South Dakota worked together to create the Rapid Assessment of Mental Health Needs of Refugees, Displaced and Other Populations Affected by Conflict and Post-Conflict Situations Available Resources (RAMH). This document debuted at the International Consultation on Mental Health of Refugees and Displaced Populations in Conflict and Post-Conflict Situations conference in Geneva. RAMH is a diagnostic tool for mental health professionals and other personnel working in refugee support roles in order to more effectively assess the mental health needs of refugees and other displaced persons in emergency situations.

Research has shown that community programs, particularly in a refugee's native language, can be effective at bridging some cultural gaps and addressing other social and psychological needs, including mental health care. Compulsory screenings help detect potential mental health problems, but they do not provide programs that are tailored to the unique needs of refugee

experiences and conditions. Addressing this concern continues to be a difficulty in U.S. schools.

Resources

BOOKS

Carranza, Mirna E. "Refugee Mothers." *Encyclopedia of Motherhood.* Ed. Andrea O'Reilly. Vol. 3. Thousand Oaks, CA: Sage Reference, 2010.

"Extreme Weather and Health: Hurricanes and Floods." *Health and Disease.*Diane Andrews Henningfeld. Ed. Michael E. Mann. Detroit: Greenhaven Press, 2011.

Nthakomwa, Martin. "Refugee Policy." *Encyclopedia of Disaster Relief.* Ed. K. Bradley Penuel and Matt Statler. Vol. 2. Thousand Oaks, CA: Sage Reference, 2011.

"Rapid Assessment of Mental Health Needs of Refugees, Displaced and Other Populations Affected by Conflict and Post-Conflict Situations Available Resources (RAMH)." *The Encyclopedia of Trauma and Traumatic Stress Disorders.* Ronald M. Doctor and Frank N. Shiromoto. New York: Facts on File, 2010.

"Refugee." *An Encyclopedia of Human Rights in the United States.* H. Victor Condé. 2nd. ed. Vol. 1. Amenia, NY: Grey House Publishing, 2011.

Weine, Stevan. "Refugees and Family Health." *Encyclopedia of Family Health.* Ed. Martha Craft-Rosenberg and Shelley-Rae Pehler. Vol. 2. Thousand Oaks, CA: Sage Reference, 2011.

WEBSITES

United Nations High Commissioner for Refugees "Programme Overview Fact Sheets: Refugee Public Health 2007."

http://www.unhcr.org/cgi-bin/texis/vtx/homeAccessed September 27, 2012.

ORGANIZATIONS

United Nations High Commissioner for Refugees, Case Postale 2500, CH-1211Genève 2 Dépôt, Suisse, 41 22 739 8111, Fax: 41 22 739 7377, www.unhcr.org

Andrea Nienstedt, MA

Reproductive health

Definition

The **World Health Organization (WHO)** defines reproductive health as going beyond the absence of disease and infirmity to include a complete physical, mental, and social state of well-being that allows a person to have a safe, satisfying, and responsible sexual life at all stages of their lives with the potential for reproduction and the freedom to choose whether, when, and how to reproduce. The term refers to a very wide range of elements that range from the earliest introduction to sexual activity, through the decision to become pregnant or not, through childbirth, and into the postpartum period of pregnancy.

Description

Pregnancy

Pregnancy is a state in which a woman carries a fertilized egg inside her body. Due to technological advances, pregnancy is increasingly occurring among older women in the United States.

FIRST MONTH. At the end of the first month, the embryo is about a third of an inch long, and its head and trunk—plus the beginnings of arms and legs—have started to develop. The embryo receives nutrients and eliminates waste through the umbilical cord and placenta. By the end of the first month, the liver and digestive system begin to develop, and the heart starts to beat.

SECOND MONTH. In this month, the heart starts to pump, and the nervous system (including the brain and spinal cord) begins to develop. The 1 in (2.5 cm) long fetus has a complete cartilage skeleton, which is replaced by bone cells by month's end. Arms, legs, and all of the major organs begin to appear. Facial features begin to form.

THIRD MONTH. By now, the fetus has grown to 4 in (10 cm) and weighs a little more than an ounce (30 g).

The major blood vessels and the roof of the mouth are almost completed, and the face starts to take on a more recognizably human appearance. Fingers and toes appear. All the major organs are now beginning to form; the kidneys are now functional, and the four chambers of the heart are complete.

FOURTH MONTH. The fetus begins to kick and swallow, although most women still can not feel the baby move at this point. Now 4 oz (100 g), the fetus can hear and urinate, and has established sleep-wake cycles. All organs are now fully formed, although they will continue to grow for the next five months. The fetus has skin, eyebrows, and hair.

FIFTH MONTH. Now weighing up to a 1 lb (450 g) and measuring 8–12 in (20–30 cm), the fetus experiences rapid growth as its internal organs continue to grow. At this point, the mother may feel her baby move, and she can hear the heartbeat with a stethoscope.

SIXTH MONTH. Even though its lungs are not fully developed, a fetus born during this month can survive with intensive care. Weighing 1–1.5 lbs (450–700 g), the fetus is red, wrinkly, and covered with fine hair all over its body. The fetus will grow very fast during this month as its organs continue to develop.

SEVENTH MONTH. There is a better chance that a fetus born during this month will survive. The fetus continues to grow rapidly and may weigh as much as 3 lb (1.3 kg) by now. Now the fetus can suck its thumb and look around its watery womb with open eyes.

EIGHTH MONTH. Growth continues but slows down as the baby begins to take up most of the room inside the uterus. Now weighing 4–5 lbs (1.8–2.3 kg) and measuring 16–18 in (40–45 cm) long, the fetus may at this time prepare for delivery next month by moving into the head-down position.

NINTH MONTH. Adding 0.5 lb (225 g) a week as the due date approaches, the fetus drops lower into the mother's abdomen and prepares for the onset of labor, which may begin any time between the 37th and 42nd week of gestation. Most healthy babies will weigh 6–9 lb (2.7–4 kg) at birth and will be about 20 in (50 cm) long.

Causes and symptoms

The first sign of pregnancy is usually a missed menstrual period, although some women bleed in the beginning. A woman's breasts swell and may become tender as the mammary glands prepare for eventual breastfeeding. Nipples begin to enlarge, and the veins over the surface of the breasts become more noticeable.

Common prenatal tests

Test	What it is	How it is done
Amniocentesis (AM-nee-oh-sen-TEE-suhss)	This test can diagnosis certain birth defects, including: • Down syndrome • Cystic fibrosis • Spina bifida It is performed at 14 to 20 weeks. It may be suggested for couples at higher risk for genetic disorders. It also provides DNA for paternity testing.	A thin needle is used to draw out a small amount of amniotic fluid and cells from the sac surrounding the fetus. The sample is sent to a lab for testing.
Biophysical profile (BPP)	This test is used in the third trimester to monitor the overall health of the baby and to help decide if the baby should be delivered early.	BPP involves an ultrasound exam along with a nonstress test. The BPP looks at the baby's breathing, movement, muscle tone, heart rate, and the amount of amniotic fluid.
Chorionic villus (KOR-ee-ON-ihk VIL-uhss) sampling (CVS)	A test done at 10 to 13 weeks to diagnose certain birth defects, including: • Chromosomal disorders, including Down syndrome • Genetic disorders, such as cystic fibrosis CVS may be suggested for couples at higher risk for genetic disorders. It also provides DNA for paternity testing.	A needle removes a small sample of cells from the placenta to be tested.
First trimester screen	A screening test done at 11 to 14 weeks to detect higher risk of: • Chromosomal disorders, including Down syndrome and trisomy 18 • Other problems, such as heart defects It also can reveal multiple births. Based on test results, your doctor may suggest other tests to diagnose a disorder.	This test involves both a blood test and an ultrasound exam called nuchal translucency (NOO-kuhl trans-LOO-sent-see) screening. The blood test measures the levels of certain substances in the mother's blood. The ultrasound exam measures the thickness at the back of the baby's neck. This information, combined with the mother's age, help doctors determine risk to the fetus.
Glucose challenge screening	A screening test done at 26 to 28 weeks to determine the mother's risk of gestational diabetes. Based on test results, your doctor may suggest a glucose tolerance test.	First, you consume a special sugary drink from your doctor. A blood sample is taken one hour later to look for high blood sugar levels.
Glucose tolerance test	This test is done at 26 to 28 weeks to diagnose gestational diabetes.	Your doctor will tell you what to eat a few days before the test. Then, you cannot eat or drink anything but sips of water for 14 hours before the test. Your blood is drawn to test your "fasting blood glucose level." Then, you will consume a sugary drink. Your blood will be tested every hour for three hours to see how well your body processes sugar.
Group B streptococcus (STREP-tuh-KOK-uhss) infection	This test is done at 36 to 37 weeks to look for bacteria that can cause pneumonia or serious infection in newborn.	A swab is used to take cells from your vagina and rectum to be tested.
Maternal serum screen (also called quad screen, triple test, triple screen, multiple marker screen, or AFP)	A screening test done at 15 to 20 weeks to detect higher risk of: • Chromosomal disorders, including Down syndrome and trisomy 18 • Neural tube defects, such as spina bifida Based on test results, your doctor may suggest other tests to diagnose a disorder.	Blood is drawn to measure the levels of certain substances in the mother's blood. [continued]

(Table by PreMediaGlobal. © 2013 Cengage Learning)

Nausea and vomiting are very common symptoms and are usually worse in the morning and during the first trimester of pregnancy. They are usually caused by hormonal changes, in particular, increased levels of progesterone. Women may feel worse when their stomach is empty, so it is a good idea to eat several small meals throughout the day and to keep things like crackers on hand to eat even before getting out of bed in the morning.

Many women also feel extremely tired during the early weeks. Frequent urination is common, and there may be a creamy white discharge from the vagina. Some women crave certain foods, and an extreme sensitivity to smell may worsen the nausea. Weight begins to increase.

In the second trimester (13–28 weeks), a woman begins to look noticeably pregnant, and the enlarged uterus is easy to feel. The nipples get bigger and darker,

Common prenatal tests

Test	What it is	How it is done
Nonstress test (NST)	This test is performed after 28 weeks to monitor your baby's health. It can show signs of fetal distress, such as your baby not getting enough oxygen.	A belt is placed around the mother's belly to measure the baby's heart rate in response to its own movements.
Ultrasound exam	An ultrasound exam can be performed at any point during the pregnancy. Ultrasound exams are not routine. But it is not uncommon for women to have a standard ultrasound exam between 18 and 20 weeks to look for signs of problems with the baby's organs and body systems and confirm the age of the fetus and proper growth. It also might be able to tell the sex of your baby. Ultrasound exam is also used as part of the first trimester screen and biophysical profile (BPP). Based on exam results, your doctor may suggest other tests or other types of ultrasound to help detect a problem.	Ultrasound uses sound waves to create a "picture" of your baby on a monitor. With a standard ultrasound, a gel is spread on your abdomen. A special tool is moved over your abdomen, which allows your doctor and you to view the baby on a monitor.
Urine test	A urine sample can look for signs of health problems, such as: • Urinary tract infection • Diabetes • Preeclampsia If your doctor suspects a problem, the sample might be sent to a lab for more in-depth testing.	You will collect a small sample of clean, midstream urine in a sterile plastic cup. Testing strips that look for certain substances in your urine are dipped in the sample. The sample also can be looked at under a microscope.

SOURCE: U.S. Department of Health and Human Services Office on Women's Health. womenshealth.gov, 2010.

(Table by PreMediaGlobal. © 2013 Cengage Learning)

FDA categories for drugs during pregnancy

Category A Adequate and well-controlled (AWC) studies in pregnant women have failed to demonstrate a risk to the fetus in the first trimester of pregnancy (and there is no evidence of a risk in later trimesters).

Category B Animal reproduction studies have failed to demonstrate a risk to the fetus and there are no AWC studies in humans, AND the benefits from the use of the drug in pregnant women may be acceptable despite its potential risks. OR animal studies have not been conducted and there are no AWC studies in humans.

Category C Animal reproduction studies have shown an adverse effect on the fetus, there are no AWC studies in humans, AND the benefits from the use of the drug in pregnant women may be acceptable despite its potential risks. OR animal studies have not been conducted and there are no AWC in humans.

Category D There is positive evidence of human fetal risk based on adverse reaction data from investigational or marketing experience or studies in humans, BUT the potential benefits from the use of the drug in pregnant women may be acceptable despite its potential risks (for example, if the drug is needed in a life-threatening situation or serious disease for which safer drugs cannot be used or are ineffective).

Category X Studies in animals or humans have demonstrated fetal abnormalities OR there is positive evidence of fetal risk based on adverse reaction reports from investigational or marketing experience, or both, AND the risk of the use of the drug in a pregnant woman clearly outweighs any possible benefit (for example, safer drugs or other forms of therapy are available).

SOURCE: U.S. Food and Drug Administration.

(Table by PreMediaGlobal. © 2013 Cengage Learning)

skin may darken, and some women may feel flushed and warm. Appetite may increase. By the 22nd week, most women have felt the baby move. During the second trimester, nausea and vomiting often fade away, and the pregnant woman often feels much better and more energetic. Heart rate increases as does the volume of blood in the body.

By the third trimester (29–40 weeks), many women begin to experience a range of common symptoms. Stretch marks may develop on abdomen, breasts, and thighs, and a dark line may appear from the navel to pubic hair. A thin fluid may be discharged from the nipples. Many women feel hot, sweat easily, and often find it hard to get comfortable. Kicks from an active baby may cause sharp pains, and lower backaches are common. More rest is needed as the woman copes with the added **stress** of extra weight. Braxton Hicks contractions may get stronger.

At about the 36th week in a first pregnancy (later in repeat pregnancies), the baby's head drops down low into the pelvis. This may relieve pressure on the upper abdomen and the lungs, allowing a woman to breathe more easily. However, the new position places more pressure on the bladder.

A healthy weight gain for most women is between 25 and 35 pounds. Women who are overweight should gain less, and women who are underweight should gain

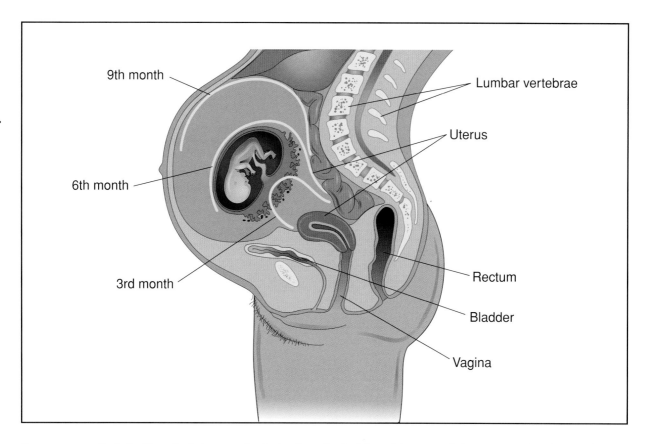

9th month

Lumbar vertebrae

Uterus

6th month

3rd month

Rectum

Bladder

Vagina

Pregnancy usually lasts 40 weeks in humans, beginning from the first day of the woman's last menstrual period, and is divided into three trimesters. The illustration above depicts the position of the developing fetus during each trimester.
(Illustration by Electronic Illustrators Group. © 2013 Cengage Learning)

more. On average, pregnant women need an additional 300 calories a day. Generally, women will gain three to five pounds in the first three months, and then add one to two pounds a week until the baby is born. An average, healthy full-term baby at birth weighs 7.5 lb (3.4 kg), and the placenta and fluid together weigh another 3.5 lb. The remaining weight that a woman gains during pregnancy is mostly due to water retention and fat stores. Her breasts, for instance, gain about 2 lb. in weight, and she gains another 4 lb due to increased blood volume.

In addition to the typical, common symptoms of pregnancy, some women experience other problems that may be annoying, but which usually disappear after delivery. Constipation may develop as a result of food passing more slowly through the intestine. Hemorrhoids and heartburn are fairly common during late pregnancy. Gums may become more sensitive and bleed more easily, and eyes may dry out, making contact lenses feel painful. Pica (a craving to eat substances other than food) may occur. Swollen ankles and varicose veins may be a problem in the second half of pregnancy, and chloasma may appear on the face.

Chloasma, also known as the "mask of pregnancy" or melasma, is caused by hormonal changes that result in blotches of pale brown skin appearing on the forehead, cheeks, and nose. These blotches may merge into one dark mask. It usually fades gradually after pregnancy, but it may become permanent or recur with subsequent pregnancies. Some women also find that the line running from the top to the bottom of their abdomen darkens. This is called the linea nigra.

While the above symptoms are all considered to be normal, there are some symptoms that could be a sign of a more dangerous underlying problem. A pregnant woman with any of the following signs should contact her doctor immediately:

• abdominal pain

• rupture of the amniotic sac or leaking of fluid from the vagina

• bleeding from the vagina

• no fetal movement for 24 hours (after the fifth month)

• continuous headaches

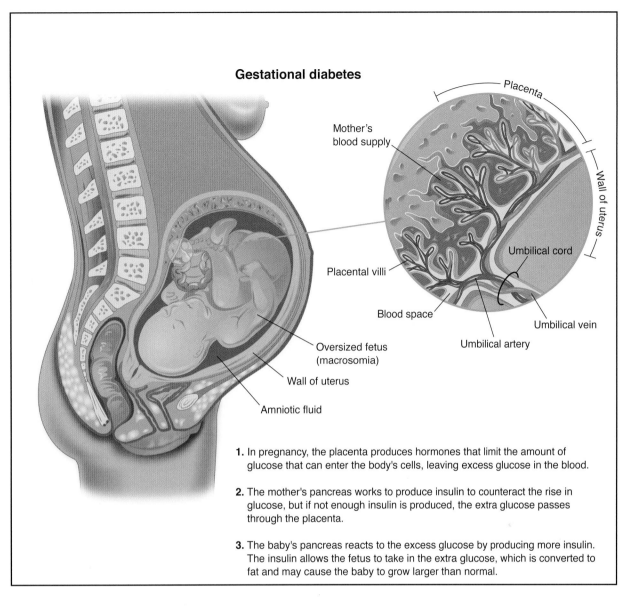

Gestational diabetes

Placenta

Mother's blood supply

Wall of uterus

Umbilical cord

Placental villi

Blood space

Umbilical vein

Umbilical artery

Oversized fetus (macrosomia)

Wall of uterus

Amniotic fluid

1. In pregnancy, the placenta produces hormones that limit the amount of glucose that can enter the body's cells, leaving excess glucose in the blood.

2. The mother's pancreas works to produce insulin to counteract the rise in glucose, but if not enough insulin is produced, the extra glucose passes through the placenta.

3. The baby's pancreas reacts to the excess glucose by producing more insulin. The insulin allows the fetus to take in the extra glucose, which is converted to fat and may cause the baby to grow larger than normal.

(Illustration by Electronic Illustrators Group. Reproduced by permission of Gale, a part of Cengage Learning.)

• marked, sudden swelling of eyelids, hands, or face during the last three months

• dim or blurry vision during last three months

• persistent vomiting

Diagnosis

Many women first discover they are pregnant after a positive home pregnancy test. Pregnancy urine tests check for the presence of human chorionic gonadotropin (hCG), which is produced by a placenta. The newest home tests can detect pregnancy on the day of the missed menstrual period.

Home pregnancy tests are more than 97% accurate if the result is positive, and about 80% accurate if the result is negative. If the result is negative, and there is no menstrual period within another week, the pregnancy test should be repeated. While home pregnancy tests are very accurate, they are less accurate than a pregnancy test conducted at a lab. For this reason, women may want to consider having a second pregnancy test conducted at their doctor's office to be sure of the accuracy of the result.

Blood tests to determine pregnancy are usually used only when a very early diagnosis of pregnancy is needed. This more expensive test, which also looks for hCG, can produce a result within nine to 12 days after conception.

Once pregnancy has been confirmed, there are a range of screening tests that can be done to screen for **birth defects**, which affect about 3% of unborn children. Two tests are recommended for all pregnant women: alpha-fetoprotein (AFP) and the triple marker test.

Other tests are recommended for women at higher risk for having a child with a birth defect. This includes women over age 35, who had another child or a close relative with a birth defect, or who have been exposed to certain drugs or high levels of **radiation**. Women with any of these risk factors may want to consider amniocentesis, chorionic villus sampling (CVS), or ultrasound.

OTHER PRENATAL TESTS. There are a range of other prenatal tests that are routinely performed, including:

- PAP test
- gestational diabetes screening test at 24–28 weeks
- tests for sexually transmitted diseases
- urinalysis
- blood tests for anemia or blood type
- screening for immunity to various diseases, such as German measles

Treatment

Prenatal care is vitally important for the health of the unborn baby. A pregnant woman should be sure to eat a balanced, nutritious diet of frequent, small meals. Women should begin taking 400 mcg of folic acid several months before becoming pregnant, as folic acid has been shown to reduce the risk of spinal cord defects, such as spina bifida.

No medication (not even a nonprescription drug) should be taken except under medical supervision, since it could pass from the mother through the placenta to the developing baby. Some drugs, called teratogens, have been proven harmful to a fetus, but no drug should be considered completely safe (especially during early pregnancy). Drugs taken during the first three months of a pregnancy may interfere with the normal formation of the baby's organs, leading to birth defects. Drugs taken later on in pregnancy may slow the baby's growth rate, or they may damage specific fetal tissue (such as the developing teeth), or cause preterm birth. Herbal supplements and other "natural" remedies can also be extremely harmful to an unborn baby and should not be taken during pregnancy without close supervision by a physician.

To have the best chance of having a healthy baby, a pregnant woman should avoid:

- smoking
- alcohol
- street drugs

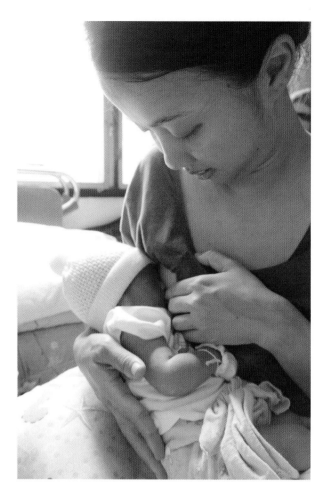

Breastfeeding an infant. *(Criminalatt/Shutterstock.com)*

- large amounts of caffeine
- artificial sweeteners

NUTRITION. Women should begin following a healthy diet even before they become pregnant. This means cutting back on high-calorie, high-fat, high-sugar snacks and increasing the amount of fruits, vegetables, and whole grains in her diet. Once she becomes pregnant, she should make sure to eat at least six to 11 servings of breads and other whole grains, three to five servings of vegetables, two to four servings of fruits, four to six servings of milk and milk products, and three to four servings of meat and protein foods, and to drink six to eight glasses of water each day. She should limit caffeine to no more than one soft drink or cup of coffee per day.

Prognosis

Pregnancy is a natural condition that usually causes little discomfort, provided the woman takes care of herself and gets adequate prenatal care. Childbirth education

Global breastfeeding rates: percentage of infants younger than 6 mos. who are breastfed exclusively, by region, 2006–2010

Eastern and Southern Africa	49%
South Asia	45%
Latin America and Caribbean	42%
Middle East and North Africa	34%
East Asia and Pacific	30%
West and Central Africa	29%
Central Eastern Europe	24%
United States	16%

SOURCE: UNICEF, "Current Status: Breastfeeding," http://www.childinfo.org/breastfeeding_status.html, and U.S. Centers for Disease Control and Prevention, "Breastfeeding Report Card—United States, 2012," http://www.cdc.gov/breastfeeding/data/reportcard.htm.

(Table by PreMediaGlobal. © 2013 Cengage Learning)

classes for the woman and her partner help prepare the couple for labor and delivery.

Prevention

There are many ways to avoid pregnancy. A woman has a choice of many methods of contraception which will prevent pregnancy, including (in order of least to most effective):

• spermicide alone

• natural (rhythm) method

• diaphragm or cap alone

• condom alone

• diaphragm with spermicide

• condom with spermicide

• intrauterine device (IUD)

• contraceptive pill

• sterilization (either a man or woman)

• avoiding intercourse

Breastfeeding

An important health issue faced by parents with newborn children is breastfeeding.

Definition

Breastfeeding is the practice of feeding an infant milk through the mother's breast. According to La Leche League International (LLLI), human milk is "a living fluid that protects babies from disease and actively contributes to the development of every system in baby's body." Breastfeeding stimulates the immune systems of babies and helps to protect against diarrhea and infection.

Purpose

The purpose of breastfeeding is to provide healthy **nutrition** for a newborn infant at low cost.

Description

The mother's body prepares for breastfeeding while she is pregnant. The fatty tissue of the breast is replaced by glandular tissue that is necessary to produce milk. When baby suckles, the breast the hormone oxytocin is released. This causes the muscle cells of the breast to squeeze milk from the milk ducts to the nipple.

Demographics

In 1982, the United States experienced a resurgence in breastfeeding, and rates have continued to increase. A 2012 report by the Surgeon General noted that three-quarters of infants age 19 to 35 months were breastfed at birth, 43% were still being breastfed at six months, and 22% at one year.

The developing world has experienced a decline in breastfeeding rates, largely due to urbanization, social change, and the promotion of formula. Mothers who choose to feed their babies formula often encounter unsafe hygienic conditions in which to prepare the bottles, or they cannot afford to purchase the fuel needed to heat the water to sterilize the bottle and preparation equipment. Two of the major causes of infant mortality in developing countries are diarrhea and acute respiratory infections. Both are conditions that breastfeeding can protect against.

The **World Health Organization** (**WHO**) and the United Nations Children's Fund (UNICEF) are working together to bring about a change in the global breastfeeding culture. In 2002, they developed "The Global Strategy for Infant and Young Child Feeding," which recommends that all babies be exclusively breastfed for the first six months of life with continued breastfeeding up to two years or beyond. Exclusive breastfeeding means that breast milk is the child's only source of nutrition for the first six months of life and that no other solids or liquids, such as formula or water, are introduced at this time, with the exception of liquid **vitamins** or medicines. Current studies suggest that the rate of breastfeeding varies dramatically from country to country. The lowest rate of breastfeeding during the first six months of a child's life currently varies from less than 5% in countries like Djibouti (1%), Chad (2%), and the Dominican Republic (4% to as high as 80% in Kiribati, 65% in North Korea, and 63% in Peru.

Composition of breast milk

Breast milk is the perfect food for an infant. It contains all the nutrients a baby needs to grow and stay healthy, such as:

Alpha-fetoprotein—A substance produced by a fetus's liver that can be found in the amniotic fluid and in the mother's blood. Abnormally high levels of this substance suggests there may be defects in the fetal neural tube, a structure that will include the brain and spinal cord when completely developed. Abnormally low levels suggest the possibility of Down's syndrome.

Braxton Hicks contractions—Short, fairly painless uterine contractions during pregnancy that may be mistaken for labor pains. They allow the uterus to grow and help circulate blood through the uterine blood vessels.

Celiac disease—A condition in children and adults where the body is unable to tolerate wheat protein (gluten).

Chloasma—A skin discoloration common during pregnancy, also known as the "mask of pregnancy" or melasma, in which blotches of pale brown skin appear on the face. It is usually caused by hormonal changes. The blotches may appear in the forehead, cheeks, and nose, and may merge into one dark mask. It usually fades gradually after pregnancy, but it may become permanent or recur with subsequent pregnancies. Some women may also find that the line running from the top to the bottom of their abdomen darkens. This is called the linea nigra.

Eczema—A disease in which the skin becomes dry, red, itchy, and thickened.

Foremilk—Thin, watery milk found at the beginning of breast feeding.

Embryo—An unborn child during the first eighth weeks of development following conception (fertilization with sperm). For the rest of pregnancy, the embryo is known as a fetus.

Fetus—An unborn child from the end of the eighth week after fertilization until birth.

Galactosemia—A rare genetic disorder where an infant cannot metabolize the sugar in breast milk and therefore cannot breastfeed.

Human chorionic gonadotropin (hCG)—A hormone produced by the placenta during pregnancy.

Hyperemesis—Severe vomiting during pregnancy. Hyperemesis appears to increase a woman's risk of postpartum depression.

Immunoglobulin (Ig)—A substance made by B cells that neutralizes specific disease–causing substances and organisms. Also called "antibody." Immunoglobulins are divided into five classes: IgA, IgD, IgE, IgG, and IgM.

Lactose—A sugar found in milk that provides energy.

Omega-3 fatty acids—A class of fatty acids which lowers the level of cholesterol in the blood. Omega-3 fatty acids are also essential for the growth and development of the brain and nerve tissue.

Osteoporosis—A condition found in older individuals in which bones decrease in density and become fragile and more likely to break. It can be caused by lack of vitamin D and/or calcium in the diet.

Oxytocin—A hormone that stimulates contractions during child labor and the production of breast milk.

Placenta—The organ that develops in the uterus during pregnancy that links the blood supplies of the mother and baby.

Postpartum—Following childbirth.

Rhythm method—The oldest method of contraception, with a very high failure rate, in which partners periodically refrain from having sex during ovulation. Ovulation is predicted on the basis of a woman's previous menstrual cycle.

Spina bifida—A congenital defect in which part of the vertebrae fail to develop completely, leaving a portion of the spinal cord exposed.

Taurine—An amino acid that is important in the development of brain tissue. Taurine is a key component of bile, which is needed to digest fats.

Type 1 diabetes—A chronic immune system disorder in which the pancreas does not produce sufficient amounts of insulin, a hormone that enables cells to use glucose for energy. Also called juvenile diabetes, it must be treated with insulin injections.

Type 2 diabetes—Formerly called adult-onset diabetes. In this form of diabetes, the pancreas either does not make enough insulin or cells become insulin resistant and do not use insulin efficiently.

- Fats. Breast milk contains omega-3 fatty acids essential for the growth and development of the brain and nerve tissue. The amount of fat a baby receives depends on the length of the feeding. The milk at the beginning of the feeding is called the foremilk. It is the low-fat milk. The hindmilk that comes at the end of the feeding contains higher concentrations of fat. Therefore, the longer the baby nurses, the higher the fat content.

- Proteins. The whey proteins found in breast milk are easier to digest than formula. Taurine, an amino acid that is important in the development of brain tissue, is found in breast milk but not in cow's milk.

- Sugars. Breast milk contains lactose, a milk sugar that provides energy. Breast milk contains 20%–30% more lactose than cow's milk.

- Vitamins and minerals. Breast milk provides the most balanced source of vitamins and minerals for an infant.

- Immune system boosters. White blood cells and immunoglobulins are responsible for fighting and destroying infection.

The content of breast milk varies from feeding to feeding, at different times of day, and as the baby grows.

Benefits

BENEFITS FOR BABY. There are many benefits for the breastfeeding baby, including:

- Increased immunity. Breast milk contains antibodies that are relayed by the mother and help to protect the baby from bacteria and viruses. These immunoboosters are not found in formula.

- Lower incidence of ear infections and respiratory infections.

- Potentially higher intelligence. Several studies have found higher levels of brain-boosting docosahexaenoic acid (DHA) in the blood levels of breastfed babies than in formula-fed babies.

- Improved digestion and less constipation.

- Decreased risk of diarrhea, pneumonia, urinary tract infections, and certain types of spinal meningitis.

- Decrease in food allergies and eczema.

- More normal weight gain. Breastfed babies are less likely to be overweight than formula-fed babies.

- Reduced risk of type 1 (juvenile) and type 2 (adult onset) diabetes, celiac disease, cancer, rheumatoid arthritis, multiple sclerosis, liver disease, and acute appendicitis.

- Lower risk of sudden infant death syndrome (SIDS).

- Reduced risk of breast cancer (in daughters who have been nursed).

- Better development of jaw and facial structure

- Strong bonding between mother and child.

BENEFITS FOR MOTHER. Breastfeeding women also enjoy many benefits:

- Reduced risk of breast, ovarian, and uterine cancers.

- Natural contraceptive. Many women who breastfeed exclusively for six months experience a delay of fertility.

- Faster postpartum recovery. Breastfeeding uses up extra calories, so it is easier for moms to lose their pregnancy weight. Nursing also helps the uterus shrink back to its normal size faster.

- Relaxation. When a mother is breastfeeding, her body produces oxytocin, a hormone that induces a calm, content feeling.

- Protection from osteoporosis.

- Savings in time and money. Breast milk is cheaper than formula and the mother does not have to spend time preparing bottles.

- Better stewardship of the environment, as there are no bottles to wash or cans to dispose of.

Precautions

Almost every substance that a breastfeeding mother puts into her body has the potential to pass to her baby through her breast milk. This includes food, medicine, alcohol, and cigarettes.

- Foods: Foods such as dairy products, caffeine, grains and nuts, gassy foods, and spicy foods may cause the baby to fuss if they upset the baby's stomach. If this occurs, the mother should eliminate the suspect food from her diet for 10–14 days to see if the trouble stops.

- Medications: Any medication taken while breastfeeding should be approved by a doctor.

- Birth control pills: The high-estrogen type of birth control pills may decrease a breastfeeding mother's milk supply and are not recommended. A progestin-only pill such as the "mini-pill" is the least likely to cause milk supply issues.

- Alcohol: Infants have a hard time detoxifying from the alcohol that passes through their mother's breast milk to them. It is recommended to limit alcohol consumption while breastfeeding.

- Cigarettes: Cigarettes contain toxins that can pass through to the baby and are not recommended for breastfeeding women.

When breastfeeding is not an option

Although breastfeeding is the optimal way to feed an infant, sometimes it is not possible or feasible. A small percentage of women have conditions that prevent breast milk production, such as insufficient development of milk production glands, and cannot breastfeed. Women with HIV infection are advised against breastfeeding, as the virus may be passed to their babies. Women who are newly diagnosed with infectious **tuberculosis** should not breastfeed unless they are on medication. Other health conditions may require that the woman take medication that prevents them from breastfeeding. Babies with galactosemia, a rare genetic disorder that prevents them from metabolizing the sugar in breast milk, cannot breastfeed.

Postpartum depression

One of the most common health problems with which a new mother has to deal is postpartum depression. Postpartum depression is a mood disorder that begins after childbirth and usually lasts at least six weeks.

Postpartum depression, or PPD, affects approximately 15% of all childbearing women. The onset of postpartum depression tends to be gradual and may persist for many months or develop into a second bout following a subsequent pregnancy. Mild to moderate cases are sometimes unrecognized by women themselves. Many women feel ashamed and may conceal their difficulties. This is a serious problem that disrupts women's lives and can have effects on the baby, other children, partners, and other relationships. Levels of depression for fathers can also increase significantly.

Postpartum depression is often divided into two types: early onset and late onset. Early-onset PPD most often seems like the "blues," a mild brief experience during the first days or weeks after birth. During the first week after the birth, up to 80% of mothers experience the "baby blues." This period is usually a time of extra sensitivity; symptoms include tearfulness, irritability, anxiety, and mood changes, which tend to peak between three to five days after childbirth. The symptoms normally disappear within two weeks without requiring specific treatment apart from understanding, support, skills, and practice. In short, some depression, fatigue, and anxiety may fall within the "normal" range of reactions to giving birth.

Late-onset PPD appears several weeks after birth. It involves slowly growing feelings of sadness, depression, lack of energy, chronic fatigue, inability to sleep, change in appetite, significant weight loss or gain, and difficulty caring for the baby.

Causes and symptoms

The cause of postpartum depression has been extensively studied. Alterations of hormone levels of prolactin, progesterone, estrogen, and cortisol are not significantly different from those of patients who do not suffer from postpartum depression. However, some research indicates a change in a brain chemical that controls the release of cortisol.

Research seems to indicate that postpartum depression is unlikely to occur in a patient with an otherwise psychologically uncomplicated pregnancy and past history. There is no association of postpartum depression with marital status, social class, or the number of live children born to the mother. However, there seems to be an increased chance of developing this disorder after pregnancy loss.

Certain characteristics have been associated with increased risk of developing postpartum depression. These risk factors include:

• medical indigence—being in need of health care and not being able to receive it, possibly due to lack of medical insurance

• being younger than 20 years old at time of delivery

• being unmarried

• having been separated from one or both parents in childhood or adolescence

• receiving poor parental support and attention in childhood

• having had limited parental support in adulthood

• poor relationship with husband or boyfriend

• economic problem with housing or income

• dissatisfaction with amount of education

• low self-esteem

• past or current emotional problem(s)

• family history of depression

Experts cannot always say what causes postpartum depression. Most likely, it is caused by a combination of factors that vary from person to person. Some researchers think that women are vulnerable to depression at all major turning points in their reproductive cycle, childbirth being only one of these markers. Factors before the baby's birth that are associated with a higher risk of PPD include severe vomiting (hyperemesis), premature labor contractions, and psychiatric disorders in the mother. In addition, new mothers commonly experience some degree of depression during the first weeks after birth. Pregnancy and birth are accompanied by sudden hormonal changes that affect emotions. Additionally, the 24-hour responsibility for a newborn infant represents a major psychological and lifestyle adjustment for most mothers, even after the first child. These physical and emotional stresses are usually accompanied by inadequate rest until the baby's routine stabilizes, so fatigue and depression are not unusual.

In addition to hormonal changes and disrupted sleep, certain cultural expectations appear to place women from some cultures at increased risk of postpartum depression. For example, women who bear daughters in societies with a strong preference for sons (such as China) are at increased risk of postpartum depression. In other cultures, a strained relationship with the husband's family is a risk factor. In Western countries, domestic **violence** is associated with a higher rate of PPD.

Experiences of PPD vary considerably but usually include several symptoms.

Feelings:

• persistent low mood
• inadequacy, failure, hopelessness, helplessness
• exhaustion, emptiness, sadness, tearfulness
• guilt, shame, worthlessness
• confusion, anxiety, and panic
• fear for the baby and of the baby
• fear of being alone or going out

Behaviors:

• lack of interest or pleasure in usual activities
• insomnia or excessive sleep, nightmares
• not eating or overeating
• decreased energy and motivation
• withdrawal from social contact
• poor self-care
• inability to cope with routine tasks

Thoughts:

• inability to think clearly and make decisions
• lack of concentration and poor memory
• running away from everything
• fear of being rejected by the partner
• worry about harm or death to partner or baby
• ideas about suicide

Some symptoms may not indicate a severe problem. However, persistent low mood or loss of interest or pleasure in activities, along with four other symptoms occurring together for a period of at least two weeks, indicate clinical depression and require adequate treatment.

There are several important risk factors for postpartum depression, including the following:

• stress
• lack of sleep

• poor nutrition
• lack of support from one's partner, family, or friends
• family history of depression
• labor/delivery complications for mother or baby
• premature or postmature delivery
• problems with the baby's health
• separation of mother and baby
• a difficult baby (temperament, feeding, sleeping problems)
• pre-existing neurosis or psychosis

Physical and emotional stress during delivery in conjunction with great demands for infant care may cause the patient to neglect other family members, increasing the woman's feelings of self-worthlessness, isolation, and being trapped. Patients may also feel as if they are inadequate mothers, causing them guilt and embarrassment.

Demographics

There is a 20% to 30% risk of postpartum depression for women who had a previous depressive episode that was not associated with pregnancy. Additionally, there is an increased risk of recurrence in subsequent pregnancies, since more than half of patients will have more than one episode.

Diagnosis

Diagnosis of postpartum depression entails a clinical interview with the patient to assess symptoms. A doctor or other professional healthcare provider may ask the mother about thoughts and feelings, and take a detailed personal history. Clinical assessment may be conducted by a psychologist or psychiatrist, who can determine the risk factors and diagnose the condition. A comprehensive psychological assessment interview could reveal a previous depressive cycle or a family history of depression—important risk factors. The most widely used standard for diagnosis is the Edinburgh Postnatal Depression Scale (EPDS). This is a simple and short 10-question scale. A score of 12 or greater on the EPDS is considered high risk for postpartum depression.

Treatment

Several treatment options exist, including medication, psychotherapy, counseling, and group treatment and support strategies. Treatment should begin as soon as the diagnosis is established. One effective treatment combines antidepressant medication and psychotherapy. These types of medication are often effective when used for three to four weeks. Any medication use must be carefully considered if the woman is breastfeeding, but with some medications, continuing breastfeeding is safe. There are many classes of antidepression medications. Two of the most commonly prescribed for PPD are selective serotonin reuptake inhibitors (SSRIs), such as citalopram (Celexa), escitalopram (Lexapro), fluoxetine (Prozac), paroxetine (Paxil, Pexeva), and sertraline (Zoloft), and tricyclids, such as amitriptyline (Elavil), desipramine (Norpramin), imipramine (Tofranil), and nortriptyline (Aventyl, Pamelor). Nevertheless, medication alone is never sufficient and should always be accompanied by counseling or other support services. Also, many women with postpartum depression feel isolated. It is important for these women to know that they are not alone in their feelings. There are various postpartum depression support groups available in local communities, often sponsored by non-profit organizations or hospitals. For women who have thoughts of **suicide**, it is imperative to seek help immediately.

When medications are combined with psychological therapy, the rates for successful treatment are increased. Interpersonal therapy and cognitive-behavioral therapy have been found to be effective.

Adjunct therapies such as acupuncture, traditional Chinese medicine, yoga, meditation, and herbs may be considered to help the mother suffering from postpartum depression.

Some strategies that may help new mothers cope with the stress of becoming a parent include:

• Valuing her role as a mother and trusting her own judgment.

• Making each day as simple as possible.

• Avoiding extra pressures or unnecessary tasks.

• Trying to involve her partner more in the care of the baby from the beginning.

• Discussing with her partner how both can share the household chores and responsibilities.

• Scheduling frequent outings, such as walks and short visits with friends.

• Sharing her feelings with her partner or a friend who is a good listener.

• Talking with other mothers to help keep problems in perspective.

• Trying to sleep or rest when the baby is sleeping.

• Taking care of her health and well being.

Exercise, including yoga, can help enhance a new mother's emotional wellbeing. New mothers should also try to cultivate good sleeping habits and learn to rest when they feel physically or emotionally tired. It is important for a woman to learn to recognize her own warning signs of fatigue and respond to them by taking a break.

Expected results

When a woman has supportive friends and family, mild postpartum depression usually disappears quickly. If depression becomes severe, and a mother cannot care for herself and the baby, hospitalization may be necessary. Medication, counseling, and support from others usually resolve even severe depression in three to six months. The prognosis for postpartum depression is better if it is detected early during its clinical course, and a combination of SSRIs and psychotherapy is available and initiated.

Prevention

Mothers should be advised prior to hospital discharge that if the "maternity blues" last longer than two weeks or pose tough difficulties with family interactions, they should call the hospital where their baby was delivered and pursue a referral for a psychological evaluation. Education concerning risk factors and reduction of these is important. Prophylactic (preventive) use of SSRIs is indicated two to three weeks before delivery to prevent the disorder in a patient with a past history of depression, since recurrence rates are high if the mother had a previous depressive episode.

Resources

BOOKS

Bayram, Güliz Onat, Mezihe Kizilkaya Beji, and Sule Gokyildiz. *Reproductive Health*. New York: Nova Science Publishers, 2011.

Hussein, J., A. McCaw-Binns, and R. Webber. *Maternal and Perinatal Health in Developing Countries*, 2nd ed. Willingford, UK: CABI, 2012.

Reichenbach, Laura, and Mindy Jane Roseman. *Reproductive Health and Human Rights: The Way Forward*. Philadelphia: University of Pennsylvania Press, 2011.

Reitz, Gladys. *Reproductive Health Handbook*. Delhi: Library Press, 2012.

PERIODICALS

Chuang, C.H., et al. "Primary Care Physicians' Perceptions of Barriers to Preventive Reproductive Health Care in Rural Communities." *Perspectives on Sexual and Reproductive Health* 44, 2. (2012): 78–83.

Edouard, E., and L. Edouard. "Application of Information and Communication Technology for Scaling Up Youth Sexual and Reproductive Health." *African Journal of Reproductive Health*. 16, 2. (2012): 197–205.

Saewyc, E.M. "What About the Boys? The Importance of Including Boys and Young Men in Sexual and Reproductive Health Research." *The Journal of Adolescent Health* 51, 1. (2012): 1–2.

Shrikhande, Laxmi, et al. "2015: Year of Goals in Reproductive Health." *Journal of SAFOG* 4. (2012): 1–4.

WEBSITES

"Improving Reproductive Health." United Nations Population Fund. http://www.unfpa.org/rh/index.htm. Accessed December 3, 2012.

"Reproductive Health." Centers for Disease Control and Prevention. http://www.cdc.gov/reproductivehealth/. Accessed December 3, 2012.

"Reproductive Health." U.S. Department of Health and Human Services. http://www.hhs.gov/opa/reproductive-health/. Accessed December 3, 2012.

"Reproductive Health." World Health Organization. http://www.who.int/topics/reproductive_health/en/. Accessed December 3, 2012.

ORGANIZATIONS

Association of Reproductive Health Professionals - East, 1901 L St., N.W., Suite 300, Washington, DC 20036, 1 (202) 466–3825, ARHP@arhp.org, http://www.arhp.org/.

David E. Newton, Ed.D.

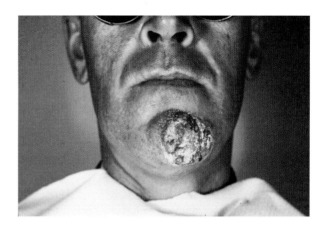

Ringworm on a man's chin. These infections are most common on the feet, scalp, or in toenails, but they can infect any part of the skin. *(Custom Medical Stock Photo, Inc. Reproduced by permission.)*

Ringworm

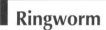

Definition

Ringworm is a common fungal infection of the skin. The name is a misnomer, however, since the disease is not caused by a worm. Ringworm may also be referred to as dermatophyte infection or dermatophytosis. Dermatophytes are parasitic fungi that live on keratin, a fibrous structural protein found in hair, nails, and the outer layer of skin.

Ringworm is often classified as a **zoonosis** because humans can contract it from infected animals (as well as from other humans).

Demographics

Ringworm is a common fungal infection found in all countries around the world. It is estimated that between 14% and 20% of the world's population has some form of ringworm at any given time. There are an estimated 4.3 million outpatient visits in the United States each year for treatment of ringworm infections; 22% of these visits are for infections of the nails, 20% for body ringworm, 19% for athlete's foot, 15% for ringworm of the scalp, and 9% for ringworm of the groin (**jock itch**).

The single most common type of ringworm worldwide is infection of the feet, sometimes called tinea pedis or athlete's foot. This type of ringworm is characterized by **itching**, scaly patches, and a burning sensation between the toes; itchy blisters; or unusually dry skin on the sides and soles of the feet.

Some forms of ringworm are more common in certain age groups than in others. As noted below, ringworm of the scalp and hair commonly affects children but is rare after **puberty**. One study of schoolchildren in the American Midwest reported in 2010 that rates of scalp ringworm in schoolchildren range from 1% in some schools to as high as 30% in others. African American children are at particularly high risk of this type of ringworm. One reason why younger children are more susceptible to ringworm of the scalp is that sebum, a waxy substance secreted by skin glands that protects the skin and hair against fungi and some bacteria, is not produced in humans in significant quantities until puberty. Tinea pedis, tinea cruris (jock itch), and nail infections are much more common in adults. About 3% of adult males worldwide and 1.4% of females have fungal nail infections.

Description

Ringworm is characterized by itchy patches of rough, reddened skin. Raised eruptions usually form the circular pattern that gives the condition its name. As the lesions grow, the centers start to heal. The inflamed borders expand and spread the infection. Ringworm is usually a superficial infection confined to the upper layers of the skin or scalp. In some cases, however, it can invade deeper layers of tissue, producing raised areas of boggy and reddened skin known as kerion.

Types of ringworm

Ringworm is a term that is commonly used to encompass several types of fungal infection. Sometimes, however, only body ringworm is classified as true ringworm.

Body ringworm (tinea corporis) can affect any part of the body except the scalp, feet, and facial area where a man's beard grows (tinea barbae). The well–defined flaky sores can be dry and scaly or moist and crusty.

Scalp ringworm (tinea capitis) is most common in children. It causes scaly, swollen blisters or a rash that looks like black dots. Sometimes inflamed and filled with pus, scalp ringworm lesions can cause crusting, flaking, and round bald patches. Most common in black children, scalp ringworm can cause scarring and permanent hair loss.

Ringworm of the groin (tinea cruris or jock itch) produces raised red sores with well-marked edges. It can spread to the buttocks, inner thighs, and external genitals.

Ringworm of the nails (tinea unguium) generally starts at the tip of one or more toenails, which gradually thicken and discolor. The nail may deteriorate or pull away from the nail bed. Fingernail infection is far less common than toenail infection.

Risk factors

Risk factors for ringworm infections include:

- Living in a hot, humid climate or having a personal tendency to heavy sweating.

- Participating in contact sports, particularly wrestling, football, or rugby.

- Wearing closely fitted clothes or clothing made from synthetic fabrics that do not "breathe."

- Pet ownership. According to the American Academy of Family Physicians (AAFP), there are about two million cases each year in the United States of ringworm acquired from a pet cat or dog.

- Living in a college dormitory, military barracks, or other group housing situation.

- Having AIDS or any other disorder that weakens the immune system.

- Having diabetes mellitus.

- Having cuts, scrapes, or minor breaks in the skin.

- Using greasy hair gels or oils to groom the hair.

- Male sex. Men are more likely than women to contract ringworm infections, particularly athlete's foot and jock itch. Fungal nail infections are twice as common in men as in women.

Causes and symptoms

Causes

Ringworm is caused by parasitic fungi belonging to one of three genera: *Trichophyton*, *Microsporum*, or *Epidermophyton*. Humans can acquire the parasites through any of three routes of transmission: person–to–person contact, including contact with sheets, towels, sports equipment, or other personal items used by an infected person; contact with an infected animal; or contact with contaminated soil, including garden soil. *Trichophyton rubrum* and *Trichophyton tonsurans* are most commonly spread from person to person, while *Microsporum canis* is most commonly transmitted to humans from infected household pets. Cats are the most common carriers of *Microsporum canis*, but the fungus is also frequently carried by dogs, horses, pet mice and rabbits, and farm animals.

When dermatophytes are transmitted to a human or animal's skin, fur, nails, or hair, they obtain nutrients from keratin, a protein found in these tissues. The rash and other symptoms of ringworm are caused by the immune system's reaction to the metabolic byproducts of the fungi.

Symptoms

The symptoms of ringworm typically begin between 4 and 14 days after exposure and include one or more of the following:

- Itchy red patches of scaly skin that may also blister and ooze tissue fluid. The patches are often ring-shaped, with normal-appearing skin in the center of the ring.
- Nearby skin may appear darker or lighter than normal.
- Ringworm infections of the scalp or beard area (in adult males) typically produce bald spots or areas of hair loss. In some cases, the hair loss may be permanent. Severe cases of ringworm on the scalp may be marked by raised nodules or pustules.
- Infections of the nails may produce thickened, discolored, and crumbly nails. In some cases, the entire nail may detach from the underlying nail bed. Infections of the toenails are more common than infections of the fingernails.
- It is possible for a secondary bacterial infection to develop in areas of the body infected by the ringworm fungi, often as a result of scratching itchy areas. The person may then develop a fever along with increased reddening of the affected area, a discharge of pus, and swelling. *A doctor should be contacted at once if these symptoms of bacterial infection develop.*

Household pets carrying dermatophytes often do not have any noticeable symptoms, although they may develop circular bare patches of skin.

KEY TERMS

Dermatologist—A doctor who specializes in diagnosing and treating diseases of the skin.

Dermatophyte—The medical name for three genera of fungi that cause ringworm in humans and domestic pets. The name is derived from two Greek words that mean "skin" and "plant."

Keratin—A type of protein that provides structure to the nails, hair, and outer layer of skin.

Kerion—A raised boggy or swollen patch of reddened skin that develops as a complication of ringworm.

Pustule—A small elevation of the skin containing pus or cloudy tissue fluid.

Sebum—An oily or waxy substance secreted by certain glands in the skin that protects hair and skin against fungi and some bacteria.

Tinea—The general medical term for a fungal infection of the skin. It is often used as a synonym for ringworm.

Wood's lamp—A special ultraviolet lamp used by dermatologists to diagnose ringworm and other skin disorders.

Zoonosis (plural, zoonoses)—Any disease that can be transmitted to humans by animals. Ringworm is a zoonosis caused by fungi.

Diagnosis

Diagnosis of ringworm is based on a combination of patient history, an office examination, and laboratory tests.

Examination

In many cases the diagnosis of ringworm can be made by a primary care physician, but the patient may also be referred to a dermatologist (a doctor who specializes in treating skin disorders). The doctor will usually ask some questions about the patient's living situation (including pets); school or work history; participation in sports or other outdoor activities; and any history of immune disorders.

Tests

The doctor will begin with a visual examination of the patient's skin or other affected areas of the body. He or she may also use a Wood's lamp, which is a special kind of ultraviolet lamp named for the doctor who invented it in 1903. The patient sits in a darkened room while the doctor shines the ultraviolet light about four or five inches away from the affected area. Normal skin or hair will not change color under the lamp. While ringworm caused by *Trichophyton tonsurans* will not fluoresce under a Wood's lamp, ringworm caused by *Microsporum canis* will appear as blue–green or greenish patches.

Procedures

The doctor may also take a scraping of material from the affected area and dissolve it in a solution of potassium hydroxide. The resultant mixture can be examined under a microscope. When dermatophytes are present, the doctor will be able to see their spores or other characteristic structures. If it is important to identify the particular species of fungus, the doctor can use a special medium called dermatophyte test medium or DTM. A scraping of material from the patient's hair or skin is embedded in the DTM and cultured at room temperature for 10–14 days. If dermatophytes are present, the DTM will turn bright red. Other fungi will not cause a color change.

The tests used by veterinarians to diagnose ringworm in pets are the same as those used in humans.

Treatment

Traditional

A person with body ringworm should wear loose clothing and check daily for raw, open sores. Wet **dressings** applied to moist sores two or three times a day can lessen inflammation and loosen scales. The doctor may suggest placing special pads between folds of infected skin, and anything the patient has touched or worn should be sterilized in boiling water. Patients should see their doctor if symptoms do not improve after four weeks of self-care.

Infected nails should be cut short and straight and carefully cleared of dead cells with an emery board.

Patients with jock itch should:

• wear cotton underwear and change it more than once a day

• keep the infected area dry

• apply antifungal ointment over a thin film of antifungal powder

Patients should wash their sheets, pillowcases, and pajamas every day while infected.

Drugs

Some ringworm infections disappear without treatment. Others respond to such topical antifungal medications as naftifine (Caldesene Medicated Powder) or tinactin (Desenex). Ringworm that covers large areas of the body is usually treated with either prescription topical or oral medications. Topical prescription drugs include butenafine (Mentax), ciclopirox (Loprox), miconazole (Monistat-Derm), oxiconazole (Oxistat), or terbinafine (Lamisil). Oral medications for ringworm include traconazole (Sporanox), fluconazole (Diflucan), and ketoconazole (Nizoral). Medications should be continued for two weeks after lesions disappear.

Oral medications for ringworm do have side effects, the most common of which are digestive upsets, abnormal liver functioning, and skin **rashes**. In addition, people taking these drugs should avoid taking **antacids** for **indigestion** or peptic ulcer disease during treatment for ringworm, as antacids interfere with the effectiveness of oral antifungal drugs.

Shampoo containing selenium sulfide can help prevent spread of scalp ringworm, but prescription shampoo or oral medication is usually needed to cure hair or scalp infections. Ketoconazole is particularly effective in treating ringworm of the hair or scalp.

The doctor will also prescribe oral **antibiotics** if the patient has developed a secondary bacterial infection.

Pets with ringworm are treated with many of the same medications used to treat the fungi in humans, particularly terbinafine and fluconazole. The veterinarian will also often recommend trimming or clipping the pet's fur during treatment. Close shaving is not recommended, however, because of the risk of causing breaks or small cuts in the cat or dog's skin. Another treatment for infected pets is twice-weekly dips in a diluted solution of lime sulfur over a three- to eight-week period to eliminate the fungal spores.

Alternative

The fungal infection ringworm can be treated with homeopathic remedies. Among the homeopathic remedies recommended are:

• *sepia* for brown, scaly patches

• *tellurium* for prominent, well-defined, reddish sores

• *graphites* for thick scales or heavy discharge

• *sulphur* for excessive itching.

Topical applications of antifungal herbs and essential oils also can help resolve ringworm. Tea tree oil (*Melaleuca* spp.), thuja (*Thuja occidentalis*), and lavender (*Lavandula officinalis*) are the most common. Two drops of essential oil in 1/4 oz of carrier oil is the dose recommended for topical application. Essential oils should not be applied to the skin undiluted. Botanical medicine can be taken internally to enhance the body's immune response. A person must be susceptible to exhibit this overgrowth of fungus on the skin. Echinacea (*Echinacea* spp.) and astragalus (*Astragalus membranaceus*) are the two most common immune-enhancing herbs. A well-balanced diet, including protein, complex carbohydrates, fresh fruits and vegetables, and good-quality fats, is also important in maintaining optimal immune function. Alternative treatments should be used with care, as the benefits of many such treatments have not been confirmed by scientific research.

Prognosis

Ringworm can usually be cured but recurrence is common. Chronic infection develops in one patient in five. Patients with weakened immune systems may develop invasive dermatophyte infections that are difficult to treat.

It can take six to 12 months for new hair to cover bald patches, and three to 12 months to cure infected fingernails. Toenail infections do not always respond to treatment.

Prevention

The following precautions may help to lower the risk of dermatophyte infections:

• Maintain good personal hygiene, including frequent handwashing.

• Do not share towels, bedding, sports equipment, hair brushes, or other similar items.

• Stay cool and dry during hot, sticky weather or when traveling to tropical climates. Wear cotton, linen, or other natural fabrics that absorb perspiration rather than holding it against the body, and wear loose rather than closely fitted garments.

• Make sure household pets have regular veterinary checkups, and vacuum the household regularly so that shed fur does not accumulate.

• Keep common areas in the house or school clean; be particularly careful about the cleanliness of locker rooms, gyms, and swimming pools.

• Notify local public health authorities if there is an outbreak of ringworm in your child's school or daycare center.

• Use a dilute solution of chlorine bleach (1/4 cup per gallon of water) to disinfect counter tops and other hard surfaces that are safe to bleach.

Resources

BOOKS

Brock, David L. *Infectious Fungi*. Philadelphia: Chelsea House Publishers, 2006.

Hall, John C., and Brian J. Hall, editors. *Skin Infections: Diagnosis and Treatment*. New York: Cambridge University Press, 2009.

PERIODICALS

Abdel–Rahman, S.M., et al. "The Prevalence of Infections with *Trichophyton tonsurans* in Schoolchildren: the CAPITIS Study." *Pediatrics* 125 (May 2010): 966–73.

Andrews, R.M., et al. "Skin Disorders, Including Pyoderma, Scabies, and Tinea Infections." *Pediatric Clinics of North America* 56 (December 2009): 1421–40.

Chait, J. " Diabetes Quiz. How Much Do You Know about Athlete's Foot?" *Diabetes Self–Management* 25 (November–December 2008): 36, 38.

Isa–Isa R., et al. "Inflammatory Tinea Capitis: Kerion, Dermatophytic Granuloma, and Mycetoma." *Clinics in Dermatology* 28 (March 4, 2010): 133–36.

Panackal, A.A., et al. "Cutaneous Fungal Infections in the United States: Analysis of the National Ambulatory Medical Care Survey (NAMCS) and National Hospital Ambulatory Medical Care Survey (NHAMCS), 1995–2004." *International Journal of Dermatology* 48 (July 2009): 704–12.

Patel, G.A., et al. "Tinea Cruris in Children." *Cutis* 84 (September 2009): 133–37.

OTHER

Centers for Disease Control and Prevention (CDC). "Dermatophytes (Ringworm)." [Accessed September 22, 2010] http://www.cdc.gov/nczved/divisions/dfbmd/diseases/dermatophytes/.

Mayo Clinic. "Ringworm (body)." [Accessed September 22, 2010] http://www.mayoclinic.com/health/ringworm/DS00489.

Rabinowitz, Peter, Zimra Gordon, and Lynda Odofin. "Pet–related Infections." *American Family Physician* 76 (November 1, 2007): 1314–1322. [Accessed September 22, 2010] http://www.aafp.org/afp/2007/1101/p1314.html.

Rashid, Rashid M., et al. "Tinea." eMedicine. (March 15, 2010). [Accessed September 22, 2010] http://emedicine.medscape.com/article/787217–overview.

Trevino, Julian, and Michael Cairns. "Tinea (Dermatophyte) Infections." [Accessed September 22, 2010] http://www.aad.org/education/students/Tineainfect.htm.

ORGANIZATIONS

American Academy of Dermatology (AAD), P.O. Box 4014, Schaumburg, IL 60168, (847) 330-0230, (866) 503-SKIN, Fax: (847) 240-1859, http://www.aad.org/

American College of Sports Medicine (ACSM), P.O. Box 1440, Indianapolis, IN 46206, (317) 637-9200, Fax: (317) 634-7817, http://www.acsm.org/

American Veterinary Medical Association (AVMA), 1931 North Meacham Rd., Suite 100, Schaumburg, IL 60173-4360, (847) 925-8070, Fax: (847) 925-1329, avmainfo@avma.org, http://www.avma.org/

Centers for Disease Control and Prevention (CDC), 1600 Clifton Rd., Atlanta, GA 30333, (800) 232-4636, cdcinfo@cdc.gov, http://www.cdc.gov

National Institute of Allergy and Infectious Diseases (NIAID), 6610 Rockledge Dr., MSC 6612, Bethesda, MD 20892-6612, (301) 496-5717, (866 284-4107, Fax: (301) 402-3573, http://www3.niaid.nih.gov

Maureen Haggerty
Rebecca J. Frey, Ph.D.

▌Risk factors and assessment

Definition

In medicine, the term *risk* is something that causes a person or group of people to be particularly vulnerable to an unwanted, unpleasant or unhealthy event that increases the incidence or severity of an undesirable event such as an infection. It can also refer to an action or habit that that increases the chance of an unwanted or unwelcome event occurring. As an example, exposure to ultraviolet (UV) **radiation** in a particular portion of the spectrum (UVB) is a risk factor for developing skin **cancer**.

Description

Knowing the risk factors for any specific medical condition is very helpful for health workers. This information allows a health worker to understand how likely it is that a certain individual or group of people is likely to develop various health problems. The risk factors for each medical condition differ, however. They must be determined by long-term **population** studies for each individual disease or health problem. As an example, years of research have resulted in the following list of risk factors for cardiovascular disease:

• Age: The older a person is, the more likely cardiovascular disease is to develop. Heart attacks are increasingly common for men over the age of 40 and women over the age of 65.

• Gender: Men tend to be at greater risk for cardiovascular disease than are women. However, the apparent advantage held by females disappears approximately five years after menopause.

- Family history: Cardiovascular disease tends to "run in families." People having a parent that had cardiovascular disease are much more likely to have the same condition than a person with no family history of the condition. When both parents had cardiovascular disease, the risk of their child developing the same condition increases significantly.
- Tobacco: People who smoke or use tobacco in other ways are more likely to develop cardiovascular disease (and a number of other health problems), compared to people who do not smoke.
- Alcohol intake: While moderate amounts of alcohol appear to protect a person against cardiovascular disease, excessive consumption is associated with increased risk for cardiovascular disease.
- Physical activity: Generally speaking, people who are physically active tend to be at lower risk for cardiovascular disease.
- Diet: The consumption of some foods (fats, for example) tends to be more highly correlated with developing cardiovascular disease than are other foods (green vegetables, for example).
- Cholesterol: High concentrations of some types of cholesterol are associated with increased risk for cardiovascular disease. Other types of cholesterol are associated with decreased risk for cardiovascular disease.
- Diabetes: Diabetics tend to be at considerably higher risk for cardiovascular disease than are non-diabetics.
- Blood pressure: High blood pressure tends to be a strong indicator of increased risk for cardiovascular disease.

There are two important points to be noted about this list. First, risk factors are conditions that are *correlated with* a medical condition, which means that as the factor increases, so does the chance of developing the medical condition: higher blood pressure means higher risk of cardiovascular disease. But a high correlation does not necessarily mean *causation*. That is, the fact that blood pressure and cardiovascular disease are closely correlated does not necessarily mean that high blood pressure *causes* cardiovascular disease. It could, but it might also be that both conditions are caused by some third factor that may or may not be known.

The second point is that some of the risk factors mentioned are under a person's control, and other are not. For example, men could theoretically reduce their risk for cardiovascular disease by becoming women. But that is not a very realistic option. Neither can people change the **aging** process or the families from whom they come. But

a person does have control over other factors, such as whether or not one chooses to smoke, drink alcohol, lead an active physical life, or eat a healthful diet.

Cultural Disparities

Another type of risk factor goes beyond personal factors such as age, gender, diet, and tobacco use. Researchers have learned that a number of other social factors can increase or decrease a person's risk for health problems. For example, religious beliefs can have both positive and negative effects on one's risk for disease. In perhaps the most extreme example, some religious groups believe that medical conditions should be treated only by prayer or other religious observances. Members of these groups decline to seek medical assistance when a child becomes ill, a decision that generally increases the risk that the child will die from the condition. Ethnicity is another cultural factor that affects the probability of a person's becoming ill. In a large study reported by researchers at the Harvard School of Public Health in 2010, for example, data showed that the United States could be subdivided into "eight Americas" whose risk for a number of medical conditions was very different, depending on race, geographic location, and socioeconomic condition. As an example, the study found that rural Blacks in the South had a much shorter **life expectancy** than did any other of the "eight Americas," while Asian Americas in any part of the country had the highest life expectancy.

Costs to Society

All medical conditions have a cost both to individuals and to society as a whole. If all persons could pay the cost of their own medical treatment, risk analysis might be less of a public health problem. But the rising costs of health care have meant that more and more of an individual's healthcare costs are now being paid by the government. So, controlling risk factors is a rapidly growing health care problem. As an example, the American Heart Association and the National Heart, Lung, and Blood Institute estimated in 2009 that annual costs for cardiovascular disease in the United States were $475.3 billion. Any progress in reducing risk factors for cardiovascular disease will then, of course, dramatically reduce costs for both individuals and society as a whole.

Effects on Public Health

Over the past hundred years, a major focus of the work of public health professionals has been discovering risk factors for a number of medical conditions and then developing programs designed to reduce those risk factors. One of the best known of these efforts has been the campaign to change personal habits in order to reduce the spread of HIV infection and **AIDS** in the United States and other parts of the world. Key features of these efforts have been educational programs aimed at getting gay and bisexual men to change their sexual behaviors by avoiding unsafe sex practices and trying to persuade illegal drug users to stop exchanging dirty needles with each other. HIV/AIDS educational programs go far beyond these two major themes, of course, but they are all essentially focused on getting people to avoid risky practices that increase their likelihood of developing the disease. Other public health programs of this type have been developed to encourage people to change their dietary habits to reduce diabetes; to wear seat belts to reduce traffic accidents; to increase their use of contraceptive devices and practices to reduce unwanted pregnancies; and to stop (or never start) **smoking** to reduce the risk of a number of debilitating and potentially fatal medical conditions.

Prevention

The concept of using risk factors to predict individual health outcomes can be traced to the late 1960s when a group of researchers involved in the now famous Framingham (Massachusetts) Study released a publication called *How to Practice Prospective Medicine*. That publication outlined a procedure that involved three steps, the first of which involved having individuals complete a questionnaire about their personal habits. This health history was a very detailed version of the type of medical history that most physicians collect from new patients. A physician then reviewed that questionnaire to identify potential health risks facing the patient, risks such as diseases present in the family, medical events in the person's own history, and lifestyle choices (diet, exercise, or tobacco use, for example) that might predispose a person toward various medical conditions. The third step of the procedure involved a conference between physician and patient in which the former outlined the potential health risks facing the latter, based on data from the questionnaire, as well as changes in the patient's lifestyle that could reduce those risks.

Over the years, use of the health risk assessment (HRA) procedure has become common practice at every level of the public health profession, from individual medical workers to county and state public health agencies to national and international bodies such as the **World Health Organization**. A key element in the growth in popularity of the HRA has been much-improved predictive estimates of the effects of various risk factors on various health outcomes. As an example, the American Heart Association (AHA) and American

Stroke Association (ASA) have developed a questionnaire that allows people to estimate their risk of heart attack. By answering a number of questions about one's age, gender, smoking habits, family history, and the like, the risk of heart attack over some given period of time can be estimated. (See https://www.heart.org/gglRisk/locale/en_US/index.html?gtype=health) The AHA/ASA then provides suggestions as to lifestyle changes that are likely to reduce people's risk for heart attack and stroke.

Quantification of Risk

Risk assessment has become a largely quantifiable process. Medical workers can now express the risks a person faces in relatively specific numerical terms. One system simply involves comparing various groups with each other by saying, for example, that women are twice as likely to develop a particular medical condition than are men. A more helpful measure is the predicted likelihood of a person's developing a specific condition over some period of time. A physician might tell a patient, for example, that based on all the data provided in a questionnaire, that person has a 4–7% chance of having a heart attack over the next five years. This information provides patients with a relatively concrete way of looking at their potential health problems in the future, provided that no changes are made in lifestyle choices. It also outlines some steps that persons can take to change their health outlook.

Advantages and Disadvantages of HRA

An HRA has both positive and negative aspects. Perhaps the most important negative aspect is the likelihood that a person will assume that the results of an HRA are reliably predictive, rather than suggestive. Seeing precise numbers may produce a certain amount of concern or despair and leave them with the conclusion that they are going to die within the next five years. Medical practitioners must be sure to remind their

QUESTIONS TO ASK YOUR DOCTOR

- What are the risk factors for [choose a medical condition]?

- What specific lifestyle changes can I make to address each of the risk factors you have mentioned?

- What kinds of questions do I have to answer for a health risk assessment in your office?

- What would be the disadvantages of completing a health risk assessment with you?

patients that the numbers provided by an HRA are probabilities that can be altered by making changes in their habits or lifestyles. As for the advantages of an HRA, the Wellness Councils of America have mentioned ten key benefits to be gained from an HRA, some of which are providing people with an accurate snapshot of their present health status; providing ways for them to keep track of changes in their health over time; helping employers monitor the health status and health changes in their employees; and helping individuals to learn about and become involved in health coaching designed to improve their overall health prospects.

Resources

BOOKS

Birley, Martin H. *Health Impact Assessment: Principles and Practice*. Abingdon, UK; New York: Earthscan, 2011.

Global Health Risks: Mortality and Burden of Disease Attributable to Selected Major Risks. Geneva: World Health Organization, 2009.

Lopez, Alan D. *Global Burden of Disease and Risk Factors*. New York: Oxford University Press, 2006.

PERIODICALS

Colkesen, Ersen B. "Initiation of Health-behaviour Change among Employees Participating in a Web-based Health Risk Assessment with Tailored Feedback." *Journal of Occupational Medicine and Toxicology*. 6. (2011): 5–16.

Mills, P.R., et al. "Impact of a Health Promotion Program on Employee Health Risks and Work Productivity." *American Journal of Health Promotion*. 22. 1. (2007): 45–53.

WEBSITES

"The 10 Benefits of Conducting a Personal Health Assessment. Wellness Council of America." http://www.welcoa.org/freeresources/index.php?category=8. Accessed September 11, 2012.

Sammer, Joanne. "Meeting the Health Risk Assessment Challenge." http://www.shrm.org/hrdisciplines/benefits/

ORGANIZATIONS

World Health Organization (WHO), Avenue Appia 20, 1211 Geneva 27, Switzerland, +41 22 791 21 11, Fax: +41 22 791 31 11, http://www.who.int/about/contact_form/en/index.html, http://www.who.int/en/

David E. Newton, Ed.D.

River blindness *see* **Onchocerciasis**

Road traffic safety

Definition

The term "Road Traffic Safety" represents a complex system designed to improve and maintain the safety of drivers, passengers, and pedestrians who travel on roadways.

Description

Road traffic safety encompasses the efforts of many industries and government departments and the scientists who test these efforts. Some of the areas included in road traffic safety are the design and construction of roads, automobiles, automobile components, traffic lights and signs, and regulatory legislation. Road traffic safety affects not only drivers, passengers, and pedestrians, but also workers involved in various types of road and municipal construction and maintenance.

In the United States, some of the government departments and organizations involved in road traffic safety and data include the U.S. **Department of Health and Human Services** (including the **Centers for Disease Control and Prevention**), the U.S. Department of Transportation (including the Federal Highway Administration, and the National Highway Traffic Safety Administration), and the National Transportation Safety Board. The federal government has the ability to make regulations for commerce that crosses state and national boundaries, but other road traffic safety laws are the responsibility of each individual state, and vary in statute and enforcement from state to state. There has been debate between state and federal governments since World War II over who has the right and the responsibility to regulate road traffic safety.

As branches of the Department of Transportation, the National Highway Traffic Safety Administration (NHTSA) oversees regulations for drivers and vehicles,

Percent of seat belt use in the United States, 2006-2011, and number of lives saved by restraint use and additional lives that would have been saved at 100% seat belt use, 2006-2010					
Year	Percent of seat belt use in the United States	Lives saved, age 4 & younger with child restraints	Lives saved, age 5 & older with seat belts	Lives saved, age 13 & older with frontal air bags	Additional Lives that would have been saved at 100% seat belt use
2006	81%	427	15,458	2,824	5,468
2007	82%	388	15,223	2,800	5,048
2008	83%	286	13,312	2,557	4,171
2009	84%	307	12,763	2,387	3,700
2010	85%	303	12,546	2,306	3,341
2011	84%				

Source: National Highway Traffic Safety Administration, U.S. Department of Transportation. 2006-2009 FARS Final Files and FARS 2010 Annual Report File and Traffic Safety Facts: Crash Stats, February 2012 and August 2012.

(Illustration by Electronic Illustrators Group. © 2013 Cengage Learning)

while the Federal Highway Administration (FHWA) oversees the roadways. The NHTSA is responsible for dictating safety standards and vehicle safety ratings and issuing safety recalls. The NHTSA also distributes grants motivating states to pass laws—like those regarding child safety seats, seat belts, motorcycle helmets, drunk driving, and teen drivers—that will, in turn, motivate changes in driver behavior. The FHWA is responsible for implementing safety measures like rumble strips, guard rails, and education programs used to train state officials in the leading safety developments.

Vehicle ownership continues to grow steadily, and roads become more crowded. One result is the number of road fatalities continues to grow. Developing countries with poorly constructed and maintained roadways have experienced the most drastic increases in fatalities. In addition to the poor condition of such roads, the variety of vehicles using the roadway—including cars, vans, trucks, scooters, motorcycles, bicycles, animal carts, and pedestrians—makes driving more complicated and dangerous.

The human factor that contributes to accidents remains the biggest road traffic safety problem in the United States, largely due to issues with enforcement and compliance. For instance, despite traffic laws and cultural shifts about drinking across recent decades, more than 40% of all deadly crashes involve impaired drivers. Additionally, despite seat belt laws and public service campaigns, more than 50% of automobile accident fatalities were not wearing seat belts. The greatest number of road deaths are associated with: lack of seat belt use, impaired drivers, cars that leave their lane—either going off the road or crossing the median—and young drivers.

Recent efforts to improve road traffic safety include minimizing **distracted driving**. Distracted driving includes the completion of another task while driving; these alternate tasks include: reading a book or map, or sending and receiving text messages; eating, drinking, applying makeup, or **smoking**; and talking on a cell phone or with other passengers. Teen drivers are especially prone to distracted and reckless driving and have been the target of much road traffic safety legislation, education, and public service advertisements.

Road traffic safety programs should address the five Es of roadway safety: engineering, enforcement, education, emergency response, and everyone else (i.e., driver behavior, cultural influence). Road traffic safety efforts that include all of these points are the most comprehensive and are more likely to see success.

Demographics

Roughly 1.2 million lives are lost worldwide in road accidents every year. By 2025, it is estimated that that annual figure will rise to 2 million.

According to the **World Health Organization (WHO)**, nearly 3,500 people internationally, are killed on the roads each day.

There are over 40,000 road fatalities annually in the United States. Motor vehicle crashes are the leading cause of death for persons age 34 and younger.

In the U.S., driver condition and behavior is a factor in 95% of crashes and the primary factor in 67% of crashes. This includes distracted driving, which accounts for roughly 15-25% of all accidents. Weather and

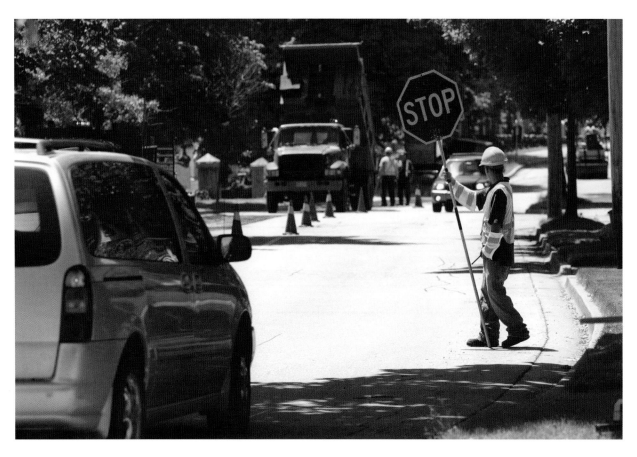

A worker controlling traffic. *(© iStockphoto.com/Mike Clarke)*

Fatalities, by Role, in Crashes Involving at Least One Driver with a Blood Alcohol Content (BAC) of .08 or Higher, 2010		
Role	**Number**	**Percent of Total**
Driver with BAC of .08+ Passenger Riding with Driver with BAC of .08+	6,627	65%
Subtotal	8,348	82%
Occupants of Other Vehicles	1,151	11%
Nonoccupants	729	7%
Total Fatalities	10,228	100%

Source: National Highway Traffic Safety Administration, U.S. Department of Transportation. Traffic Safety Facts: 2010 Data, April 2012. Available at http://www-nrd.nhtsa.dot.gov/Pubs/811606.pdf

(Illustration by Electronic Illustrators Group. © 2013 Cengage Learning)

roadway design are contributing factors in only 28% of accidents and the primary factor in only 4% of crashes. The condition of the vehicle involved is a contributing factor in only 8% of crashes.

Effects on Public Health

The loss of life and peripheral results of serious injury from road crashes are a worldwide public epidemic—as declared by the **World Health Organization (WHO)** in 2004. Cultural and technological advances continue to change the landscape of road traffic safety as they will probably continue to do in the future. In the United States, drivers can check with the various divisions of the Department of Transportation or the Centers for Disease Control and Prevention to check on the latest road traffic safety concerns and statistics.

Costs to Society

Road traffic safety is essential for saving lives and money—the annual cost of road fatalities globally is estimated at 518 billion U.S. dollars. When road traffic safety efforts are successful, society reaps the benefits. For example, in 2010 (the most recent data available), the NHTSA reports just under 33,000 deaths, which is a nearly 3% decline from the year before. After reaching all-time highs in the 1990s, traffic injuries have also been on the decline. This same report also showed a decline in all alcohol-impairment-related traffic accidents from 2009 to 2010.

Efforts and Solutions

The World Bank now funds road safety programs in the same manner as it already funds other responses to epidemics. These funds help countries around the world find the capital to improve their road traffic safety efforts.

The Work Zone Safety and Mobility Rule (Rule) was published in 2004 in the Federal Register, requiring all local and state governments receiving federal aid to reach compliance by October 2007. The Rule was designed to help improve safety in construction and work zones for workers and drivers.

In 2005, the United States passed the Safe, Accountable, Flexible, Efficient, Transportation Equity Act: A Legacy for Users (SAFETEA-LU). This legislation aimed to reduce serious injuries and fatalities as well as increase involvement in the planning and enforcement of strategies to this effect. This law resulted in a national discussion hosted by the American Automobile Association entitled, *Improving Traffic Safety Culture in the United States: The Journey Forward.*

KEY TERMS

Compliance—the degree to which a population obeys public safety standards or obeys the statutes of laws.

Enforcement—the degree to which a population is held to the statutes of a particular law.

Public service announcements (PSAs)—media including television or radio commercials, brochures, and posters gained at affecting change on behalf of the public good. PSAs may try to enhance compliance with existing laws, like obeying seat belt or child safety seat laws). PSAs may also attempt to improve consumer behavior in ways that will increase safety—for instance, PSAs discouraging text messaging while driving preceded legislation that made this behavior illegal.

Resources

BOOKS

"Transportation Department." *Gale Encyclopedia of American Law.* Ed. Donna Batten. 3rd ed. Vol. 10. Detroit: Gale, 2010.

"Traffic Safety." *Governing America: Major Decisions of Federal, State, and Local Governments from 1789 to the Present.* Paul J. Quirk and William Cunion. Vol. 1.: Economic Policies. New York: Facts on File, 2011.

Welch, Thomas M. "Highway Safety." *Encyclopedia of Science and Technology Communication.* Ed. Susanna Hornig Priest. Vol. 1. Thousand Oaks, CA: Sage Reference, 2010.

PERIODICALS

Johnson, Teddi Dineley. "Distracted driving: stay focused when on the road." *The Nation's Health* Feb. 2012: 28.

WEBSITES

Federal Highway Administration "Work Zone Mobility and Safety Program." http://www.ops.fhwa.dot.gov/wz/resources/final_rule.htm Accessed September 27, 2012.

National Highway Traffic Safety Administration. "Traffic Safety Facts."http://www-nrd.nhtsa.dot.gov/Pubs/811552.pdf Accessed September 27, 2012.

World Health Organization "Road traffic injuries." http://www.who.int/violence_injury_prevention/road_traffic/en/ Accessed September 27, 2012.

ORGANIZATIONS

U.S. Department of Transportation, 1200 New Jersey Avenue Southeast, Washington, DC 20590, 1 (202) 366-4542, www.dot.gov

Andrea Nienstedt, MA

Rotavirus

Definition

Rotavirus is the major cause of diarrhea and vomiting in young children worldwide. The infection is highly contagious and may lead to severe dehydration (loss of body fluids) and even death. Before a vaccine became available for U.S. infants in 2006, nearly all children in the United States were infected with rotavirus by the time they reached five years old.

EFFECTS ON PUBLIC HEALTH. Until 2006, rotavirus infections resulted in more than 400,000 visits to the doctor, more than 200,000 visits to the emergency room, 55,000–70,000 hospitalizations; and 20–60 deaths in the United States each year, according to the **Centers for Disease Control and Prevention (CDC)**. Worldwide, and especially in developing countries where babies might not have access to the vaccine, rotavirus infection continues to cause more than 500,000 deaths each year in children younger than five years of age.

Adults may also become infected with rotavirus, but they usually have milder symptoms, and some experience no symptoms at all. Among immunocompromised adults, however, rotavirus infections can cause severe symptoms.

Description

Viral gastroenteritis, or inflammation of the stomach and the intestine, is the second most common illness in the United States, after the **common cold**. Many different viruses can cause gastroenteritis, but the most common cause of infectious gastroenteritis in infants and young children worldwide is rotavirus.

The name "rotavirus" comes from the Latin word "rota" for wheel. It describes the viruses' distinct wheel-like shape. Rotavirus infection is also known as "infantile diarrhea," or "winter diarrhea," because it mainly targets infants and young children. Rotavirus outbreaks usually occur in the cooler months of winter.

The virus is classified into different groups, depending on the type of protein marker (antigen) that is present on its surface. Group A, B, and C rotaviruses pose problems for people. The Group A rotaviruses cause diarrheal infection of children. Group B rotaviruses have caused major epidemics of adult diarrhea in China. Group C rotavirus has been associated with rare cases of diarrheal outbreaks in Japan and England. Other groups of the virus cause infections in various species of animals, including cows and monkeys.

Origins

In the 1940s, six epidemics of diarrhea in newborns occurred in three hospitals in the Baltimore–Washington,

QUESTIONS TO ASK YOUR DOCTOR

- When should my baby begin receiving the rotavirus vaccine?
- Is the rotavirus vaccine safe?
- My child has a rotavirus infection. What measures can I take to ensure that the other members of the family will not become infected?
- My child has a rotavirus infection. How long will he or she remain contagious?

D.C., area. A 1943 study (by Jacob S. Light and Horace L. Hodes of Johns Hopkins Hospital, Johns Hopkins University, and Sydenham Hospital, Baltimore City Health Department) revealed a "filtrable agent" in the stools of the patients. When they exposed the stool from these patients to the nasal passage of a calf, the calf developed diarrhea, leading the scientists to conclude that the agent was the cause of the symptoms. In a 1976 study in the journal *Infection and Immunity*, researchers reported that the agent was rotavirus. A 2008 analysis conducted by a research team from the Institute for the Promotion of Innovation through Science and Technology in Flanders, Belgium, and the National Institutes of Health indicated a possible animal origin for the common human strains of rotavirus.

Causes

Rotavirus infection is highly contagious, because the stool of infected individuals contains considerable quantities of the virus (100–1,000 particles of virus per milliliter of feces), and this virus spreads by the "fecal-oral route." In other words, a person can become infected by touching the mouth after handling toys, soiled diapers, door knobs, or other contaminated things. Because rotavirus can survive on an object for several days and on the hands for a few hours, and because it is also is resistant to most disinfectant cleaners, the virus can spread rapidly. Outbreaks may occur in daycare facilities, in hospitals, and at playgrounds, and usually result from children neglecting to wash their hands after using the toilet or before eating food.

The viruses can also spread by way of contaminated food and **drinking water**. Infected food handlers who prepare salads, sandwiches, and other foods that require no cooking can spread the disease. Symptoms appear within 4–48 hours after exposure to the contaminated food or **water**.

Children between the ages of six months and two years, especially in a daycare setting, are the most susceptible to this infection. Breastfed babies may be less likely to become infected, because breast milk contains antibodies (proteins produced by the white blood cells of the immune system) that fight the illness.

Children who have been infected once can be infected again, but second infections are less severe than the first infections. By the time a child has had two infections, the chances of subsequent severe infection are remote.

Adults often pick up the virus while caring for their infected children but also may get it as a result of travel-related infection or epidemic outbreak. Individuals who are elderly and those who have weak immune systems experience a higher incidence of symptoms from rotavirus infection than the overall adult population.

Symptoms

The main symptoms of the rotavirus infection in children are fever, stomach cramps, vomiting, and frequent, watery diarrhea. Children with rotavirus infection may become dehydrated. The symptoms usually appear about two days after becoming infected but may appear sooner. When symptoms occur, they usually last from three to eight days. Rotavirus infection is rarely fatal to American children. In third-world countries, where quality healthcare may be lacking, rotavirus infection causes more than a half million deaths to children every year.

Adults with rotavirus infection typically have similar symptoms to those in children—nausea, run-down feeling, headache, abdominal cramping, diarrhea, and fever—but the symptoms are usually milder, and some may have no symptoms at all. Among immunocompromised adults and those who are elderly, the infection may be sustained, and the symptoms more severe.

Diagnosis

Rotavirus infection in children is often initially diagnosed upon a report of dehydration, extremely watery diarrhea, vomiting, fever, and abdominal **pain**. Signs of dehydration include: dry lips and tongue, dry skin, sunken eyes, lack of tears when crying, extreme thirst, and wetting fewer than six diapers a day. The rotavirus infection is positively diagnosed by identifying the virus in the patient's stool. Immunological tests, such as ELISA (enzyme-linked immunosorbent assay), are widely used for diagnosis, and several commercial kits are available. In addition, screening with electron microscopy, polyacrylamide gel electrophoresis, and reverse transcription-polymerase chain reaction are sometimes used to detect and identify rotavirus infection.

KEY TERMS

Intussusception—A type of bowel blockage that results from one portion of the bowel sliding into another. It is more common in children than adults.

Vaccine—A preparation that is derived from an agent that confers immunity to a disease. The agent may be a dead virus, for instance, that prompts the body's immune system to recognize the virus so that it can mount a quick response to future infection.

Treatment

The primary aim of treatment is "oral rehydration therapy," or drinking enough fluids to replace those lost through bowel movements and vomiting. Electrolyte and fluid replacement solutions are available over the counter in food and drug stores. Dehydration is one of the greatest dangers for infants and young children. If the diarrhea becomes severe, it may be necessary to hospitalize the patient so that fluids can be administered intravenously.

Parents should not give anti-diarrheal medications to a child unless directed to do so by the physician. Antibiotic therapy is not useful in viral illness. Specific drugs for the virus are not available.

Prognosis

Most of the infections resolve spontaneously. Dehydration due to severe diarrhea is one of the major complications.

Prevention

The best way to prevent the disease is through proper food handling and thorough hand washing after using the toilet, whenever hands are soiled, and before eating. In childcare centers and hospital settings, the staff should be educated about personal and environmental **hygiene**. All dirty diapers should be regarded as infectious and disposed of in a sanitary manner. In addition, all children should be vaccinated.

EFFORTS AND SOLUTIONS. Two rotavirus vaccines are licensed for use in the United States and became available in 2006. According to the **CDC**, both vaccines have been shown to be safe and effective. Clinical trials demonstrated that the vaccines prevented 85–98% of severe rotavirus episodes and 74–87% of all rotavirus illness episodes.

The vaccine is intended to be given orally (by mouth) at two, four, and six months of age, although the first dose of the vaccine can be given when the child is as young as six weeks old.

Some studies have shown a small rise in cases of intussusception (a type of bowel blockage that requires hospital care), which occurs in about one infant out of 100,000 who are vaccinated. In these rare cases, intussusception occurs within a week after the first dose of rotavirus vaccine. Medical professionals recommend the vaccine because its benefits far outweigh the slight risk of intussusception.

Resources

WEBSITES

"BBB—Rotavirus." U.S. Food and Drug Administration. http://www.fda.gov/Food/FoodSafety/FoodborneIllness/FoodborneIllnessFoodbornePathogensNaturalToxins/BadBugBook/ucm071331.htm (accessed August 20, 2012).

"Protect Your Child From Rotavirus Disease." Centers for Disease Control and Prevention. http://www.cdc.gov/features/rotavirus/ (accessed August 20, 2012).

"Resources for Consumers." National Foundation for Infectious Diseases. http://www.nfid.org/idinfo/rotavirus/Rotavirus-Information-for-Consumers/consumer.html (accessed August 20, 2012).

"Rotavirus." Centers for Disease Control and Prevention. http://www.cdc.gov/vaccines/pubs/pinkbook/downloads/rota.pdf (accessed August 20, 2012).

"Rotavirus." Centers for Disease Control and Prevention. http://www.cdc.gov/vaccines/vpd-vac/rotavirus/downloads/PL-dis-rotavirus-color-office.pdf (accessed August 20, 2012).

Medline Plus. "Rotavirus Infections." U.S. National Library of Medicine and National Institutes of Health. http://www.nlm.nih.gov/medlineplus/rotavirusinfections.html (accessed August 20, 2012).

ORGANIZATIONS

Centers for Disease Control and Prevention (CDC), 1600 Clifton Road, Atlanta, GA 30333, (800) 232-4636, cdcinfo@cdc.gov, http://www.cdc.gov

National Foundation for Infectious Diseases, 4733 Bethesda Ave., Suite 750, Bethesda, MD 20814, (301) 656-0003, http://www.nfid.org/

Lata Cherath, Ph.D.
Leslie Mertz, Ph.D.

Rubella

Definition

Rubella is a highly contagious viral disease, spread through contact with discharges from the nose and throat of an infected person. Although rubella causes only mild

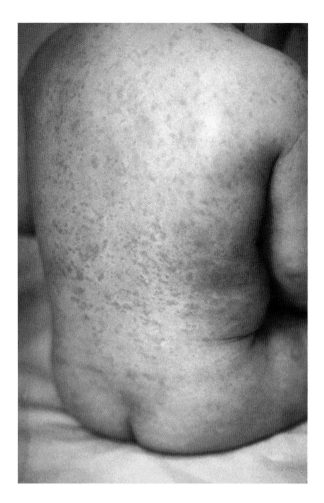

Rash of rubella on skin of child's back. *(© CDC)*

symptoms of low fever, swollen glands, joint **pain**, and a fine red rash in most children and adults, it can have severe complications for women in their first trimester of pregnancy. These complications include severe **birth defects** or death of the fetus.

Description

Rubella, also known as German **measles** or three-day measles, is spread through contact with fluid droplets expelled from the nose or throat of an infected person. A person infected with the rubella virus is contagious for about seven days before any symptoms appear and continues to be able to spread the disease for about one to two weeks after the rubella-caused rash disappears. Rubella has an incubation period of 12–23 days.

Although rubella is generally considered a childhood illness, people of any age who have not been vaccinated or previously caught the disease can become infected. Having rubella once or being immunized against it normally gives lifetime immunity. This is why **vaccination** is so effective in reducing the number of rubella cases.

Women of childbearing age who do not have immunity against rubella should be the most concerned about getting the disease. Rubella infection during the first three months of pregnancy can cause a woman to miscarry or can cause her baby to be born with birth defects.

Origins

Originally thought to be a type of measles, because the rash it produces is similar to measles. German scientists ultimately determined that it was not measles but a separate disease entirely, in 1814. This disease was once a common childhood illness, and a worldwide rubella epidemic occurred from 1963 to 1965. Some 11,000 babies died, and 20,000 more developed birth defects. Its occurrence has been drastically reduced since a vaccine against rubella became available in 1969.

Rubella's nickname of "German measles" arose because the rubella rash looks much like measles, and the disease was first discovered in Germany.

Demographics

Thanks to the rubella vaccine, rubella has been practically eradicated in the United States and other developed countries. It is still common in less-developed countries because of poor **immunization** penetration.

Causes and symptoms

Causes

Rubella is caused by the rubella virus (*Rubivirus*).

Symptoms

Symptoms are generally mild, and complications are rare in anyone who is not pregnant. The first visible sign of rubella is a fine red rash that begins on the face and rapidly moves downward to cover the whole body within 24 hours. The rash lasts about three days, which is why rubella is sometimes called the three-day measles. A low fever and swollen glands, especially in the head (around the ears) and neck, often accompany the rash. Joint pain, sometimes accompanied by joint swelling, can occur. This occurs more often in women. About 50% of people who contract rubella, however, do not show any symptoms (subclinical infection).

Symptoms disappear within three to four days, except for joint pain, which may linger for a week or two. Most people recover fully with no complications. However, severe complications may arise in the unborn children of women who get rubella during the first three months of their pregnancy. These babies may be miscarried or stillborn. A high percentage of these children are born with birth defects. Birth defects are reported to occur in 50% of women

---

who contract the disease during the first month of pregnancy, 20% of those who contract it in the second month, and 10% of those who contract it in the third month.

The most common birth defects resulting from congenital rubella infection are eye defects, such as cataracts, glaucoma, and blindness; deafness; congenital heart defects; and mental retardation. Taken together, these conditions are called congenital rubella syndrome (CRS). The risk of birth defects drops after the first trimester, and by the 20th week, complications rarely occur.

Diagnosis

The rash caused by the rubella virus and the accompanying symptoms are so similar to other viral infections that it is impossible for a physician to make a confirmed diagnosis on visual examination alone. The only sure way to confirm a case of rubella is by isolating the virus with a blood test or in a laboratory culture.

A blood test is done to check for rubella antibodies. When the body is infected with the rubella virus, it produces both immunoglobulin G (IgG) and immunoglobulin M (IgM) antibodies to fight the infection. Once IgG exists, it persists for a lifetime, but the special IgM antibody usually wanes over six months. A blood test can be used either to confirm a recent infection (IgG and IgM) or determine whether a person has immunity to rubella (IgG only). The lack of antibodies indicates that a person is susceptible to rubella.

All pregnant women should be tested for rubella early in pregnancy, regardless of whether they have a history of vaccination. If the woman lacks immunity, she is counseled to avoid anyone with the disease and to get a vaccination after giving birth.

There is no drug treatment for rubella. Bed rest, fluids, and acetaminophen for pain and temperatures over 102°F (38.9°C) are usually all that is necessary.

Babies born with suspected CRS are isolated and cared for only by people who are sure they are immune to rubella. Congenital heart defects are treated with surgery.

Alternative treatment

Rather than vaccinating a healthy child against rubella, many alternative practitioners recommend allowing the child to contract the disease naturally at the age of five or six years, since the immunity conferred by contracting the disease naturally lasts a lifetime. It is, however, difficult for a child to contract rubella naturally when everyone around him or her has been vaccinated.

Ayurvedic practitioners recommend making the patient comfortable and giving them ginger or clove tea to hasten the progress of the disease. Traditional Chinese medicine uses a similar approach. Believing that inducing the skin rash associated with rubella hastens the progress of the disease, traditional Chinese practitioners prescribe herbs, such as peppermint (*Mentha piperita*) and *chai-hu* (*Bupleurum chinense*). Cicada is often prescribed as well. Western herbal remedies may be used to alleviate rubella symptoms. Distilled witch hazel (*Hamamelis virginiana*) helps calm the itching associated with the skin rash, and an eyewash made from a filtered diffusion of eyebright (*Euphrasia officinalis*) can relieve eye discomfort.

Prognosis

Complications from rubella infection are rare in children, pregnant women past the 20th week of pregnancy, and other adults. For women in the first trimester of pregnancy, however, a high likelihood exists for the child to be born with one or more birth defects. Unborn children exposed to rubella early in pregnancy are also more likely to be miscarried or stillborn or to have a low birth weight. Although the symptoms of rubella pass quickly for the mother, the consequences to the unborn child can last a lifetime.

Prevention

Vaccination is the best way to prevent rubella and is normally required by law for children entering school. Rubella is usually given in conjunction with measles and **mumps** vaccines in a shot referred to as MMR (mumps, measles, and rubella). Children receive one dose of MMR vaccine at 12–15 months and another dose before entering school at 4–6 years. An alternate MMRV (measles, mumps, rubella, and varicella) vaccination has also been available since 2004.

The U.S. Centers for Disease Control and Prevention recommends that all persons born during or after 1957 who have not had rubella or been vaccinated against the disease should get at least one dose of MMR vaccine. In cases where a person is unsure about the need for a vaccine, his or her health professional can test the blood to check for disease immunity.

QUESTIONS TO ASK YOUR DOCTOR

- My child has mild symptoms due to rubella infection. What symptoms might warrant medical attention?
- Which over-the-counter medications do you recommend to treat mild symptoms?
- I had the vaccine two months ago but just found out that I'm pregnant. Is this cause for concern?
- Which do you recommend for my child: the MMR (mumps, measles, and rubella) vaccine or the MMRV (measles, mumps, rubella, and varicella) vaccine?

Pregnant women should not be vaccinated, and health professionals typically recommend that women who are not pregnant avoid conceiving for at least three months following vaccination. Women may be vaccinated while they are breastfeeding. People whose immune systems are compromised, either by the use of drugs such as steroids or by disease, should discuss possible complications with their doctor before being vaccinated.

Effects on public health

Rubella has been nearly eradicated in the United States, but it persists in some less-developing countries. This poses a risk to susceptible travelers. Some countries have chosen to target rubella vaccination to females only, and outbreaks in foreign-born males have occurred on cruise ships and at U.S. summer camps.

Costs to society

Rubella infection just before conception and in early pregnancy can result in harm and possibly death to the fetus. Newborns may experience a range of birth defects, including cataracts, glaucoma, blindness, deafness, congenital heart defects, and mental retardation. Depending on the defect, these children may experience many social and physical challenges throughout their childhood and into their adult lives. Their limitations may also make it difficult for them to find employment and earn a living. Since rubella is most common in developing countries, the healthcare for affected children may cause financial hardship, and in some cases, the child may have to go without proper care.

Efforts and solutions

Many health organizations and government agencies around the world are promoting the administration of the rubella vaccination, because its use can nearly eliminate the disease. Some countries are still not strongly advocating the vaccine, although measles-vaccination programs are routine. The **World Health Organization** recommends that these countries consider adding a rubella vaccine to their current measles program so their citizens are protected against both diseases.

Resources

WEBSITES

MedlinePlus. "Rubella." U.S. National Library of Medicine, National Institutes of Health. http://www.nlm.nih.gov/medlineplus/rubella.html (accessed November 11, 2012).

PubMedHealth. "Rubella." U.S. National Library of Medicine. http://www.ncbi.nlm.nih.gov/pubmedhealth/PMH0002541/ (accessed November 11, 2012).

"Rubella and Pregnancy." March of Dimes. http://www.marchofdimes.com/pregnancy/complications_rubella.html (accessed November 11, 2012).

"Rubella: Make Sure Your Child Gets Vaccinated." U.S. Centers for Disease Control and Prevention. http://www.cdc.gov/Features/Rubella/ (accessed November 11, 2012).

"Rubella." U.S. Centers for Disease Control and Prevention. http://www.cdc.gov/vaccines/vpd-vac/rubella/downloads/PL-dis-rubella-bw-office.pdf (accessed November 11, 2012).

"Rubella" World Health Organization. http://www.who.int/immunization/topics/rubella/en/index.html (accessed November 11, 2012).

ORGANIZATIONS

Centers for Disease Control and Prevention (CDC), 1600 Clifton Road, Atlanta, GA 30333, (800) 232-4636, cdcinfo@cdc.gov, http://www.cdc.gov/std/

March of Dimes Birth Defects Foundation, 1275 Mamaroneck Ave., White Plains, NY 10605, (914) 997-4488, http://www.modimes.org

Tish Davidson, A.M.
Leslie Mertz, Ph.D.

Rural health

Definition

A rural area is defined by the United States Census Bureau as one with open country as well as settlements that have less than 2,500 residents. Rural health concerns the physical and mental well-being and health care services for persons that live in rural areas.

Demographics

Approximately one-quarter of the population of the United States lives in a rural community. Rural-based hospitals provide health care for approximately 72 million people in the United States. Rural hospitals face issues such as staff shortages, lack of funds for capital improvements, and diminishing revenues from Medicare.

In 2005, there were 55 primary care physicians for each 100,000 people living in rural areas compared with 72 who served the same number of people in urban areas. In very small and isolated rural areas, the number falls to 36 primary care physicians per 100,000 residents. Care from specialists is also scarce, with half the number of medical specialists per 100,000 rural residents when compared with the number of specialists available in urban areas.

Description

Patients and health care providers in rural settings face circumstances that differ from their counterparts in urban areas. Factors such as educational deficiencies, economic issues, lack of legislative voice, and sheer isolation serve as obstacles for living a healthy everyday life. Rural residents have limited choices in medical care and must travel longer distances to obtain the care that is available.

Life in rural areas is different from that of urban environments. The National Rural Health Association points out these differences:

• One-fourth of the United States population lives in rural settings, but only 10% of physicians in the nation practice medicine in these communities.

• One-third of motor vehicle accidents take place on rural roads but two-thirds of motor vehicle accident deaths happen on these roads.

• People living in rural areas are poorer than those living in urban settings. The average per capita income in rural areas is $7,417 lower than it is for urban dwellers. The differences are more significant for minorities living in rural areas. Almost 24% of rural children are impoverished.

• Individuals living in rural areas are almost two times more likely to die from unintentional injuries (other than motor vehicle accidents) when compared with persons living in urban communities.

• Youth in rural communities have serious problems with alcohol abuse and the utilization of smokeless tobacco. While 25% of urban youth report that they use alcohol while driving, that figure jumps to 40% for rural youth. Just over 12% of youth in urban settings smoke cigarettes in the eighth grade, while more than 26% of rural youth engage in this behavior.

• Emergency medical care personnel do not have the same level of training in rural settings as they do in urban areas. In rural settings, the percentage of first responders who serve on a volunteer basis ranges from 57% to 90%.

In 2012, researchers from the University of Florida and University of Kansas reported on their study, which found that almost 40% of adults in rural communities are obese, compared to 33% of their urban counterparts. The researchers cited less access to healthy foods and ingesting large meals as the primary causes behind this finding.

The patient population of rural hospitals is such that they are especially vulnerable to cuts in Medicare reimbursement. The American Hospital Association advocates for Medicare reimbursements at a level that is appropriate for the rural facilities.

If a facility is designated as a Critical Access Hospital (CAH), Medicare covers reasonable care provided there at 101% of reasonable cost. A hospital may receive CAH designation if it meets the certain criteria such as location in a state that has a rural health plan; location in a rural community 35 miles from the nearest hospital or CAH (or more than 15 miles in areas with mountain roads or rugged terrain); and provides emergency services seven days a week around the clock. The American Hospital Association is working toward ensuring that payment programs for rural hospitals, such as the CAH designation, are updated as needed.

Effect on public health

Health status tends to be poorer in rural areas when compared with urban communities. For example, the South Carolina Rural Research Center reports that rates of diabetes are higher in rural settings (9.6% compared with 8.4% in urban areas) and that **obesity** is more prevalent (27% compared to 23.9%).

Women living in rural sections of the nation obtain **women's health** care services less often than females living in urban areas. While 78% of urban women have regular mammograms, that number falls to 71% when applied to rural women.

A study published in *BMC Public Health* in 2012 found that people living in rural settings were less likely to be knowledgeable about the symptoms of a heart attack. The researchers asked 13 questions regarding the early symptoms of heart attack and **stroke**. One hundred three million adults living in both rural and urban sections of the United States participated in the research during 2005, 2007, and 2009. Those with the lowest scores lived in rural communities and tended to be men ages 65 and up, of Hispanic or other multi-racial origin,

---

with an education level of high school or less, unmarried, with a household income less than $50,000. The researchers pointed out that knowledge of early symptoms of a heart attack is especially critical in the rural population because of the long distances these individuals must travel for health care.

Costs to society

The Center for Rural Affairs reports that persons who live in rural areas are less likely to have health insurance. Additionally, they tend to maintain their non-insured status for longer periods of time than people who live in urban environments. While 69% of urban employees have employer-sponsored health insurance, that figure drops to 59% for persons living in rural counties. A major reason behind this is that workers in rural areas are more likely to be employed by small businesses and earn low wages. On a national basis, more than one-quarter of children who live in remote rural areas have Medicaid coverage.

Families who live on ranches or farms may need to purchase private health insurance, which is costly.

Georgetown University's Center on **Aging** points out that "The rural population is consistently less well-off than the urban population with respect to health."

Efforts and solutions

The Office of Rural **Health Policy** (ORHP) is the group that coordinates rural health activities within the United States **Department of Health and Human Services**. The office advises the Secretary of Health and Human Services and administers grants designed to enhance health care in rural communities. These grants bring to rural America improvements in health care, such as better emergency medical programs. The office's Hospital State Division is dedicated to improving rural health care via activities such as the management of grants.

The National Health Service Corps (NHSC) is a government agency that provides scholarships and loan repayment programs for health care professionals who practice in underserved areas such as small towns in the western portion of the United States as well as inner-city communities.

Resources

BOOKS

Bennet, Kevin J., Ph.D., Olatosi Bankole, Ph.D., and Janice C. Probst, Ph.D. *Health Disparities: A Rural-Urban Chartbook* Columbia, SC: South Carolina Rural Health Research Center, 2008.

Mason, Diana J., RN, Ph.D., FAAN *Policy & Politics in Nursing and Health Care 6th Ed.* St. Louis, MO: Elsevier Saunders, 2012.

PERIODICALS

Befort, C.A., N. Nazir, and M.G. Perri. "Prevalence of Obesity Among Adults from Rural and Urban Areas of the United States: Findings from NHANES (2005-2008)." *Journal of Rural Health* Fall (2012).

Swanoski, M.T., et al. "Knowledge of Heart Attack and Stroke Symptomology: A Cross-Sectional Comparison of Rural and Non-Rural U.S. Adults." *BMC Public Health* 12, no. 1 (2012): 283.

WEBSITES

American Hospital Association. http://www.ers.usda.gov/topics/rural-economy-population/rural-classifications.aspx (accessed September 28, 2012).

Health Care in Rural America. http://www.cfra.org/Health-Care-in-Rural-America (accessed September 28, 2012).

Office of Rural Health Policy. http://www.hrsa.gov/ruralhealth/about/index.html (accessed September 28, 2012).

USDA Economic Research Service. http://www.aha.org/advocacy-issues/rural/index.shtml (accessed September 28, 2012).

ORGANIZATIONS

American Hospital Association, 155 N. Wacker Drive, Chicago, IL 60606, (312) 422-3000, (800) 424-4301, www.aha.org

Center for Rural Affairs, 145 Main Street, P.O. Box 136, Lyons, NE 60606, (402) 687-2100, info@crfa.org, www.cfra.org

National Rural Health Association, 1108 K Street NW, 2nd Floor, Washington DC, 20005-4094, (202) 639-0550, Fax: (202) 639-0559, dc@NRHArural.org, www.ruralhealthweb.com

Rhonda LAST, RN

S

Safe sex

Definition

Safe sex refers to sexual intercourse or other consensual sexual activity conducted by people who have taken precautions to protect themselves against sexually transmitted infections (STIs). It should not be confused with contraception, which refers to prevention of pregnancy.

As of 2012, some public health workers prefer to use the terms *safer sex* or *protected sex* when referring to sexual risk reduction practices, on the grounds that no sexual activity apart from abstinence is completely free of the risk of disease transmission.

Description

Safe sex covers a range of practices and behaviors intended to reduce the risk of STIs.

Barrier methods

Barrier methods of safe sex refer to the use of protective devices to reduce the risk of disease transmission by preventing contact with body fluids that can carry STIs, including blood, saliva, and vaginal fluid as well as semen.

MALE CONDOMS. Male condoms are thin sheaths of latex (rubber), polyurethane (plastic), or animal tissue that are rolled onto an erect penis immediately prior to intercourse. They are commonly called "safes," "rubbers," or "prophylactics," from their use in preventing disease.

Because many men and women are allergic to latex, the Food and Drug Administration (FDA) approved the use of Vytex for condoms sold in the United States in May 2009. Vytex is a form of latex that has been treated to remove 90% of the proteins that cause allergic reactions. A completely allergen-free condom made of polyisoprene, a synthetic latex, is also available. Polyisoprene is more expensive than standard latex but has the advantages of being as flexible and soft as latex without triggering allergic reactions.

Most condoms made of animal tissue as of 2012 are made from sheep intestines and are labeled as lambskin. They provide more sensation than latex and are also less likely to trigger allergic reactions. They are also significantly more expensive than latex condoms and offer less protection against STDs. The reason for this difference is that sheep intestine is a porous material whose pores are large enough to permit the HIV virus and other infectious organisms to pass through, even though the pores are small enough to block sperm.

Male condoms may be purchased lubricated, ribbed, or studded on the outside. Studded condoms should not be used for anal intercourse, however, because they can irritate the tissues lining the rectum and increase the risk of HIV transmission. To be effective, condoms must be removed carefully so as not to "spill" the contents into the vaginal canal. Condoms that leak or break do not provide complete protection against pregnancy or disease, although they are more effective than completely unprotected intercourse.

An important fact to keep in mind when reading statistics about condom effectiveness is the distinction between "perfect" or "method effectiveness" use rates and "actual" or "typical" use rates. Perfect or method effectiveness rates include only consumers who use condoms properly and consistently. Typical or actual use rates include all persons who use condoms, including those who use them incorrectly or do not use them during every act of intercourse. With regard to disease transmission, in 2000 the National Institutes of Health (NIH) reported that correct and consistent use of latex condoms reduces the risk of HIV/AIDS transmission by approximately 85% relative to a person's risk when unprotected. In 2007 the **World Health Organization (WHO)** reported a similar risk reduction rate of 80% to 95%. The **CDC** states that "Latex condoms, when used consistently and correctly, are highly effective in preventing the sexual transmission of HIV, the virus that causes **AIDS**. In addition, consistent and correct use of latex condoms reduces the risk of other **sexually transmitted diseases** (STDs), including diseases transmitted by genital secretions, and to a lesser degree, genital ulcer diseases." Incorrect or inconsistent use of condoms, however, reduces their effectiveness in preventing STIs to as low as 60%.

FEMALE CONDOMS. Female condoms are thin, loose sheaths with flexible rings at both ends, one end being open and the other closed. The female condom is inserted into the vaginal canal before sexual relations. The open end covers the outside of the vagina, and the ring at the closed end fits over the cervix (opening into the uterus). The first female condoms were made of polyurethane, but most female condoms are now made of nitrile, a synthetic rubber that is also used to make disposable surgical gloves. Nitrile is as flexible as latex but is more resistant to puncture.

Female condoms come in various sizes; most women find the medium sizes easiest to use, but women who have recently given birth should try the larger sizes first. Female condoms can be used for anal as well as vaginal intercourse.

DENTAL DAMS. Dental dams are thin squares of latex rubber that were originally developed for use in dentistry to isolate a tooth from the saliva and bacteria in the patient's mouth during the placement of fillings and similar procedures. The tooth being operated on protrudes through a hole punched in the dam by the dentist. Unpunctured dams are used during oral sex to prevent transmission of saliva or vaginal fluid; the dam is placed over the vulva or anus prior to oral stimulation. Silicone dams are available for persons allergic to latex.

Surgical gloves made from nitrile, latex, or polyurethane may be used in place of dental dams to provide barrier protection during oral sex. They may also be used during masturbation to protect the user's hands, as broken skin on the hands can be infected by body fluids from the self or the partner.

Nonpenetrative sex

Nonpenetrative sex refers to sexual practices that do not involve the use of anal, vaginal, or oral penetration by the male penis or a sex toy. This form of safe sex includes autoeroticism, also known as self-stimulation, solitary sex, or masturbation. Masturbation is relatively safe, provided there is no contact with another person's bodily fluids.

"Outercourse." Outercourse is an informal term for sexual activities with a partner that do not involve

penetration. They include kissing, fondling, and mutual masturbation. Although these practices are effective in preventing pregnancy and most STIs, they do not protect against genital **herpes**, genital warts, or other infections that can be transmitted by skin-to-skin contact.

Abstinence

Abstinence refers to avoiding or refraining from some or all forms of sexual activity for medical, psychological, legal, social, or religious reasons. Abstinence should not be confused with asexuality, which refers to the absence of interest in sex or the lack of sexual desire for or attraction to others.

Abstinence is a highly effective form of protection against STIs, although it is possible for an abstinent person to contract an STI as a result of rape or occupational exposure to contaminated needles.

Other behavioral precautions

Other behavioral practices and precautions associated with safe sex include:

• Avoidance of drug and alcohol use. This precaution has been recommended since the 1980s to reduce the

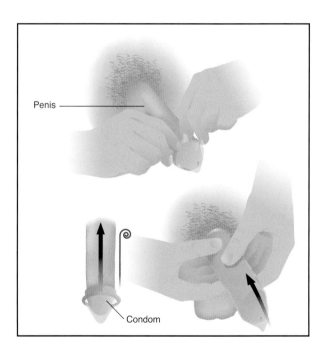

A condom is most effective when it is placed on the penis correctly without trapping air between the penis and the condom. *(Illustration by Electronic Illustrators Group. © 2013 Cengage Learning)*

risk of STIs on the grounds that alcohol intoxication or a drug high affects a person's judgment and reduces their inhibitions against risky sexual practices.

• Careful selection of partners. One study recommended that people who choose to be sexually active should avoid the following types of partners: those who have had an STI in the past year; those who have a drug or alcohol problem; and those who have had sex with multiple partners in the past year.

• Monogamy/limiting the number of partners. Monogamy refers to marriage or a faithful relationship with only one partner. Although it is true that a monogamous person can still be infected by an unfaithful or previously infected partner, monogamy is a very safe sexual practice when both partners are uninfected.

• Periodic testing for STIs. Periodic testing for STIs is recommended for people who have a variety of sexual partners. It is particularly useful in detecting asymptomatic infections or infections producing nonspecific symptoms.

• Immunization against sexually transmitted viral diseases. Women can be immunized against the human papilloma virus (HPV); and homosexual males can be immunized against hepatitis B.

• Clear communication between partners prior to sexual activity. Open and frank conversation before sexual activity reduces the risk of misunderstandings about appropriate precautions or taking unnecessary risks when passion takes over. Sexual assertiveness on the part of women appears to be an important factor in protecting them against high-risk practices (such as the male partner's refusal to use a condom).

Origins

Safe sex as a term for reducing the risk of STI transmission originated in the United States in the mid-1980s as a result of the AIDS epidemic. The term appears to have been first used in a 1984 paper describing the psychological impact of the disease on homosexual men. "Safe sex" then began appearing in newspaper articles and brochures about sexual risk reduction for the gay community in 1985. In 1986 the term was incorporated in sexual health materials intended for college students. By the early 2000s, "safe sex" was widely used on the Internet as well as print publications in most developed countries; it now appears in materials aimed at adults over 65 as well as those intended for younger readers.

KEY TERMS

Abstinence—Intentional refraining from some or all forms of sexual activity.

Asexuality—Lack of interest in sexual activity or lack of sexual attraction to others. It should not be confused with abstinence, which is a behavioral choice.

Contraception—The use of a device, sexual practice, or chemical intended to prevent conception; birth control. It should not be confused with safe sex.

Expedited partner therapy (EPT)—A preventive measure that allows a doctor to prescribe or give medications to an infected patient's partner without having to first examine the partner for an STI.

Monogamy—Being married to only one person or having only one sexual partner at a time.

Post-exposure prophylaxis (PEP)—In the context of HIV, a course of antiretroviral drugs given immediately after a risky sexual encounter to reduce the risk of HIV infection. PEP should ideally be started within an hour after exposure; it is ineffective after 72 hours' delay.

Prophylactic—A drug, medical device, or technique intended to prevent (rather than treat) disease. Condoms are sometimes called prophylactics.

Semen—The thick whitish liquid released from the penis during sexual intercourse. It contains sperm and other secretions.

Sexual tourism—The practice of traveling to other countries for the purpose of paid sexual encounters.

Demographics

Information about reducing one's risk of contracting an STI is now almost universal, in the sense that brochures and medical office handouts, school-based education programs, social media, television special presentations, and medical websites on the Internet are available to persons of all age groups, genders, and sexual preferences in the developed countries. In Africa and other underdeveloped regions, education about safe sex is particularly aimed at women, because of the spread of HIV infections among heterosexual adults. China appears to be an exception in regard to availability of safe sex education as of 2012.

In spite of the fact that such information has been available since the late 1980s, STIs continue to be a major public health concern worldwide. It has been estimated that about half of all sexually active people will contract an STI at some point in their lifetime. The CDC's 2010 report on trends in the United States for three specific STIs (gonorrhea, chlamydia, and **syphilis**) identified three new public health concerns. With regard to gonorrhea, the number of cases is relatively low, but the infectious agent (the gonococcus) is increasingly resistant to all known **antibiotics**. With regard to chlamydia, rates continue to increase; 1.3 million new cases were reported in 2010. In the case of syphilis, there are fewer new cases in the general population but an explosive increase among young African American males. As of 2012, sexually active teenagers and young adults remain at much higher risk for STIs than adults over 30; some recent studies indicate that American teenagers still have a low level of knowledge about STIs in spite of sex education in public schools.

Effects on public health

Safe sex has become a major topic of public **health education** campaigns as well as treatment and prevention of STIs. The CDC has established a new center, the National Center for HIV/AIDS, Viral **Hepatitis**, STD, and TB Prevention (NCHHSTP) to deal with the ongoing threats to the health of the general population posed by STIs.

Efforts and solutions

In addition to education campaigns and the funding of a new center at the CDC, efforts to encourage safer sexual practices include the distribution of "Safe in the City," a 23-minute HIV/STD prevention video designed for STD clinics that requires no setup time or small-group discussions. According to the CDC, the video has lowered STI recurrence among clinic patients by 10%. The video can be ordered in DVD format or downloaded from the CDC website at the link provided. Another preventive measure undertaken by the CDC since 2005 is expedited partner therapy or EPT. EPT allows a doctor treating a patient for an STI to provide prescriptions or medications for the infected person to take to his or her partner without the partner's being required to undergo a physical examination first.

One important ongoing public health problem with regard to safe sex is the close connection between drug

---

QUESTIONS TO ASK YOUR DOCTOR

- What is your opinion of safe sex education materials for adolescents? For older adults?
- Where do you usually refer patients for more information about safe sex?
- What is your opinion of expedited partner therapy? Have you ever participated in EPT?

---

or alcohol abuse and risky sexual behaviors. In addition to facilitating unsafe sex between casual sexual partners, substance abuse is frequently associated with paid sex. Many addicts engage in prostitution in order to pay for their drugs or alcohol. One approach that is being used with homosexual men who use **methamphetamine** is post-exposure prophylaxis (PEP); however, this approach was still in its pilot-study phase as of 2012.

Another ongoing public health concern worldwide is sexual tourism; that is, the practice of traveling to other countries for paid sexual encounters, often those that are illegal in the home country (such as child prostitution, which is illegal in the United States). Sexual tourism contributes to the spread of STIs as well as encouraging **human trafficking** and child prostitution. This particular public health problem, however, requires cooperation and enforcement at the international level.

Resources

BOOKS

Ambrose, Marylou, and Veronica Deisler. *Investigating STDs (Sexually Transmitted Diseases): Real Facts for Real Lives.* Berkeley Heights, NJ: Enslow Publishers, 2011.

Larsen, Laura, ed. *Sexually Transmitted Diseases Sourcebook*, 4th ed. Detroit, MI: Omnigraphics, 2009.

Lord, Alexandra M. *Condom Nation: The U.S. Government's Sex Education Campaign from World War I to the Internet.* Baltimore, MD: Johns Hopkins University Press, 2010.

PERIODICALS

Brown, G., et al. "HIV Risk among Australian Men Travelling Overseas: Networks and Context Matter." *Culture, Health and Sexuality* 14 (June 2012): 677-690.

Crosby, R., and S. Bounse. "Condom Effectiveness: Where Are We Now?" *Sexual Health* 9 (March 2012): 10-17.

Kennedy, B.R., and C.C. Jenkins. "Promoting African American Women and Sexual Assertiveness in Reducing HIV/AIDS:

An Analytical Review of the Research Literature." *Journal of Cultural Diversity* 18 (Winter 2011): 142-149.

Kurkowski, J.P., et al. "Knowledge of Sexually Transmitted Infections among Adolescents in the Houston Area Presenting for Reproductive Healthcare at Texas Children's Hospital." *Journal of Pediatric and Adolescent Gynecology* 25 (June 2012): 213-217.

Landovitz, R.J., et al. "A novel combination HIV prevention strategy: post-exposure prophylaxis with contingency management for substance abuse treatment among methamphetamine-using men who have sex with men." *AIDS Patient Care and STDs* 26 (June 2012): 320-328.

Shang, H., et al. "HIV Prevention: Bring Safe Sex to China." *Nature* 485 (May 30, 2012): 576-577.

WEBSITES

"2010 Sexually Transmitted Diseases Surveillance." Centers for Disease Control and Prevention (CDC). http://www.cdc.gov/std/stats10/default.htm (accessed October 8, 2010).

"All about Condoms." American Social Health Association (ASHA). http://www.ashastd.org/sexual_health/condoms.html (accessed October 7, 2012).

"Condoms and STDs: Fact Sheet for Public Health Personnel." Centers for Disease Control and Prevention (CDC). http://www.cdc.gov/condomeffectiveness/latex.htm (accessed October 6, 2012).

"Frequently Asked Questions: How to Prevent Sexually Transmitted Diseases." American Congress of Obstetricians and Gynecologists (ACOG). www.acog.org/~/media/For Patients/faq009.pdf (accessed October 6, 2012).

National Center for HIV/AIDS, Viral Hepatitis, STD, and TB Prevention. (NCHHSTP)/Centers for Disease Control and Prevention. http://www.cdc.gov/nchhstp/Default.htm (accessed October 7, 2012).

"Protecting Yourself: Barrier to Barrier." GMHC. http://www.gmhc.org/protect/protecting-yourself/barrier-to-barrier (accessed October 7, 2012).

"Safe in the City STD Videos." Centers for Disease Control and Prevention (CDC). http://www.cdc.gov/std/safe-in-the-city/default.htm (accessed October 6, 2012).

"Safe Sex." Medline Plus (National Library of Medicine). www.nlm.nih.gov/medlineplus/ency/article/001949.htm (accessed October 7, 2012).

"Your Safer Sex Toolbox." American Social Health Association (ASHA). http://www.ashastd.org/sexual_health/your-safer-sex-toolbox.html (accessed October 7, 2012).

ORGANIZATIONS

American Congress of Obstetricians and Gynecologists (ACOG), PO Box 70620, Washington, DC United States 20024-9998, (202) 638-5577, (800) 673-8444, http://www.acog.org/

American Social Health Association (ASHA), P.O. Box 13827, Research Triangle Park, NC United States 27709, (919) 361-8400, Fax: (919) 361-8425, info@ashastd.org, http://www.ashastd.org/

Centers for Disease Control and Prevention (CDC), 1600 Clifton Road, Atlanta, GA United States 30333, (800) CDC-INFO (232-4636), http://www.cdc.gov/cdc-info/requestform.html, http://www.cdc.gov/

GMHC [formerly Gay Men's Health Crisis], 446 West 33rd Street, New York, NY United States 10001-2601, (212) 367-1000, (800) 243-7692, http://www.gmhc.org/about-us/contact-us, http://www.gmhc.org/

Rebecca J. Frey, Ph.D.

Salmonella

Definition

Salmonellosis is a type of food **poisoning** that is caused by bacteria in the genus *Salmonella*. Also known as *Salmonella* enterocolitis or non-typhoidal *Salmonella*, salmonellosis results in the swelling of the lining of the stomach and intestines (gastroenteritis). While domestic and wild animals, including poultry, pigs, cattle; and pets such as turtles, iguanas, chicks, dogs, and cats; can transmit this illness, most people become infected by ingesting foods that are contaminated with significant amounts of *Salmonella*. Swallowing contaminated **water** can also cause salmonellosis.

DESCRIPTION. Improperly handled or undercooked poultry and eggs are the foods that most frequently cause salmonellosis. Chickens are a major carrier of *Salmonella* bacteria. Infected chickens rarely show any signs or symptoms indicating that they are carrying the

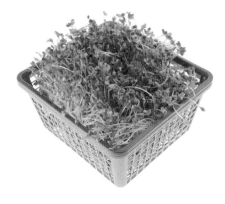

Young sprouts. When contaminated, they've caused Salmonella outbreaks. (© *Gregory Gerber/Shutterstock.com*)

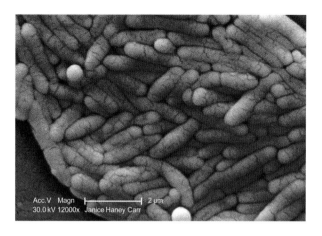

Gram-negative Salmonella typhimurium bacteria that had been isolated from a pure culture. *(CDC/ Bette Jensen)*

bacterium, so their eggs or meat may wind up at the grocery store, and go on to cause food poisoning among consumers.

Anyone may contract salmonellosis. Typical symptoms include diarrhea, fever, and abdominal cramps that may last for several days, but most people recover on their own. The disease is most serious in infants, the elderly, and individuals with weakened immune systems. In these individuals, the infection may spread from the intestines to the bloodstream, and then to other body sites, causing death unless the person is treated promptly with **antibiotics**. In addition, people who have had part or all of their stomach or their spleen removed, or who have sickle cell anemia, cirrhosis of the liver, leukemia, lymphoma, **malaria**, louse-borne relapsing fever, or acquired immunodeficiency syndrome (**AIDS**) are particularly susceptible to *Salmonella* food poisoning.

ORIGINS. The genus *Salmonella* is named for Daniel Elmer Salmon, a veterinary surgeon who studied animal disease for the U.S. Department of Agriculture and its new Bureau of Animal Industry from the late 1800s to the early 1900s. Actually, it was his research assistant, Theobald Smith, who actually isolated the first *Salmonella* bacterium in 1885. Smith originally (and erroneously) thought the bacterium was responsible for hog **cholera** and named it *Salmonella cholera suis*.

At one time, scientists believed that *Salmonella* bacteria were only found in eggs that had cracked shells, thus allowing the bacteria to enter. Ultimately, it was learned that egg shells are riddled with tiny pores through which bacteria can enter, so even uncracked eggs that sit for a time on a surface (such as a nest) contaminated with *Salmonella* can themselves become contaminated.

Demographics

Salmonella food poisoning occurs worldwide, however it is most frequently reported in North America and Europe. Only a small proportion of infected people are tested and diagnosed, and as few as 1% of cases are actually reported. Salmonellosis typically occurs in small, localized outbreaks in the general population or in large outbreaks in hospitals, restaurants, or institutions for children or the elderly. In the United States, *Salmonella* is responsible for about 35% of all cases of foodborne illnesses that result in hospitalization.

Causes and symptoms

Causes

Salmonella food poisoning can occur when someone drinks unpasteurized milk or contaminated water or eats undercooked chicken, eggs, or salad dressings or desserts that contain raw eggs.

Even if *Salmonella*-containing foods such as chicken are thoroughly cooked, any food can become contaminated during preparation if conditions and equipment for food preparation are unsanitary. For example, other foods can become accidentally contaminated if they come into contact with infected surfaces.

In addition, children have become ill after playing with turtles or iguanas, and then eating without washing their hands. Because the bacteria are shed in the feces for weeks after infection with *Salmonella*, poor **hygiene** can allow such a carrier to spread the infection to others.

Symptoms

Symptoms appear about one to two days after infection and include fever (in about half of patients), nausea and vomiting, diarrhea, and abdominal cramps and **pain**. The diarrhea is usually very liquid and rarely contains mucus or blood. Diarrhea usually lasts for about four days. Most people fully recover from the illness in about five to seven days.

Serious complications are rare, occurring most often in individuals with other medical illnesses, and result when the *Salmonella* bacteria make their way into the bloodstream (bacteremia). Once there, the bacteria can enter any organ system throughout the body, causing disease. The infections that can be caused by *Salmonella* include:

- bone infections (osteomyelitis)
- joint infections (arthritis)
- infection of the sac containing the heart (pericarditis)
- infection of the tissues which cover the brain and spinal cord (meningitis)
- infection of the liver (hepatitis)
- lung infections (pneumonia)

- infection of aneurysms (abnormal outpouchings which occur in weak areas of the walls of blood vessels)
- infections in the center of existing tumors or cysts.

Diagnosis

Health professionals may check patients for a tender abdomen or for the presence of "rose spots," which are small, pink splotches on the skin, or may test the patient for specific antibodies that are indicative of the presence of *Salmonella*. Under appropriate laboratory conditions, *Salmonella* can be grown and then viewed under a microscope for identification. Early in the infection, the blood is far more likely to positively show a presence of the *Salmonella* bacterium when a sample is grown on a nutrient substance (culture) for identification purposes. Eventually, however, positive cultures can be obtained from the stool and, in some cases, from a urine culture.

Prevention

Prevention of *Salmonella* food poisoning involves the proper handling and cooking of foods likely to carry the bacteria. This means that recipes utilizing uncooked eggs (e.g., Caesar salad dressing, meringue toppings, and mousses) need to be modified to eliminate the raw eggs. Not only should poultry be cooked thoroughly (to 165°F internal temperature), but all leftovers should also be cooked to the same temperature. In addition, surfaces and utensils used on raw poultry must be carefully cleaned to prevent *Salmonella* from contaminating other foods. The **CDC** recommends disinfecting these food-contact surfaces with a freshly prepared solution of 1 tablespoon unscented liquid chlorine bleach to 1 gallon of water.

Careful **handwashing** is a must before, during, and after all food preparation involving eggs and poultry. Handwashing is also important after handling and playing with pets such as turtles, iguanas, chicks, dogs, and cats.

Some individuals are more susceptible to salmonellosis. They include people who work in a health facility; have a weakened immune system; regularly take medications to reduce stomach acid; have recently taken antibiotics; or have Crohn's disease or ulcerative colitis. These individuals should ensure that they take all preventative measure to prevent exposure to the bacteria.

Treatment

General care for salmonellosis is rehydration in the form of water or other liquids to counter the fluid loss caused by diarrhea. For infants, healthcare professionals may suggest electrolyte replacement solutions.

Even though *Salmonella* food poisoning is a bacterial infection, most practitioners do not treat simple cases with

KEY TERMS

Culture—a nutrient substance on which bacteria or other organisms can be grown.

Gastroenteritis—Inflammation of the stomach and intestines. Usually causes nausea, vomiting, diarrhea, abdominal pain, and cramps.

antibiotics. Studies have shown that using antibiotics does not usually reduce the length of time that the patient is ill. Paradoxically, it appears that antibiotics do, however, cause the patient to shed bacteria in their feces for a *longer* period of time. In order to decrease the length of time that a particular individual is a carrier who can spread the disease, antibiotics are generally not given.

In situations where an individual has a more severe type of infection with *Salmonella* bacteria, a number of antibiotics may be used. The bacteria, however, are becoming resistant to many of the antibiotics in the anti-*Salmonella* arsenal. A 2012 study in the *Journal of Infectious Diseases*, for instance, reported that one form, or serotype, of the bacteria, known as *Salmonella* Kentucky (or *Salmonella enterica* serotype Kentucky ST198-X1), had become resistant to fluoroquinolones, which are some of the most commonly prescribed antibiotics to treat salmonellosis. Usually transmitted by eating chicken, *Salmonella* Kentucky has been causing human illness in the United States and other countries since 2002.

Antibiotics are administered orally or, for very ill patients, intravenously. With effective antibiotic therapy, patients feel better in 24 to 48 hours, the temperature returns to normal in three to five days, and the patient has generally recovered by 10 to 14 days.

Research on *Salmonella* is ongoing. A 2012 study by a research team from the Yale School of Medicine and the Yale Microbial Diversity Institute, for instance, is trying to learn more about how the bacterium becomes pathogenic to humans. In the team's study, it learned that the pathway toward virulence begins when internal cellular sensors in the bacterium pick up cues from the surroundings. Specifically, changes in the acidity in the environment trigger an increase in levels of adenosine triphosphate (ATP), which is often described as a cell's energy currency. The boost in ATP activates genes that ultimately make the bacterium virulent. Studies like this one are helping scientists understand the bacterium and may help in the development of new treatments.

Alternative treatment

A number of alternative treatments have been recommended for food poisoning. One is supplementation

Salmonella

with *Lactobacillus acidophilus*, *L. bulgaricus*, and/or *Bifidobacterium* to restore essential bacteria in the digestive tract. These preparations are available as powders, tablets, or capsules from health food stores; yogurt with live *L. acidophilus* cultures can also be eaten.

Fasting or a liquid-only diet is often used for food poisoning. Homeopathic treatment can be effective in the treatment of *Salmonella* food poisoning. Some examples of remedies commonly used are *Chamomilla*, *Nux vomica*, *Ipecac*, and *Colchicum*.

Juice therapy, including carrot, beet, and garlic juices, is sometimes recommended, although it can cause discomfort for some people. Charcoal tablets can help absorb toxins and remove them from the digestive tract through bowel elimination. A variety of herbs with antibiotic action, including citrus seed extract, goldenseal (*Hydrastis canadensis*), and Oregon grape (*Mahonia aquifolium*), may also be effective in helping to resolve cases of food poisoning.

Of course, individuals should consult a physician about homeopathic treatments to ensure their safety and to ensure that no drug interactions exist. All individuals with severe salmonellosis symptoms should see a physician immediately.

PROGNOSIS. The prognosis for uncomplicated cases of *Salmonella* food poisoning is excellent. Most people recover completely within a week's time. In cases where other medical problems complicate the illness, prognosis depends on the severity of the other medical conditions, as well as the specific organ system infected with *Salmonella*.

EFFECTS ON PUBLIC HEALTH. Salmonellosis outbreaks occur with some frequency. In 2011, for instance, the **Centers for Disease Control and Prevention** worked with other agencies to investigate a multistate outbreak of the serotype of the bacteria known as *Salmonella* Heidelberg. Affected states included Michigan, Ohio, California, Texas, Illinois, Pennsylvania, South Dakota, and Kentucky. More than a third of the ill persons were hospitalized, and one died, and the CDC determined that the ingestion of undercooked ground turkey was a likely culprit. That same year, salmonellosis outbreaks occurred with the suspected sources being grape tomatoes and papaya. In 2010, nearly 2,000 persons became ill, prompting the recall of more than a half billion suspect eggs; and in 2009, a large outbreak tied tainted peanut butter to more than 22,000 cases of salmonellosis and up to nine deaths.

COSTS TO SOCIETY. According to the CDC, salmonellosis caused more than one million illnesses, more than 19,300 hospitalizations, and 378 deaths in the United States in 2011. A 2012 Ohio State University

---

QUESTIONS TO ASK YOUR DOCTOR

- What are the side effects, if any, of antibiotics?
- How effective are alternative treatments?
- Which liquids should I give my child to aid the recovery, and how often should I give them?

---

study put the total annual cost associated with *Salmonella* food poisoning in the United States at $11.4 billion.

EFFORTS AND SOLUTIONS. Some *Salmonella* serotypes are quickly adapting and becoming resistant to many of the antibiotics currently used to treat severe salmonellosis. In response, considerable research is under way to develop new antibiotics and to understand alternate pathways to impede resistance. At the same time, health agencies and medical professionals are re-evaluating their administration of antibiotics as well as recommendations for antimicrobial agents in cleaning and other applications, because their overuse has been implicated as promoting bacterial resistance.

Resources

BOOKS

Russell, Scott M.*Controlling Salmonella in Poultry Production and Processing.* Boca Raton, FL: CRC Press, 2012.

PERIODICALS

Groisman E.A., and E-J Lee. "Control of a *Salmonella* virulence locus by an ATP-sensing leader messenger RNA." *Nature* 486, no. 7402 (2012): 271–2785.

Scharff R.L. "Economic Burden from Health Losses Due to Foodborne Illness in the United States." *Journal of Food Protection* 75, no. 1 (2012): 123–131.

WEBSITES

CDC Estimates of Foodborne Illness in the United States "Drug-Resistant *Salmonella*," World Health Organization. http://www.cdc.gov/foodborneburden/2011-foodborne-estimates.html (accessed August 20, 2012).

'Drug-Resistant *Salmonella*,' World Health Organization. http://www.who.int/mediacentre/factsheets/fs139/en/ (accessed August 20, 2012).

"Foodborne Illness Costs $77.7 Billion a Year," Ohio State University. http://extension.osu.edu/news-releases/archives/2012/january/ohio-state-researcher-foodborne-illness-costs-77.7-billion-a-year (accessed August 20, 2012).

'Investigation Announcement: Multistate Outbreak of Human *Salmonella* Heidelberg Infections,' Centers for Disease Control and Prevention. http://www.cdc.gov/salmonella/heidelberg/080111/ (accessed August 20, 2012).

Yale News. 'Internal Cellular Sensors Make *Salmonella* Dangerous, Yale Researchers Find,' Yale University.

http://news.yale.edu/2012/06/14/internal-cellular-sensors-make-salmonella-dangerous-yale-researchers-find (accessed August 20, 2012).

ORGANIZATIONS

Center for Food Safety and Applied Nutrition, U.S. Food and Drug Administration, 5100 Paint Branch Parkway, College Park, MD 20740, (888) 723-3366, consumer@fda .gov, http://www.fda.gov/AboutFDA/CentersOffices/ OfficeofFoods/CFSAN/default.htm.

Centers for Disease Control and Prevention (CDC), 1600 Clifton Road, Atlanta, GA 30333, (800) 232-4636, cdcinfo@cdc.gov, http://www.cdc.gov.

Lata Cherath, Ph.D.
Rosalyn Carson-DeWitt, M.D.
Laura Jean Cataldo, RN, Ed.D.
Leslie Mertz, Ph.D.

Sanitation

Definition

Sanitation refers to any process designed to prevent disease and promote good health by the proper treatment of **water** supplies, human and other types of waste, and, in some cases, other procedures, such as the handling of foods in commercial operations.

Purpose

The purpose of sanitation is to remove the factors, such as waterborne pathogens, that tend to cause disease and reduce the health of a **population**.

Description

Virtually every human society has been aware of the health advantages of good sanitary procedures and has developed technologies designed to promote good sanitation. Archaeologists have traced some of the earliest sanitary sewer systems, for example, to the Babylonian civilization of the fourth millennium BCE. Virtually every society since that time has made use of some form of toilets and sewer systems to remove human wastes from homes and other habitable areas. As civilizations became more technologically complex, and urban areas became more crowded, such efforts were much more difficult to accomplish. As a result, by the early modern age, sanitary facilities were often not available to people living in large cities who were forced to dispose of their wastes simply by throwing them out of the window or into the closest street. Finally, in 1842,

English social reformer Edwin Chadwick produced a now-classic report, "An Inquiry into the Sanitary Condition of the Labouring Population of Great Britain," describing the execrable conditions in which most urban dwellers and many rural residents lived at the time. Chadwick's report eventually led to the adoption of the Public Health Act of 1848, the first national legislation of the modern era designed to provide for proper sanitation of a nation's population. In general, the act provided for the establishment of sewer systems for the removal of wastes and the development of systems for the delivery of safe water to urban residents.

The term *sanitation* refers, first and foremost, to these two considerations: pure water and removal of human and other wastes. The reason for these priorities is that impure water and wastes are a primary cause of illness and death wherever they occur. Poor sanitation in the modern world, for example, is thought to be responsible for at least 10% of the global disease burden, largely in the form of diarrheal diseases. Such diseases are thought to be the second leading cause of disease among children under the age of five around the world, accounting for 1.5 million child deaths each year. The **World Health Organization** estimates that about two billion cases of diarrheal diseases occur worldwide annually. Even when such diseases are not fatal, they tend to cause such severe dehydration problems that normal growth and development are interrupted, with long-term health defects the eventual result.

One of the fundamental issues with which sanitation programs must deal is waterborne diseases. A waterborne disease is one caused by pathogens that live in water and are capable of infecting humans and other animals. Some examples of waterborne diseases are **amebiasis** (caused by the *Entamoeba histolytica* parasite), **campylobacteriosis** (*Campylobacter jejuni* bacterium), cryptosporidiosis *Cryptosporidium* parasite), **cholera** (*Vibrio cholerae* bacterium, giardiasis (*Giardia lamblia* parasite), legionellosis (*Legionella pneumophila* bacterium), and salmonellosis (*Salmonella* bacteria). Signs and symptoms of these waterborne diseases are broadly similar and include diarrhea, nausea, vomiting, bloody stools, abdominal **pain**, fever, chills, and cramps.

A second challenge for sanitation systems is fecal-to-oral transmission of disease. In this case, pathogens pass through an animal body and into the surrounding environment, where they may become part of the water or food supply. Some of the diseases listed above are also transmitted via the fecal-to-oral route. Other such diseases include a number of foodborne infections, diseases that are transmitted when a person eats food that has been contaminated by some type of pathogen. Examples of foodborne illnesses include botulism

(*Clostridium botulinum* bacterium), **brucellosis** (*Brucella* bacteria), **shigellosis** (*Shigella* bacteria), staphylococcus food **poisoning** (*Staphylococcus aureus* bacterium), and trichinellosis/trichinosis (*Trichinella* parasite). The signs and symptoms of foodborne illnesses (also called "food poisoning") are similar to those of waterborne diseases.

Foodborne diseases can be spread through a number of specific pathways, as:

• failure of individuals, especially workers in the food service industry, to wash their hands adequately after using toilet facilities

• practices that cause food products to come into contact with feces as, for example, when human wastes are used to fertilize a crop grown for commercial consumption

• use of certain types of sexual behavior, such as analingus (oral-anal contact)

• consumption of water that has come into contact with animal wastes and then used to wash food items

Disease can also be transmitted through the soil. A number of members of the genus **Clostridium**, for example, can survive in the soil and be consumed along with foods that have been in contact with that soil. The bacillus *Clostridium tetani*, for example, is responsible for the disease known as **tetanus** (lockjaw), and its cousin, *Clostridium perfringens*, can survive in oxygen-free conditions and cause typical gastrointestinal symptoms. A number of fungi, such as *Histoplasma capsulatum*, *Aspergillus spp*, and *Cryptococcus neoformans*, are also common disease-causing pathogens that live in the soil.

Efforts and Solutions

Efforts to improve sanitation can take two general directions, aimed either at a community as a whole or individual members of the community. In the former category are programs to construct large water treatment and sewage disposal systems, to create food inspection programs, and to establish other initiatives that involve monitoring and control of potential disease-causing events on a widespread scale. All developed countries and many developing countries, for example, now have relatively sophisticated solid waste disposal systems that involve the regular collection of garbage, trash, junk, litter, yard wastes, recyclable materials, and other solid waste products from residences and industrial sites. These materials are then transported to storage sites, such as landfills or garbage sites; to incineration plants, where they may be burned to produce useable energy; or to recycling center, where their components may be separated and processed for reuse. Water purification

plants are also standard in most developed countries, but not necessarily in most developing countries, where residents may have to rely on wells, rivers, or other natural sources for their water supplies. Water purification plants carry out a number of operations on water drawn from natural sources, like lakes and rivers, to remove sediments and other solid impurities and to kill pathogens present in the water. The most common methods of treatment are the addition of chlorine and chlorine derivatives to the water, **radiation** of the water with ultraviolet radiation, and exposure of the water to oxygen in the air. Another method of sanitation monitoring is the use of food inspectors to monitor the storage and preparation of food in commercial establishments along with the inspection of facilities themselves and individuals who work in the facilities. Throughout most developing countries, food inspectors visit restaurants, grocery stores, food distribution centers, and other locations where food is handled to check on dozens of specific items, such as the temperature at which foods are stored, facilities available for **handwashing** and other hygienic practices, and possession of food handler certificates by employees at a facility.

Public health agencies have also established a number of recommendations for acceptable and desirable sanitation practices in individual residences. Such recommendations are particularly important in regions where commercial water purification and sewage treatment plants and routine monitoring of food handling practices are not available. For example, the Joint Monitoring Programme for Water Supply and Sanitation of the **World Health Organization (WHO)** and the United Nations Children's Fund (UNICEF) recognizes a number of possible so-called improved sanitation devices and practices, such as:

• pit latrine with a slab

• ventilated improved latrine

• mechanical pull or flush-pull toilet connected to pit latrine

• composting toilet

• flush toilet

• piped sewage system

• septic tank

These "improved" sanitation devices and practices contrast with "unimproved" sanitation devices and practices such as use of a bucket, toilets that flush to places other than a pit latrine or other controlled site, or use of a natural setting, such as a river, lake, or wooded area.

Some of the "improved" sources of **drinking water** include

- rainwater
- a protected spring
- a protected dug well
- water piped into a dwelling or yard from a sanitary source
- water from a public standpipe or tap

These "improved" water sources compare to "unimproved" sources, such as

- tanker trucks
- water carts
- water from unprotected springs or wells
- bottled water
- surface water, such as ponds, lakes, or rivers

Demographics

The nonprofit organization Water.org has accumulated statistics about the type of sanitation facilities that are available to people worldwide, and the diseases that result from inadequate water treatment and santiation practices. Among those statistics are the following:

- An estimated 1.2 billion people have no facilities whatsoever for treating human wastes or separating wastes from food and water supplies.
- If sanitation facilities could be provided to these individuals, deaths from diarrheal disease could be reduced by one-third.
- An estimated 1.1 billion people practice open defecation into wooded areas, open fields, lakes and rivers, or other natural settings.
- An estimated 780 million people lack access to any type of improved water system of the types described above.
- As much as 10% of the world's disease burden would be eliminated by better sanitation devices and practices.
- Ninety percent of childhood deaths due to diarrheal diseases are caused by poor sanitation.

In developed countries, where water and sewage treatment facilities are generally available to the vast majority of individuals, foodborne diseases are more likely to be the major sanitary concerns. In the United States, for example, millions of people become ill and thousands die from food that has been improperly grown, harvested, transported, processed, stored, and prepared. The U.S. **Centers for Disease Control and Prevention (CDC)** estimated for 2011, for example, that foodborne pathogens were responsible for 47.8 million illnesses in the United States, 127,839 hospitalizations, and 3,037 deaths. Norovirus was responsible for the largest number of illnesses; while nontyphoidal *Salmonella*, norovirus,

KEY TERMS

Burden of disease—A measure of the impact of disease as measured by mortality, morbidity, financial cost, or other measures.

Foodborne disease—An illness caused by consuming a food or drink infected with pathogens.

Latrine—A type of toilet, often one used by a number of individuals.

Pathogen—A microorganism (e.g., bacterium, virus, fungus) capable of causing a disease in a plant or animal.

Sanitarian—A person who has been trained in the sanitary sciences and is qualified to work in some aspect of that field.

Toilet—A device, usually a bowl of some kind, for receiving urine and feces.

Waterborne disease—An illness caused by ingesting water contaminated with some type of pathogen.

Campylobacter spp., and *Toxoplasma gondii* caused the most hospitalizations; and nontyphoidal *Salmonella*, *Toxoplasma gondii*, *Listeria monocytogenes*, and norovirus were responsible for the largest number of deaths.

Prevention

As noted above, virtually every human civilization has devised practices to encourage better sanitation as a way of improving and maintaining as high a level of public health as possible. Individuals who work in this field are known as *sanitarians*. Historians of sanitary practices trace the origins of their profession in the United States to the earliest years of the Colonial period. For example, some experts point to a 1640 law adopted in Virginia that required all residents to keep their homes "sweet and clean" and that prohibited specific unhygienic practices, such as throwing soapy water into the streets or cleaning pots and pans near a well. Today, sanitarians can belong to a variety of professional organizations that may certify their qualifications for holding jobs in the field, providing training and educational programs in the field of sanitation, or otherwise promote the profession and the interests of its members. Examples of such organizations include the American Academy of Sanitarians and sanitarian councils, associations, boards, and other organizations in most of the states. Individuals interested in pursuing a career in sanitation can earn the title of Registered Sanitarian by taking certain prescribed courses and passing a special examination in the field.

They are then qualified to work in a number of fields of sanitation, including water and food sanitation, disaster programs, recreational water facilities, sewage treatment, milk supply, infectious medical wastes, body piercing, child care centers, disease surveillance, manufactured home inspection, industrial **hygiene**, and air quality.

Resources

BOOKS

Davis, Mackenzie, and David Cornwell. *Introduction to Environmental Engineering*, 5th ed. New York: McGraw-Hill Science/Engineering/Math, 2012.

Marriott, Norman G., and Robert B. Gravani. *Principles of Food Sanitation*, 5th ed. New York: Springer, 2010.

Selendy, Janine M.H., ed. *Water and Sanitation Related Diseases and the Environment: Challenges, Interventions and Preventive Measures*. New York: Wiley-Blackwell, 2011.

Stanga, Mario. *Sanitation*. New York: Wiley-VCH, 2010.

PERIODICALS

Fink, G., I. Günther, and K. Hill. "The Effect of Water and Sanitation on Child Health: Evidence from the Demographic and Health Surveys 1986–2007." *International Journal of Epidemiology* 40, 5. (2011): 1196–204.

Groce, N., et al. "Water and Sanitation Issues for Persons with Disabilities in Low- and Middle-Income Countries: A Literature Review and Discussion of Implications for Global Health and International Development." *Journal of Water and Health* 9, 4. (2011): 617–27.

Minh, Hong Van, and Nguyen-Viet Hung. "Economic Aspects of Sanitation in Developing Countries." *Environmental Health Insights* 5. (2011): 63–70.

Pink, R. "Child Rights, Right to Water and Sanitation, and Human Security." *Health and Human Righs* 14, 1. (2012): E78–87.

WEBSITES

"Global Water, Sanitation & Hygiene." Centers for Disease Control and Prevention. http://www.cdc.gov/healthywater/global/sanitation/. Accessed October 16, 2012.

Mara, Duncan, et al. "Sanitation and Health." PLOS Medicine. http://www.ncbi.nlm.nih.gov/pmc/articles/PMC2981586/. Accessed October 15, 2012.

"Sanitation." World Health Organization. http://www.who.int/topics/sanitation/en/. Accessed October 16, 2012.

"Welcome to the JMP Website!" Joint Monitoring Programme. http://www.wssinfo.org/about-the-jmp/introduction/. Accessed October 16, 2012.

ORGANIZATIONS

World Health Organization (WHO), Avenue Appia 20, 1211 Geneva 27, Switzerland, +41 22 791 21 11, Fax: +41 22 791 31 11, http://www.who.int/about/contact_form/en/index.html, http://www.who.int/en/.

David E. Newton, Ed.D.

Scarlet fever

Definition

Scarlet fever is an infection that is caused by group A streptococcus bacteria, in particular, *S. pyogenes*. The disease is characterized by fever, a sore throat, and a sandpaper-like rash on reddened skin. It is primarily a childhood disease. If scarlet fever is untreated, serious complications, such as rheumatic fever (a **heart disease**) or kidney inflammation (glomerulonephritis) can develop.

Description

Scarlet fever, also known as scarlatina, gets its name from the fact that the patient's skin, especially on the cheeks, is flushed. A sore throat and raised rash over much of the body are accompanied by fever and sluggishness (lethargy). The fever usually subsides within a few days, and recovery is complete by two weeks. After the fever is gone, the skin on the face and body flakes; the skin on the palms of the hands and soles of the feet peels more dramatically.

This disease affects primarily children ages two to ten. It is highly contagious and is spread by sneezing, coughing, or direct contact. The incubation period is three to five days, with symptoms usually beginning on the second day of the disease, and lasting from four to ten days.

Early in the twentieth century, severe scarlet fever epidemics were common. Today, the disease is rare. Although this decline is due in part to the availability of **antibiotics**, that is not the entire reason, since the decline began before the widespread use of antibiotics. One theory is that the strain of bacteria that causes scarlet fever has become weaker with time.

Demographics

Scarlet fever has largely been brought under control in the world today. In one of the latest studies conducted (2004), a total of 24 deaths worldwide from the disease were reported, six in Mexico, four in Egypt, two in the United States, and one in each of 12 other nations. Outbreaks continue to occur, however. For example, an antibiotic-resistant strain of group A streptococcal bacteria in China was blamed for an outbreak that infected more than 500 children, causing two deaths in 2011. The deaths were the first from scarlet fever reported in the country in more than a decade. The spread of bacteria resistant to the streptococcal bacteria is a possible source of concern for future outbreaks of the disease.

GLADYS DICK (1881–1963)

Before 1922, not much was known about the then-endemic disease of scarlet fever, which primarily affected children in Europe and North America, killing about 25% of the children who contracted it. Additionally, scarlet fever had many complications, some of which were severe and could be crippling. Gladys Dick, with her husband, George Dick, successfully isolated the bacteria which caused scarlet fever, developed a test for human vulnerability to the disease, and devised preventive methods. The couple patented their findings, specifically the way their scarlet fever toxin and antitoxin were prepared, although this decision was controversial at the time.

In 1923, the Dicks published papers in which they proved that scarlet fever was caused by hemolytic streptococcus. Within a few years, the Dicks also published papers on how to prevent, test, diagnose, and treat scarlet fever. Their groundbreaking work ensured that the disease was finally understood and brought under control.

Dick and her husband announced the development of what came to be known as the Dick test in 1924. This skin test showed whether the patient was susceptible or immune to scarlet fever. The test involved injecting a toxin-containing substance in the arm and determining if the skin around the area became inflamed. If it did, the patient was vulnerable to scarlet fever. This test was also useful in predicting if pregnant women would develop puerperal infection during childbirth.

Causes and symptoms

Scarlet fever is caused by group A streptococcal bacteria, most commonly by *S. pyogenes*. Group A streptococci can be highly toxic microbes that can cause strep throat, wound or skin infections, **pneumonia**, and serious kidney infections, as well as scarlet fever. Group A streptococci are hemolytic bacteria, which means that the bacteria can lyse or break open red blood cells. The strain of streptococcus that causes scarlet fever is slightly different from the strain that causes most strep throats. The scarlet fever strain of bacteria produces a toxin, called an erythrogenic toxin, which is what causes the skin to flush.

The main symptoms and signs of scarlet fever are fever, lethargy, sore throat, and a bumpy rash that blanches under pressure. The rash appears first on the upper chest and spreads to the neck, abdomen, legs, arms, and folds of skin, such as under the arm or groin. In scarlet fever, the skin around the mouth tends to be pale, while the cheeks are flushed. The patient usually has a "strawberry tongue," on which inflamed bumps rise above a bright red coating. Finally, dark red lines (called Pastia's lines) may appear in the creases of skin folds.

Diagnosis

Cases of scarlet fever are usually diagnosed and treated by pediatricians or family medicine practitioners. The chief diagnostic signs of scarlet fever are the characteristic rash, which spares the palms and soles of the feet, and the presence of a strawberry tongue in children. Strawberry tongue is rarely seen in adults.

The doctor will take note of the signs and symptoms to eliminate the possibility of other diseases. Scarlet fever can be distinguished from **measles**, a viral infection that is also associated with a fever and rash, by the quality of the rash, the presence of a sore throat in scarlet fever, and the absence of the severe eye inflammation and severe runny nose that usually accompany measles.

The doctor will also distinguish among a strep throat, a viral infection of the throat, and scarlet fever. With a strep infection, the throat is sore and appears beefy and red. White spots appear on the tonsils. Lymph nodes under the jawline may swell and become tender. However, none of these symptoms is specific for strep throat and may also occur with a viral infection. Other signs are more characteristic of bacterial infections. For example, inflammation of the lymph nodes in the neck is typical in strep infections, but not viral infections. On the other hand, cough, laryngitis, and stuffy nose tend to be associated with viral infections rather than strep infections. The main feature that distinguishes scarlet fever from a mere strep throat is the presence of the sandpaper-red rash.

Laboratory tests are needed to make a definitive diagnosis of a strep infection and to distinguish a strep throat from a viral sore throat. One test that can be performed is a blood cell count. Bacterial infections are associated with an elevated white blood cell count. In viral infections, the white blood cell count is generally below normal.

A throat culture can distinguish between a strep infection and a viral infection. A throat swab from the infected person is brushed over a nutrient gel (a sheep blood agar plate) and incubated overnight to detect the presence of hemolytic bacteria. In a positive culture, a clear zone will appear in the gel surrounding the bacterium, indicating that a strep infection is present.

Treatment

Although scarlet fever will often clear up spontaneously within a few days, antibiotic treatment with either

KEY TERMS

Clindamycin—An antibiotic that can be used instead of penicillin.

Erythrogenic toxin—A toxin or agent produced by the scarlet fever-causing bacteria that causes the skin to turn red.

Erythromycin—An antibiotic that can be used instead of penicillin.

Glomerulonephritis—A serious inflammation of the kidneys that can be caused by streptococcal bacteria; a potential complication of untreated scarlet fever.

Hemolytic bacteria—Bacteria that are able to burst red blood cells.

Lethargy—The state of being sluggish.

Pastia's lines—Red lines in the folds of the skin, especially in the armpit and groin, that are characteristic of scarlet fever.

Penicillin—An antibiotic that is used to treat bacterial infections.

Procaine penicillin—An injectable form of penicillin that contains an anesthetic to reduce the pain of the injection.

Rheumatic fever—A heart disease that is a complication of a strep infection.

Sheep blood agar plate—A petri dish filled with a nutrient gel containing red blood cells that is used to detect the presence of streptococcal bacteria in a throat culture. Streptococcal bacteria will lyse or break open red blood cells, leaving a clear spot around the bacterial colony.

Strawberry tongue—A sign of scarlet fever in which the tongue appears to have a red coating with large, raised bumps.

oral or injectable penicillin is usually recommended to reduce the severity of symptoms, prevent complications, and prevent spread to others. Antibiotic treatment will shorten the course of the illness in small children but may not do so in adolescents or adults. Nevertheless, treatment with antibiotics is important to prevent complications.

Since penicillin injections are painful, oral penicillin may be preferable. If the patient is unable to tolerate penicillin, alternative antibiotics such as erythromycin or clindamycin may be used. However, the entire course of antibiotics, usually 10 days, will need to be followed for

the therapy to be effective. Because symptoms subside quickly, there is a temptation to stop therapy prematurely. It is important to take all of the pills in order to kill the bacteria. Not completing the course of therapy increases the risk of developing rheumatic fever and kidney inflammation.

If the patient is considered too unreliable to take all of the pills or is unable to take oral medication, daily injections of procaine penicillin can be given in the hip or thigh muscle. Procaine is an anesthetic that makes the injections less painful.

Bed rest is not necessary, nor is isolation of the patient. Aspirin or Tylenol (acetaminophen) may be given for fever or relief of **pain**.

Prognosis

If treated promptly with antibiotics, full recovery is expected. Once a patient has had scarlet fever, he or she develops immunity and cannot develop it again.

Prevention

Avoiding exposure to children who have the disease will help prevent the spread of scarlet fever.

Resources

BOOKS

Berger, Stephen A. *Rheumatic Fever and Scarlet Fever: Global Status*. Los Angeles: Gideon Informatics, 2011.

Schwartz, M. William, et al. *The 5-minute Pediatric Consult*. Philadelphia: Wolters Kluwer Health/Lippincott Williams & Wilkins, 2012.

Von Liebermeister, Carl. *Infectious Diseases, Part 2: Measles, Scarlet Fever, Small-pox, Vaccinia, Varicella, Rubella, Diphtheria*. Charleston, SC: Bibliobazaar, 2011.

PERIODICALS

Chen, Mingliang, et al. "Outbreak of Scarlet Fever Associated With emm12 Type Group A Streptococcus in 2011 in Shanghai, China." *The Pediatric Infectious Disease Journal* 31, 9. (2012): e158–62.

Lau, Eric H.Y., et al. "Scarlet Fever Outbreak, Hong Kong, 2011." *Emerging Infectious Diseases* 18, 10. (2012): 1700–02.

Wong, Samson S.Y., and Kwok-Yung Yuen. "Streptococcus Pyogenes and Re-emergence of Scarlet Fever as a Public Health Problem." *Emerging Microbes & Infections* 1, 7. (2012): e2.

OTHER

"Scarlet Fever." PubMed Health. http://www.ncbi.nlm.nih.gov/pubmedhealth/PMH0001969/. Accessed November 2, 2012.

"Understanding Scarlet Fever: The Basics." WebMD. http://www.webmd.com/a-to-z-guides/understanding-scarlet-fever-basics. Accessed November 2, 2012.

Zabawski, Edward J., Jr. "Scarlet Fever." Medscape Reference. http://emedicine.medscape.com/article/1053253-overview. Accessed November October 2, 2012.

ORGANIZATIONS

Centers for Disease Control and Prevention, 1600 Clifton Rd., N.E., Atlanta, GA 30333, 1 (800) 232–4636, cdcinfo@ cdc.gov, www.cdc.gov

Sally J. Jacobs, Ed.D.

Schistosomiasis

Definition

Schistosomiasis, also known as bilharziasis or snail fever, is a primarily tropical parasitic disease caused by the larvae of one or more of five types of flatworms or blood flukes known as schistosomes.

DESCRIPTION. Infections associated with worms present some of the most universal health problems in the world. In fact, only **malaria** accounts for more diseases than schistosomiasis. The **World Health Organization (WHO)** estimates that 240 million people are infected and that another 700 million people are at risk of infection because they live in areas where schistosomes thrive.

Intestinal schistosomiasis, caused by *Schistosoma japonicum*, *S. mekongi*, *S. mansoni*, and *S. intercalatum*, can lead to serious complications of the liver and spleen. Urinary schistosomiasis is caused by *S. haematobium*.

It is difficult to know how many individuals die of schistosomiasis each year, because death certificates and patient records seldom identify schistosomiasis as the primary cause of death. The **World Health Organization** estimates that several million people around the world suffer from severe morbidity as a consequence of schistosomiasis.

ORIGINS. The name bilharziasis comes from Theodor Bilharz, a German pathologist, who identified the worms in 1851.

DEMOGRAPHICS. Five species of schistosomes are prevalent in different areas of the world:

• *Schistosoma mansoni* is widespread in Africa, the Eastern-Mediterranean, the Caribbean, and South America.

• *S. mekongi* is prevalent Cambodia and Laos.

• *S. japonicum* is found in Indonesia, parts of China, and Southeast Asia.

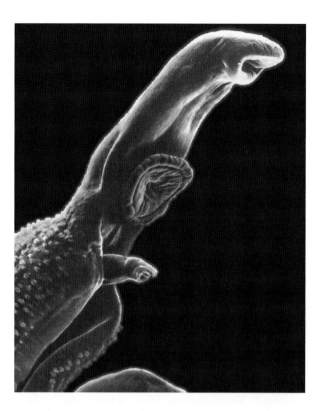

Schistosomiasis, bilharzia fluke, male and female. (© SPL/ Photo Researchers, Inc. Reproduced bypermission.)

• *S. intercalatum* is found in central and western Africa.

• *S. haematobium* occurs predominantly in Africa and the Middle East.

It is most common in developing countries that have poor **sanitation**, and predominantly affects children, who may play or swim in infested **water**.

Causes and symptoms

Causes

All five species are contracted in the same way: through direct contact with fresh water infested with the free-living form of the parasite. This form is known as cercariae. The building of dams, irrigation systems, and reservoirs, and the movements of refugee groups can introduce and spread schistosomiasis.

Infected persons excrete the worms in the urine and feces and, in areas with poor sanitation, contaminate freshwater sources. The eggs break open to release a form of the parasite called miracidium. Freshwater snails become infested with the miracidium, which multiply inside the snail and mature into multiple cercariae that the snail ejects into the water. The cercariae, which survive outside a host for 48 hours, quickly penetrate unbroken skin, the lining of the mouth, or the gastrointestinal tract. Once inside the human body, the worms break through the wall of the nearest vein and travel to the liver, where they grow and sexually mature. Mature male and female worms pair and migrate either to the intestines or the bladder, where egg production occurs. One female worm may lay an average of 200 to 2,000 eggs per day for up to 20 years. Most eggs leave the bloodstream and body through the intestines. Some of the eggs are not excreted, however, and can lodge in the tissues. It is the presence of these eggs, rather than the worms themselves, that causes the disease.

Symptoms

Early symptoms of infection

Many individuals do not experience symptoms. In those that do, the first symptom of the disease may be a general ill feeling. Within 12 hours of infection, an individual may complain of a tingling sensation or light rash, commonly referred to as "swimmer's itch," due to irritation at the point of entrance. (This is not the same as the swimmer's itch or duck itch that is common to swimmers in U.S. lakes. Duck itch, which does not have lasting effects, produces a burning, itching rash of short duration.) The rash that from schistosomiasis may develop can mimic scabies and other types of rashes. Other symptoms can occur two to 10 weeks later, and can include fever, aching, cough, diarrhea, or gland enlargement. These symptoms can also be related to avian schistosomiasis, which does not cause any further symptoms in humans.

Katayama fever

Another primary condition, called Katayama fever, may also develop from infection with these worms, and it can be very difficult to recognize. Symptoms include fever, lethargy, the eruption of pale temporary bumps associated with severe itching (urticarial) rash, liver and spleen enlargement, and bronchospasm.

Intestinal schistosomiasis

In intestinal schistosomiasis, eggs become lodged in the intestinal wall and cause an immune system reaction called a granulomatous reaction. This immune response can lead to obstruction of the colon and blood loss. The infected individual may have what appears to be a potbelly. Eggs can also become lodged in the liver, leading to high blood pressure through the liver, enlarged spleen, the build-up of fluid in the abdomen (ascites), and potentially life-threatening dilations or swollen areas in the esophagus or gastrointestinal tract that can tear and bleed profusely (esophageal varices). Rarely, the central nervous system may be affected. Individuals with chronic active schistosomiasis might not complain of typical symptoms.

KEY TERMS

Ascites—The condition that occurs when the liver and kidneys are not functioning properly and a clear, straw-colored fluid is excreted by the membrane that lines the abdominal cavity (peritoneum).

Cercariae—The free-living form of the schistosome worm that has a tail, swims, and has suckers on its head for penetration into a host.

Miracidium—The form of the schistosome worm that infects freshwater snails.

Urinary tract schistosomiasis

Urinary tract schistosomiasis is characterized by blood in the urine, **pain** or difficulty urinating, and frequent urination and are associated with *S. haematobium*. The loss of blood can lead to iron deficiency anemia. A large percentage of persons, especially children, who are moderately to heavily infected experience urinary tract damage that can lead to blocking of the urinary tract and bladder **cancer**.

DIAGNOSIS. Proper diagnosis and treatment may require a tropical disease specialist because the disease can be confused with malaria or typhoid in the early stages. The healthcare provider should do a thorough history of travel in endemic areas. The rash, if present, can mimic scabies or other rashes, and the gastrointestinal symptoms may be confused with those caused by bacterial illnesses or other intestinal **parasites**. These other conditions will need to be excluded before an accurate diagnosis can be made. As a result, clinical evidence of exposure to infected water along with physical findings, a negative test for malaria, and an increased number of one type of immune cell, called an eosinophil, are necessary to diagnose acute schistosomiasis.

Eggs may be detected in the feces or urine. Repeated stool tests may be necessary to concentrate and identify the eggs. Blood tests may be used to detect a particular antigen or particle associated with the schistosome that induces an immune response. Persons infected with schistosomiasis might not test positive for six months, and as a result, tests may need to be repeated to obtain an accurate diagnosis. Blood can be detected visually in the urine or with chemical strips that react to small amounts of blood.

Imaging techniques, such as ultrasound, computed tomography scan (CT scan), and magnetic resonance imaging (MRI), can detect damage to the blood vessels in

---

the liver, and can visualize polyps and ulcers of the urinary tract, for example, that occur in the more advanced stages. *S. haematobium* is difficult to diagnose with ultrasound in pregnant women.

TREATMENT. The typically used medication to treat schistosomiasis is praziquantel. Praziquantel is effective against all forms of schistososmiasis and has few side effects. If the infection is severe or involves the brain, the health professional may prescribe corticosteroids. This drug is given in either two or three doses over the course of a single day. The medicine oxamniquine treats intestinal schistosomiasis and is typically administered in Africa and South America to to fight this infection. Research has shown that another medicine, metrifonate, is safe and effective in the treatment of urinary schistosomiasis.

Patients are typically checked for the presence of living eggs at three and six months after treatment. If the number of eggs excreted has not significantly decreased, the patient may require another course of medication.

As of 2012, the development of a potential vaccine for schistosomiasis is continuing.

PROGNOSIS. If treated early, prognosis is very good, and complete recovery is expected. People can, however, die from the effects of untreated schistosomiasis. The severity of the disease depends on the number of worms, or "worm load," in addition to how long the person has been infected. With treatment, the number of worms can be substantially reduced, and the secondary conditions can be treated.

People have little natural immunity to reinfection. Treated individuals do not usually require retreatment for two to five years in areas of low transmission.

PREVENTION. Prevention of the disease involves several targets and requires long-term community commitment. Infected patients require diagnosis, treatment, and education about how to avoid reinfecting themselves and others. Adequate healthcare facilities need to be available, water systems must be treated to kill the worms and control snail populations, and sanitation must be improved to prevent the spread of the disease.

To avoid schistosomiasis in endemic areas:

- Contact the CDC for current health information on travel destinations.

- Upon arrival, ask an informed local authority about the infestation of schistosomiasis before being exposed to freshwater in countries that are likely to have the disease.

- Do not swim, stand, wade, or take baths in untreated water.

QUESTIONS TO ASK YOUR DOCTOR

- Should I be concerned about schistosomiasis, given my travel plans?
- What precautions can I take to avoid the infection during my trip?
- I swam in a body of water that I later discovered was contaminated with schistosomes. What should I do now?

- Treat all water used for drinking or bathing. Water can be treated by letting it stand for three days, heating it for five minutes to around 122°F (around 50°C), or filtering or treating water chemically, with chlorine or iodine, as with drinking water.

- Should accidental exposure occur, infection can be prevented by hastily drying off or applying rubbing alcohol to the exposed area.

EFFECTS ON PUBLIC HEALTH. With nearly a quarter of a billion people infected with schistosomiasis, and many more at risk, schistosomiasis is a worldwide health concern. Travelers to areas where schistosomiasis is prevalent may inadvertently contract the infection by drinking contaminated water or swimming in contaminated areas.

COSTS TO SOCIETY. Chronic schistosomiasis reduces the capacity of infected to work and contribute to their family's finances. Since the infections are common in developing countries, any decrease in income can severely impact the family's basic living expenses. In some cases, schistosomiasis can also result in death. The World Health Organization estimates that 200,000 people per year die due to schistosomiasis in sub-Saharan Africa alone.

EFFORTS AND SOLUTIONS. The World Health Organization is targeting schistosomiasis and has issued recommendations for the use of anthelminthic drugs to control schistosomiasis in poor and marginalized communities. It recommends treatment with praziquantel at least three times during childhood (no younger than four years of age) to prevent disease in adulthood. It also recommends treatment for other at-risk populations, including entire communities living in endemic areas. It does not recommend treatment for children younger than four years of age, although medical professionals may recommend treatment for these young children on an individual basis.

Other organizations are also developing strategies to fight schistosomiasis. The Carter Center, for example, is undertaking a large initiative to provide both education about the illness, and schistosomiasis treatment in Nigeria, where the illness is very common. The Carter Center estimated the cost of preventative treatment at approximately 18 cents per dose, an inexpensive alternative to what may otherwise become a debilitating and perhaps deadly infection.

Resources

BOOKS

Carvalho E.M., and A.A.M. Lima. "Schistosomiasis (Bilharziasis)." In: Goldman L., A.I. Schafer, eds. *Cecil Medicine*. 24th edition. Philadelphia, PA: Saunders Elsevier (2011): chapter 363.

WEBSITES

"Epidemiological Situation." World Health Organization. http://www.who.int/schistosomiasis/epidemiology/en/ (accessed November 11, 2012).

"Initiative for Vaccine Research." World Health Organization. http://www.who.int/vaccine_research/diseases/soa_parasitic/en/index5.html (accessed November 11, 2012).

MedlinePlus"Schistosomiasis." U.S. National Library of Medicine, National Institutes of Health. http://www.nlm.nih.gov/medlineplus/ency/article/001321.htm (accessed November 11, 2012).

"Parasites—Schistosomiasis." U.S. Centers for Disease Control and Prevention. http://www.cdc.gov/parasites/schistosomiasis/ (accessed November 11, 2012).

PubMedHealth. "Schistosomiasis." U.S. National Library of Medicine. http://www.ncbi.nlm.nih.gov/pubmedhealth/PMH0002298/ (accessed November 11, 2012).

"Schistosomiasis Control Program." Carter Center. http://www.cartercenter.org/health/schistosomiasis/index.html (accessed November 11, 2012).

"Schistosomiasis Strategy." International Association for Medical Assistance to Travelers. http://www.iamat.org/disease_details.cfm?id=139 (accessed November 11, 2012).

"Schistosomiasis Strategy." World Health Organization. http://www.who.int/schistosomiasis/strategy/en/ (accessed November 11, 2012).

"Schistosomiasis." World Health Organization. http://www.who.int/schistosomiasis/en/ (accessed November 11, 2012).

ORGANIZATIONS

Carter Center, 1 Copenhill, 453 Freedom Parkway, Atlanta, GA 30307, (800) 550-3560, carterweb@emory.edu, http://www.cartercenter.org

World Health Organization, Avenue Appia 20, 1211 Geneva 27, Switzerlandhttp://www.who.int/

Ruth E. Mawyer, R.N.
Leslie Mertz, Ph.D.

School health

Definition

The American School Health Association (ASHA) defines school health as "all the strategies, activities, and services offered by, in, or in association with schools that are designed to promote students' physical, emotional, and social development make up a school's health program."

Purpose

The purpose of school health programs is to educate children about the types of behavior that will result in a healthy life both at the present time and throughout one's adult life.

Description

Public health officials generally agree that it is easier and more efficient to teach good health habits early in life than to trying to correct incorrect health habits later in life. For that reason, schools have a special role in establishing the types of behavior that will lead to a healthier and safer life for most individuals. More than 95% of adolescents in the United States spend an average of six hours a day for up to 13 years in schools, so the educational environment is an ideal setting in which to provide instruction and education about good health practices.

A school health program is, ideally, a mixture of a number of programs and activities, one of which is formal classes in **health education**. Health education can be offered as stand-alone classes or as units in other types of classes in every grade from kindergarten through grade 12. Among the topics typically included in such classes are alcohol, tobacco, and other drug use and abuse, proper **nutrition**, mental and emotional health, personal health and wellness, **physical activity**, safety and injury prevention, sexual health, and **violence** prevention. In 1995, a group of federal agencies and private organizations met to develop a set of eight National Health Education Standards (NHES) that serve as a framework for an effective school health education program. Those standards are:

• Students will comprehend concepts related to health promotion and disease prevention to enhance health.

• Students will analyze the influence of family, peers, culture, media, technology, and other factors on health behaviors.

• Students will demonstrate the ability to access valid information, products, and services to enhance health.

Minimum nutrient and calorie levels for school lunches*

[traditional menu planning approach]

Nutrient and energy allowances	Preschool	Grades K–3	Grades 4–12	Optional Grades 7–12
Calories	517	633	785	825
Total fat	1	1	1	1
Saturated fat	2	2	2	2
Protein (g)	7	9	15	16
Calcium (mg)	267	267	370	400
Iron (mg)	3.3	3.3	4.2	4.5
Vitamin A (RE)³	150	200	285	300
Vitamin C (mg)	14	15	17	18

*School week averages
[1]Total fat not to exceed 30 percent of calories
[2]Saturated fat to be less than 10 percent of calories
[3]Retinol equivalent (1 mcg of retinol or 6 mcg of beta carotene)

SOURCE: U.S. Department of Agriculture, "Chapter 1: Nutrient Standards," *Nutrient Analysis Protocols: How to Analyze Menus for USDA's School Meals Programs.*

(Table by PreMediaGlobal. © 2013 Cengage Learning)

- Students will demonstrate the ability to use interpersonal communication skills to enhance health and avoid or reduce health risks.

- Students will demonstrate the ability to use decision-making skills to enhance health.

- Students will demonstrate the ability to use goal-setting skills to enhance health.

- Students will demonstrate the ability to practice health-enhancing behaviors and avoid or reduce health risks.

- Students will demonstrate the ability to advocate for personal, family, and community health.

The NHES also provide specific performance indicators at each grade level to assess an individual's success in accomplishing each of the eight goals. As an example, a performance indicator for standard 1 at the grades K–2 level is that the student should be able to describe why it is important to seek health care, while a performance indicator for the same standard at grades 9–12 is that the student should be able to analyze the potential severity of injury or illness if engaging in unhealthy behaviors. The NHES are available online on a number of sites, including that of the **Centers for Disease Control and Prevention (CDC)** at http://www.cdc.gov/healthyyouth/sher/standards/index.htm.

A second element of a sound school health program is the presence of specially trained school health professionals who perform a wide variety of functions, including:

- Conduct various types of health assessments, such as individual health histories and screenings for vision, hearing, and other physical problems;

- Interpret the meaning of specific health tests for students, parents, teachers, and other school personnel;

- Initiate referrals for student health problems to parents, school personnel, and other health professionals;

- Provide individualized health counseling for students, parents, and school personnel;

- Make available individualized health care for certain types of health problems that can be handled at the school level;

- Design and develop procedures for dealing with emergency health problems that may develop at a school;

- Serve as a resource and consultant for in-school health education classes and programs;

- Participate in programs for the control of communicable diseases;

- Make home visits where appropriate and necessary to deal with individual health issues;

- Counsel with individual students about specialized health issues, such as pregnancy, gender orientation issues, and drug abuse;

- Advise and acts as a resource on possible health career choices for students; and

- Act as a coordinator among home, school, and community programs and activities.

Historically, these functions have often been performed by a designated school nurse, although other trained health professionals may also be responsible for the overall school health program.

In many schools, some of the responsibilities are performed by one or more individuals with special training in counseling and other psychological and social services. These staff members work not only with individual students, but also with the school community as a whole in dealing with personal, emotional, social, occupational, educational, community, and other types of psychological and sociological issues.

A third element of an effective school health program is the provision of nutritious lunches and other meals for students who would not otherwise have access to such meals. The concept of free or low-cost nutritious meals provided by state or federal governments for students has a very long history, dating back to at least 1790 in Europe and to about 1890 in the United States. The current school lunch program in the United States was created by the National School Lunch Act of 1946 and signed by President Harry S Truman. The National School Lunch Program (NSLP) currently operates in more than 100,000 public and private schools and other residential child care institutions. Although the program is paid for by the federal government, it is usually administered by state or local authorities. More than 31 million children receive at least one free or low-cost meal each school day through the program. Meals provided under the plan must meet certain federal standards for nutritional value, based on the latest version of the U.S. Department of Agriculture's (USDA) *Dietary Guidelines for Americans.* According to the most recent rules, children from families with incomes at or below 130% of the **poverty** level are eligible for free meals, while those with families with incomes between 130 and 185% of poverty level are eligible for meals at reduced price, which in no case can exceed 40 cents per meal. The federal government reimburses schools for these meals according to a scale that is adjusted from time to time. For the period July 1, 2012, to June 30, 2012, that reimbursement amounted to $2.86 for free lunches, $2.46 for reduced price lunches, and $0.27 for fully paid lunches. The government also reimburses schools for approved after-school snacks at a rate ranging from $0.07 to $0.78 per snack. These rates are adjusted for schools in Alaska and Hawaii and for school with especially high rates of students from low-income families. As part of the NSLP, the federal government also offers schools so-called entitlement and bonus foods available through special arrangement between the USDA and farmers, often as the result of surpluses in various types of crops. These foods may be provided to schools at no cost or at costs significantly less than market value.

Although devised and administered with the best possible objectives in mind, NSLP sometimes falls short of the best health program that it might be. The 2010 documentary film "Lunch" said that the average elementary school lunch averages 821 calories and that 80% of nation's schools do not meet federal standards for fat intake. One problem is that the so-called entitlement and bonus foods do not meet the nutritional standards established for the program. Red meats that make up a significant share of the bonus foods, for example, are generally higher in fat than generally considered best for school-age children. The Physicians Committee for Responsible Medicine (PCRM) annually conducts a national survey to assess the nutritional value of school lunch meals. It consistently finds that schools range from very high to very low on their School Lunch Report Card. In its 2008 report, for example, schools across the nation ranged from a low score of 42 points (out of 100) to a high of 99 points. These scores are based on a group of criteria associated with **obesity** and chronic disease prevention (55 points in all) and nutrition and healthy eating initiatives.

A school's lunch program is only one part of its overall school food environment, the complete set of food experiences to which a student is exposed at her or his school. Another part of many school food environments is vending machines, through which students can select additional foods and drinks to supplement their regular meals. According to the "Lunch" documentary, 43% of all U.S. elementary schools and 74% of all secondary schools contain at least one vending machine. And research has shown that students, when given the choice, tend to select sugary drinks at a far greater rate than any other item offered in the vending machine.

As a consequence, a number of states have now adopted relatively severe regulations as to the types of foods and drinks that may be offered in school vending machines. These regulations vary from state to state. For example, in Arkansas at least half of all drinks offered in vending machines or other school facilities must be 100% fruit juice, low-fat or fat-free milk, unflavored or unsweetened water; Connecticut prohibits the sale of any beverage not approved by the state, excluding virtually all sugary drinks; Mississippi permits the sale of bottled water, milk products, and pure fruit juices only at the elementary level, with some additional drinks permitted at the seconday level. Some states, such as Alaska and Montana, have no restrictions on the sale of food products through vending machines.

Yet another element of school health is a program of physical education that, in the words of the **CDC**, enables a person "to enjoy a lifetime of healthful physical activity." As with health education, a physical education program should involve a well-planned curriculum that includes formal instruction from grades K–12. The components of that program are outlined in a document, *Moving into the Future: National Standards for Physical Education*, revised most recently in 2004. The standards listed in that document are:

• Competency in motor skills and movement patterns needed to perform a variety of physical activities.

• Understanding of movement concepts, principles, strategies, and tactics as they apply to the learning and performance of physical activities.

• Regular participation in physical activity.

• Achievement and maintainenance of a health-enhancing level of physical fitness.

• Responsible personal and social behavior that respects self and others in physical activity settings.

• An appreciation of physical activity for health, enjoyment, challenge, self-expression, and/or social interaction.

Concern for school health also extends beyond student issues; it also involves the physical, mental, and emotionl health of teachers, administrators, parents, and other adults who are stakeholders in the educational process. A strong and healthy student body cannot achieve its maximum potential if any one of these additional elements is dealing with significant health problems of one kind or another of its own.

Finally, a healthy school population also depends on a healthy physical environment. Students and staff can not be expected to live a healthy existence in buildings that are old and decrepit or filled with hazardous materials and physical settings.

Demographics

The CDC conducts periodic surveys of the nation's schools to determine the extent to which they are meeting the goals for effective school health programs established by experts in the field. Some of the findings of the most recent survey (2006) are as follows:

• The most common health topics taught in formal classes or units at the elementary level were violence prevention (86.6% of all schools), nutrition and dietary behavior (84.6%), and injury prevention and safety (83.3%). The least popular topics were pregnancy prevention (16.4%), sexually transmitted infection prevention (21.7%), and suicide prevention (25.5%).

• The most common health topics in middle schools were alcohol and drug use prevention (84.6%), tobacco use prevention (84.0%), and nutrition and dietary behavior

(82.3%). The least popular topics were asthma awareness (47.0%), suicide prevention (54.4%), and foodborne illness prevention (60.0%).

• The most popular health topics at the senior-high level were alcohol and other drug use prevention (91.8%), tobacco use prevention (91.0%), and HIV prevention (88.4%), while the least popular topic was asthma awareness (53.8%), with all other topics scoring in the high 70% and 80% range.

• Daily physical education equivalent to 150 minutes per week for elementary students and 225 minutes per week for secondary students was provided by 3.8% of elementary schools, 7.9% of middle schools, and 2.1% of senior high schools.

• Just over 35% (35.7%) of all schools had a full-time (at least 30 hours a week) nurse, and an additional 50.6% had a part-time nurse.

• A part-time or full-time counselor was available at 77.9%, while 61.4% had a part-time or full-time school psychologist, and 41.7% had a part-time or full-time school social worker.

• Among a list of specific foods offered in a school cafeteria, the item most commonly offered to students at all levels, elementary, middle, and senior high school was fruit, and the least common, deep-fried potatoes.

• The areas in which most respondents appeared to be deficient was in faculty and staff care and community involvement. In the former case, just under a quarter of all school districts offered employee assistance programs designed to promote health efforts, and fewer than a third of all districts offered any type of health screening for their employees.

Resources

BOOKS

Gilbert, Glen G., Robin G. Sawyer, and Ellisa Beth McNeill. *Health Education: Creating Strategies for School & Community Health*, 3rd ed. Sudbury, MA: Jones & Bartlett Learning, 2009.

Meeks, Linda, Phillip Heit, and Randy Page. *Comprehensive School Health* 8th ed. New York: McGraw Hill, 2012.

Samdal, Oddrun, and Louise Rowling, eds. *The Implementation of Health Promoting Schools: Exploring the Theories of What, Why and How*. London: Routledge, 2013.

PERIODICALS

Clayton, S., et al. "Different Setting, Different Care: Integrating Prevention and Clinical Care in School-Based Health Centers." *American Journal of Public Health* 100, 9. (2010): 1592–96.

Keeton, V., S. Soleimanpour, and C.D. Brindis. "School-Based Health Centers in an Era of Health Care Reform: Building on History." *Current Problems in Pediatric and Adolescent Health Care* 42, 6. (2012): 132–56.

Tang, K.C., et al. "Schools for Health, Education and Development: A Call for Action." *Health Promotion International* 24, 1. (2009): 68–77.

WEBSITES

"Adolescent and School Health." Centers for Disease Control and Prevention. http://www.cdc.gov/healthyyouth/. Accessed September 30, 2012.

"Healthy School Lunches." Physicians Committee for Responsible Medicine. http://www.healthyschoollunches .org/. Accessed September 30, 2012.

"National School Lunch Program." United States Department of Agriculture. http://www.fns.usda.gov/cnd/lunch/. Accessed September 30, 2012.

"School Health." Medline Plus. http://www.nlm.nih.gov/ medlineplus/schoolhealth.html. Accessed September 30, 2012.

ORGANIZATIONS

American School Health Association (ASHA), 4340 East West Hwy., Suite 403, Bethedsa, MD USA 20814, 1 (301) 652–8072, Fax: 652–8077, info@ashaweb.org, http://www .ashaweb.org/

David E. Newton, Ed.D.

Scurvy

Definition

Scurvy is a condition caused by a lack of vitamin C (ascorbic acid) in the diet. Signs of scurvy include

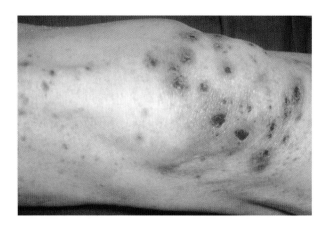

Scurvy, seen in secondary stage as bleeding wounds on limbs. *(BIOPHOTO ASSOCIATES/PRI/Gettyimages.com)*

tiredness, muscle weakness, joint and muscle aches, a rash on the legs, and bleeding gums. In the past, scurvy was common among sailors and other people deprived of fresh fruits and vegetables for long periods of time.

Description

Scurvy is very rare in countries where fresh fruits and vegetables are readily available and where processed foods have vitamin C added. Vitamin C is an important antioxidant vitamin involved in the development of connective tissues, lipid and vitamin metabolism, biosynthesis of neurotransmitters, immune function, and wound healing. It is found in fruits, especially citrus fruits like oranges, lemons, and grapefruit, and in green leafy vegetables like broccoli and spinach. In adults, it may take several months of vitamin C deficiency before symptoms of scurvy develop.

Currently, the recommended dietary allowance (RDA) for vitamin C is 50–60 milligrams per day (mg/ day) for adults; 35 mg/day for infants; 40–45 mg/day for children 1–14; 70 mg/day during pregnancy; and 90–95 mg/day during lactation. The body's need for vitamin C increases when a person is under **stress**, **smoking**, or taking certain medications.

Origins

The name "scurvy" is derived from the Latin word *scorbutus*. Humans have known about scurvy since ancient Greek and Egyptian times, as early as the middle of the second century B.C. It is commonly associated with sailors from the sixteenth to eighteenth centuries who frequently died from the condition while on long sea voyages. French explorer Jacques Cartier (1491–1557) first described scurvy in 1541 A.D. References to scurvy first appeared in print within the Oxford English

Dictionary in 1565. In the twenty-first century, cases of scurvy are rare.

Demographics

Hundreds of cases are reported each year in the United States, and even more are reported worldwide.

Causes and symptoms

There is one main cause of scurvy, but it can cause numerous symptoms.

Causes

A lack of vitamin C in the diet is the primary cause of scurvy. This can occur in people on very restricted diets, who are under extreme physiological stress (for example, during an infection or after an injury), and in chronic alcoholics. Infants can develop scurvy if they are weaned from breast milk and switched to cow's milk without an additional supplement of vitamin C. Babies of mothers who took extremely high doses of vitamin C during pregnancy can develop infantile scurvy.

Symptoms

In children, the deficiency can cause painful swelling of the legs along with fever, diarrhea, and vomiting. In adults, early signs of scurvy include feeling weak, tired, and achy. The appearance of tiny red blood-blisters to larger purplish blotches on the skin of the legs is a common symptom. Wound healing may be delayed, and scars that had healed may start to break down. The gums swell and bleed easily, eventually leading to loosened teeth. Muscle and joint **pain** may also occur.

Diagnosis

Scurvy is often diagnosed based on the symptoms present. A dietary history showing few or no fresh fruits or vegetables may help to diagnose vitamin C deficiency. A blood test can also be used to check the level of ascorbic acid in the body.

Prevention

Eating foods rich in vitamin C every day prevents scurvy. A supplement containing the recommended dietary allowance (RDA) of vitamin C will also prevent a deficiency. Infants who are being weaned from breast milk to cow's milk need a supplement containing vitamin C. People who eat the following foods, which have plenty of vitamin C, are unlikely to get scurvy:

- bell peppers
- blackcurrants

- broccoli
- cabbage
- carrots
- guava
- kiwifruit
- lemons
- liver
- oranges
- oysters
- papaya
- potatoes
- spinach
- strawberries
- tomatoes

Treatment

Adult treatment is usually 300–1,000 milligrams (mg) of ascorbic acid per day. Infants should be treated with 50 mg of ascorbic acid up to four times per day.

Prognosis

Treatment with vitamin C is usually successful if the deficiency is recognized early enough. Left untreated, the condition can cause death.

Precautions

Bottle-fed infants should be given orange juice. However, what should be given to breast-fed infants depends on the mother's diet. Ask professional advice from a pediatrician. In the elderly, eating adequate fruit and vegetables is the best way to avoid scurvy. Caregivers should carefully monitor elderly people who live alone. Ascorbic acid supplements can be given on a regular basis.

Risks

Because humans are unable to synthesize vitamin C, they must obtain it from external sources, such as citrus fruits. The risk comes when people do not obtain sufficient amounts of vitamin C from fruits and vegetables that contain or are fortified with vitamin C. When this happens, the vitamin C deficiency known as scurvy occurs. Though it is a rare disease, it still occurs in some high-risk patients such as alcoholics, the elderly, or those on diets lacking fresh fruits and vegetables. Infants and children on special or poor diets may also be at a higher risk for contracting scurvy.

Resources

BOOKS

Bown, Stephen R. *Scurvy: How a Surgeon, a Mariner, and a Gentleman Solved the Greatest Medical Mystery of the Age of Sail.* New York: Thomas Dunne Books, 2004.

Carpenter, Kenneth J. *The History of Scurvy and Vitamin C.* Cambridge: Cambridge University Press, 1988.

Frankenburg, Frances Rachel. *Vitamin Discoveries and Disasters: History, Science, and Controversies.* Westport, CT: Praeger, 2009.

WEBSITES

Scurvy. eMedicine, Medscape. (August 8, 2011). http://emedicine.medscape.com/article/125350-overview. (accessed August 15, 2012).

What Is Scurvy? What Causes Scurvy? Medical News Today. (June 30, 2009). http://www.medicalnewstoday.com/articles/155758.php. (accessed August 15, 2012).

ORGANIZATIONS

American Medical Association, 515 N. State St., Chicago, IL (800) 621-8335, http://www.ama-assn.org/

Altha Roberts Edgren
William A. Atkins, B.B., B.S., M.B.A.

Secondhand smoke

Definition

Secondhand smoke is tobacco smoke that is inhaled involuntarily or passively by a person who is not **smoking**. That person may inhale smoke that is either exhaled by a person who is smoking a cigarette, cigar, or pipe (exhaled smoke is known as "mainstream" smoke), or generated from smoldering tobacco (known as "sidestream" smoke). Secondhand smoke contains at least 69 chemicals that are known to cause lung **cancer**, even in nonsmokers. Secondhand smoke increases the likelihood of **heart disease**, including heart attacks, and various breathing problems.

DESCRIPTION. Secondhand smoke, also known as "passive smoking" or "environmental tobacco smoke" causes disease and premature death for nonsmoking adults and children, because tobacco smoke contains toxic chemicals that increase health risks. The amount of smoke created by a tobacco product is related to the amount of tobacco in that product. According to the National Cancer Institute, secondhand smoke emitted from one large cigar is similar to that of an entire pack of cigarettes. Because of tobacco's effects on both smokers and nonsmokers, smoking constitutes a universal public health risk.

Babies and young children are especially susceptible to the effects of secondhand smoke. According to the **Tobacco Control** Research Branch of the National Cancer Institute through its smokefree.gov website:

- Babies who are exposed to secondhand smoke after birth, or whose mothers smoked while pregnant, are more likely to die from sudden infant death syndrome than babies who do not breathe secondhand smoke.

- Mothers who breathe secondhand smoke while pregnant are more likely to have a baby weighing 5.5 pounds or less. Underweight babies often experience serious health problems.

- Bronchitis, pneumonia, and other lung problems, as well as middle-ear infections, are more common among children who have smoking parents.

DEMOGRAPHICS. Secondhand smoke can affect anyone anywhere. Approximately 126 million Americans are exposed to secondhand smoke at home and at work.

Studies show that secondhand smoke exposure has, however, declined. To determine exposure, scientists measure the level of a substance called cotinine in bodily fluids. Cotinine is a byproduct produced as the body breaks down nicotine inhaled from tobacco smoke. During 1988–1991, about 87.9% of nonsmokers had

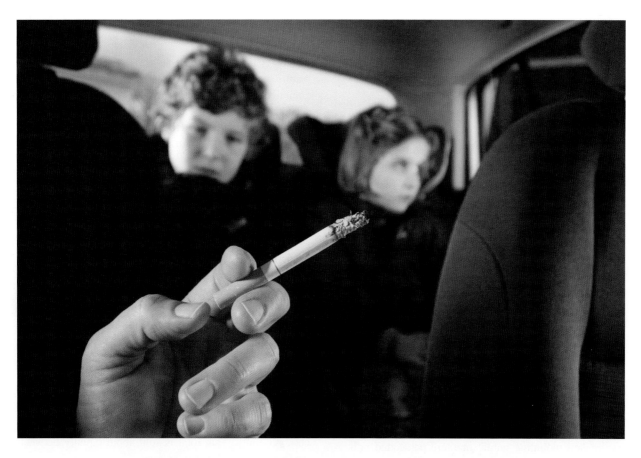

Children ingesting second hand smoke as a parent smokes in the car. *(© iStockphoto.com/Richard Clark)*

measurable levels of cotinine. The proportion dropped to 52.5% in 1999–2000, and to 40.1% in 2007–2008, according to a report from the **Centers for Disease Control and Prevention (CDC)**. Those declines are correlated with the increasing number of smoking restrictions (bans) in the workplace and in public places, such as restaurants; the decline in smoking rates overall, and the rise in the number of private citizens who restrict smoking in their own homes.

Cotinine levels are detected at higher levels in certain racial and ethnic groups. While the cotinine levels of 40.1% of non-Hispanic whites reveal exposure to secondhand smoke, the proportion of exposed Mexican Americans is just 28.5%. Among non-Hispanic blacks, however, the proportion is 55.9%. In addition, second-hand smoke exposure is high—60.5%—among low-income individuals.

CAUSES AND SYMPTOMS.

Causes

Secondhand smoke contains dozens of cancer-causing chemicals. These include arsenic, benzene, nickel, and vinyl chloride. It also contains about 7,000 other chemicals, hundreds of which are known to be toxic. Some of these include formaldehyde and toluene.

Symptoms

Many patients experiencing effects of secondhand smoke report coughing, increased phlegm production, and breathing problems. Those who have other conditions associated with secondhand smoke, such as heart disease, bronchitis, or cancer, have various symptoms indicative of those illnesses.

DIAGNOSIS. Secondhand smoke exposure may be measured by checking the indoor air for nicotine or other chemicals that are found in tobacco smoke. The urine, blood, or saliva of a nonsmoker may also be tested for levels of cotinine.

PREVENTION. The most effective way to prevent the dangers of secondhand smoke is to avoid those places where smoking occurs. This can be difficult, especially if a family member smokes at home, a friend lights up in a car, or if a coworker puffs a cigarette at a workplace. Although restrictions are now in place to prohibit smoking in many public places, secondhand smoke is common in the everyday environment, and neither air-cleaning systems nor ventilation can fully eliminate secondhand smoke exposure, according to the **CDC**.

Origins

Takeshi Hirayama published the first study that examined the relationship between passive smoking and lung cancer in 1981, concluding that wives of heavy smokers were more likely to develop lung cancer than wives of nonsmokers. This discovery spurred an increase in scientific research on secondhand smoke in the following decades. Although many scientists supported Hirayama's conclusions, others countered his claim. The most notable opponents were those funded by the tobacco industry and related businesses.

Scientific findings often gained attention through news media. The sustained interest in secondhand smoke remained in media headlines following claims proposed by nonsmokers' rights groups such as Americans for Nonsmokers' Rights (ANR), the U.S. Surgeon General, and other advocates, in conjunction with counterclaims made by the tobacco industry.

The argument of secondhand smoke as a public health issue convinced employees of smoking establishments, as well as the general public, that passive smoking posed a serious health risk. Shortly thereafter, interested parties and mounting public pressure persuaded policymakers to take legal action against smoking in public places.

Despite the general public's contribution to tobacco-control policies, many people rejected the scientific findings and did not support public smoking bans. Antagonists presented their opinions through legal, moral, and economic frameworks. First, smokers were upset by bans because many believed that smoking is a First Amendment right. Second, establishments that depend on a high proportion of smoking clientele argued that their businesses would suffer from the legal restriction. Similarly, the tobacco industry also fought smoking bans on grounds it would hurt their industry.

In particular, the tobacco industry challenged a 1993 report issued by the **Environmental Protection Agency (EPA)** stating that 3,000 lung cancer deaths result from passive smoking each year. This report encouraged many private establishments and communities to pass smoking bans. Representatives of tobacco companies claimed that **EPA** manipulated scientific findings by selecting only cases that supported their hypothesis. In 1998, U.S. District Court Judge William Osteen sided with the tobacco industry, declaring that EPA did not follow accepted scientific procedures. Nonetheless, the U.S. Court of Appeals for the Fourth Circuit overturned this decision in 2002 on technical grounds. As of 2012, many

states have mandated bans to reduce exposure to secondhand smoke.

EFFECTS ON PUBLIC HEALTH. Secondhand smoke results in nearly 50,000 deaths in adult nonsmokers annually, including about 3,400 due to lung disease and 46,000 due to heart disease. Nonsmokers who are exposed to secondhand smoke at home or at work have a 25–30% higher risk for heart disease, and a 20–30% higher risk for lung cancer.

Infants and children are more susceptible to the effects of secondhand smoke, yet among those aged six or younger, almost 3 million (11%) are exposed to secondhand smoke at least four days per week. As many as 300,000 children and infants experience **pneumonia**, bronchitis and other respiratory infections as a result, and up to 15,000 are hospitalized each year. Secondhand smoke also can cause severe attacks among children who already have **asthma**. More than 40% of all children who are rushed to an emergency room for severe asthma attacks live in homes with smokers. In addition, according to the **Environmental Protection Agency**, secondhand smoke can cause new cases of asthma in children who have not previously shown symptoms.

COSTS TO SOCIETY. According to a 2005 study, secondhand smoke is a $10 billion per year drain on the U.S. economy. That total is split about equally between medical costs and lost wages.

Efforts and solutions

Smoking Bans

The first smoking bans in the United States, in the late 1980s, restricted smoking on domestic flights. In the following decade, EPA, the U.S. National Institute of Occupational Safety and Health, and other government agencies joined the U.S. Surgeon General in the fight against secondhand smoke. In 1995, New York City and California became the first major regions to enact tobacco restrictions in restaurants; several years later they extended the ban to other public places.

One of the strongest arguments that pushed public smoking bans was from employees who worked in establishments where smoking was allowed. Workers argued that their health was in jeopardy from constant exposure to the secondhand smoke of coworkers or patrons in their establishments. Proponents for smoking bans argued that the removal of environmental tobacco smoke is necessary for several reasons. Aside from the danger in certain establishments, where smoking would interfere with flammable materials or general cleanliness, workers claimed that passive smoking increased health risks of heart disease, cancer, and respiratory-related problems. For example, in New York City, Mayor Michael Bloomberg supported employees who framed passive smoking as a safety issue. As a former smoker himself, Mayor Bloomberg advocated for the New York City Clean Air Act of 2003, which then expanded to a statewide ban several months later.

In the United States, each state has jurisdiction to enact smoking bans. From 2000 to 2010, the number of states (including the District of Columbia) that had enacted laws to prohibit smoking in indoor areas of worksites, restaurants, and bars increased from zero to 26, according to the CDC's April 22, 2011, Morbidity and Mortality Weekly Report. It went on to state, "However, regional disparities remain in policy adoption, with no southern state having adopted a smoke-free law that prohibits smoking in all three venues."

In its 2011 report "Saving Lives, Saving Money," the American Cancer Society's Cancer Action Network made several policy recommendations, including one stipulating that smoke-free laws should cover all workplaces, including such places as casinos, hookah bars, and tobacco retail stores, which are often exempt. It also recommended that each of these locations should be 100% smoke-free, and that state smoke-free laws should not preclude local authorities from taking even stronger action.

Other

Besides public smoking bans, additional efforts may contribute to reducing secondhand smoke. These include taxation, media campaigns, increasing law enforcement for underage users, advertisement restrictions, youth education, cessation services, and other programs, laws, and policies that focus on prevention and helping current smokers to quit. A reduction in smoking is also a reduction in secondhand smoke.

Research Perspectives

Research on secondhand smoke covers a variety of perspectives. Chemical and biological scientists evaluate the health effects of environmental tobacco smoke and the chemical composition of emitted fumes. Policy analysts decipher the level of public support of smoking bans, if businesses comply with legislation, and what additional policies aid overall effectiveness (e.g., media campaigns, tobacco taxes). Social scientists study patterns of smoking use by social identities (e.g., age, race/ethnicity, gender, class, national origin, religion), psychological factors (e. g., mental history, **addiction**), or family and neighborhood characteristics. However, so far little research evaluates the effect of legislation on particular social groups.

Researchers find that smoking bans, taxation, and media campaigns have the greatest deterrent effect on

---

KEY TERMS

Mainstream smoke—The tobacco smoke exhaled by a smoker

Nicotine—A substance found in tobacco and other plants of the nightshade family (Solanaceae) that acts as a stimulant. Nicotine is highly addictive.

Sidestream smoke—The smoke emitted from burning tobacco (not exhaled by a smoker).

---

smoking rates. They argue that states with smoking bans use cigarettes less per capita than states without similar legislation. Businesses that implement smoking bans report reductions in quantity and frequency of cigarettes smoked. Studies in countries outside the United States show similar usage patterns. Research also suggests that smoking bans affect youth smoking.

The effect of smoking bans varies by the strictness of legislation. Policies that do not ban smoking completely but include areas specifically designated for smokers affect smoking rates far less than total bans. Enforcement also influences policy success. Government involvement to enact legislation is more successful than private organization policies. Therefore, individual compliance is more likely under public laws compared to private rules. However, businesses do not always agree with government policy. Widespread legislation imposes policies that some private businesses often disfavor or zealously challenge.

Resources

BOOKS

Committee on Secondhand Smoke Exposure and Acute Coronary Events. *Secondhand Smoke Exposure and Cardiovascular Effects: Making Sense of the Evidence.* Washington, D.C.: National Academies Press, 2010.

U.S. Department of Health and Human Services. *How Tobacco Smoke Causes Disease: The Biology and Behavioral Basis for Smoking-Attributable Disease: A Report of the Surgeon General..* Atlanta, GA: U.S. Department of Health and Human Services, Centers for Disease Control and Prevention, National Center for Chronic Disease Prevention and Health Promotion, Office on Smoking and Health, 2010.

PERIODICALS

Centers for Disease Control and Prevention. "Vital Signs: Nonsmokers' Exposure to Secondhand Smoke—United States, 1999–2008." *Morbidity and Mortality Weekly Report* 59, no. 35 (2010): 1141–1146.

WEBSITES

"Fact Sheet: National Survey on Environmental Management of Asthma and Children's Exposure to Environmental

---

Tobacco Smoke." Environmental Protection Agency. http://www.epa.gov/smokefre/pdfs/survey_fact_sheet.pdf (accessed August 28, 2012).

"Health Effects of Exposure to Secondhand Smoke." Environmental Protection Agency. http://www.epa.gov/smokefre/healtheffects.html (accessed August 28, 2012).

"Saving Lives, Saving Money: A State by State Report on the Health and Economic Impact of Comprehensive Smoke-Free Laws." Cancer Action Network, American Cancer Society. http://www.acscan.org/pdf/tobacco/reports/acscan-smoke-free-laws-report.pdf (accessed August 28, 2012).

"Secondhand Smoke and Cancer." National Cancer Institute. http://www.cancer.gov/cancertopics/factsheet/Tobacco/ETS (accessed August 28, 2012).

Smoke-Free.gov. "Secondhand Smoke." Tobacco Control Research Branch of the National Cancer Institute. http://smokefree.gov/topic-secondhand_smoke.aspx (accessed August 28, 2012).

U.S. Department of Health and Human Services. "The Health Consequences of Involuntary Exposure to Tobacco Smoke: A Report of the Surgeon General." http://www.surgeongeneral.gov/library/reports/secondhandsmoke/index.html (accessed August 28, 2012).

ORGANIZATIONS

Americans for Nonsmokers' Rights, 2530 San Pablo Avenue, Suite J, Berkeley, CA 94702, (510) 841-3032, http://www.no-smoke.org/index.php

Centers for Disease Control and Prevention (CDC), 1600 Clifton Road, Atlanta, GA 30333, (800) 232-4636, cdcinfo@cdc.gov, http://www.cdc.gov

National Cancer Institute, 6116 Executive Boulevard, Suite 300, Bethesda, MD 20892-8322, (800) 422-6237, http://www.cancer.gov/

Leslie Mertz, Ph.D.

Senior health

Definition

Seniors health refers to the physical and mental conditions of senior citizens, those who are in their 60s and older.

DESCRIPTION. For seniors, the **aging** process and an individual's lifestyle will affect health. People who maintain a healthy weight, exercise regularly, and eat nutritionally reduce the risk for many health conditions. This wellness allows people to live longer and to remain independent for more years. **Smoking**, **obesity** (excess weight), and lack of exercise shorten **life expectancy** and increase the risk for many health conditions.

According to the **Centers for Disease Control and Prevention**, about 80% of people in the United States age 65 and older have at least one chronic (long-lasting) condition and 50% have two.

Diet and exercise

Proper diet and regular exercise form the foundation of senior health. A nutritional diet and **physical activity** can help prevent diseases such as **cancer**, **stroke**, **heart disease**, and diabetes. A healthy diet also can help manage diabetes, high blood pressure, and heart disease.

As people age, regular exercise is especially important. According to the U.S. Department of Health and Human Services' Agency for Healthcare Research and Quality, the inactive person loses from 3–5% of muscle fiber each decade after age 30. Yet, nearly 40% of people over the age of 55 report having no leisure-time physical activity.

Exercise can help to

• boost muscle strength

• improve balance and coordination

• prevent falls

• prevent bone loss (osteoporosis)

• lower the risk of conditions such as heart disease, type 2 diabetes, colon cancer, stress, and depression

• extend the lives of people with conditions such as diabetes, high blood pressure, and high cholesterol

• prevent serious illness or death from common infections.

Demographics

The U.S. Administration on Aging, in its report "A Profile of Older Americans: 2011," noted that the **population** aged 65 and older numbered 40.4 million in 2010, an increase of 5.4 million or 15.3% since 2000. In addition, that number is projected to rise to 55 million by 2020 (a 36% increase for that decade).

PROGNOSIS. A number of health problems begin to occur as an individual ages. Early recognition of these conditions and proper treatment can improve a senior's health and longevity.

Osteoporosis

Osteoporosis is a condition in which bones become less dense (solid). Bones become brittle and thinner and break easily. The risk of osteoporosis increases as a person ages. According to the U.S. Department of Health and Human Services' Healthy People initiative, an estimated 5.3 million Americans aged 50 years and older have osteoporosis. Of that total, 4.5 million are women.

Another 34 million additional Americans, people—22 million women and 12 million men—have low bone mass and are therefore at increased risk for developing osteoporosis. Approximately half of all women and as many as a quarter of all men will experience a fracture related to osteoporosis in their lifetimes.

Osteoarthritis

Osteoarthritis is a joint disease in which cartilage wears out, and bones rub against each other. This condition can occur gradually over time as activities performed throughout the years cause wear on joints. In addition, bones thin as a person ages. About one in five Americans experiences some form of arthritis, and it is the most common cause of disability, according to the Health People initiative. It generally affects the neck, fingers, lower back, knees, and toes. Symptoms include **pain**, stiffness, swelling, and creaking. The pain may disrupt sleep, and joint stiffness may make it difficult for a person to dress.

Falls

Each year, a third of all adults aged 65 or older will fall, according to the Centers for Disease Control and **Prevention**. For seniors, fall-related injuries can reduce mobility and hinder independence. Falls are an issue with older individuals, because as people age, slower reflexes, combined with deteriorating vision and hearing, and other health issues may increase the likelihood of a fall. Falls can result in broken bones or fractures, especially in bones that are weakened by osteoporosis. Head injuries can affect sight and hearing. Because healing takes longer in older people, injuries sustained during falls have the potential to reduce an active person's mobility and independence.

Vision

Eyesight changes as people age. Generally, people are in their 40s when they experience presbyopia, a form of farsightedness. This is a progressive condition involving a decrease in the eye's ability to focus on close objects (near vision). By age 65, little near-focusing ability remains.

Glaucoma is a condition caused by pressure from the build-up of a large amount of fluid in the eye. This progressive condition is often seen in people in their 50s. It starts with the gradual loss of peripheral vision. If not treated, it can lead to vision loss.

People in their 60s may experience the first signs of age-related macular degeneration (AMD), a progressive condition that can result in blindness.

More than half of people age 65 or older will be diagnosed with cataracts. Cataract refers to the loss of the transparency in the lens of the eye. As the loss progresses, the person is able to see less detail. This condition generally affects both eyes.

Hearing

Presbycusis, age-related **hearing loss**, is a progressive condition that usually starts with a difficulty in hearing high-frequency sound such as people talking. Background noise makes it even more difficult to hear. Presbycusis affects approximately 40%–66% of people older than 75, and more than 80% of those older than 85. Many people diagnosed with this condition report feelings of dizziness and a ringing in their ears.

Sleep disorders

Many people in their 60s and 70s experience less time in the stages of deep sleep known as "delta sleep." Despite this change, many healthy older people do not experience sleep disorders. Overall health plays a role in whether a senior experiences trouble sleeping.

Some seniors' sleep is affected by snoring and sleep apnea. A person with apnea stops breathing for up to one minute until the brain restarts the breathing process. This action can be repeated several hundred times each night.

Furthermore, a senior's sleep can be disrupted by conditions such as arthritis, osteoporosis, and Alzheimer's disease. Insomnia, or the inability to stay asleep, is a symptom of conditions including depression, anxiety, chronic pain, and restless leg syndrome (movement of legs when a person is at rest).

Mental health

While age has little effect on the mind, social and emotional factors affect an older person's health. For instance, after a lifetime of work, a person who has been identified for years by a profession may experience a sense of lost identity. A senior may find that their thinking process has changed. Learning something new may take longer. However, older people have excellent recall of new information. Memory loss, on the other hand, may be a concern, particularly since this is a symptom of Alzheimer's disease.

Dementia

Alzheimer's disease is a form of dementia, a condition in which mental abilities decline. Symptoms of dementia include memory loss that goes beyond forgetting a word or where an item was placed. The person with dementia may no longer recognize family members or remember how to perform everyday functions, such as preparing a meal. Sometimes they experience a change in personality, with some uncharacteristic aggression or paranoia.

Alzheimer's disease is the most prevalent form of dementia. The risk of Alzheimer's increases as a person ages. The condition affects one in eight people over the age of 65. As of 2012, 5.4 million Americans had Alzheimer's disease, and by 2050, that number will climb as high as 30 million, according to the Alzheimer's Association.

PRECAUTIONS. A health condition may result in a doctor recommending against some forms of exercise. Even if a person cannot jog, other forms of exercise include those designed for people in wheelchairs and those who are bedridden.

TREATMENT. Costs of medical treatments vary, depending on the condition and the individual's health.

Vision and hearing

A senior should schedule periodic vision exams because early treatment helps prevent or lessen a risk of cataracts or glaucoma. Eye exams can also diagnose presbyopia and provide a prescription for bifocals or reading glasses.

Seniors are sometimes reluctant to acknowledge a hearing difficulty. This is unfortunate, because a wide range of always-improving hearing aids are available. An audiologist administers tests to determine the amount of hearing loss and can help the patient make a choice of an aid that works well.

Sleep disorders

For seniors who experience snoring and sleep apnea, a doctor may advise the individual to quit smoking, to lose weight, to reduce alcohol consumption, or to sleep on his or her side. In some cases, a doctor may refer the senior to a sleep-disorder clinic. The senior may be prescribed a continuous positive airway pressure device, known as a CPAP, that is placed over the nose and administers a continuous flow of air.

Insomnia treatments include exercising and treating depression, **stress**, and other causes of sleeplessness. Restless leg syndrome may be treated with prescription drugs.

Mental health

After retirement, a senior must find activities and interests to provide a sense of fulfillment and to avoid feelings of loneliness and isolation that can lead to depression and susceptibility to poor health. A senior may opt to start an exercise program, take up hobbies, take classes, or volunteer. Senior centers offer numerous activities. Lunch programs provide nutritional meals and companionship.

A doctor can assist with other mental-health issues, such as a diagnosis of Alzheimer's disease or depression.

PROGNOSIS. Seniors should maintain a schedule of regular exercise in order to remain mobile and continue living independently. Regular exercise can also help shorten recovery time following surgery, prevent falls, and bring other quality-of-life benefits. If mobility becomes limited due to a condition such as osteoarthritis, seniors should discuss options with a doctor and work with a physical or occupational therapist to remain as active and independent as possible.

Seniors who stay active and eat healthy are at less risk for many health conditions, such as diabetes. Mental stimulation and social interaction provide enjoyment, boost self-esteem, and help reduce feelings of isolation and depression. Although eyesight and hearing may weaken, glasses and hearing aids can help seniors keep their sight and hearing.

PREVENTION. Overall, the best course of action for a healthy life is regular exercise, proper **nutrition**, and a socially active lifestyle. In addition, men and women should consult their doctors about important screening exams, such as bone density, **hepatitis** C, or colonoscopies, to help maintain good health and catch any health conditions as early as possible. Women may also wish to consult a doctor about issues arising from menopause and the options afforded through natural remedies or hormone replacement therapy.

Exercise

Physical activity should be rhythmic and repetitive and should challenge the circulatory system. It also should be enjoyable so that a senior gets in the habit of exercising regularly for 30 minutes each day. It may be necessary to check with a doctor to determine the type of exercise that can be done.

Walking is recommended for weight loss, stress release, and many other conditions. Brisk walking is said to produce the same benefits as jogging. Other forms of exercise can include gardening, bicycling, hiking, swimming, dancing, or ice skating. If the weather prohibits outdoor activities, a person can work out indoors with an exercise video.

Exercise also offers a chance to socialize. In some cities, groups of seniors meet for regular walks at shopping malls. Senior centers offer exercise classes ranging from line dancing to belly dancing.

Fall prevention starts with regular exercise such as walking. This improves balance and muscles. The walk route should be on level ground. Other methods for preventing falls include:

- moving slowly when rising from a chair or bed to avoid dizziness
- quitting smoking
- wearing shoes with low heels and rubber soles
- monitoring medications because of side effects that increase the probability of a fall
- checking vision and hearing periodically
- fall-proofing the home, including the installation of lighting, especially on stairways, clearing clutter and electrical cords that can cause falls, and installing handrails and strips in bathtubs as well as rails on stairs

Nutrition

Nutrition plays an important role in senior health. Not only does a well-balanced diet keep a person from becoming obese, that same diet is a safeguard against health conditions that seniors face. Proper diet can help prevent a condition like diabetes or keep it from worsening.

The senior diet should consist of foods that are low in fat, particularly saturated fat and cholesterol. A person should choose foods that provide nutrients such as iron and calcium. Other healthy menu choices include:

- fish, skinless poultry, and lean meat
- proteins such as dry beans (red beans, navy beans, and soybeans), lentils, chickpeas, and peanuts
- low-fat dairy products
- vegetables, especially those that are dark green and leafy
- citrus fruits or juices, melons, and berries
- whole grains like wheat, rice, oats, corn, and barley
- whole grain breads and cereals

DESCRIPTION. Elder abuse can take place anywhere, but the sites of the abuse are often the elder's home, the caregiver's home, or an institutional setting, such as a nursing home or group home. Elder abuse can be divided into five basic types:

- Physical. Physical abuse refers to physical force that causes bodily harm to an elderly person, such as slapping, pushing, kicking, pinching, or burning.
- Sexual. Any kind of non-consensual sexual contact with an elderly person that takes place without his or her consent is considered sexual abuse. It may also include forcing an individual to view or to pose for suggestive photographs, or any other inappropriate activities.
- Emotional or psychological. The National Center on Elder Abuse defines emotional and psychological abuse

of a senior as causing anguish, pain, or distress through verbal or nonverbal acts, such as verbal assaults, insults, intimidation, and humiliation. Isolating elderly persons from their friends and family as well as giving them the silent treatment are two other forms of emotional and psychological abuse.

- Financial. Financial exploitation is defined as the use of an elderly person's resources without his or her consent.
- Neglect. Neglect occurs when a caretaker deprives an elderly person of the necessary care needed in order to avoid physical or mental harm. Sometimes the behavior of an elderly person threatens his or her own health; in those cases, the abuse is called "self-neglect." Depending on the specific definition of elder abuse used by an agency, self-neglect might not be included as a form of neglect.

Elder abuse

Although much elder abuse remains unreported, estimates suggest that about 10–14.1% of non-institutionalized Americans aged 60 and older are victims or elder abuse in any given year. Women, especially those over 80 years of age, tend to be victimized more than men. Other factors associated with a greater likelihood of an individual being subjected to elder abuse are: physical, cognitive, or mental impairment; clinical depression; limited or no social support; and previous exposure to a traumatic event.

Family members, usually spouses or adult children, are usually the perpetrators. Women are just as likely as men to be abusers. Additional factors associated with those inflicting elder abuse include: clinical depression; substance abuse; social isolation; and heightened stress caused by being a caregiver, especially of an elderly person who is cognitively impaired.

Causes and symptoms

Causes

Elder abuse is a complex problem that can be caused by many factors. According to the National Center on Elder Abuse, social isolation and mental impairment are two factors of elder abuse. Studies show that people advanced in years, such as in their eighties, with a high level of frailty and dependency are more likely to be victims of elder abuse than those who are younger and better equipped to stand up for themselves.

The risk of elder abuse appears to be especially high when adult children live with their elderly parents for financial reasons or because they have personal problems, such as drug dependency or mental illness. More research in this very important area is needed in order to illuminate the relationship between these factors.

Symptoms

The National Center on Elder Abuse identifies the following as signs of elder abuse:

- Bruises, pressure marks, broken bones, abrasions, and burns may indicate physical abuse or neglect.
- Unexplained withdrawal from normal activities and unusual depression may be indicators of emotional abuse.
- Bruises around the breasts or genital area, as well as unexplained bleeding around the genital area, may be signs of sexual abuse.
- Large withdrawals of money from an elder's bank account, sudden changes in a will, and the sudden disappearance of valuable items may be indications of financial exploitation.
- Bedsores, poor hygiene, unsanitary living conditions, and unattended medical needs may be signs of neglect.
- Failure to take necessary medicines, leaving a burning stove unattended, poor hygiene, confusion, unexplained weight loss, and dehydration may all be signs of self-neglect.

EFFECTS ON PUBLIC HEALTH. Everyone ages, and although individuals tend to develop chronic conditions as they get older, a healthy lifestyle can help them avoid disabilities that can affect their quality of life and their independence.

The graying of America—the increasing average age of individuals—is a cause for concern, because older people do and will need care. A 2009 U.S. Centers for Disease Control and Prevention Report Card stated that 35.3% of older adults reported that they were limited in their activities by a physical, mental, or emotional problem or that they used assistive equipment, such as a cane, wheelchair, or special telephone. New Jersey and Hawaii reported the lowest percentages at 29.5% and 29.9%, respectively. Alaska, Mississippi, and Oklahoma reported the highest percentages with 43.1%, 41.3%, and 41.3%, respectively. The average number of days that individuals reported feeling unwell in the previous month was 5.3. The average percentage of surveyed older adults who reported frequent mental distress was 6.7%.

COSTS TO SOCIETY. According to the U.S. Administration on Aging report "A Profile of Older Americans: 2011," consumers aged 65 or older had average out-of-pocket healthcare expenditures in 2010 of $4,843 (65% for insurance, 18% for medical services, 17% for drugs, and 3% for medical supplies). That total represented an increase of 49% since 2000. In addition, this population spent more than 13% of its total expenditures on health, about twice that spent (6.6%) by all consumers.

Falls alone are expensive. They are the leading cause of injury death for persons aged 65 and older, and about a third of adults in that population will fall each year, according to the **CDC**. In 2010, emergency departments treated 2.3 million nonfatal fall injuries among older adults, and more than 662,000 of those patients were hospitalized. The direct medical costs of falls, adjusted for inflation, was $30.0 billion in 2010.

EFFORTS AND SOLUTIONS. Federal, state, and local governments, along with a variety of organizations, encourage healthy living for older individuals. For instance, the U.S. **Department of Health and Human Services** in March 2012 awarded $1.3 billion in grants for programs "that help older adults live healthy, safely, and independently in their communities." These programs are designed to help this population avoid institutional care by emphasizing prevention and wellness, nutrition, family caregiver, and respite services. The department's Administration on Aging provides funding for nutrition and supportive home and community-based services; disease-prevention/health promotion services; elder-rights programs (long-term care ombudsman program, legal services, and elder-abuse prevention efforts); the National Family Caregiver Support Program; and the Native American Caregiver Support Program.

The National Council on Aging, which works with thousands of organizations across the country to help seniors improve their health, live independently, and maintain an active lifestyle, is a major organization advocating for senior health. A directory of many of the national health and aging organizations, as reviewed by the National Institute on Aging, is available at http://www.nia.nih.gov/health/resources.

Resources

BOOKS

Burton, John R., and William J. Hall *Taking Charge of Your Health*. Baltimore, MD: The Johns Hopkins University Press, 2010.

PERIODICALS

U.S. Administration on Aging. "A Profile of Older Americans: 2011." U.S. Department of Health and Human Services. http://www.aoa.gov/aoaroot/aging_statistics/Profile/2011/docs/2011profile.pdf (accessed September 17, 2012).

U.S. Centers for Disease Control and Prevention. "The State of Aging and Health in America Report." (2007). http://apps.nccd.cdc.gov/SAHA/Default/Default.aspx (accessed September 17, 2012).

WEBSITES

"2012 Alzheimer's Disease Facts and Figures." Alzheimer's Association. http://www.alz.org/documents_custom/2012_facts_figures_fact_sheet.pdf (accessed September 17, 2012).

AoA Press Office. "$1.3 billion to improve the health and independence of America's older adults." U.S.

Administration on Aging, Department of Health and Human Services. http://www.aoa.gov/AoARoot/Press_Room/For_The_Press/pr/archive/2012/March/2012_03_02.aspx (accessed September 17, 2012).

"Benefits of Physical Activity for Older Americans." American Heart Association. http://www.heart.org/HEARTORG/GettingHealthy/PhysicalActivity/StartWalking/Benefits-of-Physical-Activity-for-Older-Americans_UCM_308037_Article.jsp (accessed September 17, 2012).

"Falls Among Older Americans: An Overview." Centers for Disease Control and Prevention. http://www.cdc.gov/homeandrecreationalsafety/falls/adultfalls.html (accessed September 17, 2012).

Healthy People Initiative. "Arthritis, Osteoporosis, and Chronic Back Conditions." U.S. Department of Health and Human Services. http://www.healthypeople.gov/2020/topicsobjectives2020/overview.aspx?topicid=3 (accessed September 17, 2012).

National Institute on Aging Newsroom. "CDC recommends that all baby boomers get hepatitis C test." U.S. National Institutes of Health. http://www.nia.nih.gov/newsroom/announcements/2012/08/cdc-recommends-all-baby-boomers-get-hepatitis-c-test (accessed September 17, 2012).

National Institute on Aging. "Featured Health Topic: Healthy Aging/Longevity." U.S. National Institutes of Health. http://www.nia.nih.gov/health/featured/healthy-aging-longevity (accessed September 17, 2012).

National Institute on Aging. "Exercise and Physical Activity: Getting Fit for Life." U.S. National Institutes of Health. http://www.nia.nih.gov/health/publication/exercise-and-physical-activity-getting-fit-life (accessed September 17, 2012).

National Institute on Aging. "Health & Aging Organizations Directory." U.S. National Institutes of Health. http://www.nia.nih.gov/health/resources (accessed September 17, 2012).

ORGANIZATIONS

Division of Aging and Seniors, Health Canada, Public Health Agency of Canada, 1015 Arlington Street, Winnipeg, CanadaManitobaR3E 3R2, (204) 789-2000, ph-sp-info@phac-aspc.gc.ca, http://www.phac-aspc.gc.ca/seniors-aines/

Foundation for Health in Aging, 40 Fulton Street, 18th Floor, New York, NY 10038, (212) 308-1414, http://www.healthinaging.org

National Institute on Aging, Building 31, Room 5C27, 31 Center Drive, MSC 2292, Bethesda, MD 20892, (800) 222-2225, niaic@nia.nih.gov, http://www.nia.nih.gov

U.S. Administration on Aging, 1 Massachusetts Avenue NW, Washington, DC 20001, (202) 619-07240, aoainfo@aoa.hhs.gov, http://www.aoa.gov

National Council on Aging (NCOA), 1901 L Street NW, 4th Floor, Washington, DC 20036, (202) (301) 479-1200, http://www.ncoa.org/

Liz Swain
Ken R. Wells
Laura Jean Cataldo, RN, Ed.D.
Leslie Mertz, Ph.D.

Severe acute respiratory syndrome (SARS)

Definition

Severe acute respiratory syndrome (SARS) is the first emergent and highly transmissible viral disease to appear during the twenty-first century.

Description

Patients with SARS develop flu-like fever, headache, malaise, dry cough and other breathing difficulties. Many patients develop **pneumonia**, and in 5–10% of cases, the pneumonia and other complications are severe enough to cause death. SARS is caused by a virus that is transmitted usually from person to person—predominantly by the aerosolized droplets of virus infected material.

The first known case of SARS was traced to a November 2002 case in Guangdong province, China. By mid-February 2003, Chinese health officials tracked more than 300 cases, including five deaths in Guangdong province from what was at the time described as an acute respiratory syndrome. Many flu-causing viruses have previously originated from Guangdong province because of cultural and exotic cuisine practices that bring animals, animal parts, and humans into close proximity. In such an environment, pathogens can more easily genetically mutate and make the leap from animal hosts to humans. The first cases of SARS showed high rates among Guangdong food handlers and chefs.

Chinese health officials initially remained silent about the outbreak, and no special precautions were taken to limit travel or prevent the spread of the disease. The world health community, therefore, had no chance to institute testing, isolation, and quarantine measures that might have prevented the subsequent global spread of the disease.

On February 21, Liu Jianlun, a 64-year-old Chinese physician from Zhongshan hospital (later determined to have been "super-spreader," a person capable of infecting unusually high numbers of contacts) traveled to Hong Kong to attend a family wedding despite the fact that he had a fever. Epidemiologists subsequently determined that, Jianlun passed on the SARS virus to other guests at the Metropole Hotel where he stayed—including an American businessman en route to Hanoi, three women from Singapore, two Canadians, and a Hong Kong resident. Jianlun's travel to Hong Kong and the subsequent travel of those he infected allowed SARS to spread from China to the infected travelers' destinations.

Johnny Chen, the American businessman, grew ill in Hanoi, Vietnam, and was admitted to a local hospital.

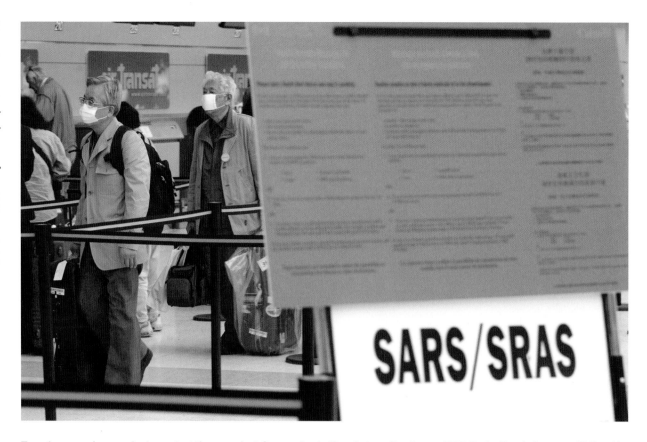

Travelers wearing masks to protect them against Severe Acute Respiratory Syndrome (SARS). (© iStockphoto.com/EdStock)

Chen infected 20 health care workers at the hospital including noted Italian epidemiologist Carlo Urbani who worked at the Hanoi **World Health Organization (WHO)** office. Urbani provided medical care for Chen and first formally identified SARS as a unique disease on February 28, 2003. By early March, 22 hospital workers in Hanoi were ill with SARS.

Unaware of the problems in China, Urbani's report drew increased attention among epidemiologists when coupled with news reports in mid-March that Hong Kong health officials had also discovered an outbreak of an acute respiratory syndrome among health care workers. Unsuspecting hospital workers admitted the Hong Kong man infected by Jianlun to a general ward at the Prince of Wales Hospital because it was assumed he had a typical severe pneumonia—a fairly routine admission. The first notice that clinicians were dealing with an unusual illness came—not from health notices from China of increasing illnesses and deaths due to SARS—but from the observation that hospital staff, along with those subsequently determined to have been in close proximity to the infected persons, began to show signs of illness. Eventually, 138 people, including 34 nurses, 20 doctors, 16 medical students, and 15 other health care workers, contracted pneumonia.

One of the most intriguing aspects of the early Hong Kong cases was a cluster of more than 250 SARS cases that occurred in a cluster of high-rise apartment buildings—many housing health care workers—that provided evidence of a high rate of secondary transmission. Epidemiologists conducted extensive investigations to rule out the hypothesis that the illnesses were related to some form of local contamination (e.g., sewage, bacteria on the ventilation system). Rumors began that the illness was due to cockroaches or rodents, but no scientific evidence supported the hypothesis that the disease pathogen was carried by insects or animals.

Hong Kong authorities then decided that those suffering the flu-like symptoms would be given the option of self-isolation, with family members allowed to remain confined at home or in special camps. Compliance checks were conducted by police.

One of the Canadians infected in Hong Kong, Kwan Sui-Chu, return to Toronto, Ontario, and died in a Toronto hospital on March 5. As in Hong Kong, because there were no alert from China about the SARS outbreak, Canadian officials did not initially suspect that Sui-Chu had been infected with a highly contagious virus, until Sui-Chu's son and five health care workers showed similar symptoms. By mid-April, Canada reported more than 130 SARS cases and 15 fatalities.

Increasingly faced with reports that provided evidence of global dissemination, on March 15, 2003, the **World Health Organization** (**WHO**) took the unusual step of issuing a travel warning that described SARS is a "worldwide health threat." WHO officials announced that SARS cases, and potential cases, had been tracked from China to Singapore, Thailand, Vietnam, Indonesia, Philippines, and Canada. Although the exact cause of the "acute respiratory syndrome" had not, at that time, been determined, WHO officials issuance of the precautionary warning to travelers bound for Southeast Asia about the potential SARS risk served as notice to public health officials about the potential dangers of SARS.

Within days of the first WHO warning, SARS cases were reported in United Kingdom, Spain, Slovenia, Germany, and the United States.

WHO officials were initially encouraged that isolation procedures and alerts were working to stem the spread of SARS, as some countries reporting small numbers of cases experienced no further dissemination to hospital staff or others in contact with SARS victims. However, in some countries, including Canada, where SARS cases occurred before WHO alerts, SARS continued to spread beyond the bounds of isolated patients.

WHO officials responded by recommending increased screening and quarantine measures that included mandatory screening of persons returning from visits to the most severely affected areas in China, Southeast Asia, and Hong Kong.

In early April 2003, WHO took the controversial additional step of recommending against non-essential travel to Hong Kong and the Guangdong province of China. The recommendation, sought by **infectious disease** specialists, was not controversial within the medical community, but caused immediate concern regarding the potentially widespread economic impacts.

Mounting reports of SARS showed a increasing global dissemination of the virus. By April 9, the first confirmed reports of SARS cases in Africa reached WHO headquarters, and eight days later, a confirmed case was discovered in India.

Causes and symptoms

In mid-April 2003, Canadian scientists at the British Columbia **Cancer** Agency in Vancouver announced that they that sequenced the genome of the coronavirus most likely to be the cause of SARS. Within days, scientists at the Centers for Disease Control (**CDC**) in Atlanta,

Georgia, offered a genomic map that confirmed more than 99% of the Canadian findings.

Both genetic maps were generated from studies of viruses isolated from SARS cases. The particular coronavirus mapped had a genomic sequence of 29,727 nucleotides—average for the family of coronavirus that typically contain between 29,000–31,000 nucleotides.

Proof that the coronavirus mapped was the specific virus responsible for SARS would eventually come from animal testing. Rhesus monkeys were exposed to the virus via injection and inhalation and then monitored to determine whether SARS like symptoms developed, and then if sick animals exhibited a histological pathology (i.e., an examination of the tissue and cellular level pathology) similar to findings in human patients. Other tests, including polymerase chain reaction (PCR) testing helped positively match the specific coronavirus present in the lung tissue, blood, and feces of infected animals to the exposure virus.

Identification of a specific pathogen can be a complex process, and positive identification requires thousands of tests. All testing is conducted with regard to testing Koch's postulates—the four conditions that must be met for an organism to be determined to the cause of a disease. First, the organism must be present in every case of the disease. Second, the organism must be able to be isolated from the host and grown in laboratory conditions. Third, the disease must be reproduced when the isolated organism is introduced into another, healthy host. The fourth postulate stipulates that the same organism must be able to be recovered and purified from the host that was experimentally infected.

Early data indicates that SARS has an incubation period range of two to 10 days, with an average incubation of about four days. Much of the inoculation period allows the virus to be both transported and spread by an asymptomatic carrier. With air travel, asymptotic carriers can travel to anywhere in the world. The initial symptoms are non-specific and common to the flu. Infected cases then typically spike a high fever 100.4°F (38°C) as they develop a cough, shortness of breath, and difficulty breathing. SARS often fulminates (reaches it maximum progression) in a severe pneumonia that can cause respiratory failure and death in about 10% of its victims.

Diagnosis

Currently, initial tests include blood cultures, Gram stain, chest radiograph, and tests for other viral respiratory pathogens such as **influenza** A and B. Other serologic techniques are used, and if SARS is suspected, samples are forwarded to state/local public **health departments** and/ or the CDC for coronavirus antibody testing.

Treatment

As of May 1, 2003, no therapy was demonstrated to have clinical effectiveness against the virus that causes SARS, and physicians could offer only supportive therapy (e.g., administration of fluids, oxygen, ventilation).

Prognosis

By late April/early May 2003, WHO officials had confirmed reports of more than 3,000 cases of SARS from 18 different countries with 111 deaths attributed to the disease (about a 5–10% death rate). United States health officials reported 193 cases with no deaths. Significantly, all but 20 of the U.S. cases were linked to travel to infected areas, and the other 20 cases were accounted for by secondary transmission from infected patients to family members and health care workers.

Information on countries reporting SARS and the cumulative total of cases and deaths is updated each day on the WHO SARS web site at http://www.who.int/csr/sarscountry/en/.

Prevention

Until a vaccine is developed, isolation and quarantine remain potent tools in the modern public health arsenal. Both procedures seek to control exposure to infected individuals or materials. Isolation procedures are used with patients with a confirmed illness. Quarantine rules and procedures apply to individuals who are not currently ill but are known to have been exposed to the illness (e.g., been in the company of a infected person or come in contact with infected materials).

Isolation and quarantine both act to restrict movement and to slow or stop the spread of disease within a community. Depending on the illness, patients placed in isolation may be cared for in hospitals, specialized health care facilities, or in less severe cases, at home. Isolation is a standard procedure for TB patients. In most cases, isolation is voluntary; however, isolation can be compelled by federal, state, and some local law.

States governments within the United States have a general authority to set and enforce quarantine conditions. At the federal level, the Centers for Disease Control and Prevention's (CDC) Division of Global Migration and Quarantine is empowered to detain, examine, or conditionally release (release with restrictions on movement or with a required treatment protocol) individuals suspected of carrying certain listed communicable diseases.

As of April 27, 2003, the CDC in Atlanta recommended SARS patients be voluntarily isolated, but had not recommended enforced isolation or quarantine. Regardless, CDC and other public heath officials, including the Surgeon General, sought and secured increased powers to deal with SARS. On April 4, 2003, U.S. President George W. Bush signed Presidential Executive Order 13295, which added SARS to a list of quarantinable communicable diseases. The order provided health officials with the broader powers to seek "... apprehension, detention, or conditional release of individuals to prevent the introduction, transmission, or spread of suspected communicable diseases...."

Travel advisories issued by WHO should be reviewed and people who must travel to areas with SARS outbreaks should follow such preventative measures as frequent hand washing and avoidance of large crowds. Likewise, family members caring for suspected and/or confirmed SARS patients should wash hands frequently, avoid direct contact with the patient's bodily fluids, and monitor their own possible development of symptoms closely.

Brenda Wilmoth Lerner
K. Lee Lerner

Sexual assault

Definition

Sexual assault occurs when an individual is forced to engage in sexual activity without that person's explicit consent. The United States Code defines two types of sexual assault: sexual abuse and aggravated sexual abuse. Sexual abuse includes acts in which an individual is forced to engage in sexual activity by use of threats or other fear tactics (and when the individual does not, or is unable to provide, consent), or instances in which an individual is physically unable to decline. Aggravated sexual abuse occurs when an individual is forced to submit to sexual acts by use of physical force; threats of death, injury, or kidnapping; or substances that render that individual unconscious or impaired. In both cases, the act may be completed or may only be only attempted, but it still considered a sexual assault.

DESCRIPTION. Many misconceptions exist about sexual assault, and especially rape. Often, people assume that rape victims are all women who have been attacked by a total stranger and forced into having sexual intercourse. In reality, sexual assault can take many forms—it may be violent or nonviolent; the victim may be male or female, child or adult; the offender may be a stranger, relative, friend, authority figure, or spouse.

The number of sexual assaults reported depends on how those abuses are defined. The United States Code uses two terms to distinguish between different sexual activities:

• Sexual act: contact between penis and vulva, or penis and anus that involves penetration; contact between the mouth and genitals or anus; penetration of the vagina or anus with an object; or direct touching (not through clothing) of the genitals of an individual under the age of 16 years.

• Sexual contact: intentional touching of the genitals, breasts, buttocks, anus, inner thigh, or groin (even through the clothing) without sexual penetration.

Rape means slightly different things in different states. In some, sexual assault and rape are synonymous. In others, rape is used to describe sexual assaults that occur under the use of or threat of physical force.

DEMOGRAPHICS. Rape or sexual assault can happen to anyone—women, men, or children. The attacker can be anyone—a stranger, friend or acquaintance, family member, former or current partner, or person that is in a position of trust, confidence, authority, or power (such as clergies, teachers, or superiors). Typically, the offenders are men, and the victims are women, but the opposite may occur. Rape performed by a man onto another man, or by a woman onto another woman, is also a type of sexual assault. Such instances typically occur in closed environments, such as in prisons.

The **Centers for Disease Control and Prevention** is conducting an ongoing telephone survey, called the National Intimate Partner and Sexual **Violence** Survey that collects data on sexual assault. In late 2011, it released the data for the previous year. According to the findings, women are disproportionately affected by sexual assault. The survey estimated that nearly one in five women had been raped in their lifetime. The survey defined rape as completed forced penetration; attempted forced penetration; or alcohol-facilitated or drug-facilitated completed penetration. In this group of women, 80% were first raped before the age of 25, about 30% between the ages of 11 and 17, and 12% at age 10 or younger. Among men, one in 71 men had been raped in their lifetime, and 28% were first raped at age 10 or younger.

The prevalence of sexual assault varies among ethnic groups, according to the survey. The percentage of women in different ethnic groups who had experienced rape/physical violence/stalking in their lifetime by ethnicity are:

• 43.7% of black women

• 34.6% of white, non–Hispanic women

• 37.1% of Hispanic women

• 46% of American Indian or Alaska Native

• 53.8% of multiracial, non–Hispanic

The percentage of men in different ethnic groups who had experienced rape/physical violence/stalking in their lifetime by ethnicity are:

• 38.6% of black men

• 28.2% of white, non–Hispanic men

• 26.6% of Hispanic men

• 45.3% of American Indian or Alaska Native

• 39.3% of multiracial, non–Hispanic

Causes and symptoms

Causes

No conclusive, single reason is behind the reason that offenders commit sexual assault. Some explanations include: desire for power and dominance; anger and hostility; need to inflict **pain**; and sexual gratification. Some **sociologists** point to the evolution of males in their role to propagate the species as one reason for sexual assault; that is, if they cannot convince a woman to copulate (have sexual intercourse), then they attempt violent means to accomplish the act.

Symptoms

Victims of sexual assault experience varying symptoms. Some of the more common symptoms include:

• confusion

• withdrawing from social events

• nervousness

• crying without apparent reason

• hostilities

• fearfulness

• inappropriate behaviors

DIAGNOSIS. Sometimes a rape or sexual assault victim will not initially tell the medical profession of the attack, and instead will visit the doctor for other stated reasons. In other cases, the victim will state that he or she has been attacked. In the former case, the assault may never be known by the doctor, or may be identified as the examination progresses. In the latter case, the medical professional should be supportive of the victim and help in any way possible. Many larger medical facilities possess special teams to deal with the emotional, physical, and legal issues involved with such assaults.

Law enforcement officials recommend that rape and sexual assault victims go to a medical facility immediately after the attack, and without changing clothing, showering, or urinating so that evidence left by the perpetrator will not be removed. Psychologists recommend that a friend be present to help support the victim. If that is not possible, a nurse or other professional is often provided to assist.

Medical professionals, and often members of the local law enforcement agency, will gather details about the attack. The medical professional typically asks about any existing or previous illnesses or injuries, along with any current medications, and conducts a complete physical examination, including analysis of any suspected trauma or injury to the body. Samples of clothing, pubic hair, and fingernail scrapings may be taken. Evidence of sperm within the body's orifices may also be collected by the doctor. Tests for **sexually transmitted diseases** will also be taken. For women, the medical professional will also ask the date of the last menstrual period and gynecological history and will consider the possibility of pregnancy both before and after the attack. A number of options are available for women if they choose to use emergency contraceptives to prevent pregnancy following a sexual assault, and the medical professional can provide guidance.

PREVENTION. Awareness that sexual assault can happen to anyone is a key to prevention. The police suggest the following to minimize the risk of sexual assault:

- Secure all home windows and doors with sturdy locks and other safety devices, and consider installing a home-security system.
- Stay away from isolated or secluded areas when alone and outside (especially at night).
- Lock all car doors while driving. Be aware of the immediate surroundings while driving, and while getting into and out of the vehicle.
- Sit as near to the driver as possible when taking public transportation.
- Carry items that can help to alert others (such as whistles and personal alarms).
- Carry items that can provide defense if attacked (such as pepper spray).
- Do not hitchhike in any situation.
- If having vehicle problems, call for assistance and wait inside the vehicle until help arrives.
- Take a course in self-defense; know how to defend oneself.

TREATMENT. Once a victim of sexual assault reports the crime to local authorities, calls a rape-crisis hotline, or arrives at the emergency room to be treated for injuries, a multidisciplinary team is often formed to address his or her physical, psychological, and judicial needs. This team usually includes law enforcement officers, physicians, nurses, mental-health professionals, victim advocates, and/or prosecutors.

The victim of sexual assault may continue to feel fear and anxiety for some time after the incident, and in some instances this may significantly impact his or her personal or professional life. Follow-up counseling should therefore be provided for the victim, particularly if symptoms of post-traumatic stress disorder (PTSD) become evident.

If the attacker is potentially infected with HIV (human immunodeficiency virus), the doctor may recommend that an antiretroviral medication, generally called a post-exposure prophylaxis (PEP), be used to reduce the chance of infection in the victim.

After the examination is complete, the medical professional may also recommend the victim be referred to a local rape-crisis center for further advice, counseling, and information. Medications to relieve symptoms of such conditions as depression and anxiety are often also prescribed.

Forensic medical examination

Because sexual assault is a crime, certain requirements exist for medical evaluation of the patient and for recordkeeping. The forensic medical examination is an invaluable tool for collecting evidence against a perpetrator that may be admissible in court. Since the great majority of victims know their assailant, the purpose of the medical examination is often not to establish identity but to establish nonconsensual sexual contact. Many hospitals and clinics use the Sexual Assault Nurse Examiner (SANE) program, which is an effective model to collect and document evidence, evaluate and treat for STDs and pregnancy, and refer victims to follow-up medical care and counseling. The "Sexual Assault Nurse Examiner Development and Operation Guide," prepared by the Sexual Assault Resource Service, describes the ideal protocol for collecting evidence from a sexual assault victim. This includes:

- performing the medical examination within 72 hours of the assault
- taking a history of the assault
- documenting the general health of the victim, including menstrual cycle, potential allergies, and pregnancy status
- assessment for trauma and taking photographic evidence of injuries
- taking fingernail clippings or scrapings
- taking samples for sperm or seminal fluid
- combing head/pubic hair for foreign hairs, fibers, and other substances

- collection of bloody, torn, or stained clothing
- taking samples for blood typing and DNA screening

PROGNOSIS. The prognosis for rape and sexual assault victims varies. Its outcome is more positive when the victim realizes that the fault lies with the attacker, not themselves, and seeks counseling to help cope with any emotional or health problems that may arise after the attack has occurred.

Two phases commonly occur after the assault: the acute phase that occurs immediately following the attack, and the reorganization phase that comes later. In the acute phase, the victim feels the physical pain and the mental emotions of the attack, and begins to cope with the situation. The reorganization phase, which occurs about a week or so after the attack, may last for several months or even years. In this phase, the victim continues to cope with the reality of the attack and its effects on everyday life. Psychological studies have shown that victims do better in both phases when they participate in psychotherapy and other forms of counseling.

Many victims may need many months, even years, to emotionally recover from the attack, and some may never recover. Approximately 31% of rape victims develop PTSD as a result of their assault. Complications from PTSD often occur, such as nightmares, flashbacks, depression and anxiety, and inappropriate or deadened emotions. Persons who have been sexually assaulted have an increased risk for developing other mental health problems. Compared to those who have not been victimized, rape victims are:

- three times more likely to have a major depressive episode
- four times more likely to have contemplated suicide
- thirteen times more likely to develop alcohol dependency problems
- twenty–six times more likely to develop drug abuse problems

Effects on public health

National statistics

According to the FBI's *Uniform Crime Reports*, an estimated 84,767 forcible rapes were reported to U.S. law enforcement agencies in 2010. The FBI reports that the figure is the lowest number in the last twenty years. When compared to the 2009 estimate, the 2010 estimate was 5.0% lower. Slightly more than 54 out of every 100,000 women were reported to be victims of rape in 2010, compared to slightly more than 59 per 100,000 in 2007. The actual number of rapes and sexual assaults, however, is likely much larger. According to the National Violence Against Women Survey, 1.3 million women

---

KEY TERMS

Aggravated sexual abuse—Sexual acts forced upon an individual by use of physical force; threats of death, injury, or kidnapping; or substances that render that individual unconscious or impaired.

Forcible sodomy—Forced oral or anal intercourse.

Forensic—Pertaining to or used during legal proceedings.

Post–traumatic stress disorder (PTSD)—Also known as rape trauma syndrome, it is a mental health disorder that describes a range of symptoms often experienced by someone who has undergone a severely traumatic event.

Sexual abuse—Sexual activity forced upon an individual by use of threats or other fear tactics, or incurred by an individual who is physically unable to refuse.

Sexual assault nurse examiner (SANE)—A registered nurse who is trained to collect and document evidence from a sexual assault victim, to evaluate and treat for sexually transmitted diseases (STDs) and pregnancy, and to refer victims to follow-up medical care and counseling.

---

had been sexually assaulted in 2010, a much higher figure than the number the FBI reported.

It is difficult to obtain definitive totals for sexual assault, because many victims refrain from reporting the attacks. This happens for many reasons: fear of retaliation from the offender; worry about family members, friends, the community, or the media learning about the offense; concern about being judged or blamed by others; and apprehension that no one will believe the assault occurred.

THE VICTIMS. "Victim, Incident, and Offender Characteristics," published by the National Center for Juvenile Justice (NCJJ) back in 2000, analyzed sexual-assault data collected by law enforcement agencies over a five–year span. It found the following characteristics to be significant among victims of sexual assault:

- Age: More than two-thirds of reported victims of sexual assault were juveniles under the age of 18 years. Those between the ages of 12 and 18 represented the largest group of victims at 33%, followed by 6–11-year-olds at 20%.
- Gender: Females were more than six times more likely to be a victim of sexual assault than males; more than 86% of victims were females. The great majority (99%)

of the victims of forcible rapes were women, while men constituted the majority (54%) of the victims of forcible sodomy (oral or anal intercourse).

• Location: The residence of the victim was the most commonly noted location of sexual assault (70%). Other common locations included schools, hotels/motels, fields, woods, parking lots, roadways, and commercial/office buildings.

• Weapons: A personal weapon (hands, feet, or fists) was used in 77% of cases. Firearms were involved in 2% of cases, and other weapons (e.g., knives, clubs) were used in 6% of cases.

THE OFFENDERS. "Victim, Incident, and Offender Characteristics" also noted characteristics of the perpetrators of sexual assault:

• Age: About 77% of offenders were adults and were responsible for attacks involving 67% of juvenile victims (under the age of 12). More than 23% of offenders were under the age of 18 years; juveniles were more likely to be perpetrators of forcible sodomy and fondling. These young offenders were responsible for approximately 40% of the assaults on other juveniles.

• Gender: The great majority of all reported offenders were male (96%).

• Relationship with offender: Approximately 59% of offenders were acquaintances of their victims, compared to family members (27%) or strangers (14%). Family members were more likely to be perpetrators against juveniles (34%) than against adults (12%). In contrast, strangers accounted for assaults on 27% of adult victims and 7% of juveniles.

• Past offenses: In 19% of juvenile cases, the victim was not the only individual to be assaulted by the offender. Among adults, only 4% are repeat offenders.

COSTS TO SOCIETY. According to a study that appeared in a 2010 issue of *The Journal of Forensic Psychiatry & Psychology*, the average economic costs per rape total $138,310 in victim costs, $8,503 in criminal-justice costs, and $4,610 in offender-productivity costs. That totals $151,423. By comparison, armed robbery averages a total of $48,869 in victim, criminal-justice, and offender-productivity costs.

EFFORTS AND SOLUTIONS. Education is important in preventing sexual assault and in helping victims. In 1994, the U.S. Congress passed the Violence Against Women Act, which established the Rape Prevention and Education (RPE) program at the **CDC**. RPE-funded efforts include educational seminars, professional training, and other evidence-informed and culturally relevant prevention strategies conducted by state **health departments**,

QUESTIONS TO ASK YOUR DOCTOR

• Are there any post–assault symptoms—physical or emotional—I should watch for?

• What impact will the assault have on my chances to become pregnant?

• I need a safe house. How can I find one?

• How can I be certain that I have not acquired a sexually transmitted disease?

• How long after the attack can I resume sexual relations safely with my partner?

rape-crisis centers, state sexual-assault coalitions, and other public and private nonprofit entities. The program also funds statewide and community hotlines that assist callers who have experienced a sexual assault.

The RPE program employs the CDC's social ecological model to develop comprehensive prevention strategies. The model takes into account the roles of the age, education, income, and other factors, such as family or other relationships, that may increase an individual's risk of becoming a victim or offender. By considering these various factors, the program is designed to encourage prevention activities that are most likely to prevent sexual violence.

Individual states, communities, schools, businesses, and other entities across the country have also developed their own programs to prevent sexual assault, as well as other forms of violence. One example is Men Can Stop Rape, a national, nonprofit organization based in Washington, D.C., that has developed several programs, including a Men of Strength Club (MOSC) that reaches boys aged 11–18 years old. MOSC is a 22-week curriculum that teaches healthy-dating relationship skills, and encourages the boys to choose positive ways to show their strength.

Resources

BOOKS

Ferguson, Christopher J., ed. *Violent Crime: Clinical and Social Implications.* Los Angeles: SAGE, 2010.

Ullman, Sarah E. *Talking about Sexual Assault: Society's Response to Survivors.* Washington, DC: American Psychological Association, 2010.

PERIODICALS

DeLisi, M., et al. "Murder by Numbers: Monetary Costs Imposed by a Sample of Homicide Offenders." *The Journal of Forensic Psychiatry & Psychology.* 21, no. 4 (2010): 501–513.

WEBSITES

"The National Intimate Partner and Sexual Violence Survey." Centers for Disease Control and Prevention. http://www.cdc.gov/violenceprevention/nisvs/index.html (accessed October 21, 2012).

"Emergency Contraception After Sexual Assault: Five Key Facts for Survivors." Massachusetts Department of Public Health. http://www.mass.gov/eohhs/docs/dph/quality/healthcare/ec-patient-fact-sheet.pdf (accessed October 21, 2012).

"Sexual Assault Nurse Examiner (SANE) Development & Operation Guide." Sexual Assault Resource Service, Minneapolis, Minnesota, and Office for Victims of Crime. http://www.ojp.usdoj.gov/ovc/publications/infores/sane/saneguide.pdf (accessed October 21, 2012).

"Rape Prevention and Education (RPE) Program." U.S. Centers for Disease Control and Prevention. http://www.cdc.gov/ViolencePrevention/RPE/index.html (accessed October 21, 2012).

"Men Can Stop Rape: What We Do." Men Can Stop Rape. http://www.mencanstoprape.org/What-We-Do/ (accessed October 21, 2012).

ORGANIZATIONS

American Psychiatric Association, 1000 Wilson Boulevard, Suite 1825, Arlington, VA 22209-3901, (888) 357-7924, apa@psych.org, http://www.psych.org

Federal Bureau of Investigation, J. Edgar Hoover Building, 935 Pennsylvania Avenue NW, Washington, DC 20535-0001, (202) 324-3000, http://www.fbi.gov

Men Can Stop Rape, 1003 K Street NW, Suite 200, Washington, DC 20001, (202) 265-6530, (800) 656-4673, info@mencanstoprape.org, http://www.mencanstoprape.org/

Office for Victims of Crime, U.S. Department of Justice, 810 7th Street NW, 8th Floor, Washington, DC 20531, (202) 307-1034, (800) 656-5983, http://www.ojp.usdoj.gov/ovc/

Rape, Abuse, and Incest National Network, 2000 L Street NW, Suite 406, Washington, DC 20036, (202) 544-1034, (800) 656-4673, info@rainn.org, http://www.rainn.org/

Rebecca J. Frey, Ph.D.
Leslie Mertz, Ph.D.

▌Sexually transmitted diseases

Definition

Sexually transmitted disease (STD) is a term used to describe more than 20 different infections that are transmitted through exchange of semen, blood, and other body fluids, or by direct contact with the affected body areas of people with an STD. Sexually transmitted diseases are also called venereal diseases.

Demographics

The **Centers for Disease Control and Prevention (CDC)** has reported that 85% of the most prevalent infectious diseases in the United States are sexually transmitted. The rate of STDs in the U.S. is 50 to 100 times higher than that of any other industrialized nation. One in four sexually active Americans will be affected by an STD at some time in his or her life.

Description

Types of STDs

Some of the most common and potentially serious STDs in the United States include:

• Chlamydia. This STD is caused by the bacterium *Chlamydia trachomatis*, a microscopic organism that lives as a parasite inside human cells. In 2010, there were 1,307,893 reported cases of chlamydia. That means that chlamydia affects more about 426 out of every 100,000 people. Chlamydia has been increasing in frequency in the United States; between 1990 and 2010, the rate of reported chlamydial infection increased from 160.2 to 426.0 cases per 100,000 population. Infection rates are substantially higher among women than among men; among those aged 20 to 24, the group reporting the highest numbers of infections, there were 3,407.9 cases among women and 1,187 cases among men. The highest infection rates were among 19-year-old women, with 4,917.3 cases per 100,000. Because chlamydia is asymptomatic, many women do not receive treatment and subsequently develop pelvic inflammatory disease (PID) as a result of chlamydia infection, a leading cause of infertility.

• Human papillomavirus (HPV). HPV causes genital warts and is the single most important risk factor for cervical cancer in women. Over 100 types of HPV exist, but only about 30 of them can cause genital warts and are spread through sexual contact. In some instances, warts are passed from mother to child during childbirth, leading to a potentially life-threatening condition for newborns in which warts develop in the throat (laryngeal papillomatosis).

• Genital herpes. Herpes is an incurable viral infection thought to be one of the most common STDs in the United States. It is caused by one of two types of herpes simplex viruses: HSV-1 (commonly causing oral herpes) or HSV-2 (usually causing genital herpes). It is believed to affect one out of every six Americans between the ages of 14 and 49. HSV-2 infection is more common in women (20.9%) than men (11.9%) and in African Americans (39.2%) than Caucasians (12.3%). African American women are most affected, with a prevalence rate of 48%.

- Gonorrhea. Gonorrhea is the second most commonly reported notifiable disease in the United States. The bacterium *Neisseria gonorrhoeae* is the causative agent of gonorrhea and can be spread by vaginal, oral, or anal contact. The CDC reports that 309,341 new cases of gonorrhea were reported in 2010. This is about 100.8 cases per 100,000 people. This was a slight increase from a low of 98.1 cases per 100,000 that was recorded in 2009. Since 1975, reported cases of gonorrhea have declined more than 70%.

- Syphilis. Syphilis is a potentially life-threatening infection that increases the likelihood of acquiring or transmitting HIV. After a decade of decline, the rate of syphilis increased every year from 2001 to 2009 before declining again in 2010 to 7.9 cases per 100,000 among men and 1.1 cases per 100,000 among women. The rate of congenital syphilis also declined in 2010, with 377 cases reported (a rate of 8.7 cases per 100,000 live births).

- Human immunodeficiency virus (HIV) infection. The CDC estimates that there are approximately 1,106,400 people in the United States living with HIV/AIDS, and that about one-fifth of them were not aware of the HIV infection. In 2007, 35,962 diagnosed cases of AIDS were diagnosed in the United States, with 28 of them occurring in children under the age of 13. As of 2010, The World Health Organization estimated that there were 33.4 million people living with HIV worldwide. There is no cure for this STD.

STDs can have very painful long-term consequences as well as immediate health problems. They can cause:

- birth defects
- blindness
- bone deformities
- brain damage
- cancer
- heart disease
- infertility and other abnormalities of the reproductive system
- mental retardation
- death

Social groups and STDs

STDs affect certain population groups more severely than others. Women, young people, and members of minority groups are particularly affected. Women in any age bracket are more likely than men to develop medical complications related to STDs. Ethnic minorities are more likely to be affected by STDs than Caucasians, with African Americans especially at risk.

Causes and symptoms

The symptoms of STDs vary according to the disease agent (virus or bacterium), the sex of the patient, and the body systems affected. The symptoms of some STDs are easy to identify, others produce infections that may either go unnoticed for some time or are easy to confuse with other diseases. **Syphilis**, in particular, can be confused with disorders ranging from infectious mononucleosis to allergic reactions to prescription medications. In addition, the incubation periods of STDs varies. Some produce symptoms close enough to the time of sexual contact—often less than 48 hours later—for the individual to recognize the connection between the behavior and the symptoms. Others have a longer incubation period, so that the individual may not recognize the early symptoms as those of a sexually transmitted infection.

Some symptoms of STDs affect the genitals and reproductive organs:

- A woman who has an STD may bleed when she is not menstruating or have abnormal vaginal discharge. Vaginal burning, itching, and odor are common, and she may experience pain in her pelvic area while having sex.

- A discharge from the tip of the penis may be a sign that a man has an STD. Males may also have painful or burning sensations when they urinate.

- There may be swelling of the lymph nodes near the groin area.

- Both men and women may develop skin rashes, sores, bumps, or blisters near the mouth or genitals. Homosexual men frequently develop these symptoms in the area around the anus.

Other symptoms of STDs are systemic, which means that they affect the body as a whole. These symptoms may include:

- fever, chills, and similar flu-like symptoms
- skin rashes over large parts of the body
- arthritis-like pains or aching in the joints
- throat swelling and redness that lasts for three weeks or longer

Diagnosis

A sexually active person who has symptoms of an STD should be examined without delay by one of the following health care professionals:

- a specialist in women's health (gynecologist)
- a specialist in disorders of the urinary tract and the male sexual organs (urologist)

KEY TERMS

Chlamydia—A microorganism that resembles certain types of bacteria and causes several sexually transmitted diseases in humans.

Condom—A thin sheath worn over the penis during sexual intercourse to prevent pregnancy or the transmission of STDs. There are also female condoms.

Diaphragm—A dome-shaped device used to cover the back of a woman's vagina during intercourse in order to prevent pregnancy.

Pelvic inflammatory disease (PID)—An inflammation of the tubes leading from a woman's ovaries to the uterus (the Fallopian tubes), caused by a bacterial infection. PID is a leading cause of fertility problems in women.

Venereal disease—Another term for sexually transmitted disease.

• a family physician

• a nurse practitioner

• a specialist in skin disorders (dermatologist)

The diagnostic process begins with a thorough physical examination and a detailed medical history that documents the patient's sexual history and assesses the risk of infection.

The doctor or other healthcare professional will:

• Describe the testing process. This includes all blood tests and other tests that may be relevant to the specific infection.

• Explain the meaning of the test results.

• Provide the patient with information regarding high-risk behaviors and any necessary treatments or procedures.

The doctor may suggest that a patient diagnosed with one STD be tested for others, as it is possible to have more than one STD at a time. One infection may hide the symptoms of another or create a climate that fosters its growth. At present, it is particularly important that people who are HIV-positive be tested for syphilis as well.

Notification

The law in some parts of the United States requires public health officials to trace and contact the partners of people with some STDs. Minors, however, can get treatment without their parents' permission. Public **health departments** in most states can provide information about STD clinic locations, and Planned Parenthood facilities are available to provide testing and counseling. These agencies can also help with or assume the responsibility of notifying sexual partners who should be tested and may require treatment.

Treatment

Although self-care can relieve some of the **pain** of genital **herpes** or genital warts that has recurred after being diagnosed and treated by a physician, other STD symptoms require immediate medical attention.

Antibiotics are prescribed to treat gonorrhea, chlamydia, syphilis, and other STDs caused by bacteria. Although prompt diagnosis and early treatment can almost always cure these STDs, new infections can develop if exposure continues or is renewed. As of 2012, the oral antibiotic cephalosporin is no longer recommended as treatment for gonorrhea by the **CDC**. Viral infections can be treated symptomatically and possibly with antiviral medications.

Prognosis

The prognosis for recovery from STDs varies among the different diseases. The prognosis for recovery from gonorrhea, syphilis, and other STDs caused by bacteria is generally good, provided that the disease is diagnosed early and treated promptly. Untreated syphilis in particular can lead to long-term complications and disability. Viral STDs (genital herpes, genital warts, HIV) cannot be cured but must be treated on a long-term basis to relieve symptoms and prevent life-threatening complications.

Prevention

Vaccines

Vaccines for the prevention of **hepatitis** A and hepatitis B are currently available, and are recommended, especially for gay and bisexual men, users of illegal drugs, health care workers, and others at risk of contracting these diseases. A vaccine for **HPV** also is available and is recommended for young women. Vaccines to prevent other STDs are being actively researched and tested.

Research into vaccinations to prevent HIV infection are underway. Although some have undergone clinical trials, as of 2010, there were no vaccines approved by the United States Food and Drug Administration (FDA) to prevent the disease.

Lifestyle choices

The risk of becoming infected with an STD can be reduced or eliminated by making certain choices. Abstaining from sexual contact, maintaining a mutually monogamous relationship, or being informed about a partner's medical status can all reduce the risk. The risk of contracting an STD can also be reduced by avoiding sexual contact with partners who are known to be infected with an STD, whose health status is unknown, who abuse drugs, or who are involved in the sex trade.

Use of condoms and other contraceptives

Condoms are the only known contraceptive method to reduce the risk of STD transmission. It is important to make sure a new condom is used every time there is genital, oral, or anal contact. Used correctly and consistently, male condoms provide good protection against HIV and other STDs such as gonorrhea, chlamydia, and syphilis. Female condoms (lubricated sheaths inserted into the vagina) have also been shown to be effective in preventing HIV and other STDs. Condoms also provide a measure of protection against genital herpes, genital warts, and hepatitis B.

There is some evidence that spermicides and diaphragms may provide a small amount of protection from some STDs, but that claim remains extremely controversial, and it recommended that people do not use these instead of other methods of STD protection. They do not protect women from contracting HIV. Birth-control pills, patches, or injections do not prevent STDs. Neither do surgical sterilizations or hysterectomies.

Hygienic measures

Urinating and washing the genital area with soap and water immediately after having sex may eliminate some germs before they cause infection. Douching, however, can spread infection deeper. It may also increase a woman's risk of developing pelvic inflammatory disease (PID).

Public Health Concerns

The CDC estimates that about 19 million new STD infections occur in the United States each year. Almost half of these infections occur among teenagers and young adults between the ages of 15 and 24. It is estimated that STDs have an economic cost of as much as $17 billion dollars each year in the United States.

Screening is an effective tool against the spread of STDs, but it is underutilized, according to the CDC. Treatment, especially if the infections are caught early, can be relatively simple and have a tremendous impact for not only the affected individual but also for the rest of the population because it decreases the spread of disease. Left untreated, STDs can lead to further public health problems as the diseases spread from partner to partner,

potentially causing **infertility** among women, and infections among newborns.

Resources

BOOKS

Egendorf, Laura, ed. *Sexually Transmitted Diseases*. Detroit, MI: Greenhaven Press, 2007.

Grimes, Jill.*Seductive Delusions: How Everyday People Catch STDs*. Baltimore: Johns Hopkins University Press, 2008.

Marr, Lisa. *Sexually Transmitted Diseases: A Physician Tells You What You Need to Know*, 2nd ed. Baltimore: The Johns Hopkins University Press, 2007.

Nack, Adina. *Damaged Goods?: Women Living With Incurable Sexually Transmitted Diseases*. Philadelphia: Temple University Press, 2008.

WEBSITES

Morbidity and Mortality Weekly Report. Update to CDC's Sexually Transmitted Diseases Treatment Guidelines, 2010: Oral Cephalosporins No Longer a Recommended Treatment for Gonococcal Infections.http://www.cdc.gov/mmwr/preview/mmwrhtml/mm6131a3.htm?s_cid=mm6131a3_w (accessed October 20, 2012).

Centers for Disease Control. Sexually Transmitted Diseases. http://www.cdc.gov/std/default.htm (accessed October 20, 2012).

Medline Plus. Sexually Transmitted Diseases. http://www.nlm.nih.gov/medlineplus/sexuallytransmitteddiseases.html (accessed October 20, 2012).

ORGANIZATIONS

National STD and AIDS Hotline, (800) 227-8922

Centers for Disease Control and Prevention, 1600 Clifton Rd., Atlanta, GA 30333, (888) CDC-INFO, cdcinfo@cdc.gov, http://www.cdc.gov

Planned Parenthood Federation of America, 434 West 33rd St., New York, NY 10001, (212) 541-7800, (800) 230-PLAN, Fax: (212) 245-1845, http://www.planned-parenthood.org

Maureen Haggerty
Tish Davidson, AM
Fran Hodgkins

Shigellosis

Definition

Shigellosis is a bacterial infection of the intestinal tract. It is a well-known cause of travelers' diarrhea and illness throughout the world. The major symptoms are diarrhea, abdominal cramps, fever, and severe fluid loss (dehydration).

DESCRIPTION. Shigellosis results from infection with bacteria in the genus *Shigella*. These are extremely infectious bacteria: Ingestion of just 10 organisms is enough to cause severe diarrhea and dehydration. Different groups of *Shigella* can affect humans. These include:

• *Shigella sonnei*, also called "group D" Shigella, which is responsible for about two-thirds of shigellosis in the United States. Of the different types of *Shigella*, it effects are generally the mildest.

• *Shigella flexneri*, or "group B" Shigella, which causes almost all other cases.

• *Shigella dysenteriae* type 1, which is rare in the United States, but can lead to deadly outbreaks in developing countries. It generally produces the most severe attacks.

The most serious form of the disease is called **dysentery**, which is characterized by severe watery (and often blood- and mucous-streaked) diarrhea, abdominal cramping, rectal **pain**, and fever. *Shigella* is only one of several organisms that can cause dysentery, but the term bacillary dysentery is usually another name for shigellosis.

Shigellosis is sometimes known as *Shigella* gastro-enteritis or *Shigella* enteritis.

DEMOGRAPHICS. Most deaths from shigellosis occur in less-developed or developing countries, but even in the United States, shigellosis can be a dangerous and potentially deadly disease. In the United States, about 14,000 cases are reported occur each year, but since symptoms are typically mild, and cases often go unreported, the U.S. **Centers for Disease Control and Prevention (CDC)** estimated that as many as 20 times that number may actually occur. On the other hand, the **World Health Organization (WHO)** reports that shigella is responsible for about 120 million cases of severe dysentery with blood and mucus in the stools, and the overwhelming majority of these occur in developing countries, with most cases hitting children younger than five years old. The **WHO** also estimates that aproximately 1.1 million people die from shigellosis each year, and nearly two-thirds of the deaths are to children four years old and younger.

About a half million individuals report travelers' diarrhea every year, according to WHO.

ORIGINS. The genus *Shigella* is named in honor of Shiga, a Japanese researcher, who discovered the organism in 1897.

CAUSES AND SYMPTOMS.

Causes

Shigella are highly contagious. Infection spreads through food or **water** contaminated by human waste. Sources of transmission are:

• contaminated milk, ice cream, vegetables and other foods, which often cause epidemics

• household contacts

• poor hygiene and overcrowded living conditions

• day care centers

• refugee camps

• sexual practices which lead to oral-anal contact, directly or indirectly

Shigella bacteria are very resistant to the acid produced by the stomach, and this allows them to easily pass through the gastrointestinal tract and infect the colon (large intestine). The result is a colitis (inflammation of the colon) that produces multiple ulcers, which can bleed. *Shigella* bacteria also produce a number of toxins (Shiga toxin and others) that increase the amount of fluid secretion by the intestinal tract. This fluid secretion is a major cause of diarrhea symptoms.

Symptoms

Symptoms may be limited to mild diarrhea, usually lasting from one to seven days (typically three days), or may progress to full-blown dysentery. Dehydration results from the large fluid losses due to diarrhea, vomiting, and fever. Inability to eat or drink worsens the situation.

In developed countries, most infections are of the less severe type, and are often due to *S. sonnei*. The period between infection and symptoms (incubation period) varies from one to seven days. Shigellosis can last from a few days to several weeks, with an average of seven days.

Typical symptoms include:

• watery diarrhea

• sudden onset of abdominal pain, sometimes accompanied by cramping

• sudden onset of fever

• presence of blood, mucus, and/or pus in the stool

• nausea, sometimes accompanied by vomiting

Complications

Areas outside the intestine can be involved, including:

• nervous system—irritation of the meninges or meningitis, encephalitis, and seizures

• kidneys—producing **hemolytic-uremic syndrome** (or HUS), which leads to kidney failure

• joints—leading to an unusual form of arthritis called **Reiter's syndrome**

• skin—rash

One of the most serious complications of this disease is HUS, which involves the kidney. The main findings are kidney failure and damage to red blood cells. As many as 15% of patients die from this complication, and half of the survivors develop chronic kidney failure, which requires dialysis.

Another life-threatening condition is toxic megacolon. Severe inflammation causes the colon to dilate or stretch, and the thin colon wall may eventually tear. Clues to this diagnosis include sudden decrease in diarrhea, swelling of the abdomen, and worsening abdominal pain.

DIAGNOSIS. Shigellosis is one of the many causes of acute diarrhea, and *Shigella* bacteria share several of the characteristics of a group of bacteria that inhabit the intestinal tract. *E coli,* another cause of food-borne illness, can be mistaken for *Shigella* both by physicians and the laboratory. Careful testing is needed to ensure proper diagnosis and treatment.

Culture (growing the bacteria in the laboratory) of freshly obtained diarrhea fluid is the only way to be certain of the diagnosis. But even this method might not provide definitive results, especially if the patient is already on **antibiotics**. *Shigella* are identified by a combination of their appearance under the microscope and various chemical tests.

TREATMENT. The first aim of treatment is to keep up **nutrition** and avoid dehydration. Ideally, a physician should be consulted before starting any treatment. Many cases resolve before the diagnosis is established by culture. Medications that control diarrhea by slowing intestinal contractions can cause problems and should be avoided by patients with bloody diarrhea or fever, especially if antibiotics have not been started.

Rehydration

The **World Health Organization** (WHO) has developed guidelines for a standard solution taken by mouth and prepared from ingredients readily available at home. This Oral Rehydration Solution (ORS) includes salt, baking powder, sugar, orange juice, and water. Commercial preparations, such as Pedialyte, are also available. In many patients with mild symptoms, this is the only treatment needed. Severe dehydration usually requires intravenous fluid replacement. Patients who have severe nausea may require intravenous fluids. This is most common among children.

Antibiotics

In the early and mid-1990s, researchers began to realize that not all cases of bacterial dysentery needed antibiotic treatment. Therefore, these drugs are indicated only for treatment of moderate or severe disease, as found in the tropics. Choice of antibiotic is based on the type of bacteria found in the geographical area and on laboratory results. Antibiotics may include ampicillin,

---

KEY TERMS

Antibiotic—A medication that is designed to kill or weaken bacteria.

Carrier state—The continued presence of an organism (bacteria, virus, or parasite) in the body that does not cause symptoms but is able to be transmitted and infect other persons.

Colitis—Inflammation of the colon or large bowel, which has several causes. The lining of the colon becomes swollen and ulcers often develop. The ability of the colon to absorb fluids is also affected and diarrhea often results.

Dialysis—A form of treatment for patients with kidneys that do not function properly. The treatment removes toxic wastes from the body that are normally removed by the kidneys.

Dysentery—A disease marked by frequent watery bowel movements, often with blood and mucus, and characterized by pain, fever, dehydration, and urgency to have a bowel movement.

Food-borne illness—A disease that is transmitted by eating or handling contaminated food.

Meninges—Outer covering of the spinal cord and brain. Infection is called meningitis, and it can lead to damage to the brain or spinal cord and lead to death.

Oral rehydration solution (ORS)—A liquid preparation developed by the World Health Organization that can decrease fluid loss in persons with diarrhea. Originally developed to be prepared with materials available in the home, commercial preparations have recently come into use.

Stool—Fecal material.

Travelers' diarrhea—An illness due to infection from a bacteria or parasite that occurs in persons traveling to areas where there is a high frequency of the illness. The disease is usually spread by contaminated food or water.

---

sulfa derivatives such as trimethoprim/sulfamethoxazole (also known as Bactrim or Septra), ceftriaxone (Rocephin), azithromycin, or fluoroquinolones such as ciprofloxacin (Cipro). Antidiarrheal medications can make the illness worse and should be avoided.

PROGNOSIS. Many patients with mild infections need no specific treatment and recover completely. In those with severe infections, antibiotics will decrease the length of symptoms and the number of days bacteria appear in the feces. In rare cases, an individual may fail to clear the bacteria from the intestinal tract; resulting in a persistent carrier state. This may be more frequent in individuals who have **AIDS** (Acquired Immune Deficiency Syndrome). Antibiotics are about 90% effective in eliminating these chronic infections.

In patients who have suffered particularly severe attacks, some degree of cramping and diarrhea can last for several weeks. This is usually due to damage to the intestinal tract, which requires some time to heal. Since antibiotics can also produce a form of colitis, this must be considered as a possible cause of persistent or recurrent symptoms.

PREVENTION. *Shigellosis* is an extremely contagious disease; good hand-washing techniques and proper precautions in food handling will help deter the spread of infection. Children in daycare centers need to be reminded to wash their hands during an outbreak to minimize spread. *Shigellosis* in schools or daycare settings almost always disappears when holiday breaks occur, which sever the chain of transmission.

Travelers' diarrhea (TD)

Shigella accounts for about 10% of diarrhea illness in travelers to Mexico, South America, and the tropics. Most cases of TD are more of a nuisance than a life-threatening disease.

Aside from ruining vacations, these infections may also interrupt business conference schedules and, in the worst instances, lead to a life-threatening illness. The latter has driven the research to find a safe and effective way of preventing TD. One of the best means of **prevention** is to follow closely the rules outlined by the WHO and other groups regarding food and drinks in foreign lands. For instance, travelers should eat cooked hot foods and fruits that they have peeled themselves, and drink water that has been boiled or treated.

Some health professionals recommend large doses (typically two tablets four times a day) of Pepto-Bismol (bismuth subsalicylate) as a preventative measure for travelers' diarrhea. This regimen must start a few days before departure. Pepto-Bismol contains salicylate, which may be unsuitable for children, people who are allergic to aspirin, pregnant women, and other individuals with various health conditions. Patients should also be aware that Pepto-Bismol will turn bowel movements black and may cause ringing in the ears. For these reasons, individuals should consult a health professional before starting a Pepto-Bismol regimen.

Antibiotics have also proven to be highly effective in preventing TD. They can also produce significant side effects, however, so individuals should consult a

QUESTIONS TO ASK YOUR DOCTOR

- Do you recommend that I take antibiotics before my next international trip to avoid shigellosis? When should I start the antibiotics? What are the potential side effects?

- Given my health conditions and medications that I am taking, do you recommend that I take Pepto-Bismol before my next international trip to avoid shigellosis? When should I shart taking Pepto-Bismol, what is the proper dose, and how long should I take it?

- If I do get travelers' diarrhea, what symptoms will indicate that I need medical attention?

physician before use. Like Pepto-Bismol, antibiotics need to be started before beginning travel.

EFFECTS ON PUBLIC HEALTH. Shigellosis is most common among young children who live in economically disadvantaged, crowded areas in developing countries, and it can cause chronic health problems or death.

COSTS TO SOCIETY. Shigellosis typically occurs in a milder form in the United States but can still cause outbreaks in daycare centers and schools, resulting in their closure for a few days to break the cycle of infection. Travelers' diarrhea can ruin vacations, end business conferences, and otherwise disrupt normal activities. Individuals who have experienced travelers' diarrhea may be disinclined to take vacations in geographic areas where shigellosis is prevalent.

EFFORTS AND SOLUTIONS. Local and state **health departments**, along with the **CDC**, monitor and investigate *Shigella* outbreaks in the United States to help control transmission of the bacteria. In addition, the U.S. Food and Drug Administration promotes safer food-handling methods in both restaurants and food-processing plants, and inspects imported foods to help ensure their safety; and the U.S. **Environmental Protection Agency** works to maintain the safety of the drinking-water supply. Researchers around the world also continue to understand the illness, the bacteria that cause it, and means to prevent it. Work toward a shigellosis vaccine is ongoing.

Resources

BOOKS
DuPont, Herbert L. "Approach to the Patient With Suspected Enteric Infection." In: Goldman, Lee, and Andrew I.

Schafer, eds. *Cecil Medicine.* 24th ed. Philadelphia, PA: Saunders Elsevier; 2011: chap 291.

Giannella, Ralph A. "Infectious Enteritis and Proctocolitis and Bacterial Food Poisoning." In: Feldman Mark, Lawrence S. Friedman, and Lawrence J. Brandt, eds. *Sleisenger & Fordtran's Gastrointestinal and Liver Disease.* 9th ed. Philadelphia, PA: Saunders Elsevier; 2010: chap 107.

WEBSITES

MedlinePlus. "Shigellosis." U.S. National Library of Medicine, National Institutes of Health. http://www.nlm.nih.gov/medlineplus/ency/article/000295.htm (accessed November 6, 2012).

PubMedHealth. "Shigellosis." U.S. National Library of Medicine. http://www.ncbi.nlm.nih.gov/pubmedhealth/PMH0001340/ (accessed November 6, 2012).

"Shigellosis." U.S. Centers for Disease Control and Prevention. http://www.cdc.gov/nczved/divisions/dfbmd/diseases/shigellosis/ (accessed November 6, 2012).

"Shigellosis." World Health Organization. http://www.who.int/vaccine_research/diseases/diarrhoeal/en/index6.html (accessed November 6, 2012).

"Travel to Developing Countries - Travelers' Diarrhea" University of Maryland Medical School. http://www.umm.edu/patiented/articles/how_travelers_diarrhea_prevented_treated_000001_2.htm (accessed November 7, 2012).

ORGANIZATIONS

Centers for Disease Control and Prevention (CDC), 1600 Clifton Road, Atlanta, GA 30333, 800-232-4636, cdcinfo@cdc.gov, http://www.cdc.gov/std/

World Health Organization, Avenue Appia 20, 1211 Geneva 27, Switzerland 41 22 791 21 11, http://www.who.int

David Kaminstein, M.D.
Leslie Mertz, Ph.D.

Shingles

Definition

Shingles, or **herpes** zoster, is a condition caused by the reactivation of the varicella zoster virus (VZV) that causes chickenpox (varicella). After a bout of chickenpox, the virus remains dormant in the sensory nerve ganglia that are adjacent to the spinal cord and brain. Years later, the virus re-emerges, traveling along the nerves to the skin, where it causes red rashes that develop into blisters. In the process, the virus can damage nerves, leading to a very painful inflammation called postherpetic neuralgia (PHN), which can persist long after the rash disappears.

Demographics

Anyone who has had chickenpox or has been vaccinated against varicella can develop shingles. Virtually all American adults have had chickenpox, even if the disease was so mild as to pass unnoticed. Nearly one in three Americans eventually develops shingles, and there are at least one million cases in the United States each year.

Although shingles can occur at any age, even in children, the incidence increases steadily with age. About half of all cases occur in people aged 60 or older. About 20% of people with shingles develop PHN, which is more common in women than in men. In the United States, between 120,000 and 200,000 people suffer from PHN each year. It occurs more frequently among the elderly and is one of the most common causes of pain-related **suicide** in older adults. The incidence of PHN increases with age, and it tends to last longer in older patients:

• PHN is rare in those under age 30.

• By age 40, the risk of PHN lasting longer than one month is 33%.

• By age 70, the risk increases to 74%.

Some scientists believe that the incidence of shingles is likely to increase over the next 40–50 years due to the introduction of a childhood vaccine against chickenpox in 1995. With far fewer children contracting chickenpox, adults have far less exposure to the virus, which would otherwise boost the immunity they acquired during childhood and help prevent reactivation of latent virus in their bodies.

Description

The varicella zoster virus is a member of the herpes virus family. It causes chickenpox, or varicella, which is highly contagious and spreads through the air. Following the initial or primary VZV infection, which usually occurs in childhood, the virus remains in an inactive or latent state in nerve tissue. Years later—usually after age 50—VZV can be reactivated to cause herpes zoster or shingles. The name "varicella" is derived from "variola," the Latin name for **smallpox**, a now-eradicated deadly disease, which can resemble chickenpox. "Zoster" is the Greek word for "girdle," and "shingles" derives from "cingulum," the Latin word for "belt" or "girdle," which refer to the shingles lesions or blisters that form on one side of the waist. As early as 1909, scientists suspected that chickenpox and shingles were caused by the same virus—this suspicion was confirmed in 1958.

Shingles is an infection of the central nervous system, particularly the dorsal root ganglia of the spine. From there, the virus migrates through sensory nerve fibers to the skin—usually on the trunk—where it causes

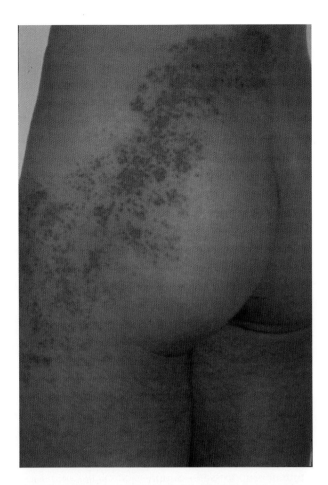

Herpes zoster is caused by a virus that affects people in a pattern characterized by erythema and pain. It follows the distribution of cutaneous nerves and is first localized in the doral ganglia of the nervous system. The virus is varicella-zoster, and the disease is often called shingles. *(© Wellcome Image Library / Custom Medical Stock Photo)*

Anyone who has ever had chickenpox or been vaccinated against it is at risk for shingles. Overall, approximately 20% of those who had chickenpox as children eventually develop shingles. Susceptibility to shingles appears to be genetically determined, and the condition runs in families. The risk of shingles increases with age and with any condition that weakens the immune system. Those at particular risk for shingles include:

- children who had chickenpox in infancy or whose mothers had chickenpox late in pregnancy
- bone marrow and other transplant recipients
- those with compromised immune systems from diseases such as HIV/AIDS
- those with suppressed immune systems from chemotherapy drugs or other medications

Causes and Symptoms

It is not clear why VZV reactivates to cause shingles, but it appears to be related to a decreased immune response due to advancing age, emotional or physical **stress**, fatigue, certain medications, chemotherapy, or diseases such as **cancer** or HIV/AIDS. Shingles is sometimes an early sign of immunodeficiency in people infected with HIV. In some cases, the virus appears to be reactivated by mechanical irritation or minor surgical procedures.

Mild cases of shingles often go unnoticed. The earliest signs may be vague and can easily be mistaken for other illnesses. The condition may begin with fever, chills, gastrointestinal discomfort, and malaise (a vague feeling of weakness or discomfort). Lymph nodes may swell. Within two to four days, localized areas of intense **pain**, itching, and numbness/tingling (paresthesia) or extreme sensitivity to touch (hyperesthesia) can develop, usually on the trunk. The second most common place is on one side of the face around the eye (ophthalmic shingles) or on the forehead. However, shingles can occur on the arms, legs, or elsewhere on the body. The pain may be continuous or intermittent, usually lasting from one to four weeks. The pain may accompany skin eruptions or precede the eruptions by days.

The red rash or oozing blisters appear along the course of the affected nerve. There is usually a vague streak or band from the spine along the path of the nerve on one side of the body. About five days after they appear, the vesicles begin to crust or scab, and the disease resolves within the next two to three weeks. There may be no visible after-effects or a slight scarring from the vesicles.

painful, fluid-filled eruptions or vesicles. Due to the fact that the sensory nerves serve sharply bounded, non-overlapping areas of the skin, called "dermatomes," the shingles lesions appear within these dermatomes and do not cross the midline of the body.

Unlike chickenpox, shingles is not contagious, because the virus is not usually in the lungs, from which it could spread through the air. However the fluid-filled eruptions on the skin contain large amounts of virus, which can be transmitted through direct contact and infect a person, often a child, who has not previously been exposed to VZV. The infected person will develop a case of primary chickenpox. A vaccine that prevents or ameliorates the symptoms of shingles became available in 2006. **Immunization** against chickenpox does not prevent shingles, although it may reduce its incidence.

Shingles can be more debilitating in the elderly or those in poor health. The eruptions may be more extensive and inflammatory; they may also include bleeding blisters, areas of skin death, secondary bacterial infection, or extensive and permanent scarring. Ophthalmic shingles can cause painful eye infections and vision loss. Shingles infections within or near the ear can cause hearing or balance problems. Sometimes shingles can cause temporary or permanent tremors or paralysis; rarely, the condition spreads to the brain or spinal cord and causes **stroke** or **meningitis**.

Shingles pain usually subsides when the rash disappears, but it may last much longer, especially in the elderly. PHN can persist for months or years. It is caused by damage to the dorsal root ganglia, with the nerves becoming either spontaneously active—which is perceived as chronic pain—or hypersensitive to slight stimuli such as light touch. In the most severe cases, PHN can cause insomnia, weight loss, depression, and disability.

Diagnosis

Examination

Diagnosis of shingles is based on a medical history and physical examination. A definite diagnosis is difficult before eruption of the characteristic vesicles or bumps on the skin. The vesicles have a clear dermatome-bounded distribution usually on the midsection of the body.

Tests

Tests for shingles are rarely necessary but may include:

• polymerase chain reaction (PCR) testing for viral DNA

• viral culture of skin lesions

• a Tzanck preparation—stained cells from a blister, which will appear under the microscope to have many very large dark nuclei if infected with VZV

• a complete blood count (CBC) to test for elevated white blood cells that are indicative of infection

• blood serum levels of antibodies against VZV

Treatment

Traditional

Shingles almost always resolves spontaneously within a few weeks. Unless complicated by conditions such as HIV/AIDS or cancer, a primary care physician can provide treatment for easing painful symptoms. Rarely, transcutaneous electrical nerve stimulation

---

KEY TERMS

Acyclovir—An antiviral drug that is available in oral, intravenous, and topical forms and that blocks replication of the varicella zoster virus.

Antibody—A specific protein produced by the immune system in response to a specific foreign protein or particle called an "antigen."

Capsaicin—An active ingredient from hot chili peppers that is used in topical ointments to relieve pain. It appears to work by reducing the levels of a chemical substance involved in transmitting pain signals from nerve endings to the brain.

Corticosteroids—A group of hormones produced by the adrenal glands or manufactured synthetically. They are often used to treat inflammation. Examples include cortisone and prednisone.

Dermatome—An area of skin which is serviced by a single ganglian from the spinal cord.

Famciclovir—An oral antiviral drug that blocks the replication of the varicella zoster virus.

Ganglion—A mass of nerve tissue outside of the central nervous system.

Immunocompromised—A weakened or poorly functioning immune system due to disease.

Immunosuppressed—Suppression of the immune system by medications during the treatment of diseases such as cancer or following an organ transplantation.

Post-herpetic neuralgia (PHN)—Long-lasting nerve pain caused by herpes zoster.

Tzanck preparation—A procedure in which skin cells from a blister are stained and examined under the microscope.

Valacyclovir—An oral antiviral drug that blocks the replication of the varicella zoster virus.

Vesicle—A small, raised lesion filled with clear fluid.

(TENS) or a permanent nerve block is used to relieve the pain of PHN.

Drugs

The antiviral drugs acyclovir, valacyclovir, and famciclovir are used to treat shingles. These drugs can shorten the course of the illness. If started within 72 hours of the onset of the rash, antiviral therapy can heal the blisters more rapidly and sometimes even halt the disease. If taken after the disease has progressed, these drugs are less effective but may still lessen the pain. Antiviral drug treatment reduces the incidence of PHN by about one-half and may also shorten its duration. Severely immunocompromised individuals, such as those with HIV/AIDS, may require intravenous administration of antiviral drugs or taking the drugs on an ongoing basis.

Various other drugs may be prescribed for shingles and PHN:

• corticosteroids, such as prednisone, to reduce inflammation from shingles, especially if the eye or other facial nerves are involved, and to reduce severe pain

• anticonvulsants such as pregabalin (Lyrica) or gabapentin to relieve pain

• the tricylcic antidepressants (TCAs) desipramine and nortriptyline

• opioid painkillers such as oxycodone, morphine, tramadol, or methadone

• tranquilizers or sedatives

• topical local anesthetics for application to the painful skin area and for post-herpetic itch; especially lidocaine, available as a cream, gel, spray, or patch

• capsaicin cream, which is available without a prescription but usually causes burning pain during application

Alternative

Alternative remedies and therapies will not cure shingles, but they may relieve pain, reduce inflammation, and speed recovery:

• The amino acid lysine has also been reported to ease the symptoms of shingles and other herpes infections. Foods that are high in lysine include soybeans, black bean sprouts, lentils, parsley, and peas.

• Vitamin B12 supplementation during the first two days of the illness and ongoing vitamin B complex, vitamin C with bioflavonoids, and calcium supplements may boost the immune system.

• Echinacea can boost the immune system and help fight viral infections.

• Red pepper (capsicum or cayenne) is an ingredient in commercial ointments including Zostrix and Capzasin-P. It should be applied only to healed blisters and is useful for treating painful PHN. Seasoning food with red pepper may also provide relief.

• Calendula or licorice (*Glycyrrhiza glabra*) ointment or lotion may help treat shingles.

• Topical applications of lemon balm (*Melissa officinalis*), licorice, or peppermint (*Mentha piperita*) may reduce pain and blistering. These can also be consumed as teas.

• Sedative herbs such as passionflower can be brewed for a tea to treat PHN.

• Vervain helps relieve pain and inflammation.

• St. John's wort, lavender, chamomile, and marjoram help relieve inflammation.

• Homeopathic remedies include *Rhus toxicodendron* for blisters, *Mezereum* and *Arsenicum album* for pain, and *Ranunculus* for itching.

• Several drops of "Rescue Remedy" placed under the tongue or taken in water throughout the day are prescribed for relieving stress.

• Ayurvedic treatments for shingles include the application of turmeric paste.

• Acupuncture and acupressure can alleviate pain and PHN.

• Biofeedback or spinal cord stimulators may help relieve PHN.

• Relaxation techniques such as hypnotherapy and yoga may help relieve pain.

• Reflexology may help balance the body.

Practitioners of traditional Chinese medicine (TCM) may recommend herbal remedies:

• Chinese gentian root is used to treat the liver.

• Skullcap root in water is a Chinese folk remedy for shingles.

• Long Dan Xie Gan Tang is used to quell the accumulation of damp, toxic heat in the liver.

• For damp, infected, painful eruptions on the torso, Huang Qin Gao can be applied to the surrounding area.

Home Remedies

Home remedies for shingles include plenty of rest, a healthy diet, regular exercise, and minimizing stress. The skin should be kept clean, and contaminated items should not be reused. Cool compresses may help reduce pain from blisters. Blisters or crusting can be treated with compresses made with one-quarter cup (60 mL) of white vinegar in two quarts (1.9 L) of lukewarm water and applied twice daily for 10 minutes. The compresses should be discontinued when the blisters have dried up. Soothing baths and lotions with colloidal oatmeal, starch, or calamine may help to relieve itching and discomfort. If the skin becomes dry, tight, and cracked as the crusts and scabs separate, a small amount of plain petroleum jelly can be applied three or four times daily. The pain of PHN may be relieved with hot and cold compresses.

Prognosis

Shingles is almost never life-threatening in otherwise healthy patients and usually resolves without treatment in a few weeks. Shingles boosts the immune response to VZV, so repeat episodes are rare, occurring in less than 4% of patients. Although PHN usually diminishes over time, it can be disabling and difficult to treat.

Shingles can be much more severe in immunocompromised patients. The condition can last for months, recur frequently, and spread to the lungs, liver, gastrointestinal tract, brain, or other vital organs. Complications of shingles in immunocompromised or immunosuppressed patients may resemble those of primary varicella infection in adults, including viral **pneumonia**, male sterility, acute liver failure, and **birth defects** in children born to infected mothers. Depletion of CD4+ T lymphocytes in HIV/AIDS patients is associated with severe and chronic or recurrent VZV infection.

Prevention

A lifestyle that promotes immune system function and overall health may help prevent shingles. Factors include a well-balanced diet rich in essential **vitamins** and minerals, adequate sleep, regular exercise, and reduced stress. Patients with shingles should avoid contact with anyone who has not had chickenpox or been vaccinated against the disease, particularly pregnant women, newborns, and those with weakened immune systems.

In the United States, it is now recommended that all children between 18 months and adolescence be immunized against chickenpox. Because a weakened (attenuated) form of the virus is used in this vaccine, it is thought that **vaccination** will reduce the likelihood of shingles later on in life.

Efforts and Solutions

A single-dose vaccine against shingles (Zostavax) became available in 2006 and is recommended for most people aged 60 and older who have previously had chickenpox. It appears to prevent shingles in about 50% of vaccinated people and reduces the pain associated with shingles in others. It also can help prevent post-herpetic neuralgia. The vaccine has been approved by the FDA for those aged 50 to 59, but the **Centers for Disease Control and Prevention (CDC)** do not have a standard recommendation for use before age 60. The vaccine is not recommended for all individuals over 60, however. Those who have a weakened immune system as a result of cancer, chemotherapy or **radiation** treatments, those with **AIDS** or other diseases affecting the immune system, and pregnant women should not receive the vaccine. In some cases, there have also been severe allergic reactions to elements of the vaccine. Those over

the age of 50 interested in the vaccine or those concerned about the appropriateness of the vaccine for their individual health concerns should talk to their healthcare professionals.

Resources

BOOKS

Kirschmann, John D. *Nutrition Almanac,* 6th ed. New York: McGraw-Hill, 2007.

Shannon, Joyce Brennfleck. *Pain Sourcebook,* 3rd ed. Detroit: Omnigraphics, 2008.

Siegel, Mary-Ellen, and Gray Williams. *Shingles: New Hope for an Old Disease,* updated ed. Lanham M. Evans and Company, Inc., 2008.

PERIODICALS

Froelich, Janis D. "How Did a Gal Like Me Come Down with Shingles?" *Tampa Tribune* (June 21, 2008): 16.

Gutpa, Sanjay. "Rash Redux." *Time* 172, no. 4 (July 28, 2008): 53.

Lang, Richard S. "Answers to questions about the shingles vaccine, cardiac devices, and epilepsy." *Men's Health Advisor* 14.3 (2012): 8. Accessed July 10, 2012.

"Herpes Zoster." *American Academy of Dermatology.* [Accessed December 3, 2010] http://www.aad.org/ public/ publications/pamphlets/viral_herpes_ zoster.htm.

CDC.Gov. "Shingles Vaccination". http://www.cdc.gov/ shingles/vaccination.html Accessed July 10, 2012.

Office of Communications and Public Liaison, National Institute of Neurological Disorders and Stroke. "Shingles: Hope Through Research." *NIH Publication No. 06-307.* [Accessed December 3, 2010] http://www.ninds. nih.gov/ disorders/shingles/detail_shingles.htm.

"Shingles." *National Institute of Allergy and Infectious Diseases.* [Accessed December 3, 2010] http://www3 .niaid.nih.gov/topics/shingles/

"Shingles & After-Shingles Pain." *AfterShingles.com.* [Accessed December 3, 2010] http://www.aftershingles .com/after-shingles-pain.aspx.

"Shingles (Herpes Zoster) Vaccination." *Vaccines & Immunizations.* [Accessed December 3, 2010] http://www.cdc .gov/vaccines/vpd-vac/shingles/default.htm.

ORGANIZATIONS

American Academy of Dermatology, PO Box 4014, Schaumburg, IL 60168, (847) 240-1280, (866) 503-SKIN (7546), Fax: (847) 240-1859, http://www.aad.org

American Botanical Council, 6200 Manor Rd., Austin, TX 78723, (512) 926-4900, Fax: (512) 926-2345, abc@ herbalgram.org, http://cms.herbalgram.org

National Institute of Allergy and Infectious Diseases (NIAID), Office of Communications and Public Liaison, 6610 Rockledge Drive, Bethesda, MD 20892-66123, (866) 284-4107, http://www3.niaid.nih.gov

National Institute of Neurological Disorders and Stroke (NINDS), NIH Neurological Institute, PO Box 5801, Bethesda, MD 20824, (301) 496-5751, (800) 352-9424, http://www.ninds.nih.gov

National Shingles Foundation, 590 Madison Ave., 21st Floor, New York, NY 10022, (212) 222-3390, Fax: (212) 222-8627, http://www.vzvfoundation.org

U.S. Centers for Disease Control and Prevention (CDC), 1600 Clifton Road, Atlanta, GA 30333, (800)-CDC-INFO (232-4636), cdcinfo@cdc.gov, http://www.cdc.gov.

Rebecca J. Frey, Ph.D.
Larry Gilman, Ph.D.
Margaret Alic, Ph.D.
Andrea Nienstedt, M.A.

Sick building syndrome

Definition

Sick building syndrome (SBS) is a term applied to an indoor environment that causes its occupants to become ill. The syndrome is usually associated with indoor air pollutants, although it has often been difficult to associate the symptoms with specific pollutants. Other issues, such as poor building management and workplace **stress**, may also be factors. Indoor air quality (IAQ) health problems fall into three categories: SBS, building-related illnesses (BRI), and multiple chemical sensitivity. Of the three, SBS accounts for about 75% of all IAQ complaints.

Description

Indoor air is a health hazard in about 30% of all buildings, according to the **World Health Organization (WHO)**. The **Environmental Protection Agency (EPA)** lists IAQ fourth among top **environmental health** threats. The problem of SBS is of increasing concern to employees and **occupational health** specialists, as well as landlords and corporations who fear the financial consequences of illnesses among tenants and employees, respectively. Respiratory diseases attributed to SBS account for about 150 million lost workdays each year, $59 billion in indirect costs, and $15 billion in medical costs.

Sick building syndrome was first recognized in the 1970s around the time of the energy crisis and the move toward conservation. Because heating and air conditioning systems accounted for a major portion of energy consumption in the United States, buildings were sealed for energy efficiency. In these buildings, occupants depend on mechanical systems rather than open windows for outside air and ventilation. There are three methods in which outside air can enter a building including infiltration, natural ventilation, and mechanical ventilation. Infiltration occurs when outside air enters a building through cracks around windows, floors, doors, and walls. Natural ventilation occurs through open doors or windows. For mechanical ventilation, outdoor-vented fans for heating, venting, and air conditioning systems (HVAC) bring outside air in and move inside air out. A building that is well insulated and sealed for energy efficiency, referred to as a tight building, can seal in and create contaminants.

According to the U.S. **Environmental Protection Agency (EPA)**, SBS is strongly identified when the following situations are present:

- Symptoms are associated with the time spent in a particular building or part of a building.
- Symptoms disappear when the individual is not in a building causing such symptoms.
- Symptoms recur seasonally (such as when a building is heated or cooled).
- Coworkers or other individuals within the particular building note similar symptoms.

Demographics

Sick building syndrome occurs when individuals occupying a certain building report similar acute health problems that seem to be related directly to the time spent in the building. No specific illness or cause is identified, and the problems may be concentrated in a particular room or area or may be widespread throughout the building.

Causes and symptoms

According to the Environmental Protection Agency, SBS is caused by four major factors:

- biological contaminants: bacteria, molds, pollen, and viruses accumulated in ducts, humidifiers, drain pans, and other sources where water has collected
- chemical contaminants from indoor sources: primarily from adhesives, carpeting, cleaning supplies, copy machines, manufactured wood products, and upholstery that emit volatile organic compounds, including formaldehyde; other contributing factors include tobacco smoke and combustion products such as carbon monoxide, nitrogen dioxide, and other particles from unvented kerosene and gas space heaters, fireplaces, gas stoves, and woodstoves
- chemical contaminants from outdoor sources: primarily from motor vehicle exhaust and from plumbing vents, and building exhausts (such as bathrooms and kitchens) that enter the building through poorly located air intake vents, windows, and other openings
- inadequate ventilation: heating, ventilating, and air conditioning systems that do not effectively distribute air throughout a building; the American Society of

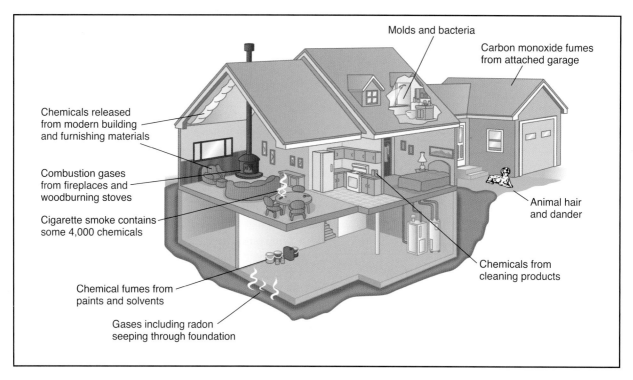

Possible causes of Sick Building Syndrome. *(Illustration by Electronic Illustrators Group. © 2013 Cengage Learning)*

Heating, Refrigerating and Air-Conditioning Engineers recommends a minimum flow of 15 cubic feet per minute (cfm) of outdoor air per person in a home and 20 cfm per person in office spaces in order to maintain the health and comfort of occupants.

Common symptoms of SBS include dizziness, skin irritation, headaches, fatigue, dry cough, sneezing, nausea, hoarseness of voice, **allergies**, **asthma** attacks, cold, flu-like symptoms, difficulty concentrating, and irritations of the eyes, nose and throat. In addition, many people have more general symptoms including personality changes, hypersensitivity reactions, and odor and taste sensations. Symptoms are caused by a range of contaminants including volatile organic compounds (VOC), which are chemicals that turn to gas at room temperature and are given off by paints, adhesives, caulking, vinyl, telephone cable, printed documents, furniture, and solvents. Most common VOCs are benzene (C_6H_6) and chloroform ($CHCl_3$), both of which have been shown to be carcinogenic. Formaldehyde (CH_2O) in building materials is also an indoor irritant. However, the concentrations of VOCs at which SBS is observed are usually well below the concentrations at which the common symptoms would be expected.

Biological agents such as viruses, bacteria, fungal spores, algae, pollen, **mold**, and dust mites add to the problems. These are produced by water-damaged carpet and furnishing or standing water in ventilation systems, humidifiers, and flush toilets.

Carbon dioxide (CO_2) levels increase as the number of people in a room increases, and too much can cause occupants to suffer hyperventilation, headaches, dizziness, shortness of breath, and drowsiness, as does carbon monoxide (CO) and the other toxins from cigarette smoke.

Schoolchildren are considered more vulnerable to SBS because schools typically have more people per room breathing the same stale air. Their size, childhood allergies, and asthmas increase their vulnerability.

Diagnosis

The diagnosis for SBS is difficult because a specific illness or cause cannot be easily identified by the medical community.

Treatment

Sick buildings can be treated by updating and cleaning ventilation systems regularly and using air cleaners and filtration devices. Also, plants spaced every 100 square feet (9.3 square meters) in offices, homes, and schools have been shown to filter out pollutants in recycled air.

A simple survey of the indoor environment can detect many SBS problems. Each room should have an air source; if windows cannot be opened, every room should have a supply vent and exhaust vent. The vents should be cleaned regularly. A tissue can be placed at each vent opening to check that air is circulating through the system. The tissue should blow out at a supply vent and be pulled in at an exhaust vent. Vents should not be blocked by partitions, file cabinets, or boxes. Supply and exhaust vents should be more than a few feet apart. Dead spaces where air stagnates and pollutants build up should be renovated. Printing and copying machines should be moved away from people and should be given adequate exhaust. The ventilation system should be checked every season for verification of full operation.

Public health role and response

The EPA enforces laws on outdoor **air pollution** but not for indoor air except for some **smoking** bans. Yet almost every pollutant, according to the EPA, is at higher levels indoors than outdoors. Help in detecting and correcting SBS is available from the National Institute of Occupational Safety and Health (NIOSH), the federal agency responsible for conducting research and making recommendations for safe and healthy work standards. The EPA and the NIOSH have developed a Building Air Quality Action plan with guidelines for improving and maintaining IAQ in public and commercial buildings.

Prognosis

The prognosis for sick building syndrome is generally good if the cause of the disorder can be identified. However, because its symptoms vary widely, and no specific illness is easily identified, the diagnosis of SBS may be lengthy.

Prevention

Important factors that can prevent and control SBS are:

- increased ventilation and air distribution
- routine maintenance of HVAC systems and replacement of water-damaged flooring and ceiling tiles
- use of open office designs and indoor plants along with skylights and scheduled filter cleaning
- education of residents and workers on the importance of ventilation
- support of legislation that bans smoking inside buildings

Resources

BOOKS

Abdul-Wahab, Sabah A, ed. *Sick Building Syndrome: In Public Buildings and Workplaces.* Berlin: Springer, 2011.

Bluyssen, Philomena M. *The Indoor Environment Handbook: How to Make Buildings Healthy and Comfortable.* London: Earthscan, 2009.

Larsen, Laura, ed. *Environmental Health Sourcebook.* Detroit: Omnigraphics, 2010.

May, Jeffrey C. *My Office Is Killing Me! The Sick Building Survival Guide.* Baltimore: Johns Hopkins University Press, 2006.

Natelson, Benjamin H. *Your Symptoms Are Real: What to Do When Your Doctor Says Nothing Is Wrong.* Hoboken, NJ: John Wiley, 2008.

Pall, Martin L. *Explaining "Unexplained Illnesses": Disease Paradigm for Chronic Fatigue Syndrome, Multiple Chemical Sensitivity, Fibromyalgia, Post-Traumatic Stress Disorder, Gulf War Syndrome, and Others.* New York: Harrington Park Press, 2007.

Preston, Flora. *Convenient, "Safe" and Deadly: The True Costs of Our Chemical Lifestyle.* Lanark, ONT: Health Risk Navigation, 2006.

Sutton, Amy L. *Allergies Sourcebook: Basic Consumer Health Information About Allergic Disorders, such as Anaphylaxis.* Detroit: Omnigraphics, 2007.

WEBSITES

Centers for Disease Control and Prevention. "Indoor Environmental Quality." (November 28, 2011). http://www.cdc.gov/niosh/topics/indoorenv/ (accessed September 21, 2012).

Environmental Illness Resource. "Sick Building Syndrome (SBS)." (March 19, 2011). http://www.ei-resource.org/illness-information/related-conditions/sick-building-syndrome-(sbs)/ (accessed September 21, 2012).

Environmental Protection Agency. "Building Air Quality: A Guide for Building Owners and Facility Managers." http://www.epa.gov/iaq/largebldgs/baqtoc.html (accessed September 21, 2012).

Environmental Protection Agency. "Consumer's Guide to Radon Reduction." http://www.epa.gov/radon/pubs/consguid.html (accessed September 21, 2012).

Environmental Protection Agency. "Indoor Air Facts No. 4 (revised) Sick Building Syndrome." (February 1999). http://www.epa.gov/iaq/pdfs/sick_building_factsheet.pdf (accessed September 21, 2012).

Environmental Protection Agency. "Indoor Air: Publications and Resources." http://www.epa.gov/iaq/pubs/ (accessed September 21, 2012).

Joshi, Sumedha M. "The Sick Building Syndrome." National Center for Biotechnology Information. (August 2008). http://www.ncbi.nlm.nih.gov/pmc/articles/PMC2796751/ (accessed September 21, 2012).

ORGANIZATIONS

Agency for Toxic Substances and Disease Registry, Centers for Disease Control and Prevention, 4770 Buford Hwy. NE, Atlanta, GA 30341, (800) 232-4636, http://www.atsdr.cdc.gov

American Academy of Environmental Medicine, 6505 E Central Ave., No. 296, Wichita, KS 67206, (316) 684-5500, Fax: (316) 684-5709, administrator@aaemonline.org, http://aaemonline.org

Environmental Protection Agency, 1200 Pennsylvania Ave., NW, Ariel Rios Bldg., Washington, DC 20460, (202) 272-0167, http://www.epa.gov

National Institute of Occupational Safety and Health, Centers for Disease Control and Prevention, 1600 Clifton Rd., Atlanta, GA 30333, (800) 232-4636, cdcinfo@cdc.gov, http://www.cdc.gov/niosh

Occupational Safety and Health Organization, U.S. Department of Labor, 200 Constitution Ave. NW, Washington, DC 20210, (800) 321-6742, http://www.osha.gov.

Linda Rehkopf

Recommended hours of sleep, by age group

Infants	
0–2 months	12–18 hours
2–12 months	14–15 hours
Toddlers/Children	
1–3 years	12–14 hours
3–5 years	11–13 hours
5–10 years	10–11 hours
Adolescents	
10–17 years	8.5–9.25 hours
Adults	
18+	7–9 hours

SOURCE: National Sleep Foundation, "How Much Sleep Do We Really Need?"

(Table by PreMediaGlobal. © 2012 Cengage Learning.)

Sleep deprivation

Definition

Sleep deprivation is an inadequate amount of sleep for a given individual.

Demographics

Sleep deprivation has become so widespread in industrialized societies that daytime drowsiness may no longer seem abnormal. Between 1998 and 2005, the number of American adults who reported getting eight or more hours of sleep on weekday nights fell from 35% to 26%. Driver fatigue causes 100,000 accidents and 1,500 deaths annually in the United States. Through a health survey, the **Centers for Disease Control and Prevention (CDC)** estimates that 7–19% of adults reported not getting enough sleep every day, with almost 40% reporting having fallen asleep without meaning to, at least once per month. The **CDC** also estimates that between 50 and 70 million Americans have some sort of chronic sleep disorder.

Sleep deprivation is considered to be a widespread chronic health problem among American teenagers. A 2006 poll found that only 20% of teens got adequate sleep on school nights: by the end of high school, they averaged fewer than seven hours, and most teens reported feeling tired during the day.

Although sleep disturbances and disorders do not necessarily result in sleep deprivation, they can contribute to it:

• About half of all people over age 65 suffer frequent sleep disturbances.

• About 60 million Americans suffer from frequent or extended periods of insomnia resulting in sleep deprivation. The incidence of insomnia increases with age, affecting about 40% of women and 30% of men.

• An estimated 18 million Americans have sleep apnea, although it usually goes undiagnosed.

• Restless leg syndrome (RLS) is one of the most common sleep disorders that causes sleep deprivation, especially among older people. RLS is estimated to affect as many as 12 million Americans.

• Narcolepsy—which affects about 250,000 Americans—can cause nighttime insomnia, resulting in sleep deprivation.

• Most people with mental disorders—including depression and schizophrenia—have sleep disturbances that cause sleep deprivation.

• Many blind people have lifelong sleeping problems, including insomnia and a type of permanent jet lag, which can result in sleep deprivation.

Description

Sleeping and wakefulness are controlled by neurotransmitters—chemical messengers in the brain—that act on different sets of nerve cells or neurons. The neurotransmitters serotonin and norepinephrine in the brainstem—the connection between the brain and the spinal cord—keep parts of the brain active during wakefulness and are switched off during sleep. Also during wakefulness, an important chemical called "adenosine" builds up in the blood to the point where it eventually causes drowsiness and is broken down during sleep.

Humans normally cycle through five stages of sleep throughout the night, with one complete sleep cycle averaging 90–120 minutes:

• Stage 1 consists of drowsiness, drifting in and out of sleep, and being easily awakened.

• Stage 2 is light sleep, which accounts for about 50% of total sleeping time.

• Stage 3 is deep sleep.

• Stage 4 is slow-wave deep sleep.

• Stages 1, 3, and 4 together account for about 30% of sleeping time.

• Stage 5 is rapid eye movement (REM) sleep, which accounts for about 20% of total sleep time.

During the first sleep cycles of the night, deep sleep is relatively long, and REM sleep short. REM periods gradually increase in length as deep sleep shortens. Towards waking, almost all sleep is stages 1, 2, and REM.

Sleep is essential for survival, and sleep deprivation can eventually result in death. However, scientists have only recently begun to understand the many functions of sleep. It is required for proper nervous system functioning. Parts of the brain that are involved in emotions, decision-making, and social interactions are less active during sleep. These neurons may need sleep to repair and replenish themselves, and sleep may also be necessary for growing new neurons and for exercising neuronal functions that are less active during wakefulness.

Other parts of the brain, however, are very active during sleep. During this period of low sensory input, the brain consolidates recently acquired memories. Nerve-signaling patterns that are generated during the day are repeated during deep sleep. REM sleep is required for learning certain mental skills, and sleep may be necessary for encoding memories and learning.

Many cells in the body produce more protein during deep and REM sleep, so sleep may be necessary for replenishing energy and repairing damage in cells throughout the body. Growth hormones in children and young adults are released during deep sleep, and sleep is required for proper immune system function and cytokines—chemicals that fight infection—are produced during sleep.

Sleep requirements

The amount of sleep required to prevent deprivation depends on a variety of factors, especially age and genetics:

• Infants need about 16 hours of sleep out of every 24 hours, with about 50% spent in REM.

• Toddlers need about 14 hours of sleep, which gradually decreases with age to a requirement of slightly over nine hours in teenagers.

• Most adults need 7–8 hours of sleep each night, although individual requirements may vary from 4 to 12 hours per night.

• Researchers have identified a gene called DEC2 that turns off some genes involved in controlling circadian rhythms—the internal clock that regulates the sleep-wake cycle. People with certain mutations in the DEC2 gene require only about six hours of sleep per night.

• Women often need several extra hours of sleep during the first three months of pregnancy.

• Although older people tend to sleep more lightly and for shorter periods, they need about the same amount of total sleep as when they were younger.

For most people, sleep deprivation accumulates as a "sleep debt," which must be made up. The ability to function relatively well—at least for short periods—under conditions of sleep deprivation appears to be genetically determined. Estimates suggest that 10%–15% of people function adequately on little or no sleep, whereas another 10%–15% cannot function at all without sleep. Most people cannot function at all after 48 hours without sleep, nor do humans appear to adapt to sleep deprivation. One study found that subjects who slept only 4–6 hours per night for 14 consecutive nights showed cognitive impairment equivalent to going without sleep for three consecutive days.

Although people may adjust to a sleep-depriving schedule, daily functioning and physical and mental health suffer, as sleep deprivation interferes with concentration, learning, and problem-solving. At least six hours of regular sleep are required for peak memory performance, and sleep deprivation is directly linked to memory loss. In addition, sleep deprivation may:

• interfere with work, school, and social interactions

• cause stress

• and slow reaction times; sleep-deprived people perform at least as poorly on driving simulators and hand-eye coordination tasks as people who are intoxicated

- disrupt the decision-making machinery of the brain, impairing judgment, increasing risky behaviors, and reducing sensitivity to loss
- increase the risk of falls and accidents
- increase the risk for many health problems, including hypertension, cardiovascular disease, diabetes, obesity, and infections
- increase appetite and inhibit weight loss, even with proper exercise and diet
- increase the effects of alcohol.
- cause sleep paralysis, a rare but frightening condition in which a person temporarily loses the ability to speak or move while falling asleep or waking up

Teenagers require an average of 9.25 hours of sleep per night for brain development, health, and optimal performance. Sleep-deprived teens are at risk for:

- impaired cognitive function and decision-making
- health problems
- poor grades and athletic performance
- emotional and behavioral problems
- depression
- substance abuse
- violence
- automobile accidents

Risk factors

Risk factors for sleep deprivation include:

- anxiety and stress
- careers with long or irregular working hours
- night or shift work
- work requiring long-distance travel
- multiple jobs
- combining full-time work and school
- being a family caregiver

Causes and symptoms

Causes

Sleep deprivation is most often caused by lifestyle choices or the requirements of work, school, or caregiving. Irregular sleep patterns that differ between weekdays and weekends can harm the quality of sleep. A new baby often results in sleep-deprived parents. Teenagers with hectic schedules of school, homework, athletics, after-school activities, jobs, and family and social obligations find themselves without enough hours for quality sleep. Furthermore, hormonal changes in adolescence set most teens' biological clocks on later schedules than those of children and adults. Teens may be wide awake—albeit exhausted—at bedtime but still have to wake up early for school.

Foods and drugs that change the balance of neurotransmitters in the brain can cause sleep deprivation, including caffeinated drinks, such as coffee, and drugs, such as diet pills and decongestants, which stimulate the brain and can cause insomnia. Many antidepressants suppress REM sleep, and substances such as alcohol and nicotine deprive the brain of REM sleep.

Changes in regions of the brain and in neurotransmitters can result in sleep deprivation. Sleeping problems in older people may be a normal part of **aging** or can be related to underlying medical conditions, medications, medical treatments, or sleep-disrupting hospital routines. Anxiety or chronic **pain** can cause sleep deprivation, which, in turn, can cause anxiety disorders or make it harder to cope with pain. Other conditions that can cause sleep deprivation include menopause, vision loss, attention deficit hyperactivity disorder (ADHD), head injury, **stroke**, **cancer**, and Alzheimer's disease.

Sleep disorders may also result in sleep deprivation. There are more than 70 known sleep disorders; the most common include:

- insomnia, which can have various causes—including stress, jet lag, diet, or an underlying medical condition—and almost always affects next-day functioning
- sleep apnea, or disrupted breathing during sleep, which causes frequent awakenings
- RLS, a condition that causes constant leg movement and insomnia and is either inherited or linked to conditions such as pregnancy, anemia, or diabetes
- periodic limb movement disorder (PLMD), which often accompanies RLS and causes repeated awakenings
- narcolepsy, which is characterized by brief attacks of daytime deep sleep and is usually caused by an inherited malfunction in the regulation of sleep-wake cycles

Symptoms of sleep deprivation include:

- difficulty awakening each morning
- daytime drowsiness
- microsleeps—very brief, often unnoticed—periods of sleep during waking hours
- falling asleep during school or work
- need for frequent naps
- routinely falling asleep within five minutes of lying down
- disrupted sleep
- parasomnias—uncontrollable actions during sleep, such as sleepwalking

- headaches
- poor school or work performance
- inability to concentrate
- inability to perform mathematical calculations
- impaired memory
- problems with decision-making
- clumsiness or impaired physical performance
- irritability or mood swings
- paranoia
- confusion
- hallucinations
- decreased consciousness

Although sleep deprivation can be an effective therapy for people with certain types of depression, it can cause depression in otherwise healthy people. Sleep deprivation can also trigger manic episodes of agitation and hyperactivity in people with bipolar disorder and seizures in patients with some types of epilepsy.

Diagnosis

Examination

Sleep deprivation is usually readily diagnosed from the symptoms accompanying the lack of sleep. Underlying medical problems resulting in sleep deprivation may require further diagnoses.

Procedures

Simple devices are available for detecting sleep apnea. Sleep apnea may be diagnosed at a specialized sleep center using polysomnography to record brain waves, heartbeat, and breathing for an entire night.

Treatment

Traditional

The usual treatment for sleep deprivation is sleep. Underlying conditions that result in sleep deprivation require more extensive treatments. For example, severe sleep apnea may require a mask—called a "continuous positive airway pressure" (CPAP) device—to keep the airways open during sleep. Surgery may be necessary to correct an airway obstruction.

Drugs

Caffeine and other stimulants cannot overcome the effects of severe sleep deprivation. However, various products are available to treat sleep disturbances that can result in sleep deprivation:

KEY TERMS

Adenosine—A nucleoside that plays multiple physiological roles in energy transfer and molecular signaling, as a component of RNA, and as an inhibitory neurotransmitter that promotes sleep.

Apnea—The transient cessation of breathing.

Circadian rhythm—A 24-hour cycle of physiological or behavioral activities.

Cytokines—A class of proteins, including interferons and interleukins, that are released by cells as part of the immune response and as mediators of intercellular communication.

Insomnia—Prolonged or abnormal inability to obtain adequate sleep.

Melatonin—A hormone involved in regulation of circadian rhythms.

Narcolepsy—A condition characterized by brief attacks of deep sleep.

Neurotransmitters—Chemicals that transmit nerve impulses from one nerve cell to another.

REM—Rapid eye movement; a stage of the normal sleep cycle characterized by rapid eye movements, increased forebrain and midbrain activity, and dreaming.

Restless leg syndrome (RLS)—A neurological disorder characterized by aching, burning, or creeping sensations in the legs and an urge to move the legs, often resulting in insomnia.

- Over-the-counter sleep aids usually contain antihistamines. Although they are sometimes effective, they have side effects, and tolerance can develop after just a few days of use.

- RLS and PLMD are often relieved with drugs that affect the neurotransmitter dopamine.

- Daily melatonin supplements may improve nighttime sleep in blind patients.

The U.S. Food and Drug Administration (FDA) has approved several sleep aids—called sedatives or hypnotics—for indefinite use. However, most sleeping pills are usually prescribed only for short-term insomnia, because they usually become ineffective after several weeks of nightly use and may be habit-forming. If sleeping pills are used for too long, they can actually cause insomnia. Some persons taking sleep aids experience next-day grogginess or engage in behaviors during sleep, such as sleep eating or sleep driving. If a medical disorder is causing the sleep deprivation, use of sleep aids may mask the underlying condition, and sleep aids may negatively interact with alcohol or other medications. In persons with sleep apnea, sleep aids may prevent them from waking up to breathe.

Alternative

Alternative treatments for insomnia and other sleep disturbances include cognitive-behavioral therapy (CBT); hypnosis; melatonin, a hormone derived from the neurotransmitter serotonin; and tryptophan, an amino acid precursor of serotonin.

Herbal remedies for insomnia include lemon balm, chamomile, valerian root, kava kava, passionflower, lavender, and St. John's wort, although the efficacy of such herbs has not been proven. Patients should discuss the use of herbal supplements with their doctor.

Home remedies

Short-term sleep deprivation may require only a night or two of additional sleep. Longer-term sleep deprivation may require a sleep vacation—a few days devoted to sleeping as much as needed. Mild sleep apnea can be treated effectively by weight loss or by not sleeping on one's back.

Prognosis

Sleep deprivation is usually readily reversible with adequate sleep.

Prevention

Sleep deprivation is preventable by getting as much sleep as an individual requires. Sleep deprivation caused by mild insomnia can often be prevented by:

- sleeping on a schedule—going to bed and rising at the same time every day, including weekends
- structuring daily activities
- exercising 20–30 minutes every day, especially 5–6 hours before sleep
- practicing stress management
- avoiding caffeine, nicotine, and alcohol
- relaxing before bed with activities such as reading or a warm bath that become routinely associated with sleep
- avoiding extreme temperatures that prevent falling or staying asleep
- avoiding lying awake in bed for more than 20 minutes since this can cause anxiety
- reading, watching television, listening to music, or performing an activity until drowsy

- sleeping until sunrise or waking with very bright lights to reset one's internal clock each day
- getting an hour of morning sun exposure

Effects on Public Health

Sleep deprivation is a serious public health concern in the United States, not only because of the vast number of Americans suffering from sleep deprivation at any given time, but also because of the serious consequences of sleep deprivation. As mentioned above, sleep deprivation can severely impair an individual's ability to safely operate a vehicle, as well as affecting their reaction time. Sleep deprivation has also been scientifically linked to many serious health problems, including **obesity**, diabetes, **heart disease**, kidney disease, high blood pressure, stroke, and depression. Promoting healthy sleeping habits, as well as promptly and effectively dealing with sleep problems, can help promote long-term health and prevent serious health complications.

Resources

BOOKS

Bellenir, Karen. *Sleep Information for Teens.* Detroit: Omnigraphics, 2008.

Chokroverty, Sudhansu. *100 Questions & Answers About Sleep and Sleep Disorders.* Sudbury, MA: Jones and Bartlett, 2008.

Epstein, Lawrence J., and Steven Mardon. *The Harvard Medical School Guide to a Good Night's Sleep.* New York: McGraw-Hill, 2007.

Mindell, Jodi A. *Sleep Deprived No More: From Pregnancy to Early Motherhood—Helping You & Your Baby Sleep Through the Night.* New York: DaCapo Press, 2007.

PERIODICALS

Bergin, Christi A., and David A. Bergin. "Sleep: The E-ZZZ Intervention." *Educational Leadership* 67, no. 4 (December 2009/January 2010): 44–47.

He, Ying, et al. "The Transcriptional Repressor DEC2 Regulates Sleep Length in Mammals." *Science* 325, no. 5942 (August 14, 2009): 866–870.

Kowalczyk, Liz. "Turns Out, There's No Magic in that Traditional Number Eight When Figuring Out How Many Hours of Shut-Eye You Need." *The Boston Globe* (December 28, 2009): G6.

Liberatore, Stephanie. "Health Wise: December 2009." *The Science Teacher* 76, no. 9 (December 2009): 62–63.

WEBSITES

Helpguide.org. "How to Stop Snoring." August 2011. http://www.helpguide.org/life/snoring.htm (accessed October 27, 2011).

MedlinePlus. "Sleep Disorders." U.S. National Library of Medicine, National Institutes of Health. http://www.nlm

.nih.gov/medline plus/tutorials/sleepdisorders/ htm/index
.htm (accessed October 27, 2011).

National Sleep Foundation. "Backgrounder: Later School Start
Times." http://www.sleepfoundation.org/article/hot-topics/
backgrounder-later-school-start-times (accessed October
27, 2011).

U.S. Department of Health & Human Services—National Heart
Lung and Blood Institute. "What Are Sleep Deprivation
and Deficiency?" http://www.nhlbi.nih.gov/health/health-
topics/topics/sdd/Accessed August 20, 2012.

U.S. National Institute of Neurological Disorders and Stroke.
"Brain Basics: Understanding Sleep." NIH Publication
No.06-3440-c. http://www.ninds. nih.gov/disorders/
brain_basics/understanding_sleep.htm (accessed October
27, 2011).

ORGANIZATIONS

American Academy of Sleep Medicine, 2510 N Frontage Rd.,
Darien, IL 60561, (630) 737-9700, Fax: (630) 737-9790,
inquiries@assmnet.org, http://www.aasmnet.org

National Institute of Neurological Disorders and Stroke, PO
Box 5801, Bethesda, MD 20824, (301) 496-5751, TTY:
(301) 468-5981, (800) 352-9424, http://www.ninds.nih
.gov

National Sleep Foundation, 1010 North Glebe Rd., Suite 310,
Arlington, VA 22201, (703) 243-1697, nsf@sleepfoun-
dation.org, http://www.sleepfoundation.org

Margaret Alic, Ph.D.
Andrea Nienstedt, M.A.

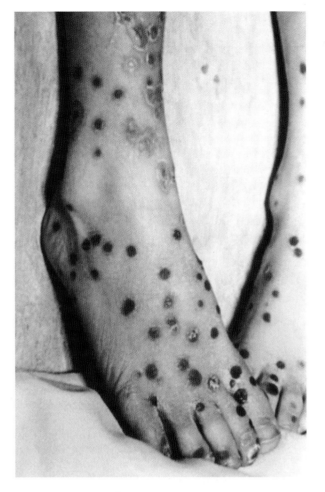

A patient with small pox. (© CDC/Dr. Robinson)

Smallpox

Definition

Smallpox is an infection caused by the variola virus
(either of two variants, Variola major or variola minor), a
member of the poxvirus family. Throughout history,
smallpox has been a greatly feared disease because it was
responsible for worldwide epidemics that resulted in
large numbers of deaths. In 1980, the **World Health
Organization (WHO)** announced that an extensive
program of **vaccination** against the disease had resulted
in the complete eradication of the virus with the
exception of samples of stored virus in two laboratories.

Description

The first appearance of smallpox is unknown in the
medical community. Smallpox probably evolved from a
rodent virus anywhere from 16,000 to 79,000 years ago.
Two clades (organisms with a common ancestor)
evolved. The variola major stain spread outward from
Asia 400–1,500 years ago. A second clade, found on the
North and South American continents and West Africa,
was known to exist roughly 1,400–6,500 years ago.

Smallpox is strictly an infection of human beings.
Animals and insects do not contract nor carry the virus in
any form. Most infections are caused by contact with a
person who has developed the characteristic skin lesions
(pox) of the disease, although a person with a less severe
infection (not symptomatic or diagnosable in the usual
way) can unknowingly spread the virus.

Risk factors

Because smallpox was eradicated in 1980, there are
no risk factors for contracting smallpox in the natural
environment. However, scientists and technicians working in laboratories and facilities with the smallpox virus
do have a minimal risk of contracting smallpox. Other
risks, though slight, include having the smallpox virus
stolen from laboratories that are holding it, and using it as
a biological weapon.

EDWARD JENNER (1749–1823)

In 1754, when Edward was five years old, both parents died within a few weeks of each other, and he came under the guardianship of his elder brother, the Reverend Stephen Jenner, who had succeeded their father as rector of Rockhampton. Jenner's first schooling was received from the Reverend Mr. Clissold at the nearby village of Wotton-under-Edge. Later, he was sent to a grammar school at Cirencester. One of his favorite boyhood activities was searching for fossils among the oolite rocks of the countryside. In 1761, Jenner was apprenticed to Daniel Ludlow, a surgeon of Sodbury, with whom he worked until 1770, when he went to London to study anatomy and surgery under John Hunter. Hunter had just taken over the large house of his brother William in Jermyn Street, and Jenner was one of Hunter's first boarding pupils. Jenner also arranged the zoological specimens brought back by Joseph Banks from the first voyage of H.S. Endeavour. In 1773, Jenner returned to Berkeley, where he lived with his elder brother and began to practice medicine.

When Jenner began medical practice at Berkeley, he was frequently asked to inoculate persons against smallpox. Smallpox inoculation had been introduced into England early in the eighteenth century. A person in good health was inoculated with matter from smallpox pustules and was thus given what was usually a mild case of the disease in order to confer immunity against further smallpox infection. The practice was dangerous, however, since smallpox thus induced could be severe or fatal, and it tended to spread smallpox among the population. Such inoculation was evidently not a common practice in the English countryside until about 1768, when it was improved by Robert Sutton of Debenham, Suffolk. Sutton required the patient to rest and maintain a strict diet for two weeks before inoculation. He inoculated by taking, on the point of a lancet, a very small quantity of fluid from an unripe smallpox pustule and introducing it between the outer and inner layers of the skin of the upper arm without drawing blood. He used no bandage to cover the incision.

Jenner began to inoculate against smallpox using Sutton's method, but he soon found some patients to be completely resistant to the disease. On inquiry, he found that these patients had previously had cowpox, the disease which produced a characteristic eruption on the teats of milk cows and was frequently transmitted to people who milked the cows. Jenner also found that among milkmen and milkmaids, it was generally believed that contraction of cowpox prevented subsequent susceptibility to smallpox, although there had apparently been instances where this had not been the case. His fellow medical practitioners in the countryside did not agree that cowpox prevented smallpox with certainty.

As early as 1780, Jenner learned that the eruptions on the teats of infected cows differed. All were called cowpox and all could be communicated to the hands of the milkers, but only one kind created a resistance to smallpox. He called this type "true cowpox." Jenner subsequently found that even true cowpox conferred immunity against smallpox only when matter was taken from the cowpox pustules before they were too old (as had been the case with Sutten's smallpox fluid). Jenner thought (mistakenly) that true cowpox was identical with a disease of the feet of horses known as "grease" and that the pox was carried from horses to cattle on the hands of milkmen who also cared for horses. He also believed at that time that the cowpox could be transmitted from person to person, serving to protect them from smallpox. But he was not able to confirm his opinions for another sixteen years.

Demographics

Vaccinations for smallpox began in the early 1800s. According to **WHO**, an estimated 50 million cases of smallpox occurred worldwide in the early 1950s. By the mid-1960s, that number dropped to between 10 and 15 million. In 1967, WHO launched an intense plan to eradicate smallpox, which continued to present serious health consequences for about 60% of the world's **population**. The global campaign to eradicate smallpox successfully decreased the area in which the infection was present. The last two outbreaks of smallpox occurred in Yugoslavia, in 1972; and in India, in 1974, where 15,000 people died of the infection. By 1977, the last natural case of smallpox occurred in Somalia, Africa. In 1980, the World Health Assembly made the official pronouncement that smallpox had been eradicated from the planet.

Causes and symptoms

Smallpox is a relatively contagious disease, which accounts for its ability to cause massive epidemics. The variola virus is acquired from direct contact with individuals infected with the disease, from contaminated air droplets, and even from objects used by a person with smallpox (books, blankets, utensils). The respiratory tract is the usual entry point for the variola virus into a human being.

After the virus enters the body, there is a 12- to 14-day incubation period during which the virus multiplies, although no symptoms are recognizable. After the incubation period, symptoms appear abruptly and include fever, chills, and muscle aches. Two to three days later, a bumpy rash begins appearing first on the face and forearms. The rash progresses—ultimately reaching the chest, abdomen, and back. Seven to ten days after the rash appears, the patient is most infectious. The individual bumps (papules) fill with clear fluid and eventually become pus-filled over the course of 10 to 12 days. These pox eventually scab over, each leaving a permanently scarred pock or pit when the scab drops off.

Initially, the smallpox symptoms and rash appear similar to chickenpox. However, unlike chickenpox, smallpox lesions develop at the same rate so that they are all visible in the same stage. Another major difference is that smallpox occurs primarily on the face and extremities, whereas chickenpox tends to be concentrate on the face and trunk area.

Complications such as bacterial infection of the open skin lesions, **pneumonia**, or bone infections are the major causes of death from smallpox. A severe and quickly fatal form called "sledgehammer smallpox," occurs in 5–10% of patients and results in massive, uncontrollable bleeding (hemorrhage) from skin lesions, as well as from the mouth, nose, and other areas of the body. This form is very infectious and usually fatal five to seven days after onset.

Fear of smallpox comes from both the epidemic nature of the disease as well as from the fact that no therapies have ever been discovered to either treat the symptoms of smallpox or shorten the course of the disease.

Diagnosis

In modern times, a diagnosis of smallpox is made using an electron microscope to identify virus in fluid from the papules, urine, or in the patient's blood prior to the appearance of the papular rash.

Treatment

No treatments have been developed to halt progression of the disease. Treatment for smallpox is only supportive, meaning that it is aimed at keeping a patient as comfortable as possible. **Antibiotics** are sometimes administered to prevent secondary bacterial infections.

Public health role and response

As of 2012, two laboratories (the U.S. **Centers for Disease Control and Prevention** (CDC) in Atlanta, Georgia, and the Russian State Centre of Virology and Biotechnology (VECTOR) in Koltsovo, Novosibirsk Region) officially retained samples of the smallpox virus. These samples, as well as stockpiles of the smallpox vaccine, are stored because some level of concern exists that another smallpox virus could undergo

---

KEY TERMS

Endemic—Occurring naturally and consistently in a particular area.

Epidemic—Occurs when the number of cases of a disease exceeds the usual or average (endemic) number for an area or region. These may occur as a large cluster of cases all occurring at about the same time within a specific community or region.

Eradicate—To completely do away with something, eliminate it, end its existence.

Hemorrhage—Bleeding that is massive, uncontrollable, and often life-threatening.

Lesion—The tissue disruption or the loss of function caused by a particular disease process.

Papules—Firm bumps on the skin.

Pox—A pus-filled bump on the skin.

Vaccine—A preparation using a non-infectious element or relative of a particular virus or bacterium that is administered with the intention of halting the progress of an infection, or completely preventing it.

---

genetic changes (mutate) and cause human infection. There is also the minute chance that smallpox virus could escape from the laboratories where it is stored. For these reasons, surveillance continues of various animal groups that continue to be infected with viruses related to the variola virus, and large quantities of vaccine are stored in different countries around the world so that response to any future threat by the smallpox virus can be swift and effective.

Of greatest concern is the potential use of smallpox as a biological weapon. Since 1980, when the WHO announced smallpox had been eradicated, essentially no one has been vaccinated against the disease. Individuals vaccinated prior to 1980 are believed to be susceptible as well because immunity only lasts 15–20 years. These circumstances, along with the nature of smallpox to spread quickly from person to person, could lead to devastating consequences.

The United States and Russia are the only two countries to officially house remaining samples of the virus. However, it is believed that other countries, such as Iraq, may have obtained samples of the smallpox virus during the Cold War (1947–1991) through their association with the Soviet Union. It is also possible that scientists with access to the virus may have sold their services and knowledge to other governments.

On June 22 and 23, 2001, four U.S. organizations (CSIS—Center for Strategic and International Studies, Johns Hopkins Center for Civilian Biodefense Studies, ANSER—Analytic Services Inc., and MIPT—Memorial Institute for the **Prevention** of Terrorism) presented a fictitious scenario of the United States' response to a deliberate introduction of smallpox titled *Dark Winter*. This exercise demonstrated that if such an event were to occur, the United States would be ill prepared on several fronts. The primary concern is an inadequate supply of vaccine, which is essential to preventing disease development in exposed persons. Between 1997 and 2001, two companies were contracted to produce additional smallpox vaccines for both military and civilian use. Through these contracts, an additional 40 million doses were made available for civilian use as of 2005. Studies were also conducted to determine if existing vaccines can be diluted in order to increase the number of doses available for immediate use. Results from a very small group of volunteers tested in 2000 found that at one-tenth strength, the existing smallpox vaccines are approximately 70% effective. In late 2001, a new study began evaluating the effectiveness of the vaccine at one-fifth strength. In 2004, the European Commission (EC) reviewed two U.S. dilution studies at one-fifth strength. It concluded that "diluting vaccine would be inadvisable." The EC states that the dilution would "increase the risk of ineffective inoculations." In addition, WHO stated that it would not consider diluting any of its stockpile of vaccine because of the risks associated with dilution.

In the event that smallpox is reintroduced into the current population, it will be imperative that doctors immediately recognize the symptoms and isolate the individual to prevent further spread of the disease. Prompt vaccination of any persons who had contact with the patient is also necessary to prevent additional cases of smallpox from developing. Controlling and containing spread of this disease is critical for prevention of a worldwide epidemic that would have a devastating impact on current populations.

Prognosis

Approximately one in three patients dies from smallpox, with the more severe, hemorrhagic form nearly 100% fatal. Patients who survive smallpox infection nearly always have multiple areas of scarring at the site of each pock.

Prevention

From about the tenth century in China, India, and the Americas, it has been noted that individuals who had

QUESTIONS TO ASK YOUR DOCTOR

- Should I be worried about smallpox if I travel to a developing country?
- How dangerous is the threat of smallpox as a terrorist attack?
- Is smallpox contagious before a rash appears?
- Is there any treatment for smallpox?
- If the vaccine for smallpox is ever given to the public, how is the vaccine given?
- Are diluted doses of smallpox vaccine as effective as the undiluted form?
- What is the smallpox vaccine made of?
- Is it possible to get smallpox from the vaccination?

even a mild case of smallpox could not be infected again. Writings from all over the world account different ways in which people tried to prevent smallpox. Material from people mildly ill with smallpox (fluid or pus from the papules, scabs over the pox) was scratched into the skin of people who had never had the illness, in an attempt to produce a mild reaction and its accompanying protective effect. These efforts often resulted in full-fledged smallpox and probably served only to help effectively spread the infection throughout a community. In fact, such crude smallpox vaccinations were against the law in colonial America.

In 1798, English physician and scientist Edward Jenner (1749–1823) published a paper in which he discussed his important observation that milkmaids who contracted a mild infection of the hands (called cowpox, and caused by a relative of the variola virus) appeared to be immune to smallpox. Jenner created an **immunization** against smallpox using the pus found in the lesions of cowpox infection. Jenner's paper led to much work in the area of vaccinations and ultimately resulted in the creation of a very effective vaccination against smallpox that utilized the vaccinia virus, another close relative of variola. The term "vaccination" is derived from *vacca*, Latin for "cow" and related to the cowpox link. Later, the term was applied to other vaccinations.

In 1967, WHO began its attempt to eradicate the smallpox virus worldwide. The methods used in the program were simple:

- Careful surveillance for all smallpox infections worldwide, to allow for quick diagnosis and immediate quarantine of patients.

- Immediate vaccination of all contacts diagnosed with infection, in order to interrupt the virus's usual pattern of infection.

WHO's program was extremely successful, and the virus was declared eradicated worldwide in May 1980.

Resources

BOOKS

Brachman, Philip S., and Elias Abrutyn, eds. *Bacterial Infections of Humans: Epidemiology and Control.* New York: Springer Science and Business Media, 2009.

Dworkin, Mark S., ed. *Outbreak Investigations Around the World: Case Studies in Infectious Disease Field Epidemiology.* Sudbury, MA: Jones and Bartlett, 2010.

Shannon, Joyce Brennfleck, ed. *Contagious Diseases Sourcebook: Basic Consumer Health Information about Diseases Spread from Person to Person.* Detroit: Omnigraphics, 2010.

PERIODICALS

Broad, William J. "U.S. Acts to Make Vaccines and Drugs Against Smallpox." *The New York Times* October 9, 2001: D1–2.

Gouvras G. "Policies in Place Throughout the World: Action by the European Union." *International Journal of Infectious Diseases* 8, Suppl. 2 (Oct 2004): S21–30.

Miller, Judith, and Sheryl Gay Stolberg. "Sept. 11 Attacks Led to Push for More Smallpox Vaccine." *The New York Times* October 22, 2001: A1.

WEBSITES

Constantine, Alex. *The Path to 9/11 (Part Five): DARK WINTER/ANSER, CSIS & Other Main Players Stage a Terror Drill in Preparation for Black Tuesday & Anthrax Attacks.* Constantine Report. May 25, 2008. http://www .constantinereport.com/allposts/the-path-to-911-part-five-dark-winteranser-csis-other-main-players-stage-a-terror-drill-in-preparation-for-black-tuesday-anthrax-attacks/ (accessed October 13, 2012).

Smallpox. World Health Organization. (2012). http://www.who .int/topics/smallpox/en/ (accessed October 13, 2012).

Smallpox: Surveillance and Investigation. Centers for Disease Control and Prevention. March 19, 2012. http://www.bt .cdc.gov/agent/smallpox/surveillance/ (accessed October 13, 2012).

ORGANIZATIONS

U.S. Centers for Disease Control and Prevention, 1600 Clifton Rd., Atlanta, GA 30333, (800) 232-4636, cdcinfo@cdc .gov, http://www.cdc.gov/

U.S. Food and Drug Administration, 10903 New Hampshire Ave., Silver Spring, MD 20993, (888) 463-6332, http:// www.fda.gov

World Health Organization, Avenue Appia 20, Geneva, Switzerland 1211 27, 41 22 791-2111, Fax: 41 22 791-3111, http://www.who.int/en/

Rosalyn Carson-DeWitt, MD
William A. Atkins, BB, BS, MBA

Smoking

Definition

Smoking is the inhalation of the smoke of burning tobacco encased in cigarettes, pipes, and cigars. Casual smoking is the act of smoking only occasionally, usually in a social situation or to relieve **stress**. A smoking habit is a physical **addiction** to tobacco products. Many health experts now regard habitual smoking as a psychological addiction, too, and one with serious health consequences. According to the **Centers for Disease Control and Prevention**, smoking is the leading cause of preventable death in the United States, accounting for approximately 443,000 deaths each year.

Description

The U.S. Food and Drug Administration has asserted that cigarettes and smokeless tobacco should be considered nicotine-delivery devices. Nicotine, the active ingredient in tobacco, is inhaled into the lungs, where most of it stays. The rest passes into the bloodstream, reaching the brain in about 10 seconds and dispersing throughout the body in about 20 seconds.

Depending on the circumstances and the amount consumed, nicotine can act as either a stimulant or tranquilizer. This can explain why some people report that smoking gives them energy and stimulates their mental activity, while others note that smoking relieves anxiety and relaxes them. The initial "kick" results in part from the drug's stimulation of the adrenal glands and resulting release of epinephrine into the blood. Epinephrine causes several physiological changes—it temporarily narrows the arteries, raises the blood pressure, raises the levels of fat in the blood, and increases the heart rate and flow of blood from the heart. Some researchers think epinephrine contributes to smokers' increased risk of high blood pressure.

Nicotine, by itself, increases the risk of **heart disease**. However, when a person smokes, he or she is ingesting far more than nicotine. Smoke from a cigarette, pipe, or cigar includes many additional toxic chemicals, including tar and carbon monoxide. Tar is a sticky substance that forms into deposits in the lungs, causing lung **cancer** and respiratory distress. Carbon monoxide limits the amount of oxygen that the red blood cells can convey throughout the body. It also may damage the inner walls of the arteries, which allows fat to build up in them.

Besides tar, nicotine, and carbon monoxide, tobacco smoke contains 4,000 different chemicals. More than 200 of these chemicals are known be toxic. Nonsmokers who are exposed to tobacco smoke also take in these toxic chemicals. They inhale the smoke exhaled by the smoker

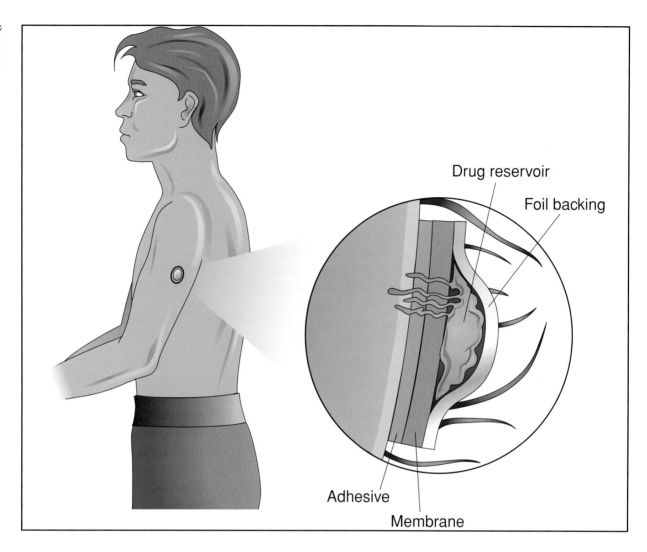

Drug reservoir

Foil backing

Adhesive

Membrane

The nicotine patch is a type of transepidermal patch designed to deliver nicotine, the addictive substance contained in cigarettes, directly through the skin and into the blood stream. The patch contains a drug reservoir sandwiched between a nonpermeable back layer and a permeable adhesive layer that attaches to the skin. The drug leeches slowly out of the reservoir, releasing small amounts of the drug at a constant rate for up to 24 hours. *(Illustration by Electronic Illustrators Group. Reproduced by permission of Gale, a part of Cengage Learning.)*

as well as the more toxic *sidestream smoke*—the smoke from the end of the burning cigarette, cigar, or pipe.

Sidestream smoke is more toxic than exhaled smoke because when a person smokes, the smoke he or she inhales, and then breathes out, leaves harmful deposits inside the body. But because lungs partially cleanse the smoke, exhaled smoke contains fewer poisonous chemicals. This is why exposure to tobacco smoke is dangerous even for a nonsmoker.

Causes and symptoms

According to the Centers for Disease Control and Prevention, nicotine dependence is the most common form of chemical dependence in the United States, and nicotine may be as addictive as alcohol, heroin, or cocaine.

No one starts smoking to become addicted to nicotine. It is not known how much nicotine may be consumed before the body becomes addicted. However, once smoking becomes a habit, the smoker faces a lifetime of health risks associated with one of the strongest addictions known.

About 70% of smokers in the United States would like to quit. In 2010, 52.4% of adult smokers stopped smoking for more than one day because they were trying to quit. In any given year, however, only about 3.6% of the country's 47 million smokers quit successfully. In 2008, the Centers for Disease Control and Prevention reported that the prevalence of smoking in the United States fell in 2007 to 19.8%, almost a full percentage point decline from 20.8% in 2006.

Researchers conjecture that genetic factors contribute substantially to developing a smoking habit. Several twin studies have led to estimates of 46–84% heritability for smoking. It is thought that some genetic variations affect the speed of nicotine metabolism in the body and the activity level of nicotinic receptors in the brain.

Smoking risks

Emphysema is a chronic respiratory disease in which there is progressive overinflation of the air sacs (alveoli) in the lungs, causing a loss of lung function and often breathlessness. Its name comes from a Greek word meaning "to blow into," hence "air-containing" or "air-inflated." Emphysema is sometimes grouped together with chronic bronchitis under the name of chronic obstructive pulmonary disease, or COPD. Many people who are diagnosed with emphysema also have chronic bronchitis. Emphysema is increasing in the United States, Canada, and other developed countries primarily because of cigarette smoking. It is almost entirely a disease of adults. About 12 million adults in the United States have been diagnosed with the disease as of 2009; however, many doctors believe emphysema is underdiagnosed. Between 4 and 6% of male adults and 1–3% of female adults in North America are estimated to have emphysema. The number of women diagnosed with the disease is rising rapidly; the year 2000 was the first year that more women than men were identified as having emphysema. In 2005, almost 66,000 females died, compared to 61,000 males. According to the American Lung Association, the cost to the United States for COPD each year is approximately $42.6 billion, including $26.7 billion in direct health care expenditures, $8.0 billion in indirect morbidity costs and $7.9 billion in indirect mortality costs. Rates of emphysema are rising worldwide as more people in the developing countries take up cigarette smoking. The Global Initiative for Chronic Obstructive Lung Disease (GOLD) estimates that 9–10% of adults around the world have either chronic bronchitis or emphysema.

Smoking is recognized as the leading preventable cause of death, causing or contributing to the deaths of approximately 440,000 Americans each year. Anyone with a smoking habit has an increased chance of cancer, particularly lung and esophageal cancers; respiratory diseases such as chronic airway obstruction and emphysema; and cardiovascular disease, such as ischemic heart disease, aortic aneurysm, and atherosclerosis (narrowing and hardening of the arteries). The risk of **stroke** is

especially high in women who smoke and take birth control pills.

Smoking makes it harder to conceive, and it can interfere with the growth of the fetus during pregnancy. It accounts for an estimated 14% of premature births and 10% of infant deaths. There is some evidence that smoking may cause impotence in some men.

Because smoking affects so many of the body's systems, smokers often have vitamin deficiencies and suffer oxidative damage caused by free radicals. Free radicals are molecules that steal electrons from other molecules, turning the other molecules into free radicals and destabilizing the molecules in the body's cells.

Smoking is recognized as one of several factors that might be related to a higher risk of hip fractures in older adults.

Studies reveal that the more a person smokes, the more likely he or she is to sustain illnesses such as cancer, chronic bronchitis, and emphysema. But even smokers who indulge in the habit only occasionally are more prone to these diseases.

Some brands of cigarettes are advertised as "low tar," but no cigarette is truly safe. If a smoker switches to a low-tar cigarette, he or she is likely to inhale longer and more deeply to get the chemicals the body craves. A smoker must quit smoking entirely for health to improve and for the chance of disease to decrease.

Although some people believe that chewing tobacco is safer than smoking, chewing tobacco has an increased risk of heart disease and mouth and throat cancer. Pipe and cigar smokers have increased health risks as well, even though these smokers generally do not inhale as deeply as cigarette smokers do. These groups have not been studied as extensively as cigarette smokers, but there is evidence that they may be at a slightly lower risk of cardiovascular problems but a higher risk of cancer and various types of circulatory conditions.

Recent research reveals that passive smokers, or those who unavoidably breathe in second-hand tobacco smoke, have an increased chance of many health problems such as lung cancer and **asthma**, and in children, sudden infant death syndrome.

Smokers' symptoms

Smokers are likely to exhibit a variety of symptoms that reveal the damage caused by smoking. A nagging morning cough may be one sign of a tobacco habit. Other symptoms include shortness of breath, wheezing, and frequent occurrences of respiratory illness, such as bronchitis. Smoking also increases fatigue and decreases the smoker's sense of smell and taste. Smokers are more likely to develop poor circulation, with cold hands and feet and premature wrinkles.

Sometimes the illnesses that result from smoking come on silently with little warning. For instance, coronary artery disease may exhibit few or no symptoms. At other times, there will be warning signs, such as bloody discharge from a woman's vagina, a sign of cancer of the cervix. Another warning sign is a hacking cough, worse than the usual smoker's cough, that brings up phlegm or blood—a sign of lung cancer.

Withdrawal symptoms

A smoker who tries to quit may expect one or more of these withdrawal symptoms: nausea, constipation or diarrhea, drowsiness, loss of concentration, insomnia, headache, nausea, and irritability.

Diagnosis

It is not easy to quit smoking, which is why it may be wise for a smoker to turn to his physician for help. For the greatest success in quitting and to help with the withdrawal symptoms, the smoker should talk over a treatment plan with his doctor or alternative practitioner. He should have a general physical examination to gauge his general health and uncover any deficiencies. He should also have a thorough evaluation for some of the serious diseases that smoking can cause.

Treatment

Research shows that most smokers who want to quit benefit from the support of other people. It helps to quit with a friend or to join a group such as those organized by the American Cancer Society. These groups provide support and teach behavior-modification methods that can help the smoker quit. The smoker's physician can often refer him to such groups.

Other alternatives to help with the withdrawal symptoms of kicking the habit include nicotine-replacement therapy in the form of gum, patches, nasal sprays, and oral inhalers. These are available by prescription or over the counter. A physician can provide advice on how to use them. They slowly release a small amount of nicotine into the bloodstream, satisfying the smoker's physical craving. Over time, the amount of gum the smoker chews is decreased, and the amount of time between applying the patches is increased. This helps wean the smoker from nicotine slowly, eventually beating the addiction to the drug. But there is one important caution: If the smoker lights up while taking a nicotine replacement, a nicotine overdose may cause serious health problems.

The prescription drug Zyban (bupropion hydrochloride) has shown some success in helping smokers to quit. This drug contains no nicotine and was originally developed as an antidepressant. It is not known exactly how bupropion works to suppress the desire for nicotine. A five-year study of bupropion reported that the drug has a very good record for safety and effectiveness in treating tobacco dependence. Its most common side effect is insomnia, which can also result from nicotine withdrawal.

Researchers are investigating two new types of drugs as possible treatments for tobacco dependence. The first is an alkaloid known as 18-methoxycoronaridine (18-MC), which selectively blocks the nicotinic receptors in brain tissue. Another approach involves developing drugs that inhibit the activity of cytochrome P450 2A6 (CYP2A6), which controls the metabolism of nicotine.

Expected results

Research on smoking shows that most smokers desire to quit, but smoking is so addictive that fewer than 20% of the people who try ever successfully kick the habit. Still, many people attempt to quit smoking over and over again, despite the difficulties—the cravings and withdrawal symptoms, such as irritability and restlessness.

For those who do quit, the benefits to health are well worth the effort. The good news is that once a smoker quits, the health effects are immediate and dramatic. After the first day, oxygen and carbon monoxide levels in the blood return to normal. At two days, nerve endings begin to grow back, and the senses of taste and smell revive. Within two weeks to three months, circulation and breathing improve. After one year of not smoking, the risk of heart disease is reduced by 50%. After 15 years of abstinence, the risks of health problems from smoking virtually vanish. A smoker who quits for good often feels a lot better, too, with less fatigue and fewer respiratory illnesses.

Prevention

The number of smokers has decreased significantly over the last few decades. In 1965, 42.4% of adults smoked; as of 2009, the figure had fallen to 20.6%. Smoking among students had reached a peak of 36.7% in 1997, but declined to 19.5% in 2009.

A combination of factors can be credited with the decline. While smoking was common in offices and restaurants in the past, many locations no longer allow smoking indoors, whether through internal policies or state and local ordinances. In November 2012, Montana's voters made their state the 30th state to require

KEY TERMS

Antioxidant—Any substance that reduces the damage caused by oxidation, such as the harm caused by free radicals.

Epinephrine—A nervous system hormone stimulated by the nicotine in tobacco. It increases heart rate and may raise smokers' blood pressure.

Free radical—An unstable molecule that causes oxidative damage by stealing electrons from surrounding molecules, thereby disrupting activity in the body's cells.

Nicotine—The addictive ingredient in tobacco, it acts on the nervous system and is both stimulating and calming.

that all public places and workplaces be smoke-free. Research has found that bars and restaurants do not suffer economically when they are made smoke-free and their employees are protected from **secondhand smoke**.

Some states have increased taxes on cigarettes, causing the cost of cigarettes to rise precipitously. As of 2012, the average state tax on a pack of cigarettes was $1.46, ranging from a high of $4.35 in New York to a low of $0.17 in Missouri.

Public **health education** programs and cessation support programs are effective in helping people to quit. However, only two states funded their anti-smoking programs at the level recommended by the **CDC**; in general, states are providing only 14% of the funding recommended, despite the fact that they collected $25.3 billion from tobacco taxes and the tobacco settlement in fiscal year 2011.

Effects on Public Health

More than 88 million nonsmokers, including 54% of children between the ages of 3 and 11, are put at risk by secondhand smoke. Each year, approximately 3,000 nonsmokers die of lung cancer, and another 46,000 die from heart disease. Smoking contributes to sudden infant death syndrome, respiratory infections, ear ailments, and asthma.

According to the CDC, the economic cost of smoking is nearly $200 billion each year, including $96 billion in medical costs.

However, as stated earlier, these tremendous losses could be prevented by two steps: If you don't smoke, don't start, or if you do smoke, quit.

Resources

BOOKS

Bevins, Rick A., and Anthony R. Caggiula. *The Motivational Impact of Nicotine and Its Role in Tobacco Use.* Nebraska Symposium on Motivation. New York: Springer, 2008.

PERIODICALS

Carlston, D.L., et al. "Exploratory analysis of patients' motivations to quit smoking and participate in smoking cessation classes." *Family Medicine* 44 (November 2012): 727–30.

Hyland, A., et al. "Predictors of cessation in a cohort of current and former smokers followed over 13 years." *Nicotine Tobacco Research* 2004 Dec. 6 Suppl. 3:S363–9.

WEBSITES

"Smoking and Tobacco Use." Centers for Disease Control. http://www.cdc.gov/tobacco/data_statistics/fact_sheets/health_effects/tobacco_related_mortality/ (accessed November 13, 2012).

"Trends in Current Cigarette Smoking Among High School Students and Adults, United States, 1965–2009." Centers for Disease Control and Prevention. http://www.cdc.gov/chronicdisease/resources/publications/aag/osh_text.htm#chart2/ (accessed November 13, 2012).

"State Cigarette Excise Tax Rates & Rankings." Campaign for Tobacco-Free Kids. http://www.tobaccofreekids.org/research/factsheets/pdf/0097.pdf (accessed November 13, 2012).

ORGANIZATIONS

American Cancer Society. Contact the local organization or call (800) 227-2345, http://www.cancer.org

American Lung Association. 1740 Broadway, New York, NY 10019, (800) 586-4872, (212) 315-8700, http://www.lungusa.org

National Heart, Lung, and Blood Institute (NHLBI). Building 31, Room 5A52, 31 Center Drive, MSC 2486, Bethesda, MD 20892, (301) 592-8573, http://www.nhlbi.nih.gov

Smoking, Tobacco, and Health Information Line. Centers for Disease Control and Prevention. Mailstop K-50, 4770 Buford Highway NE, Atlanta, GA 30341-3724, (800) 232-1311, http://www.cdc.gov/tobacco

Barbara Boughton
Fran Hodgkins

Society for Public Health Education (SOPHE)

Definition

The Society for Public **Health Education** (SOPHE) is a 501(c)(3) organization founded in 1950 to promote healthy communities, healthy behaviors, and healthy environments.

Purpose

The purpose of SOPHE is to provide global leadership to the field of public health by:

• Promoting research on the theory and practice of health education.

• Supporting high standards for health education.

• Advocating for policy and legislation aimed to improve public health education.

• Developing and promoting standards for the practice of public health education.

Description

SOPHE has almost 4,000 dues–paying members in the United States and 25 foreign countries. The organization is governed by a board of trustees of 15 members and five officers. It has chapters in 30 states, Mexico, and Canada, through which many of its activities are carried out. Members may join any of more of 13 Communities of Practice, which feature topics such as: anthropology and public health; children, adolescents and **school health** education; **emergency preparedness**; **environmental health** promotion; healthy **aging**; health communications/social marketing; health disparities/health equities; international and cross–cultural health; medical care/patient education; students/new professionals; **tobacco control** and **prevention**; university faculty; and worksite health education. Each year, the organization selects a list of advocacy priorities that constitute a major part of its activities. For 2011, those advocacy priorities included the Patient Protection and Affordable Care Act, appropriations for the National Center for Chronic Disease Prevention and Health Promotion, **health literacy**, health equity, and tobacco prevention and control. The association also develops and adopts a variety of position papers on public health education issues, such as adulterated silicone in transgender individuals, improvements in K–12 health literacy, coordinated school health, and diabetes.

Another major feature of SOPHE activities is a broad array of programs and initiatives dealing with public health education issues. Among the topics covered by current programs are chronic disease policy, emergency preparedness and environmental health, health disparities, injury prevention, school health, and capacity building in **minority health**. The aim of these programs is to raise awareness of an issue, provide knowledge and skills that health educators can use to

deal with these problems, foster partnerships through which action can be taken on the problems, improve the ability of SOPHE chapters to work on such problems, strengthen the connection between the behavioral sciences and public health in working on these problems, and improve the effectiveness with which the public health community advocates for particular positions on these issues.

SOPHE provides a number of vehicles through which its membership can improve and extend their background in the field of public health. One such element is the association's annual convention. Individual chapters also hold meetings and conferences that include training sessions on specific topics in public health. The national organization also provides a variety of online training sessions that include webinars (both live and archived), online courses, meeting webcasts, and self–study tests. The association is an approved provider of the Certificate in Public Health.

Professional Publications

SOPHE publishes two peer–reviewed journals, *Health Education & Behavior* and *Health Promotion Practice*, and two regular newsletters, the weekly *News U Can Use* and the bimonthly *News & Views*. The association also publishes and distributes a number of other publications on specific public health topics, such as *Improving Health Literacy*, *A Pregnant Woman's Guide to Quitting Smoking*, and *Social Marketing Resource Guide*.

Resources

BOOKS

Weiss, Elisa S., Rebecca Miller Anderson, and Roz Diane Lasker. *Making the Most of Collaboration: Exploring the Relationship between Partnership Synergy and Partnership Functioning*. Thousand Oaks, CA: Sage Periodicals Press, 2002.

PERIODICALS

Geiger, Brian F., et al. "Role of Health Education Specialists in Supporting Global Health and the Millennium Development Goals." *International Electronic Journal of Health Education* 14. (2011): 37–45.

Allensworth, D.D. "Addressing the Social Determinants of Health of Children and Youth: A Role for SOPHE Members." *Health Education & Behavior* 38. 4. (2011): 331–8

WEBSITES

Ohio Society for Public Health Education. http://www.ohiosophe.org/ (accessed October 13, 2012).

Southern California Society for Public Health Education. http://scsophe.org/ (accessed October 13, 2012).

ORGANIZATIONS

Society for Public Health Education (SOPHE), 10 G St., N.E., Suite 605, Washington, DC 20002, (202) 408-9804, Fax: (202) 408-9815, info@sophe.org, http://www.sophe.org

David E. Newton, Ed.D.

Sociologists

Definition

A sociologist is a person who studies human societies, social institutions, and the relationships among people.

Purpose

The purpose of sociology is to develop an understanding of how social institutions are formed, how they function, and how groups of people interact with each other. In addition to gaining knowledge about these processes, sociologists are interested in applying what they have learned to dealing with problems that arise in the social interactions among people and between people and institutions. Some sociologists focus their attention on these interactions among individuals and organizations in the field of public health.

Description

Sociology has existed in an informal sense for millennia, as some individuals have always been interested in understanding how people interact with each other and form institutions to carry out some of the functions necessary in a civilized world. Some historians suggest that the beginnings of true sociology can be dated to 1086 in England with the introduction of the Domesday Book, a careful record of the characteristics of the English people. Collecting data on the characteristics of a society has traditionally been a key activity of modern–day sociologists. Sociologists often claim the French scholar Emile Durkheim (1858–1917) as the father of modern sociology because he argued that social interactions and social structures can be studied following the same general rules of scientific research as can the physical and biological sciences.

Sociology now consists of a number of sub-disciplines:

• Sociological theory, which consists of attempts by scholars to develop theories about the fundamental features of sociological studies and to test those theories against research and observations.

• Applied sociology, in which sociologists use proven concepts in sociology to analyze, plan for, and make changes in existing institutions and interactions among individuals within an institution or within society as a whole.

• Social psychology, which studies the way in which social organizations affect individual human personalities.

• Social organization, in which the focus is on the ways in which organizations are created, the purposes for which they are established, the way in which they function, and the problems and solutions with which they may be associated.

• Demography, or population studies, which is concerned with the collection and analysis of quantitative data about groups of people, such as age, sex, ethnicity, occupations, and attitudes about particular subjects.

• Social change, which involves a study of the alterations that occur in specific social institutions or in society as a whole.

• Human ecology, which deals with the interaction between behaviors and attitudes within groups of people and the society in which they live, as in a study of drug use habits in urban or rural settings

• Sociology of specific fields, such as the sociology of sports, sociology of religion, or sociology of public health, in which the general principles of sociological theory and research are applied to the study of a particular field of human endeavor. For health workers, a field of special interest is the sociology of health and illness, often called the sociology of health and wellness. This field of study involves a study of the way social conditions affect personal and public health as, for example, how morbidity and mortality trends may differ in urban and rural areas.

Whatever speciality they select, sociologists may study or work with a number of different fields, such as culture in general, criminality, deviance, economic sociology, environment, education, family, gender, health, media, military, political sociology, race and ethnicity, religion, sexuality, social networks, urban and rural sociology, and work. An important offshoot of the field of sociology itself is social work, a profession in which individuals attempt to help people improve the quality of their personal lives by learning methods for taking control and gaining empowerment.

More than half of all sociologists are employed by colleges and universities in teaching and research positions. Federal, state, and local governments employ a much smaller number of sociologists to work on problems such as drug **addiction**, **poverty**, welfare, and housing. Another small group of sociologists are employed in private industry, where they work on issues of interest to a specific industry, such as public health or recreational therapy. Educational requirements for sociologists vary depending on the type of employer and the nature of work for which they are hired. Generally speaking, a master's degree is required, although a bachelor's degree may be sufficient in some cases. Colleges and universities and some other employers generally require a doctorate in sociology or some other closely related field.

Professional Publications

A large number of journals in sociology are published by various professional organizations in the field. A 2010 survey of the journals with the greatest impact on the profession ranked the top five journals as *Sociological Perspectives* (Pacific Sociological Association), *American Sociological Review* (American Sociological Association), *American Journal of Sociology* (University of Chicago Press), *British Journal of Sociology* (London School of Economics), and *Sociology* (British Sociological Association). A number of journals dealing with the application of sociology to health issues are also available, such as *Medical Sociology* (British Sociological Association), *Journal of Health and Social Behavior* (American Sociological Association), *Sociology of Health and Illness* (Blackwell Publishing), and *Health Sociology Review* (Australian Sociological Association).

Resources

BOOKS

Conley, Dalton. *You May Ask Yourself: An Introduction to Thinking Like a Sociologist*. New York: W.W. Norton, 2013.

Dolgon, Corey, and Chris Baker. *Social Problems: A Service Learning Approach*. Los Angeles; London: Sage/Pine Forge, 2011.

Korgen, Kathleen Odell, Jonathan M. White, and Shelley White. *Sociologists in Action: Sociology, Social Change, and Social Justice*. Thousand Oaks, CA: Pine Forge Press, 2011.

Nyeth, Philip W., Leslie H. Hossfeld, and Gwendolyn E. Nyden. *Public Sociology: Research, Action, and Change*. Thousand Oaks, CA: Pine Forge Press, 2012.

PERIODICALS

Cherney, Adrian, and Tara McGee. "Utilization of Social Science Research." *Journal of Sociology* 47. 2. (2011): 144–62

Currie, G., et al. "Let's Dance: Organization Studies, Medical Sociology and Health Policy." *Social Science & Medicine* 74. 3. (2012): 273–80.

Scambler, G. "Health Inequalities." *Sociology of Health & Illness* 34. 1. (2012): 130–46.

WEBSITES

A Day in the Life of a Sociologist. Princeton Review. http:// www.princetonreview.com/careers.aspx?cid=144 (accessed October 14, 2012).

Sociological Perspectives on Health. CliffsNotes. http://www .cliffsnotes.com/study_guide/Sociological–Perspective– on–Health.topicArticleId-26957,articleId-26936.html (accessed October 14, 2012).

Sociologists. Occupational Outlook Handbook. http://www.bls. gov/ooh/life-physical-and-social-science/sociologists.htm (accessed October 14, 2012).

Sociology in Public Health. eNotes. http://www.enotes.com/ sociology-public-health-reference/sociology-public-health (accessed October 14, 2012).

ORGANIZATIONS

American Sociological Association (ASA), 1430 K St., N.W., Suite 600, Washington, DC 20005, (202) 383-9005, Fax: (202) 638-0882, http://www.asanet.org/contactus.cfm, http://www.asanet.org/.

David E. Newton, Ed.D.

Sodium

Definition

Sodium is a mineral that exists in the body as the ion Na+. It is acquired through diet, mainly in the form of salt (sodium chloride, NaCl). Regulating the amount of Na+ in the body is absolutely critical to life and health.

Purpose

Sodium is a crucial mineral in the body. It plays a major role in controlling the distribution of fluids, maintaining blood pressure and blood volume, creating an electrical gradient that allows nerve transmission and muscle contraction to occur, maintaining the mechanisms that allow wastes to leave cells, and regulating the acidity (pH) of the blood. Many different organs working together, including the kidneys, endocrine glands, and brain, tightly control the level of Na+ in the body. Researchers estimate that between 20% and 40% of an adult's resting energy use goes toward regulating sodium. Sodium affects every cell in the body, and a major failure of sodium regulatory mechanisms results in death.

Description

In the body, sodium exists as electrolytes. Electrolytes are ions that form when salts dissolve in water or fluids. A molecule or group of molecules is an electric

Sodium

Age	Adequate Intake (mg)
Children 0–6 mos.	120
Children 7–12 mos.	370
Children 1–3 yrs.	1,000
Children 4–8 yrs.	1,200
Children 9–13 yrs.	1,500
Adolescents 14–18 yrs.	1,500
Adults 19–50 yrs.	1,500
Adults 51–70 yrs.	1,300
Adults 71≥ yrs.	1,200
Pregnant women	1,500
Breastfeeding women	1,500

Food	Sodium (mg)
Table salt, 1 tsp.	2,300
Dill pickle, 1 large	1,731
Chicken noodle soup, canned, 1 cup	850–1,100
Ham, 3 oz.	1,000
Sauerkraut, ½ cup	780
Pretzels, 1 oz.	500
Turkey breast, deli, 1 oz.	335
Soy sauce, 1 tsp.	304
Potato chips, 1 oz.	165–185

mg = milligram

(Table by PreMediaGlobal. Reproduced by permission of Gale, a part of Cengage Learning.)

charge is an ion. Positively charged ions are called "cations," and negatively charged ions are called "anions." Electrolytes are not evenly distributed within the body, and their uneven distribution allows many important metabolic reactions to occur. In addition to sodium ($Na+$), potassium ($K+$), calcium ($Ca~2+$), magnesium ($Mg~2+$), chloride ($Cl-$), phosphate ($HPO_4~2-$), bicarbonate (HCO_3-), and sulfate ($SO_4~2-$) are important electrolytes in humans.

Na+ is ten times more concentrated in fluid outside cells (i.e., extracellular fluid and blood) than it is in fluid inside cells. This difference in concentration is maintained through the expenditure of cellular energy, and it is critical to many metabolic functions, including maintaining the proportion of water that exists inside and outside of cells. When Na+ is too high or too low, it is rarely because an individual has eaten too much or too little salt. Instead, it is because organs such as the kidneys or endocrine glands, that regulate the conservation or removal of sodium from the body, have broken down.

Sodium requirements

Researchers estimate that humans can remain healthy when taking in only 500 mg of sodium daily. Salt is 40% sodium by weight, and 500 mg is slightly less than the amount of sodium found in 1/4 teaspoon of salt. Humans almost never take in too little salt; their health problems more often result from too much salt in the diet.

The United States Institute of Medicine (IOM) of the National Academy of Sciences has developed values called Dietary Reference Intakes (DRIs) for many **vitamins** and minerals, including sodium. The DRIs consist of three sets of numbers. The Recommended Dietary Allowance (RDA) defines the average daily amount of the nutrient needed to meet the health needs of 97–98% of the **population**. The Adequate Intake (AI) is an estimate set when there is not enough information to determine an RDA. The Tolerable Upper Intake Level (UL) is the average maximum amount that can be taken daily without risking negative side effects. The DRIs are calculated for children, adult men, adult women, pregnant women, and breastfeeding women.

The IOM has not set RDAs for sodium, but instead it has set AI levels for all age groups based on observed and experimental information about the amount of sodium needed to replace what is lost by a moderately active individual each day. Sodium is lost in both urine and sweat. IAs for sodium are measured in milligrams (mg). UL levels have not been set. However, the IOM recommends that adults limit their sodium intake to less than 2,400 mg per day, and the American Heart Association recommends an adult daily intake of 1,500–2,300 mg.

The daily adequte intake (AI) levels of sodium for each age group are:

- birth–6 months: AI 120 mg
- children 7–12 months: AI 370 mg
- children 1–3 years: AI 1,000 mg
- children 4–8 years: AI 1,200 mg
- children 9–13 years: AI 1,500 mg
- adolescents 14–18 years: IA 1,500 mg
- adults age 19–50: AI 1,500 mg
- adults ages 50–70 1,300 mg
- adults 71 years or older: AI 1,200 mg
- pregnant women: IA 1,500 mg
- breastfeeding women: AI 1,500 mg

Sources of sodium

Many people think that the main source of salt in their diet is what they add to food when they are cooking or at the table while eating. In reality, more than three-quarters of the sodium in the average American's diet is added to food during processing. Another 12% is already naturally in the food. For example, 1 cup of low-fat milk contains 110 mg of sodium. About 6% of sodium in the diet is added as salt during cooking and another 5% from salting food while eating.

Although most sodium in diet comes from salt, other sources of sodium include preservatives and flavor enhancers added during processing. Sodium content is required to be listed on the nutritional labels of processed foods. Some common "hidden" sources of sodium include:

• baking soda

• baking powder

• disodium phosphate

• monosodium glutamate (MSG)

• sodium nitrate or sodium nitrite

The sodium content of some common foods includes:

• table salt, 1 teaspoon:2,300 mg

• dill pickle, large: 1731 mg

• canned chicken noodle soup, 1 cup: 850–1,100 mg

• ham, 3 ounces: 1,000 mg

• sauerkraut, 1/2 cup: 780 mg

• pretzels, 1 ounce: 500 mg

• potato chips, 1 ounce: 165–185 mg

• soy sauce, 1 teaspoon: 304

• deli turkey breast, 1 ounce: 335 mg

Fresh fruits, vegetables, unsalted nuts, and rice, dried beans, and peas are examples of foods that are low in sodium.

Sodium and health

Too high a concentration of sodium in the blood causes a condition called hypernatremia. Too much sodium in the diet almost never causes hypernatremia. Causes include excessive water loss (e.g., severe diarrhea), restricted water intake, untreated diabetes (causes water loss), kidney disease, and hormonal imbalances. Symptoms include signs of dehydration such as extreme thirst, dark urine, sunken eyes, fatigue, irregular heart beat, muscle twitching, seizures, and coma.

Too low a concentration of sodium in the blood causes hyponatremia. Hyponatremia is not usually a problem in healthy individuals, although it has been known to occur in endurance athletes such as ultramarathoners. It is common in seriously ill individuals and can result from vomiting or diarrhea (extreme loss of sodium), severe **burns**, taking certain drugs that cause the kidney to selectively excrete sodium, extreme overconsumption of water (water intoxication, a

problem among the elderly with dementia), hormonal imbalances, kidney failure, and liver damage. Symptoms include nausea, vomiting, headache, tissue swelling (edema), confusion, mental disorientation, hallucinations, muscle trembling, seizures, and coma.

Hypernatremia and hyponatremia are at the extreme ends of sodium imbalance. However, high dietary intake of salt can cause less visible health damage in the form of high blood pressure (hypertension). Hypertension silently damages the heart, blood vessels, and kidney and increases the risk of **stroke**, heart attack, and kidney damage. A low-salt diet significantly lowers blood pressure in 30–60% of people with high blood pressure and a quarter to half of people with normal blood pressure. Some individuals are more sensitive to sodium than others. Those people who are most likely to see a rise in blood pressure with increased sodium intake include people who are obese; have type 2 diabetes; or are elderly, female, or African American.

The American Heart Association recommends reducing sodium in the diet to between 1,500 mg and 2,300 mg daily. Below are some suggestions for reducing salt intake.

• Eat more fresh fruits and vegetables.

• Look for processed foods that say, "No salt added."

• Limit or eliminate salty snacks such as chips and pretzels.

• Restrict processed meats such as hot dogs, pepperoni, and deli meats.

• Avoid high-sodium canned soups; choose heart-healthy lower-sodium soups instead.

• Use spices instead of salt to give foods flavor.

Interactions

Certain drugs cause large amounts of sodium to be excreted by the kidneys and removed from the body in urine. Diuretics ("water pills") are among the best-known of these drugs. Other types of drugs that may cause low sodium levels, especially in ill individuals, include nonsteroidal anti-inflammatory drugs (NSAIDs) such as Advil, Motrin, and Aleve, opiates such as codeine and morphine, selective serotonin-reuptake inhibitors (SSRIs) such as Prozac or Paxil, and tricyclic antidepressants such as Elavil and Tofranil.

Precautions

People who are salt-sensitive may need to keep their salt intake at levels below the suggested daily amounts to control their blood pressure. The Food and Drug Administration (FDA) suggests carefully reading food labels, eating fresh fruits and vegetables as much as possible, and minimizing salt intake as part of a healthy diet for all individuals. In order to determine one's appropriate daily salt intake, one should have his or her blood pressure checked regularly and consult with his or her physician. A patient's physician should be made aware of all the patient's current medications in order to properly assess the individual's sodium needs.

Salt is an acquired taste. Parents can help their children control their salt intake and discourage the development of a craving for salt by substituting low-salt foods for high-salt foods.

Effects on public health

Most problems related to high blood pressure are chronic, slow-to-develop disorders that do not cause serious complications until the second half of an individual's lifetime. Kidney failure, heart attack, and stroke are all complications of high blood pressure and potentially of high sodium intake. As instances of high blood pressure and **obesity** continue to rise, particularly in children, concern and awareness of sodium intake have increased as well. As problems like high sodium intake are contributing to health problems, such as high blood pressure, earlier on in many people's lifespans, the potential for long-term damage becomes much greater. Additionally, the medical costs related to problems like high blood pressure, heart attack, and diabetes make addressing dietary issues, like sodium intake, of the utmost importance for public health.

Efforts and solutions

In addition to the labeling requirements on processed foods, there have been many efforts to try and reduce national sodium consumption and promote healthier diets overall. On September 13, 2011, the U.S. **Department of Health and Human Services**, together with the FDA and other partners, launched the "Million Hearts" initiative, which is designed to reduce the number of heart attacks and strokes in the U.S. through efforts like improving the effectiveness of food labeling and consumer education. The FDA and **Food Safety** and Inspection Service (FSIS) have sought comments on sodium reduction and effectiveness of current approaches, as well as suggestions for improving current approaches, and are continually working to synthesize these data into workable solutions.

Resources

BOOKS

American Heart Association. *American Heart Association Low-Salt Cookbook: A Complete Guide to Reducing Sodium and Fat in Your Diet.* 3rd ed. New York: Clarkson Potter, 2006.

Hawkins, W. Rex. *Eat Right—Electrolyte: A Nutritional Guide to Minerals in Our Daily Diet.* Amherst, NY: Prometheus Books, 2006.

James, Shelly V, *The Complete Idiot's Guide to Low-Sodium Meals.* Indianapolis, IN: Alpha Books,2006.

Pressman, Alan H. and Sheila Buff.*The Complete Idiot's Guide to Vitamins and Minerals.* 3rd ed. Indianapolis, IN: Alpha Books, 2007.

WEBSITES

American Heart Association. "Sodium." September 7, 2010. (Accessed December 15, 2010) http://www.heart.org/ HEARTORG/GettingHealthy/NutritionCenter/Healthy-DietGoals/Sodium-Salt-or-Sodium-Chloride_UCM_ 303290_Article.jsp.

Mayo Clinic Staff. "Sodium: How to tame your salt habit now." May 22, 2010. (Accessed December 15, 2010) http://www.mayoclinic.com/health/sodium/ NU00284.

Medline Plus. "Dietary Sodium." U. S. National Library of Medicine. April 23, 2007. (Accessed December 15, 2010) http://www.nlm.nih/gov/medlineplus/dietary sodium.html.

Murray, Robert. "The Risk and Reality of Hyponatremia." Gatorade Sports Science Institute. 2006. (Accessed December 15, 2010) http://www.gssiweb.com/Article_ Detail.aspx?articleid=618.

United States Department of Health and Human Services and the United States Department of Agriculture. "Dietary Guidelines for Americans 2010." January 31, 2011. (Accessed August 19, 2012) http://www.health.gov/ dietaryguidelines.

U.S. Department of Health and Human Services "Million Hearts." http://millionhearts.hhs.gov/index.html. (Accessed August 19, 2012)

U.S. Food and Drug Administration "Salt Reduction." http://www.fda.gov/Food/FoodIngredients Packaging/ucm253316.htm. (Accessed August 19, 2012)

ORGANIZATIONS

American Heart Association, 7272 Greenville Avenue, Dallas, TX 75231, (800) 242-8721, http://www.americanheart .org

International Food Information Council, 1100 Connecticut Avenue, NW Suite 430, Washington, DC 20036, (202) 296-6540, Fax: (202) 296-6547, http:// ific.org

Tish Davidson, A.M.
Andrea Nienstedt, M.A.

Staphylococcal infections

Definition

Staphylococcal (staph) infections are communicable infections caused by a staphylococcal bacterium. They are generally characterized by the formation of abscesses. Staphlococcal infections are the leading cause of primary infections originating in hospitals (nosocomial infections) in the United States.

Description

Classified since the early twentienth century as among the deadliest of all disease-causing organisms, staph exists on the skin or inside the nostrils of 20–30% of healthy people. It is sometimes found in breast tissue, the mouth, and the genital, urinary, and upper respiratory tracts.

Although staph bacteria are usually harmless, when injury or a break in the skin enables the bacteria to invade the body and overcome the body's natural defenses, consequences can range from minor discomfort to death. Infection is most apt to occur in:

- newborns
- women who are breastfeeding
- individuals whose immune systems have been undermined by radiation treatments, chemotherapy, HIV/AIDS, organ transplantation, or medication
- intravenous drug users
- those with surgical incisions, skin disorders, and serious illness like cancer, diabetes, and lung disease
- the elderly, particularly those who live in nursing homes or who are hospitalized

Types of infections

Staph infections produce pus-filled pockets (abscesses) located just beneath the surface of the skin or deep within the body. Risk of infection is greatest among newborns, the very young, and the very elderly.

A localized staph infection is confined to a ring of dead and dying white blood cells and bacteria. The skin above it feels warm to the touch. Most of these abscesses eventually burst, and pus that leaks onto the skin can cause new infections.

A small fraction of localized staph infections enter the bloodstream and spread through the body. In children, these systemic (affecting the whole body) or disseminated infections frequently affect the ends of the long bones of the arms or legs, causing a bone infection called osteomyelitis. When adults develop invasive staph

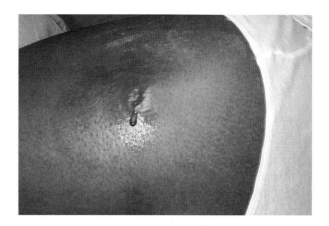

A prison inmate with an abscess caused by methicillin-resistant Staphylococcus aureus bacteria. *(CDC/ Bruno Coignard, M.D.; Jeff Hageman, M.H.S.)*

infections, bacteria are most apt to cause abscesses of the brain, heart, kidneys, liver, lungs, or spleen.

Staphylococcus aureus

Named for the golden color of the bacteria grown under laboratory conditions, *S. aureus* is a hardy organism that can survive in extreme temperatures or other inhospitable circumstances. About 70–90% of the population carry this strain of staph in the nostrils at some point in their life. Although present on the skin of only 5–20% of healthy people, as many as 40% carry the bacteria elsewhere, such as in the throat, vagina, or rectum. These people may carry the bacteria for varying periods of time (from hours to years) without developing symptoms or becoming ill.

S. aureus causes a variety of infections. Boils and inflammation of the skin surrounding a hair shaft (folliculitis) are the most common. Toxic shock (TSS) and staphylococcal scalded skin syndrome (SSSS) are among the most serious.

Methicillin-resistant Staphyloccus aureus. infections (MRSA)

S. aureus flourishes in hospitals, where it infects healthcare personnel and patients who have had surgery; who have acute dermatitis, insulin-dependent diabetes, or dialysis-dependent kidney disease; or who receive frequent allergy-desensitization injections. Staph bacteria can also contaminate bedclothes, catheters, and other objects.

Toxic shock

Toxic shock syndrome is a life-threatening infection characterized by severe headache, sore throat, fever as high as 105°F, and a sunburn-like rash that spreads from the face to the rest of the body. Symptoms appear suddenly; they also include dehydration and watery diarrhea.

Inadequate blood flow to peripheral parts of the body (shock) and loss of consciousness occur within the first 48 hours. Between the third and seventh day of illness, skin peels from the palms of the hands, soles of the feet, and other parts of the body. Kidney, liver, and muscle damage often occur.

SCALDED SKIN SYNDROME. Rare in adults and most common in newborns and other children under the age of five, scalded skin syndrome originates with a localized skin infection. A mild fever and/or an increase in the number of infection-fighting white blood cells may occur.

A bright red rash spreads from the face to other parts of the body and eventually forms scales. Large, soft blisters develop at the site of infection and elsewhere. When they burst, they expose inflamed skin that looks as if it has been burned.

MISCELLANEOUS INFECTIONS. *S. aureus* can also cause:

- arthritis
- bacteria in the bloodstream (bacteremia)
- pockets of infection and pus under the skin (carbuncles)
- tissue inflammation that spreads below the skin, causing pain and swelling (cellulitis)
- inflammation of the valves and walls of the heart (endocarditis)
- inflammation of tissue that enclosed and protects the spinal cord and brain (meningitis)
- inflammation of bone and bone marrow (osteomyelitis)
- pneumonia

Other strains of staph

S. EPIDERMIDIS. Capable of clinging to tubing (e.g., that used for intravenous feeding), prosthetic devices, and other non-living surfaces, *S. epidermidis* is the organism that most often contaminates devices that provide direct access to the bloodstream.

The primary cause of bacteremia in hospital patients, this strain of staph is most likely to infect **cancer** patients, whose immune systems have been compromised, and high-risk newborns receiving intravenous supplements.

S. epidermidis also accounts for two of every five cases of prosthetic valve endocarditis. Prosthetic valve endocarditis is endocarditis as a complication of the implantation of an artificial valve in the heart. Although contamination usually occurs during surgery, symptoms

of infection may not become evident until a year after the operation. More than half of the patients who develop prosthetic valve endocarditis die.

STAPHYLOCOCCUS SAPROPHYTICUS. Existing within and around the tube-like structure that carries urine from the bladder (urethra) of about 5% of healthy males and females, *S. saprophyticus* is the second most common cause of unobstructed urinary tract infections (UTIs) in sexually active young women. This strain of staph is responsible for 10–20% of infections affecting healthy outpatients.

Causes and symptoms

Staph bacteria can spread through the air, but infection is almost always the result of direct contact with open sores or body fluids contaminated by these organisms.

Staph bacteria often enter the body through inflamed hair follicles or oil glands. Or they penetrate skin damaged by **burns**, cuts and scrapes, infection, insect bites, or wounds.

Multiplying beneath the skin, bacteria infect and destroy tissue in the area where they entered the body. Staph infection of the blood (staphylococcal bacteremia) develops when bacteria from a local infection infiltrate the lymph glands and bloodstream. These infections, which can usually be traced to contaminated catheters or intravenous devices, usually cause persistent high fever. They may cause shock. They also can cause death within a short time.

Warning signs

Common symptoms of staph infection include:

- pain or swelling around a cut, or an area of skin that has been scraped
- boils or other skin abscesses
- blistering, peeling, or scaling of the skin; this is most common in infants and young children
- enlarged lymph nodes in the neck, armpits, or groin

A family physician should be notified whenever:

- Lymph nodes in the neck, armpits, or groin become swollen or tender.
- An area of skin that has been cut or scraped becomes painful or swollen, feels hot, or produces pus. These symptoms may mean the infection has spread to the bloodstream.
- A boil or carbuncle appears on any part of the face or spine. Staph infections affecting these areas can spread to the brain or spinal cord.

- A boil becomes very sore. Usually a sign that infection has spread, this condition may be accompanied by fever, chills, and red streaks radiating from the site of the original infection.
- Boils that develop repeatedly. This type of recurrent infection could be a symptom of diabetes.

Diagnosis

Blood tests that show unusually high concentrations of white blood cells can suggest staph infection, but diagnosis is based on laboratory analysis of material removed from pus-filled sores, and on analysis of normally uninfected body fluids, such as, blood and urine. Also, x rays can enable doctors to locate internal abscesses and estimate the severity of infection. Needle biopsy (removing tissue with a needle, then examining it under a microscope) may be used to assess bone involvement.

Treatment

Superficial staph infections can generally be cured by keeping the area clean, using soaps that leave a germ-killing film on the skin, and applying warm, moist compresses to the affected area for 20–30 minutes three or four times a day.

Severe or recurrent infections may require a 7 to 10 day course of treatment with penicillin or other oral **antibiotics**. The location of the infection and the identity of the causal bacteria determines which of several effective medications should be prescribed.

In case of a more serious infection, antibiotics may be administered intravenously for as long as six weeks. Intravenous antibiotics are also used to treat staph infections around the eyes or on other parts of the face.

Surgery may be required to drain or remove abscesses that form on internal organs, or on shunts or other devices implanted inside the body.

Alternative treatment

Alternative therapies for staph infection are meant to strengthen the immune system and prevent recurrences. Among the therapies believed to be helpful for the person with a staph infection are yoga (to stimulate the immune system and promote relaxation), acupuncture (to draw heat away from the infection), and herbal remedies. Herbs that may help the body overcome, or withstand, staph infection include:

- Garlic (*Allium sativum*). This herb is believed to have anitbacterial properties. Herbalists recommend consuming three garlic cloves or three garlic oil capsules a day, starting when symptoms of infection first appear.

- Cleavers (*Galium aparine*). This anti-inflammatory herb is believed to support the lymphatic system. It may be taken internally to help heal staph abscesses and reduce swelling of the lymph nodes. A cleavers compress can also be applied directly to a skin infection.
- Goldenseal (*Hydrastis canadensis*). Another herb believed to fight infection and reduce imflammation, goldenseal may be taken internally when symptoms of infection first appear. Skin infections can be treated by making a paste of water and powdered goldenseal root and applying it directly to the affected area. The preparation should be covered with a clean bandage and left in place overnight.
- Echinacea (*Echinacea* spp.). Taken internally, this herb is believed to have antibiotic properties and is also thought to strengthen the immune system.
- Thyme (*Thymus vulgaris*), lavender (*Lavandula officinalis*), or bergamot (*Citrus bergamot*) oils. These oils are believed to have antibacterial properties and may help to prevent the scarring that may result from skin infections. A few drops of these oils are added to water, and then a compress soaked in the water is applied to the affected area.
- Tea tree oil (*Melaleuca* spp.). Another infection-fighting herb, this oil can be applied directly to a boil or other skin infection.

Prognosis

Most healthy people who develop staph infections recover fully within a short time. Others develop repeated infections. Some become seriously ill, requiring long-term therapy or emergency care. A small percentage die.

Prevention

Healthcare providers and patients should always wash their hands thoroughly with warm water and soap after treating a staph infection or touching an open wound or the pus it produces. Pus that oozes onto the skin from the site of an infection should be removed immediately. This affected area should then be cleansed with antiseptic or with antibacterial soap.

To prevent infection from spreading from one part of the body to another, it is important to shower, rather than bathe, during the healing process. Because staph infection is easily transmitted from one member of a household to others, towels, washcloths, and bed linens used by someone with a staph infection should not be used by anyone else. They should be changed daily and laundered separately in hot water with bleach until symptoms disappear.

Children should frequently be reminded not to share:

• brushes, combs, or hair accessories

• caps

• clothing

• sleeping bags

• sports equipment

• other personal items

A diet rich in green, yellow, and orange vegetables can bolster natural immunity. A doctor or nutritionist may recommend **vitamins** or mineral supplements to compensate for specific dietary deficiencies. Drinking 8 to 10 glasses of water a day can help flush disease-causing organisms from the body.

Because some strains of staph bacteria are known to contaminate artificial limbs, prosthetic devices implanted within the body, and tubes used to administer medication or drain fluids from the body, catheters, and other devices should be removed on a regular basis, if possible, and examined for microscopic signs of staph. Symptoms might not become evident until many months after contamination has occurred, so this practice should be followed even with patients who show no sign of infection.

Resources

BOOKS

Marini, John J., and Arthur P. Wheeler. *Critical Care Medicine: The Essentials*. 2nd ed. Philadelphia: Lippincott Williams & Wilkins, 2006.

WEBSITES

American Academy of Pediatrics. "Staphylococcal Infections." http://www.healthychildren.org/English/health-issues/ conditions/infections/pages/Staphylococcal-Infections .aspx. (Accessed November 12, 2012)

Centers for Disease Control and Prevention. "Methicillin-resistant Staphylococcus Aureus (MRSA) Infections." http://www .cdc.gov/mrsa/. (Accessed November 12, 2012)

Herchline, Thomas. American Academy of Pediatrics. "Staphylococcal Infections: Treatment & Medication."

http://emedicine.medscape.com/article/228816-treatment. (Accessed November 12, 2012)

ORGANIZATIONS

Centers for Disease Control and Prevention, 1600 Clifton Rd., Atlanta, GA 30333, (800) 232-4636, www. cdc.gov.

Maureen Haggerty
Tish Davidson, A.M.
Andrea Nienstedt, M.A.

Stress

Definition

Stress is defined as an organism's total response to physical, mental, emotional, or environmental demands or pressures. A stressor is defined as the stimulus or event that provokes a stress response. Stressors can be categorized as acute or chronic and as external or internal to the organism.

Demographics

Nearly everyone experiences stress in their lives at some time. One study found that about 75% of those surveyed reported experiencing at least some stress in the previous two weeks. Occasional stress is an expected part of life for most people, and while often unpleasant, it does not lead to long-term negative outcomes. In some cases, however, severe or prolonged stress can lead to illness.

Work plays a highly visible role in the stress burden among Americans; in a 2010 survey conducted by the American Psychological Association, 70% of those surveyed included work as a top source of stress, with the other top two being money (76%) and the economy (65%). Forty-nine percent of workers cited job insecurity as a major source of stress, and only 32% felt their employers helped them attain a satisfactory work-life balance. Only one-third of respondents felt they were successful in managing their stress levels.

Description

Stress results from interactions between persons and their environment that are perceived as straining or exceeding the individuals' adaptive capacities or threatening their well-being. A certain degree of stress is a normal part of life; it comprises individuals' responses to inevitable changes in their physical or social

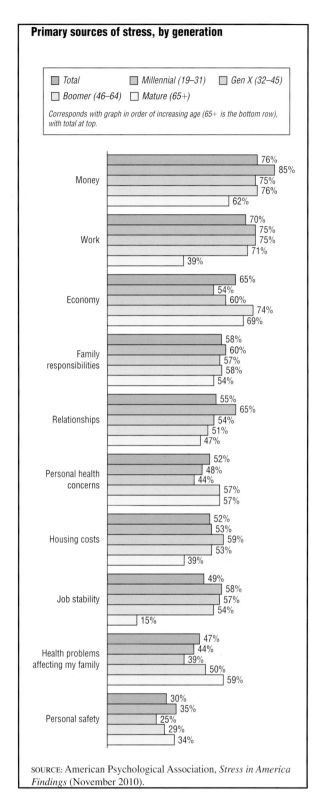

Primary sources of stress, by generation

Legend:
- Total
- Millennial (19–31)
- Gen X (32–45)
- Boomer (46–64)
- Mature (65+)

Corresponds with graph in order of increasing age (65+ is the bottom row), with total at top.

Money: 76%, 85%, 75%, 76%, 62%
Work: 70%, 75%, 75%, 71%, 39%
Economy: 65%, 54%, 60%, 74%, 69%
Family responsibilities: 58%, 60%, 57%, 58%, 54%
Relationships: 55%, 65%, 54%, 51%, 47%
Personal health concerns: 52%, 48%, 44%, 57%, 57%
Housing costs: 52%, 53%, 59%, 53%, 39%
Job stability: 49%, 58%, 57%, 54%, 15%
Health problems affecting my family: 47%, 44%, 39%, 50%, 59%
Personal safety: 30%, 35%, 25%, 29%, 34%

SOURCE: American Psychological Association, *Stress in America Findings* (November 2010).

(Table by Electronic Illustrators Group. © 2013 Cengage Learning)

environment. Moreover, positive as well as negative events can generate stress. Graduating from college, for example, is accompanied by stress related to the challenge of finding employment or saying good-bye to friends and family, as well as feelings of positive accomplishment. Some researchers refer to stress associated with positive events as eustress.

Stress may be acute or chronic. Acute stress is defined as a reaction to something believed to be an immediate threat. Acute stress reactions can occur to a falsely perceived danger as well as to a genuine threat; they can also occur in response to memories. For example, a war veteran who hears a car backfire may drop to the ground because the noise triggers vivid memories, called flashbacks, of combat experience. Common acute stressors are loud, sudden noises; being in a crowded space, such as an elevator; being cut off in heavy traffic; and being exposed to dangerous weather. Chronic stress is a reaction to a stressful situation that is ongoing, such as financial insecurity or caring for a dependent elderly parent.

Stress-related disease results from chronic stress resulting from excessive and prolonged demands on an individual's ability to cope with the stressor(s). Canadian researcher Hans Selye (1907–1982), a pioneer in studying stress, observed that an increasing number of people, particularly in developed countries, died of so-called diseases of civilization, or degenerative diseases, which are primarily caused by stress.

The role of perception in identifying stressors indicates that human stress responses reflect differences in personality, as well as differences in physical strength or general health. Selye affirmed that stress in humans depends partly on people's evaluation of a situation and their emotional reaction to it; thus, an experience that one person finds stimulating and exciting, for example, bungee jumping, may produce harmful stress in another.

One recurrent disagreement among researchers concerns the definition of stress in humans. The debate centers on whether stress is primarily an external response that can be measured by changes in glandular secretions, skin reactions, and other physical functions or a solely an internal interpretation of, or reaction to, a stressor. Perhaps, in some cases, it is both.

Risk factors

Risk factors for stress-related illnesses are a mix of personal, interpersonal, and social variables. These

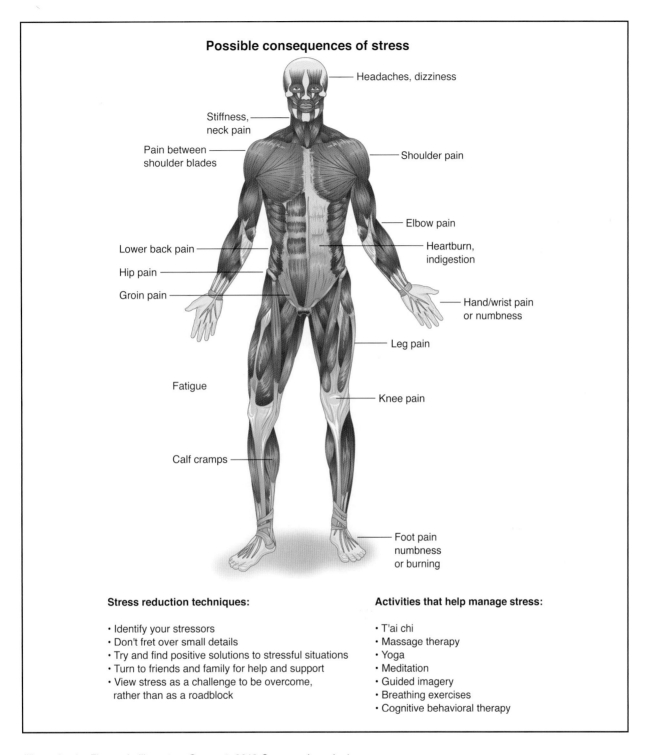

Possible consequences of stress

- Headaches, dizziness
- Stiffness, neck pain
- Pain between shoulder blades
- Shoulder pain
- Elbow pain
- Lower back pain
- Heartburn, indigestion
- Hip pain
- Groin pain
- Hand/wrist pain or numbness
- Leg pain
- Fatigue
- Knee pain
- Calf cramps
- Foot pain numbness or burning

Stress reduction techniques:

- Identify your stressors
- Don't fret over small details
- Try and find positive solutions to stressful situations
- Turn to friends and family for help and support
- View stress as a challenge to be overcome, rather than as a roadblock

Activities that help manage stress:

- T'ai chi
- Massage therapy
- Yoga
- Meditation
- Guided imagery
- Breathing exercises
- Cognitive behavioral therapy

(Illustration by Electronic Illustrators Group. © 2013 Cengage Learning)

factors include lack or loss of control over one's physical environment and lack or loss of social support networks. People who are dependent on others, such as children, the elderly, or those who are socially disadvantaged, are at greater risk of developing stress-related illnesses. Other risk factors are feelings of helplessness, hopelessness, extreme fear or anger, and cynicism or distrust of others.

Research indicates that some vulnerability to stress is genetic. Scientists at the University of Wisconsin and King's College London discovered that people who inherited a short, or stress-sensitive, version of the serotonin transporter gene were almost three times as likely to experience depression following a stressful event as people with the long version of the gene. Further research is likely to identify other genes that affect susceptibility to stress.

Stress and mental disorders

The *Diagnostic and Statistical Manual of Mental Disorders*, fourth edition, text revised (*DSM-IV-TR*) specifies two major categories of mental disorders directly related to stress: the post-traumatic syndromes and adjustment disorders. Proposed changes for the *Diagnostic and Statistical Manual of Mental Disorders*, fifth edition (*DSM-5*), scheduled for publication in 2013, combine these categories into one: trauma- and stressor-related disorders. Stress is closely associated with depression and can worsen the symptoms of most other disorders.

POST-TRAUMATIC DISORDERS. **Post-traumatic stress disorder** (PTSD) and acute stress disorder (ASD) are defined by their connection to a traumatic event in an individual's life, whether experienced or witnessed. The post-traumatic disorders are characterized by a cluster of anxiety and dissociative symptoms and by their interference with the patient's normal level of functioning. Magnetic resonance imaging (MRI) studies have shown that the high levels of sustained stress in some PTSD patients cause demonstrable damage to the hippocampus. Excessive amounts of stress hormones in brain tissue cause the nerve cells, or neurons, in parts of the hippocampus to wither and eventually die. One group of Vietnam veterans with PTSD lost as much as 8% of the tissue in the hippocampus.

SUBSTANCE ABUSE DISORDERS. Stress is related to substance abuse disorders in that chronic stress frequently leads people to self-medicate with drugs of abuse or alcohol. Substance abuse disorders are associated with a specific type of strategy for dealing with stress called emotion-focused coping. Emotion-focused coping strategies concentrate on regulating painful emotions related to stress, as distinct from problem-focused coping strategies, which involve efforts to change or eliminate the impact of a stressful event. Persons who handle stress from a problem-oriented perspective are less likely to turn to mood-altering substances when they are under stress.

ADJUSTMENT DISORDERS. The *DSM-IV-TR* defines adjustment disorders as psychological responses to stressors that are excessive given the nature of the stressor or that result in impairment of a person's academic, occupational, or social functioning. The most important difference between the post-traumatic disorders and adjustment disorders is that most people would not regard stressors involved in the latter disorder as traumatic. Adjustment disorders appear to be more common following divorce, the birth of a child, or retirement from work.

Causes and symptoms

The human stress response began as a biologically conditioned set of reactions that was necessary during earlier points in human evolution but is now less adaptive under the circumstances of modern life. In humans, the biochemical response to acute stress is known as the fight-or-flight reaction. It begins with the activation of a section of the brain called the hypothalamic-pituitary-adrenal system, or HPA. This system first activates the release of steroid hormones, which are also known as glucocorticoids. These hormones include cortisol, the primary stress hormone in humans.

Following the stress hormones, the HPA system releases a set of neurotransmitters known as catecholamines, which include dopamine, norepinephrine, and epinephrine (also known as adrenaline). Catecholamines have three important effects:

- They activate the amygdala, an almond-shaped structure in the limbic system that triggers an emotional response of fear.
- They signal the hippocampus, another part of the limbic system, to store the emotional experience in long-term memory.
- They suppress activity in parts of the brain associated with short-term memory, concentration, and rational thinking. This suppression allows a human to react quickly to a stressful situation, but it also lowers ability to deal with complex social or intellectual tasks that may be part of the situation.

In reaction to stress, heart rate, blood pressure, and breathing intake rise, allowing the lungs to take in more oxygen. Blood flow to the muscles, lungs, and brain may triple or quadruple. The spleen releases more blood cells into circulation, which increases the blood's ability to transport oxygen. The immune system redirects white blood cells to the skin, bone marrow, and lymph nodes, where injury or infection are most likely to occur.

At the same time, nonessential body systems shut down. The skin becomes cool and sweaty as blood is drawn away toward the heart and muscles. The mouth becomes dry, and the digestive system slows.

After the crisis passes, the levels of stress hormones drop, and the body's various organ systems return to normal, a process known as the relaxation response. Some people are more vulnerable to stress than others because their hormone levels do not return to normal after a stressful event. An absent or incomplete relaxation response is most likely to occur in professional athletes and in people with a history of depression.

Causes

Any event or occurrence that puts pressure on a person's coping mechanisms or resources can produce stress. Events such as a job interview, work-related presentation, or final exam can cause significant stress. Persons who dread a future event may experience an increased level of agitation and fretfulness. They may visualize the event negatively, worrying about what may go wrong. It is often hard to stop thinking about the event. This type of stress can take a significant toll if it persists for a long time.

Stress also may be caused by negative world news. Events such as the terrorist attacks on the United States, on September 11, 2001, are believed to increase stress both among Americans and people living elsewhere in the world. Events like terrorist attacks can prompt people to worry about the safety of family members and to fret about potential future attacks. These kinds of worries, when they occur over a long period of time, can produce chronic stress and related negative symptoms.

One study conducted telephone interviews following the September 11 terrorist attacks to assess stress reactions among the general U.S. **population**. The team found that the single most important factor was not geographical location relative to the attacks but the amount of time spent watching televised reports of the attacks. The interviewers discovered that 49% of the adults had watched at least eight hours of television on September 11, and the researchers considered extensive television viewing a reaction to stress.

Experiencing directly or witnessing a traumatic event such as a car accident, earthquake, or an attack of physical **violence** can cause severe stress. In these cases, an individual may mentally relive the event repeatedly. This is a normal response to a traumatic event, but if it persists for more than a short time or does not seem to get better, the individual may have PTSD or ASD.

Stress can also be caused by the presence of issues and problems that are upsetting or frustrating in day-to-day life. These can include worries about money, pressure at work, and problems in a relationship. Events such as divorce or the death of a loved one can also cause

stress for many months or years but are not generally suggestive of PTSD or ASD.

Other causes of stress can include:

- social changes, such as living far away from family members or growing apart from childhood friends
- economic issues, such as a recession or lowered socioeconomic status
- technology, including constant access to news and events or feeling tied to work via e-mail or mobile devices
- environmental changes, such as pollution or nuclear disasters apparently due to chronic emotional stress rather than physiological exposure to harmful chemicals or radioactivity
- changes in mainstream beliefs and attitudes

Symptoms

The symptoms of stress can be physical, psychological, or both. Physical symptoms may include problems sleeping, indigestion, stomach **pain** or chest pain, fatigue, headache, back or neck pain, and many others. Psychological signs of stress include anxiety, frustration, irritability, and even depression. These symptoms may not be problematic if they occur for a brief time, but in cases of chronic stress, the body's organ systems do not have the opportunity to return fully to normal functioning. Different organs become under- or overactivated on a long-term basis. In time, these abnormal levels of activity can damage an organ or organ system.

In the workplace, stress-related illness often takes the form of burnout, a loss of interest in, or ability to perform, one's job due to long-term high stress levels. For example, palliative care nurses are at high risk of burnout due to their inability to prevent their patients from dying or even to relieve their physical suffering in some circumstances.

Effects of chronic stress on body systems

CARDIOVASCULAR SYSTEM. Stress has a number of negative effects on the heart and circulatory system. Acute, sudden stress increases the heart rate but also causes the arteries to narrow, which may block the flow of blood to the heart. The emotional effects of stress can alter the rhythm of the heart. In addition, stress triggers an inflammatory response in the blood vessels that can ultimately result in injury to the lining of the arteries. Markers of inflammation, linked to the development of cardiovascular disease, are also markers of the acute-phase response to stress. Stress also can cause a change in cholesterol levels, increasing fats in the blood that can eventually lead to clogged arteries and heart attack or **stroke**.

GASTROINTESTINAL SYSTEM. The effects of chronic stress on the gastrointestinal system include diarrhea, constipation, bloating, and irritable bowel syndrome. Although stress does not cause ulcers, which arise from an infection with *Helicobacter pylori* bacteria, it can exacerbate them. Stress can also influence inflammatory bowel disease, stimulating colon spasms and possibly interacting with the immune system in producing flare-ups.

Stress is the cause of abnormal weight loss in some people and of weight gain in others, largely related to stress-related inability to eat or to control eating. It is thought that stress related to the physical and emotional changes of puberty is a major factor in the development of **eating disorders**.

REPRODUCTIVE SYSTEM. Stress affects sexual desire in both men and women and can cause impotence in men. It appears to worsen the symptoms of premenstrual syndrome (PMS) in women. Stress affects fertility because the high levels of cortisol in the blood can affect the hypothalamus, which produces hormones related to reproduction. Very high levels of cortisol can cause amenorrhea or cessation of menstrual periods.

In pregnancy, stress has been strongly associated with miscarriage during the earliest weeks of gestation; in one study, 90% of women with high cortisol levels experienced a miscarriage in the first three weeks of pregnancy, compared to 33% of women with normal cortisol levels. High stress levels of the mother during pregnancy are also related to higher rates of premature births and babies of lower-than-average birth weight; both are risk factors for infant mortality. In addition, stress during pregnancy is also associated with negative effects that persist after the baby is born.

MUSCULOSKELETAL SYSTEM. Stress intensifies the chronic pain of arthritis and other joint disorders. It also produces tension headaches, caused by the tightening of the muscles in the neck and scalp. Research indicates that people who have frequent tension headaches have a biological predisposition for converting emotional stress into muscle contraction.

BRAIN. The physical effects of stress hormones on the brain include interference with memory and learning. Acute stress interferes with short-term memory, although this effect goes away after the stress is resolved. People who are under severe stress are unable to concentrate and may become physically inefficient and accident prone. In children, the brain's biochemical responses to stress hampers the ability to learn.

Chronic stress appears to be a more important factor than **aging** in the loss of memory in older adults. Older people with low levels of stress hormones perform as well as younger people in tests of cognitive (knowledge-

---

KEY TERMS

Adjustment disorder—A psychiatric disorder marked by inappropriate or inadequate responses to a change in life circumstances. Depression following retirement from work is an example of adjustment disorder.

Biofeedback—A technique in which patients learn to modify certain body functions, such as temperature or pulse rate, with the help of a monitoring machine.

Burnout—An emotional condition, marked by fatigue, loss of interest, or frustration, that interferes with job performance. Burnout is usually regarded as the result of prolonged work-related stress.

Stress hardiness—A personality characteristic that enables persons to stay healthy in stressful circumstances. It includes belief in one's ability to influence the situation; commitment to, or full engagement with, one's activities; and a positive view of change.

Stress management—A category of popularized programs and techniques intended to help people deal more effectively with stress.

Stressor—A stimulus, or event, that provokes a stress response in an organism. Stressors can be categorized as acute or chronic and as external or internal to the organism.

---

related) skills, but those with high levels of stress hormones test between 20% and 50% lower than the younger test subjects.

IMMUNE SYSTEM. Chronic stress affects the human immune system and increases a person's risk of getting an **infectious disease**. Several research studies have shown that people under chronic stress have lower-than-normal white blood cell counts and are more vulnerable to colds and **influenza**. Men with HIV infection and high stress levels progress more rapidly to **AIDS** than infected men with lower stress levels.

Diagnosis

To identify a stress-related illness, doctors take a careful medical history that includes stressors in the patient's life (e.g., family or employment problems, other illnesses, recent major life changes). Many physicians evaluate patients' personality as well, in order to assess their coping resources and emotional response patterns. Many clinicians think that differences in attitudes toward stressful events are the single most important factor in assessing individuals' vulnerability to stress-related illnesses. The ability to cope with stress depends in part on a person's perception of the stressor. The person's resources, previous physical and psychological health, and previous life experiences all affect this interpretation. Someone who has had good experiences of overcoming hardships is more likely to develop a positive interpretation of stressful events than someone who has repeatedly faced traumas and discouragement in solving problems.

There are several personality inventories and psychological tests that doctors can use to help diagnose the amount of stress that the patient experiences and the coping strategies that the patient uses to deal with them. Doctors also try to identify what the patient perceives as threatening and stressful.

The ways in which people cope with stress can be categorized according to two different sets of distinctions. One is the distinction between emotion-focused and problem-focused styles of coping. Problem-focused coping is believed to lower the impact of stress on health; people who use problem-focused coping have fewer illnesses, are less likely to become emotionally exhausted, and report higher levels of satisfaction in their work and feelings of personal accomplishment. Emotion-focused coping, in contrast, is associated with higher levels of interpersonal problems, depression, and social isolation. Although some studies reported that men are more likely to use problem-focused coping and women to use emotion-focused coping, other research done in the early 2000s found no significant gender differences in coping styles.

The second set of categories distinguishes between control-related and escape-related coping styles. Control-related coping styles include direct-action behaviors that can be done alone, help-seeking behaviors that involve social support, and positive thinking. Escape-related coping styles include avoidance of or resignation from the stressful event and substance abuse.

Stress-related illness can be diagnosed by primary care doctors, as well as by those who specialize in psychiatry. The doctor will need to distinguish between adjustment disorders and anxiety or mood disorders, and between psychiatric disorders and physical illnesses that have psychological side effects (e.g., abnormal thyroid activity).

Treatment

Advances in the understanding of the many complex connections between the human mind and body have produced a variety of mainstream approaches to treating stress and stress-related illness. Present treatment regimens may include one or more of the following:

- Medications may include drugs to control blood pressure or other physical symptoms of stress, as well as drugs that affect the patient's mood (antianxiety drugs or tranquilizers, antidepressants).

- Stress management programs may be either individual or group treatments and usually involve analysis of the stressors in the patient's life. They often focus on job or workplace-related stress.

- Behavioral approaches include relaxation techniques, breathing exercises, and physical exercise programs, including walking.

- Cognitive therapies teach patients to reframe or mentally reinterpret the stressors in their lives in order to modify the body's physical reactions. Anger management techniques are recommended for people who have stress-related symptoms due to chronic anger.

Alternative treatment

Treatment of stress is one area in which the boundaries between traditional and alternative therapies have changed in recent years, in part because some forms of physical exercise (yoga, tai chi, aikido) that were once associated with the counterculture have become widely accepted as useful parts of mainstream stress reduction programs. Meditation, music therapy, and relaxation techniques have been clinically proven to alleviate symptoms of stress. Other alternative therapies for stress that are occasionally recommended are aromatherapy, dance therapy, biofeedback, nutrition-based treatments (including dietary guidelines and nutritional supplements), acupuncture, homeopathy, pranayama (controlled breathing), massage and other bodywork therapies, and herbal medicine. Eating a well-balanced diet, exercising regularly, and receiving adequate sleep each night promote good health in general but may also provide stress relief.

Prognosis

The prognosis for recovery from a stress-related illness is dependent on a wide variety of factors in a person's life, many of which are genetically determined (e.g., race, sex, illnesses that run in families) or beyond the individual's control (e.g., economic trends, cultural stereotypes and prejudices, death of a loved one). It is possible, however, for individuals to learn new responses to stress and, thus, change their perceptions and experiences. A person's ability to remain healthy in stressful situations is sometimes referred to as stress hardiness. Stress-hardy people have a cluster of personality traits that strengthen their ability to cope. These traits include believing in the importance of what they are doing, believing that they have some power to influence their situation, and viewing life's changes as positive opportunities rather than as threats.

Prevention

Complete **prevention** of stress is neither possible nor desirable because stress is an important stimulus of human growth and creativity, as well as an inevitable part of life. Specific strategies for stress prevention vary widely from person to person, depending on the nature and number of the stressors in an individual's life and the amount of control he or she has over these factors. In general, a combination of attitudinal and behavioral changes works well for most patients. An important form of prevention may be parental modeling of healthy attitudes and behaviors within the family.

Resources

BOOKS

Al'Absi, Mustafa. *Stress and Addiction: Biological and Psychological Mechanisms.* Boston: Academic Press, 2007.

Greenberg, Jerrold S. *Comprehensive Stress Management.* Boston: McGraw-Hill, 2010.

Miller, Allen R. *Living with Stress.* New York: Facts on File, 2010.

Romas, John A., and Sharma, Manoj. *Practical Stress Management: A Comprehensive Workbook for Managing Change and Promoting Health.* 5th ed. San Francisco: Pearson Benjamin Cummings, 2010.

Seaward, Brian Luke. *Essentials of Managing Stress.* 2nd ed. Sudbury, MA: Jones and Bartlett, 2010.

ORGANIZATIONS

American Institute of Stress, 124 Park Ave., Yonkers, NY 10703, (914) 963-1200, Fax: (914) 965-6267, Stress125@optonline.net, http://www.stress.org

Centers for Disease Control and Prevention, 1600 Clifton Rd., Atlanta, GA 30333, (404) 639-3534, 800-232-4636, inquiry@cdc.gov, http://www.cdc.gov

National Institute of Mental Health, 6001 Executive Blvd., Rm. 8184, MSC 9663, Bethesda, MD 20892-9663, (301) 443-4513, (866) 615-6464 TTY (866) 415-8051, Fax: (301) 443-4279, nimhinfo@nih.gov, http://www.nimh.nih.gov/index.shtml.

Rebecca J. Frey, Ph.D.
Tish Davidson, A.M.
Laura Jean Cataldo, R.N., Ed.D.

Stroke

Definition

Stroke is a life-threatening condition that occurs when the blood supply to a part of the brain is suddenly cut off or when brain tissue is damaged by bleeding into the brain. Stroke falls into two main types. Ischemic stroke occurs when a clot blocks an artery to the brain; this type accounts for about 87% of strokes. The other type, hemorrhagic stroke, occurs when a blood vessel in the brain bursts, allowing blood to spill out into brain tissue. The blood upsets the chemical balance that the nerve cells in the brain need to function.

Demographics

According to the American Stroke Association, stroke is the fourth leading cause of death in the United States. Each year, about 785,000 Americans have strokes, and nearly 140,000 die as a result. On average, someone in the United States has a stroke every 40 seconds. Of those 785,000, 610,000 of these are the patients' first strokes, and 185,000 are recurrent strokes.

Stroke incidence has been declining overall, dropping from 7.6 per thousand males from 1950–1977 to 5.3 from 1990–2004. Females saw a decrease from 6.2 to 5.1 over the same period. Comparing the two periods, the number of deaths occurring within 30 days of a stroke dropped from 23% to 14% for men, but only from 21% to 20% for women. In addition, women account for more than 60% of U.S. stroke deaths.

Among individuals who are black, the risk for a stroke is almost twice that for individuals who are white (among men aged 20 and older, the prevalence of stroke is 4.5% among blacks compared to 2.4% among non-Hispanic whites). Stroke incidence in the black population has remained about the same from the 1950–1977 period to the 1990–2004 period.

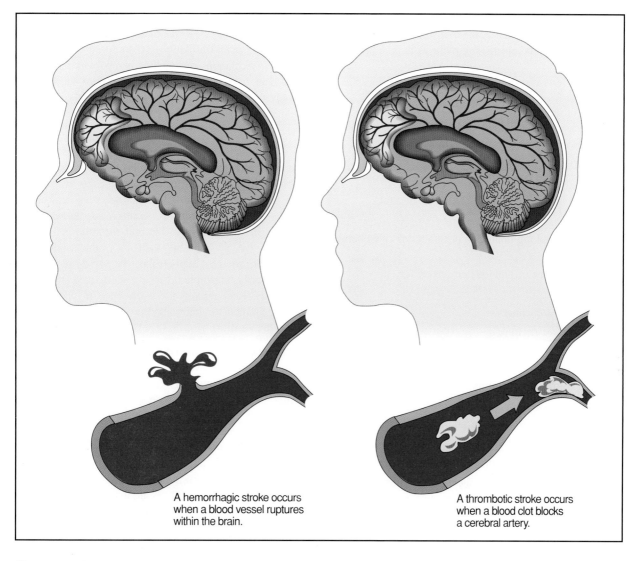

A hemorrhagic stroke occurs when a blood vessel ruptures within the brain.

A thrombotic stroke occurs when a blood clot blocks a cerebral artery.

(Illustration by Electronic Illustrators Group. © 2013 Cengage Learning)

Strokes can affect people in any age group; however, the risk increases as people age. In the 60–79-year-old age group, 7.2% of men and 8.25% of women have had a stroke. Among those 80 years old or more, 14.5% of men and 14.8% of women have had a stroke. According to the American Stroke Association, about 55,000 more women than men have a stroke each year, because women have a greater average lifespan.

According to the Children's Hemiplegia and Stroke Association, strokes do occur in children. They occur most often—at a rate of about one in 2,800—in infants up to one month of age. For children 1–18 years old, the incidence of stroke is 11 per 100,000 children.

Description

Stroke is usually a sudden occurrence. A stroke occurs when blood flow is interrupted to part of the brain.

Without blood to supply oxygen and nutrients, and to remove waste products, brain cells quickly begin to die. Depending on the region of the brain affected, a stroke may cause paralysis, speech impairment, loss of memory and reasoning ability, coma, or death. A stroke also is sometimes called a brain attack or a cerebrovascular accident (CVA).

Some people have a warning event called a transient ischemic attack (TIA) or mini-stroke. A TIA has the same symptoms as a full-blown stroke but goes away in a few minutes or hours, leaving no permanent effects. It is, however, an indication that the person is at risk of a major stroke and should see their doctor right away. A TIA offers the person an opportunity to take preventive action.

Stroke is a medical emergency requiring immediate treatment. Prompt treatment improves the chances of survival and increases the degree of recovery that may be expected. A person who may have suffered a stroke should be seen in a hospital emergency room without delay.

Risk factors

Risk factors for stroke in adults include:

- Hypertension (high blood pressure). This is the most important single risk factor for stroke.
- High blood cholesterol levels.
- Age of more than 55.
- A family history of stroke, TIA, or heart attack.
- Diabetes.
- Smoking. Smoking doubles a person's risk of ischemic stroke.
- Personal history of previous stroke or TIA.
- Obesity.
- Heavy use of cocaine.
- Irregular heart rhythm.
- Heavy drinking. Alcohol consumption raises a person's blood pressure.
- Use of birth control pills or hormone replacement therapy.

Risk factors for stroke in children include:

- Congenital (present at birth) malformations of blood vessels and other structures in the brain or heart.
- Infections of the brain like encephalitis and meningitis, and other infections, such as chicken pox.
- Head trauma.
- Metabolic disorders.
- Blood disorders, particularly sickle cell disease.

Causes and symptoms

Causes

Stroke is caused by a loss of blood supply to the brain resulting either from a clot blocking an artery or from bleeding into or around the brain. Ischemic stroke can result from two types of clots. The first is an embolus, which is a free-floating clot produced in the heart or somewhere else in the body that travels to a blood vessel in the brain. The second type of clot is called a thrombus. It is formed within an artery in the head or neck and grows there until it is large enough to block the artery. Atherosclerosis, a disease of the blood vessels in which fatty deposits build up along the walls of the vessels, is a common cause of this type of clot.

ISCHEMIC STROKE. A cerebral embolism occurs when a blood clot from elsewhere in the circulatory system breaks free. If it becomes lodged in an artery supplying the brain, either in the brain or in the neck, it can cause a stroke. The most common cause of cerebral embolism is atrial fibrillation, a disorder of the heartbeat. In atrial fibrillation, the upper chambers (atria) of the heart beat weakly and rapidly instead of slowly and steadily. Blood within the atria is not completely emptied. This stagnant blood may form clots within the atria, which can then break off and enter the circulation.

Cerebral thrombosis occurs when a blood clot, or thrombus, forms within the brain itself, blocking the flow of blood through the affected vessel. Clots most often form due to "hardening" (atherosclerosis) of brain arteries. Cerebral thrombosis occurs most often at night or early in the morning. Cerebral thrombosis is often preceded by a transient ischemic attack, or TIA, sometimes called a "mini-stroke." In a TIA, blood flow is temporarily interrupted, causing short-lived stroke-like symptoms. Recognizing the occurrence of a TIA, and seeking immediate treatment, is an important step in stroke **prevention**.

HEMORRHAGIC STROKE. Hemorrhagic stroke can occur when an aneurysm—a weak spot in the wall of an artery—suddenly bursts. High blood pressure is the most common cause of this type of hemorrhagic stroke. Hemorrhagic stroke can also occur when the walls of an artery become thin and brittle; they can then break and leak blood into the brain. Hemorrhagic stroke can take one of two forms: the blood can leak directly into brain tissue from an artery in the brain, or it can leak from an artery near the surface of the brain into the space between the skull and the membranes covering the brain.

The vessels most likely to break are those with pre-existing defects such as an aneurysm. An aneurysm is a bulge or pouch in a blood vessel caused by weakening of the arterial wall. Brain aneurysms are surprisingly common, and about 3–5 million people in the United States have them. On the positive side, most aneurysms produce no symptoms. The problems with aneurysms occur when they burst, and that is most likely to happen when blood pressure is highest. Maintaining a healthy blood pressure is an important preventive strategy.

Intracerebral hemorrhage affects vessels within the brain itself, while subarachnoid hemorrhage affects arteries at the brain's surface, just below the protective arachnoid membrane. Intracerebral hemorrhages represent about 10% of all strokes, while subarachnoid hemorrhages account for about 7%.

In addition to depriving affected tissues of blood supply, the accumulation of fluid within the inflexible skull creates excess pressure on brain tissue, which can quickly lead to death. Nonetheless, recovery may be more complete for a person who survives hemorrhage

KEY TERMS

Aneurysm—A pouch-like bulging of a blood vessel. Aneurysms can rupture, leading to stroke.

Atrial fibrillation—A disorder of the heartbeat associated with a higher risk of stroke. In this disorder, the upper chambers (atria) of the heart do not completely empty when the heart beats, which can allow blood clots to form.

Cerebral embolism—A blockage of blood flow through a vessel in the brain by a blood clot that formed elsewhere in the body and traveled to the brain.

Cerebral thrombosis—A blockage of blood flow through a vessel in the brain by a blood clot that formed in the brain itself.

Comorbid—Referring to the presence of one or more diseases or disorders in addition to the patient's primary disorder.

Deficit—In medicine, the loss or impairment of a function or ability.

Dysphagia—Difficulty in swallowing.

Embolus—A clot that forms in the heart and travels through the circulatory system to another part of the body.

Intracerebral hemorrhage—A cause of some strokes in which vessels within the brain begin bleeding.

Ischemia—Loss of blood supply to a tissue or organ resulting from the blockage of a blood vessel.

Platelets—Small irregularly shaped blood cells involved in the formation of blood clots.

Statins—A group of medications given to lower blood cholesterol levels that work by inhibiting an enzyme involved in cholesterol formation. Statins are also known as HMG-CoA reductase inhibitors.

Subarachnoid hemorrhage—A cause of some strokes in which arteries on the surface of the brain begin bleeding.

Thrombus—A blood clot that forms inside an intact blood vessel and remains there.

Tissue plasminogen activator (tPA)—A substance that is sometimes given to patients within three hours of a stroke to dissolve blood clots within the brain.

Transient ischemic attack (TIA)—A brief stroke lasting from a few minutes to 24 hours. TIAs are sometimes called mini-strokes.

than for one who survives a clot because the effects of blood deprivation usually are not as severe.

The death of brain cells triggers a chain reaction in which toxic chemicals created by cell death affect other nearby cells. This is one reason why prompt treatment can have such a dramatic effect on final recovery.

Symptoms

Stroke has five major signs or symptoms. The American Stroke Association has a quick symptom checklist called "Give Me 5" that can help identify a stroke:

- Walk: Is the person having trouble with balance or coordination?

- Talk: Is speech difficult or slurred? Is the person's face drooping?

- Reach: Is one side of the body weak or numb?

- See: Is vision partly or entirely lost?

- Feel: Does the person have a sudden severe headache with no obvious cause?

Other symptoms of stroke that some patients experience include drooling, uncontrollable eye movements, personality or mood changes, drowsiness, loss of memory, or loss of consciousness.

A person with stroke can have more than one of these symptoms at the same time. An embolic ischemic stroke come on suddenly, which helps in distinguishing stroke from other causes of dizziness, vision problems, or headache. The symptoms of a thrombotic stroke come on more gradually.

A child having a stroke may lose bladder control, have a seizure, or have nausea and vomiting as well as the symptoms associated with stroke in adults.

Diagnosis

The diagnosis of stroke includes taking the patient's history and obtaining an account of the patient's present symptoms and their time of onset. In younger patients, the doctor will ask about recent drug use, head trauma, use of oral contraceptives, or bleeding disorders. In middle-aged and older patients, the doctor will ask about such risk factors as hypertension, **diabetes mellitus**, tobacco use, high cholesterol, and a history of coronary artery disease, coronary artery bypass surgery, or atrial fibrillation.

Examination

The next step is a complete physical and neurological examination to rule out the possibility that the patient's symptoms are being caused by a brain tumor. The examination has several purposes: checking the patient's airway, breathing, and circulation; identifying any neurological deficits; identifying the potential cause(s) of the stroke; and identifying any comorbid conditions the patient may have. The neurologist may use the National Institutes of Health Stroke Scale (NIHSS), which is a checklist that allows the doctor to record the patient's level of consciousness; visual function; ability to move; ability to feel sensations; ability to move the facial muscles; and ability to talk.

Tests

Other tests used to diagnose stroke include:

• Blood tests. These can reveal the existence of blood disorders that increase a person's risk of stroke.

• Computed tomography (CT) scan. This type of imaging test is one of the first tests given to a patient suspected of having a stroke. It helps the doctor determine the cause of the stroke and the extent of brain injury.

• Magnetic resonance imaging (MRI). This imaging test is useful in pinpointing the location of small or deep brain injuries.

• Electroencephalogram (EEG). This test measures the brain's electrical activity.

• Blood flow tests. These are done to detect the location and size of any blockages in the blood vessels. One type of blood flow test uses ultrasound to produce an image of the arteries in the neck leading into the brain. Another type of blood flow test, called angiography, uses a special dye injected into blood vessels that will show up on an x ray.

• Echocardiography. This type of test uses ultrasound to produce an image of the heart. It can be useful in determining whether an embolus from the heart caused the patient's stroke.

Treatment

Traditional

Treatment of stroke depends on whether it is ischemic or hemorrhagic. Ischemic stroke is treated first with blood thinners, often aspirin or another drug known as warfarin. (Blood thinners, on the other hand, can make a hemorrhagic stroke worse.) If the patient received care from a specialized stroke team within four hours of the attack, the team may administer a drug called tissue plasminogen activator or tPA.

Ischemic stroke can also be treated through medical procedures. The two procedures most commonly used are endarterectomy, a procedure in which the surgeon removes the fatty deposits caused by atherosclerosis from the inside of one of the main arteries to the brain; and placing a tube made of metallic mesh called a stent inside the artery to prevent recurrent narrowing of the artery.

Hemorrhagic stroke is treated by removing pooled blood from the brain and repairing damaged blood vessels. To prevent another hemorrhagic stroke, the surgeon may use a procedure called aneurysm clipping. In this procedure, the surgeon clamps the weak spot in the artery away from the rest of the blood vessel, which reduces the chances that it will burst and bleed. Endovascular treatment or coil embolization may be used for aneurysms that are difficult to reach surgically. In this procedure, a catheter is guided from a larger artery up into the brain to reach the aneurysm. Small coils of wire are discharged into the aneurysm, which plug it and block off blood flow from the main artery.

Drugs

A prominent drug is the treatment of stroke is tissue plasminogen activator, or tPA, which breaks up blood clots in the arteries of the brain and both improves recovery and decreases long-term disability. For it to work, however, it must be administered within four hours of the stroke event, and earlier administration is best. tPA therapy is for the treatment of ischemic stroke only.

Emergency treatment of hemorrhagic stroke is aimed at controlling intracranial pressure. Intravenous hypertonic saline or mannitol are the most common medication regimes. If the patient is taking antiplatelet medicines or blood thinners, this use will stop.

Rehabilitation

Rehabilitation refers to a comprehensive program designed to regain function as much as possible and compensate for permanent losses.

A team of medical professionals coordinates rehabilitation. The team may include a neurologist, a physician who specializes in rehabilitation medicine (physiatrist), a physical therapist, an occupational therapist, a speech-language pathologist, a nutritionist, a mental health professional, and a social worker. A patient may receive rehabilitation services in an acute-care hospital, rehabilitation hospital, long-term care facility, at outpatient clinic or at home.

The rehabilitation program is based on the patient's individual deficits and strengths. Strokes on the left side of the brain primarily affect the right half of the body, and vice versa. In addition, in left-brain-dominant people, who constitute a significant majority of the population, left-brain strokes usually lead to speech and language deficits. Right-brain strokes may affect spatial perception, and patients with such strokes also may deny their illness, neglect the affected side of their body, and behave impulsively.

Rehabilitation may be complicated by cognitive losses, including diminished ability to understand and follow directions. Poor results are more likely in patients with significant or prolonged cognitive changes, sensory losses, language deficits, or incontinence.

PREVENTION OF COMPLICATIONS. Rehabilitation begins with prevention of stroke recurrence and other medical complications. The risk of stroke recurrence may be reduced with many of the same measures used to prevent stroke, including quitting **smoking** and controlling blood pressure.

One of the most common medical complications following stroke is deep venous thrombosis, in which a clot forms within a limb immobilized by paralysis. Clots that break free often become lodged in an artery feeding the lungs. This type of pulmonary embolism is a common cause of death in the weeks following a stroke. Resuming activity within a day or two after the stroke is an important preventive measure, along with use of elastic stockings on the lower limbs. Drugs that prevent clotting may be given, including intravenous heparin and oral warfarin.

Weakness and loss of coordination of the swallowing muscles may impair swallowing (dysphagia) and allow food to enter the lower airway. This may lead to aspiration **pneumonia**, another common cause of death shortly after a stroke. Dysphagia may be treated with retraining exercises and temporary use of pureed foods.

At 12 months post-stroke, nearly one in five stroke patients experiences depression. According to a 2012 Duke University study, younger age, greater stroke-related disability, and inability to work played a role. Although treatment in the form of antidepressants and psychotherapy are available, the study found that this depression is often left untreated.

TYPES OF REHABILITATIVE THERAPY. Brain tissue that dies in a stroke cannot regenerate. In some cases, the functions of that tissue may be performed by other brain regions after a training period. In other cases, compensatory actions may be developed to replace lost abilities.

Physical therapy is used to maintain and restore range of motion and strength in affected limbs, and to maximize mobility in walking, wheelchair use, and transferring (from wheelchair to toilet or from standing to sitting, for instance). The physical therapist advises on mobility aids such as wheelchairs, braces, and canes. In the recovery period, a stroke patient may develop muscle spasticity and contractures, or abnormal contractions. Contractures may be treated with a combination of stretching and splinting.

Occupational therapy improves such self-care skills as feeding, bathing, and dressing, and helps develop effective compensatory strategies and devices for activities of daily living. A speech-language pathologist focuses on communication and swallowing skills. When dysphagia is a problem, a nutritionist can advise alternative meals that provide adequate **nutrition**.

Mental health professionals may be involved in the treatment of depression or loss of thinking (cognitive) skills. A social worker may help coordinate services and ease the transition out of the hospital back into the home. Both social workers and mental health professionals may help counsel the patient and family during the difficult rehabilitation period. Caring for a person affected with stroke requires learning a new set of skills and adapting to new demands and limitations. Home caregivers may develop **stress**, anxiety, and depression. Caring for the caregiver is an important part of the overall stroke treatment program.

Support groups can provide an important source of information, advice, and comfort for stroke patients and for caregivers. Joining a support group can be one of the most important steps in the rehabilitation process.

First aid

If someone appears to be having a stroke, the most important first step is to call for emergency help *at once*. Stroke is a medical emergency; the sooner the person is evaluated and treated, the better their chances of recovery. The drug presently considered most useful in treating stroke must be given within four hours of the attack to be effective.

Additional measures that can be taken to help the affected person while waiting for the emergency response team include:

- administering mouth-to-mouth resuscitation if the person has stopped breathing
- tilting the head to one side if the person is vomiting
- ensuring that the person does *not* eat or drink anything

Prognosis

The prognosis of stroke depends on the person's age, the type and location of the stroke, and the amount of time elapsed between diagnosis and treatment. In general, patients with ischemic stroke have a better prognosis, including a higher survivor rate, than those with hemorrhagic stroke. Approximately 10% of stroke survivors recover without any significant disability and are able to function independently; 25% have minor impairments but can recover at home; 40% experience moderate to severe impairments that require specialized attention, but may be able to receive that care at home; 10% have serious impairments that require the services of a long-term care facility; and 15% are unable to continue their recovery and perish shortly after the stroke.

Mortality rates vary by gender and ethnicity. The death rate for stroke per 100,000 population among males is 39.0 for white males; 24.5–34.0 for Hispanic, Asian/Pacific Islander and American Indian/Alaska Native males; and 62.1 for black males. The death rates among women are 38.6 for white females, 24.0–32.1 for Hispanic, Asian/Pacific Islander and American Indian/Alaska Native females; and 53.4 for black females.

Among children, 50–80% will have serious, long-term health and other issues. These may include partial paralysis; seizures; and speech, visual, behavioral, and learning difficulties. Unlike adult survivors, children who survive strokes may develop mental retardation, epilepsy, or cerebral palsy.

Prevention

Many strokes are preventable with proper self-care. This includes:

- quitting smoking
- ceasing heavy drinking or using cocaine
- maintaining a health weight
- exercising regularly, eating a healthy diet, and taking medications for high blood pressure if applicable
- taking steps to lower the risk of diabetes or high blood cholesterol levels
- lowering the level of emotional stress or learn to manage stress more effectively
- obtaining regular checkups for abnormal heart rhythms if applicable
- seeing a doctor without delay if stroke symptoms appear

COSTS TO SOCIETY. The total cost of stroke to the American economy per year as of 2010 is approximately $74 billion. That figure includes healthcare services, medications, and lost productivity.

EFFORTS AND SOLUTIONS. Million Hearts is a national initiative that brings together communities,

---

QUESTIONS TO ASK YOUR DOCTOR

- Am I at risk for a stroke? What can I do to lessen that risk?
- I had a TIA. What can I do the reduce the chance that I will have a stroke?
- I had a stroke and have some lingering effects. What milestones should I strive for, and how can I ensure I reach them?
- I have had a stroke. Are my children at greater risk of having a stroke, too?

---

health systems, nonprofit organizations, federal agencies, and private-sector partners from around the nation to help reduce heart attacks and strokes. Launched in 2011 by the U.S. **Department of Health and Human Services**, its mission is to prevent one million heart attacks and strokes by the year 2017. It hopes to accomplish this goal by promoting health living choices and by improving healthcare for people who need it. It is targeting the second by focusing on the "ABCS":

- Aspirin for people at risk
- Blood pressure control
- Cholesterol management
- Smoking cessation

Resources

BOOKS

Brainin, Michael, and Hans-Dieter Heiss, eds. *Textbook of Stroke Medicine*. New York: Cambridge University Press, 2010.

Williams, Olajide. *Stroke Diaries: A Guide for Survivors and Their Families*. New York: Oxford University Press, 2010.

PERIODICALS

American Heart Association. "AHA Statistical Update." *Circulation* 125 (2012): e2–e220.

El Husseini, N., et al. "Depression and antidepressant use after stroke and transient ischemic attack." *Stroke* 43:6 (2012): 1609–16.

Lukovits, Timothy G., and Richard P. Goddeau Jr. "Critical Care of Patients With Acute Ischemic and Hemorrhagic Stroke: Update on Recent Evidence and International Guidelines." *Chest Journal* 139:3 (2011): 694–700.

Wanigasinghe. J., et al. "Epilepsy in hemiplegic cerebral palsy due to perinatal arterial ischaemic stroke." *Developmental Medicine & Child Neurology* 52:11(2010): 1021–7.

Substance abuse and dependence

WEBSITES

African Americans & Cardiovascular Diseases. American Heart Association/American Stroke Association. http://www.stroke.org/site/PageServer?pagename=PEDSTROKE (accessed August 10, 2012).

How Is a Stroke Diagnosed? National Heart Lung and Blood Institute. http://www.nhlbi.nih.gov/health/health-topics/topics/stroke/diagnosis.html (accessed August 10, 2012).

How Is a Stroke Treated? National Heart Lung and Blood Institute. http://www.nhlbi.nih.gov/health/health-topics/topics/stroke/treatment.html (accessed August 10, 2012).

Kids and Stroke. National Stroke Association. http://www.heart.org/idc/groups/heart-public/@wcm/@sop/@smd/documents/downloadable/ucm_319568.pdf (accessed August 10, 2012).

May Is Stroke Awareness Month; Know Your Risks. Centers for Disease Control and Prevention. http://www.cdc.gov/features/stroke/ (accessed August 10, 2012).

Men & Cardiovascular Diseases. American Heart Association/American Stroke Association. http://www.heart.org/idc/groups/heart-public/@wcm/@sop/@smd/documents/downloadable/ucm_319573.pdf (accessed August 10, 2012).

Million Hearts. Department of Health and Human Services. http://www.nhlbi.nih.gov/health/health-topics/topics/stroke/diagnosis.html (accessed August 10, 2012).

Pediatric Stroke. Children's Hemiplegia and Stroke Association. http://www.chasa.org/medical/pediatric-stroke/ (accessed August 10, 2012).

Rehabilitation Therapy After Stroke. National Stroke Association http://www.stroke.org/site/PageServer?pagename=REHABT (accessed August 10, 2012).

Women & Cardiovascular Diseases. American Heart Association/American Stroke Association. http://www.heart.org/idc/groups/heart-public/@wcm/@sop/@smd/documents/downloadable/ucm_319576.pdf (accessed August 10, 2012).

ORGANIZATIONS

American Academy of Neurology (AAN), 201 Chicago Avenue South, Minneapolis, MN 55415, (800) 879-1960, http://www.aan.com/

American Stroke Association (ASA), 7272 Greenville Avenue, Dallas, TX 75231, (888) 478-7653, strokeinfo@heart.org, http://www.strokeassociation.org/

Brain Aneurysm Foundation (BAF), 269 Hanover Street, Building 3, Hanover, MA 02339, (781) 826-5556, (888) 272-4602, office@bafound.org, http://www.bafound.org/

Children's Hemiplegia and Stroke Association (CHASA), 4101 W. Green Oaks, Suite 305, no. 149, Arlington, TX 76016, http://www.chasa.org/

National Heart, Lung, and Blood Institute (NHLBI), Health Information Center, P.O. Box 30105, Bethesda, MD 20824-0105, (301) 592-8573, nhlbiinfo@nhlbi.nih.gov, http://www.nhlbi.nih.gov/

National Institute of Neurological Disorders and Stroke (NINDS), P.O. Box 5801, Bethesda, MD 20824, (800) 352-9424, http://www.ninds.nih.gov/index.htm

National Stroke Association (NSA), 9707 E. Easter Lane, Suite B, Centennial, CO 80112, (800) STROKES, info@stroke.org, http://www.stroke.org/site/PageNavigator/HOME.

Richard Robinson
Teresa G. Odle
Rebecca J. Frey, Ph.D.
Leslie Mertz, Ph.D.

Substance abuse and dependence

Definition

Substance abuse refers to any continued pathological use of a medication, nonmedically indicated drug (called "drugs of abuse") or toxin. It is any pattern of substance use that results in repeated adverse social consequences related to drug-taking—for example, interpersonal conflicts; failure to meet work, family, or school obligations; or legal problems. Substance dependence, commonly known as **addiction**, is characterized by the physiological and behavioral symptoms related to substance use. These symptoms include the need for increasing amounts of the substance to maintain desired effects, withdrawal if drug-taking ceases, and a great deal of time spent in activities related to substance use.

Substance abuse is more likely to be diagnosed among those who have just begun taking drugs and is often an early symptom of substance dependence. However, it can appear without substance abuse, and substance abuse can persist for extended periods of time without a transition to substance dependence.

DESCRIPTION. Substance abuse and dependence are disorders that affect all **population** groups, but specific patterns of abuse and dependence vary with age, gender, culture, and socioeconomic status. According to data from the National Longitudinal Alcohol Epidemiologic Survey, 13.3% of a survey group of Americans exhibited symptoms of alcohol dependence during their lifetime, and 4.4% exhibited symptoms of alcohol dependence during the past 12 months.

In addition to being an individual health disorder, substance abuse and dependence may be viewed as a public health problem with far-ranging health, economic, and social implications. Substance-related disorders are associated with teen pregnancy and the transmission of **sexually transmitted diseases** (STDs), as well as failure in school, unemployment, domestic **violence**, homelessness, and crimes such as rape and **sexual assault**,

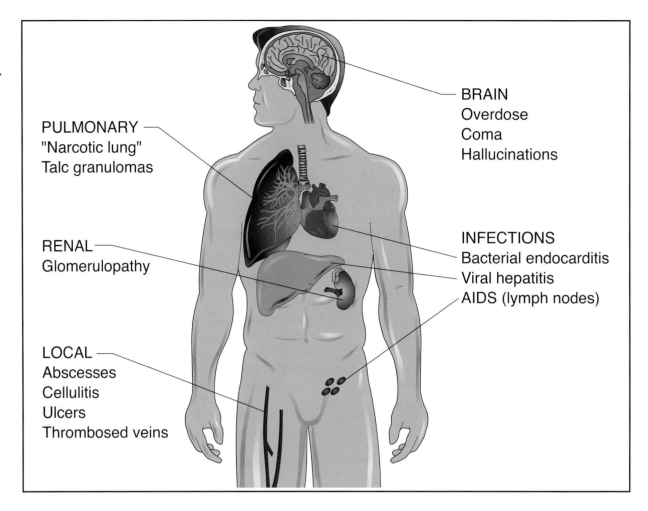

PULMONARY
"Narcotic lung"
Talc granulomas

RENAL
Glomerulopathy

LOCAL
Abscesses
Cellulitis
Ulcers
Thrombosed veins

BRAIN
Overdose
Coma
Hallucinations

INFECTIONS
Bacterial endocarditis
Viral hepatitis
AIDS (lymph nodes)

Effects of substance abuse on the human body. *(Illustration by Electronic Illustrators Group. © 2013 Cengage Learning)*

aggravated assault, robbery, burglary, and larceny. Many different estimates have been made for the economic cost of substance abuse and dependence, and most estimate it at tens or hundreds of billions of dollars annually.

The term "substance," when discussed in the context of substance abuse and dependence, refers to medications, drugs of abuse, and toxins. These substances have an intoxicating effect, desired by the user, which can have either stimulating (speeding up) or depressive/sedating (slowing down) effects on the body. Substance dependence and/or abuse can involve any of the following 10 classes of substances:

• alcohol

• amphetamines (including "crystal meth," some medications used in the treatment of attention deficit disorder [ADD], and amphetamine-like substances found in appetite suppressants)

• cannabis (including marijuana and hashish)

• cocaine (including "crack")

• hallucinogens (including LSD, mescaline, and MDMA ["ecstasy"])

• inhalants (including compounds found in gasoline, glue, and paint thinners)

• nicotine (including that found in cigarettes and smokeless tobacco)

• opioids (including morphine, heroin, codeine, methadone, oxycodone [Oxycontin (TM)])

• phencyclidine (including PCP, angel dust, ketamine)

• sedative, hypnotic, and anxiolytic (anti-anxiety) substances (including benzodiazepines such as valium, barbiturates, prescription sleeping medications, and most prescription anti-anxiety medications)

Substances of abuse may thus be illicit drugs, readily available substances such as alcohol or glue, over-the-counter drugs, or prescription medications. In many cases, a prescription medication that becomes a substance of abuse may have been a legal, medically indicated prescription for the user, but the pattern of use diverges from the use prescribed by the physician.

Caffeine has been identified as a substance in this context, but as yet it is generally not considered a drug of abuse.

Demographics

Drugs (non-alcohol)

According to the United States Department of Health and Human Services' National Survey on Drug Use and Health, in 2010 8.9% of the population age 12 or older (about 22.6 million people) were classified as having used illicit drugs during the month prior to the survey interview. About 7.7% (18.7 about million people) were classified as having alcohol abuse or dependence. The number of persons 12 and older with substance dependence or abuse was 22.1 million in 2010. This number has remained quite stable between 2002 and 2010, ranging from a low of 22.0 million in 2002 to 22.6 million in 2006.

Although substance dependence can begin at any age, higher substance abuse and dependency rates occur among those who began using drugs at a younger age. The 2010 National Survey on Drug Use and Health, estimated that 3 million individuals aged 12 or older used an illicit drug for the first time within the past 12 months, which translates to about 8,100 initiates per day on average. For nearly 62% of them, the initial drug was marijuana. The remaining initiates used psychotherapeutics (26.2%, including 17.3% with **pain** relievers, 4.6% with tranquilizers, 2.5% with stimulants, and 1.9% with sedatives); inhalants (9.0%); and hallucinogens (3.0%) as their first-used illicit drug.

In 2010, the National Survey on Drug Use and Health also gathered information on when 12- to 49-year-olds first used drugs. It found that the average age among those whose first illicit drug was marijuana was 18.4 years, a significant rise from 2002, when the age was 17.0.

Initial drug use varies. In 2010, the number of past-year initiates of the following drugs among persons aged 12 or older was:

- methamphetamine, 105,000. This compares to 157,000 in 2007 and 299,000 in 2002.

- Ecstasy, 937,000. This compares to 1.1 million in 2009, and 615,000 in 2005.

- cocaine, 637,000 (83,000 crack cocaine). This compares 1.0 million (337,000 crack) in 2002.

- heroin, 140,000. This fell within the range fro 2002–2009 of 91,000–180,000.

Gender proportions vary according to the class of drugs, but substance abuse and dependence is almost twice as likely to occur in men than in women. According to the National Survey on Drug Use and Health, the rate of illicit drug use among persons aged 12 or older has remained about the same from year to year at a rate of about 11.2% for males and 6.8% for females. The use of specific illicit drugs by males vs. females in 2010 was: marijuana, 9.1 males vs. 4.7% females; nonmedical use of psychotherapeutic drugs, 3.0 vs. 2.5%; cocaine, 0.8 vs. 0.4%; and hallucinogens, 0.6 vs. 0.3%. The 2010 rates for both males and females aged 12 or older were similar to those reported in 2009.

Among those aged 12–17, however, the rate of illicit drug use in 2010 was 10.4% for males and 9.8% for females. Males in this age group were more likely to use marijuana (8.3 vs. 6.4%), but females were more likely to use non-medical psychotherapeutic drugs (3.7 vs. 2.3%) and nonmedical pain relievers (3.0 vs. 2.0%).

Alcohol

More than 131 million people, or nearly 52%, of Americans aged 12 and older consumed alcohol, according to the 2010 National Survey on Drug Use and Health. About 23% of them participated in binge drinking, or drinking five or more drinks on the same occasion, during the month prior to the survey; and almost 7% reported that they were heavy drinkers.

Among the subset of individuals aged 18–25, the 2010 survey revealed that the rates of binge drinking and heavy drinking were 40.6% and 13.6%, respectively. For teens aged 12–17, the rate of alcohol use was 13.6%, binge drinking was 7.8%, and heavy drinking was 1.7%.

Causes and symptoms

Causes

The causes of substance dependence are not well established, but four factors are believed to contribute to substance-related disorders: genetic factors, the action of the drug, psychopathology, and social learning.

In genetic epidemiological studies of **alcoholism**, the probability of identical twins both exhibiting alcohol dependence was significantly greater than with fraternal twins, thus suggesting a genetic component in alcoholism. It is unclear, however, whether the genetic factor is related to alcoholism directly or whether it is linked to other psychiatric disorders that are known to be associated with substance abuse. For example, there is evidence that alcoholic males from families with depressive disorders tend to have more severe courses of substance dependence than alcoholic men from families without such family histories.

These and other findings suggest that substance abuse may be a way to relieve the symptoms of a psychological disorder. In this model, unless the underlying pathology is treated, attempts to permanently stop substance dependence are ineffective. Psychopathologies that are associated with substance dependence include antisocial personality disorder, bipolar disorder, depression, anxiety disorder, and schizophrenia.

Drug abuse may also be a socially learned behavior. Local social norms determine the likelihood that a person is exposed to the substance and whether continued use is reinforced. For example, individuals may, by observing family or peer role models, learn that substance use is a normal way to relieve daily stresses. Conversely, social or legal sanctions may reduce the likelihood of substance abuse among some individuals.

Symptoms

Symptoms of substance abuse include one or more of the following:

- continued substance use despite negative health, school, work, social and relationship consequences
- episodes of violence
- hostile response or making of excuses when confronted about substance abuse
- inability to control use of a substance, and/or need for a dose in order to function on a daily basis
- loss of normal appetite
- decline in physical appearance
- falling interest in activities that the person once enjoyed
- substance use even when alone
- overall state of confusion

In addition to the general symptoms, there are other physical signs and symptoms of substance abuse that are related to specific drug classes:

- Signs and symptoms of alcohol intoxication include slurred speech, lack of coordination, unsteady gait, memory impairment, and stupor, as well as behavior changes shortly after alcohol ingestion, including inappropriate aggressive behavior, mood volatility, and impaired functioning.
- Amphetamine users may exhibit rapid heartbeat, elevated or depressed blood pressure, dilated (enlarged) pupils, weight loss, excessively high energy levels, inability to sleep, confusion, and occasional paranoid psychotic behavior.

- Cannabis users may exhibit red eyes with dilated pupils, increased appetite, dry mouth, and rapid pulse. They may also be sluggish and slow to react.
- Cocaine users may exhibit rapid heart rate, elevated or depressed blood pressure, dilated pupils, and weight loss, in addition to wide variations in their energy level, severe mood disturbances, psychosis, and paranoia.
- Users of hallucinogens may exhibit anxiety or depression, paranoia, and unusual behavior in response to hallucinations (imagined sights, voices, sounds, or smells that appear real). Signs include dilated pupils, rapid heart rate, tremors, lack of coordination, and sweating. Flashbacks, or the re-experiencing of a hallucination long after stopping substance use, are also a symptom of hallucinogen use.
- Users of inhalants may experience dizziness, spastic eye movements, lack of coordination, slurred speech, and slowed reflexes. Associated behaviors may include belligerence, tendency toward violence, apathy, and impaired judgment.
- Opioid drug users exhibit slurred speech, drowsiness, impaired memory, and constricted (small) pupils. They may appear slowed in their physical movements.
- Phencyclidine users exhibit spastic eye movements, rapid heartbeat, decreased sensitivity to pain, and lack of muscular coordination. They may show belligerence, predisposition to violence, impulsiveness, and agitation.
- Users of sedative, hypnotic, or anxiolytic drugs show slurred speech, unsteady gait, inattentiveness, and impaired memory. They may also display inappropriate behavior, mood volatility, and impaired functioning.

Other signs are related to the form in which the substance is used. For example, heroin, certain other opioid drugs, and certain forms of cocaine may be injected. A person using an injectable substance may have "track marks" (outwardly visible signs of the site of an injection, with possible redness and swelling of the vein in which the substance was injected). Furthermore, poor judgment brought on by substance use can result in the injections being made under dangerously unhygienic conditions. These unsanitary conditions and the use of shared needles are risk factors for major infections of the heart, as well as infection with HIV (the virus that causes **AIDS**), certain forms of **hepatitis** (a liver infection), and **tuberculosis**.

Cocaine is often taken as a powdery substance, which is "snorted" through the nose. This can result in frequent nosebleeds, sores in the nose, and even erosion (an eating away) of the nasal septum (the structure that separates the two nostrils).

Overdosing on a substance is a frequent complication of substance abuse. Drug overdose can be purposeful (with **suicide** as a goal), or due to carelessness, the unpredictable strength of substances purchased from street dealers, the mixing of more than one type of substance, or as a result of the increasing doses that a person must take to experience a similar level of effect. Substance overdose can be a life-threatening emergency, with the specific symptoms depending on the type of substance used. Substances with depressive effects may dangerously slow the breathing and heart rate, drop the body temperature, and result in general unresponsiveness. Substances with stimulatory effects may dangerously increase the heart rate and blood pressure, produce abnormal heart rhythms, increase body temperature, induce seizures, and cause erratic behavior.

DIAGNOSIS. Tools used in the diagnosis of substance dependence include screening questionnaires and patient histories, physical examination and laboratory tests. The CAGE questionnaire is a simple and popular screening tool. CAGE refers to the first letters of each word that forms the basis of each of the four questions of the screening exam:

• Have you ever tried to Cut down on your substance use?

• Have you ever been Annoyed by people trying to talk to you about your substance use?

• Do you ever feel Guilty about your substance use?

• Do you ever need an Eye opener (use of the substance first thing in the morning) in order to start your day?

A "Yes" answer to two or more of these questions is an indication that the individual should be referred for a more thorough work-up for substance dependency or abuse.

In addition to CAGE, other screening questionnaires are available. Some are designed for particular population groups, such as pregnant women, and others are designed to more thoroughly assess the severity of substance dependence.

Patient history, as taken through the direct interview, is important for identifying physical symptoms and psychiatric factors related to substance use. Family history of alcohol or other substance dependency is also useful for diagnosis.

A physical examination may reveal signs of substance abuse. These signs are specific to the substances used, and may include needle marks, tracks, or nasal erosion.

Laboratory testing of blood, urine, or hair—toxicology screens—can also reveal substance abuse, but this may be limited by the sensitivity and specificity of the testing method, by the time elapsed since the person last used the drug, and by the type of drug used by the individual.

One of the most difficult aspects of diagnosis involves overcoming the patient's denial. Denial is a psychological state during which a person is unable to acknowledge the (usually negative) circumstances of a situation. In this case, denial leads a person to underestimate the degree of his or her substance use and of the problems associated with the substance use.

TREATMENT. According to the American Psychiatric Association, there are three goals for the treatment of people with substance use disorders: (1) the patient abstains from or reduces the use and effects of the substance; (2) the patient reduces the frequency and severity of relapses; and (3) the patient develops the psychological and emotional skills necessary to restore and maintain personal, occupational, and social functioning.

In general, before treatment can begin, many treatment centers require that the patient undergo detoxification. Detoxification is the process of weaning the patient from his or her regular substance use. Detoxification can be accomplished "cold turkey," by complete and immediate cessation of all substance use, or by slowly decreasing (tapering) the dose the individual is taking, to minimize the side effects of withdrawal. Some substances must be tapered because "cold turkey" methods of detoxification are potentially life-threatening. In some cases, medications may be used to combat the physical and psychological symptoms of withdrawal. For example, methadone is used to help patients adjust to the tapering off of heroin use.

Treatment itself consists of three parts: (1) assessment; (2) formulation of a treatment plan; (3) psychiatric management. The first step in treatment is a comprehensive medical and psychiatric evaluation of the patient. This evaluation includes:

• a history of the patient's past and current substance use, and its cognitive, psychological, physiological, and behavioral effects

• a medical and psychiatric history and examination

• a history of psychiatric treatments and outcomes

• a family and social history

• screening of blood, breath, or urine for substances

• other laboratory tests to determine the presence of other conditions commonly found with substance use disorders

After the assessment is made, a treatment plan is formulated. Treatment plans vary according to the needs of the specific patient and can change for the same patient as it is seen how he or she responds to different elements of treatment. Plans typically involve the following elements: (1) a strategy for the psychiatric management of the patient; (2) a strategy for reducing effects or use of substances, or for abstinence; (3) efforts to ensure compliance with the treatment program and to prevent relapse; (4) treatments for other conditions associated with substance use. Initial therapy and treatment setting (hospital, residential treatment, partial hospitalization, or outpatient) decisions are made as part of the treatment plan, but because substance use disorders are considered a chronic condition requiring long-term care, these plans can and do change through the course of treatment.

The third step, psychiatric management of the patient, is the implementation of the treatment plan. Psychiatric management of the patient includes establishing a trusting relationship between clinician and patient; monitoring the patient's progress; managing the patient's relapses and withdrawal; diagnosing and treating associated psychiatric disorders; and helping the patient adhere to the treatment plan through therapy and the development of skills and social interactions that reinforce a drug-free lifestyle.

As part of the treatment process, patients typically undergo psychosocial therapy and, in some cases, pharmacologic treatment. Psychosocial therapeutic modalities include cognitive-behavioral therapy, behavioral therapy, individual psychodynamic or interpersonal therapy, group therapy, family therapy, and self-help groups. Pharmacologic treatment may include medications that ease withdrawal symptoms, reduce cravings, interact negatively with substances of abuse to discourage drug-taking, or treat associated psychiatric disorders.

PROGNOSIS. Recovery from substance use is notoriously difficult, even with exceptional treatment resources. Relapse rates are high, estimated at 50 to 90% depending on the study and how relapse is defined.

Relapses are most likely to occur within the first 12 months of having discontinued substance use. Triggers for relapses can include any number of life stresses (problems on the job or in the marriage, loss of a relationship, death of a loved one, financial stresses), in addition to seemingly mundane exposure to a place, situation, or acquaintance associated with previous substance use.

The development of adaptive life skills and ongoing drug-free social support are believed to be two important factors in avoiding relapse. The effect of the support group Alcoholics Anonymous has been intensively studied, and many studies have found that long-term sobriety appears to be positively related to Alcoholics Anonymous attendance and involvement. Support for family members in addition to support for the individual

KEY TERMS

Addiction—The state of being both physically and psychologically dependent on a substance.

Dependence—A state in which a person requires a steady concentration of a particular substance to avoid experiencing withdrawal symptoms.

Detoxification—A process whereby an addict is withdrawn from a substance.

Intoxication—The mental, physical, or emotional state produced by a substance.

Street drug—A substance purchased from a drug dealer; may be a legal substance, sold illicitly (without a prescription, and not for medical use), or it may be a substance that is illegal to possess.

Tolerance—A phenomenon whereby a drug user becomes physically accustomed to a particular dose of a substance and requires increasing dosages in order to obtain the same effects.

Withdrawal—Those side effects experienced by a person who has become physically dependent on a substance, upon decreasing the substance's dosage or discontinuing its use.

in recovery is also important. Because substance dependence has a serious impact on family functioning, and because family members may inadvertently maintain behaviors that initially led to the substance dependence, ongoing therapy and support for family members should not be neglected.

EFFECTS ON PUBLIC HEALTH. Substance abuse and dependency have wide-ranging effects that go beyond the individual who is using the drugs or alcohol. For instance, since children learn from older family members, parents and older siblings who abuse drugs or alcohol, may have an influence on children to experiment with these substances at an early age, possibly setting the stage for their own addictions.

Abuse can have a number of safety implications. One is automobile accidents related to drug or alcohol use. According to estimates from the 2010 National Survey on Drug Use and Health, 11.4% of persons aged 12 or older had driven under the influence of alcohol at least once in the past year, and the rate was highest among the subset of individuals aged 21–25 at 23.4%. Among persons aged 12 years or older, 4.2% had driven under the influence of illicit drugs in the past year, and the rate was highest among persons aged 18–25 at 12.7%. Overall, more than 1.4 million drivers were arrested in 2010 for driving under the influence of alcohol or narcotics.

In addition, studies have shown that a child's risk of experiencing physical or sexual abuse increases if a parent or other family member is a drug or alcohol addict. That increase may result from a family member or from another person who is brought into the home. Even if the child does not experience any violence himself or herself, exposure to it can have lasting psychological effects.

COSTS TO SOCIETY. Estimates of the total overall costs of substance abuse in the United States exceed $400 billion annually. This total, which includes about $200 billion for illicit drugs and $235 billion for alcohol, takes into account health-related costs, declines in productivity, and costs arising due to addiction-associated crimes.

EFFORTS AND SOLUTIONS. Because higher substance abuse and dependency rates occur among those who began using drugs at a younger age, many **prevention** programs are aimed at teenagers and young adults 24 years old and younger. This group is at high risk for substance experimentation, and that experimentation can open the door to eventual addiction.

For example, the National Institute on Drug Abuse showcased its new initiative, called PEERx, in 2012. PEERx uses a variety of tools, including interactive videos, blogs, activity guides, and free downloads, to help teens understand the dangers of prescription drug abuse. The institute also provides tools for teachers and parents to help them learn about currently used drugs, and help their children and students avoid alcohol and illicit drug use.

Many non-government organizations (NGOs) are also trying to curtail the use of alcohol and illicit drugs. One of the most well-known organizations is Mothers Against Drunk Driving (MADD), which has been pushing hard for a nationwide mandate that all convicted drunk drivers must have an ignition-interlock device on their vehicles. To start a vehicle, an individual must demonstrate they are safe to drive by blowing into the device to have his or her alcohol level tested. As of August 2012, 17 states had mandated the devices for convicted drunk drivers.

A 2012 study by RAND Corp. a nonprofit think tank, reported that voluntary after-school programs can be very effective at reducing alcohol use among middle-school children. According to the study, successful programs share three characteristics: they are built with the direction of prevention researchers; they contain developmentally relevant content, which is presented in an engaging, confidential and non-judgmental way. Programs such as these can supplement the many mandatory school-based programs that are already aimed at teaching students about the perils of alcohol and illicit drugs.

Resources

BOOKS

Newton, David E. *Substance Abuse: A Reference Handbook.* Santa Barbara, CA: ABC–CLIO, 2010.

Kuhar, Michael J. *The Addicted Brain: Why We Abuse Drugs, Alcohol, and Nicotine.* Upper Saddle River, NJ: FT Press, 2011.

PERIODICALS

D'Amico, Elizabeth, et al. "Preventing Alcohol Use with a Voluntary After-School Program for Middle School Students: Results from a Cluster Randomized Controlled Trial of CHOICE." *Prevention Science*, 13, no. 4 (2012): 415–425.

WEBSITES

MedlinePlus. "Drug Dependence." U.S. National Library of Medicine. http://www.nlm.nih.gov/medlineplus/ency/article/001522.htm (accessed August 27, 2012).

"Results from the 2010 National Survey on Drug Use and Health: Summary of National Findings." Substance Abuse and Mental Health Services Administration, U.S. Department of Health and Human Services. http://www.samhsa.gov/data/NSDUH/2k10ResultsRev/NSDUHresults-Rev2010.htm (accessed August 27, 2012).

PEERx. "NIDA for Teens." National Institute for Drug Abuse. http://teens.drugabuse.gov/peerx/ (accessed August 27, 2012).

ORGANIZATIONS

National Institute on Drug Abuse, 6001 Executive Blvd., Room 5213, Bethesda, MD (301) 443-1124, information@nida.nih.gov, http://drugabuse.gov

Mothers Against Drunk Driving, 511 E. John Carpenter Freeway, Suite 700, Irving, TX 75062, (877) 275-6233, http://www.madd.org/

Substance Abuse and Mental Health Services Administration, P.O. Box 2345, Rockville, MD 20847-2345, (877) 726-4727, SAMHSAInfo@samhsa.hhs.gov, http://www.samhsa.gov/

Genevieve Pham-Kanter
Teresa G. Odle
Leslie Mertz, Ph.D.

Suicide

Definition

Suicide is defined as the intentional taking of one's own life. In some European languages, including German, the word for suicide translates into English as "self-murder." In Latin, suicide is derived from *suicidium*, or "to kill oneself." Until approximately the end of the twentieth century, suicide was considered a criminal act; legal terminology used the Latin phrase *felo-de-se*, which means "a crime against the self." Much of the social stigma that is still associated with suicide derives from its former connection with legal judgment as well as with religious condemnation.

Demographics

In the United States, the rate of suicide has continued to rise since the 1950s. More people in the general population die from suicide than homicide in North America. There are 11.3 suicide deaths each year for every 100,000 people living in the United States, according to the **National Institute of Mental Health** (NIMH), and for every suicide, there are approximately 11.5 attempts. In any given year, there are approximately 40,000 suicide-based deaths, along with up to 500,000 suicide attempts. The most recent statistics for the U.S. **Centers for Disease Control and Prevention (CDC)** state that suicide was the tenth-leading cause of death in the United States. According to the U.S. Department of Defense/Veterans Affairs website, more years of life are lost due to suicide than to any other single cause except for **heart disease** and **cancer**. Substance abuse is a major factor associated with suicide. Statistics show that substance abuse is thought to be involved in as many as one-half of all suicide cases. In fact, the abuse of alcohol is involved with about 20% of all suicide attempts. Completed suicides are most likely to involve a man over the age of 45 years who is suffering from depression or **alcoholism**.

By state, region

The demographics of suicide in the United States vary considerably from state to state, with rates higher than the national average in the West and lower in the Midwest and Northeast. Some states, like Alaska, have suicide rates that are almost twice the national average; others, such as Massachusetts, have notably lower rates.

Age and gender

These variations from state to state, and region to region, result in part from differences in age and ethnic distributions and gender ratios among the states. Recent statistics show that suicide is the eighth-leading cause of death among males and sixteenth-leading cause of death among females. Males are four times more likely than females to succeed in their suicide attempts, but females report attempting suicide at some point in their lives three times as often as men do. An increase in the overall suicide rate in the United States between 1999 and 2009 (the most recent data available) was due primarily to an increase in suicides among Caucasians aged 40–64 years,

with white middle-aged women experiencing the largest annual increases.

In terms of age, the highest number of suicides are committed by people under age 40 years, but suicide rates (percentages in a given group) increase with age. People over age 65 years have high suicide rates, with men outnumbering women who commit suicide nearly four to one.

SENIORS. The incidence of suicide and attempted suicide among seniors is widely perceived as a growing public health problem in the United States. Statistically, older adults represent about 13% of the U.S. population but account for 20% of suicides. According to the NIMH, the highest suicide rate in the nation is for Caucasian men aged 85 years and older, at 65.3 deaths per 100,000 persons—about six times the national U.S. rate of 10.8 per 100,000.

The ratio of attempted suicides to completed suicides among people over 65 is thought to be around 4:1. According to the National Strategy for Suicide **Prevention** (NSSP), seniors are more likely than are younger persons to use highly lethal means of suicide. According to a Canadian study published in 2008, seniors are most likely to use firearms to commit suicide, followed by hanging, self-poisoning, and leaping from heights.

YOUNG PEOPLE. The overall rate of suicide among young people has declined slowly since 1992, but it still remains the third-leading cause of death in age groups spanning children 10 years old to young adults up to age 24. Suicidal behavior is rare in prepubertal children, probably because of their relative inability to plan and execute a suicide attempt. Children as young as five years old, however, have succeeded in killing themselves by leaping out of windows or shooting themselves—as happened with one five-year-old who witnessed his mother killing herself with a gun and imitated her behavior several months later. According to the NIMH, the rates of suicide for American youth in 2007 (the most recent data available) were as follows:

- children between the ages of 10 and 14: 0.9 suicides per 100,000
- teenagers between the ages of 15 and 19: 6.9 per 100,000
- young adults between the ages of 20 and 24: 12.7 per 100,000

Race or ethnicity

In 2007, the NIMH reported the highest suicide rates among American Indians and Alaska Natives, at 14.3 per 100,000, and non-Hispanic whites, at 13.5 per 100,000. The lowest suicide rates were found among Hispanics, at

6.0 per 100,000; non-Hispanic blacks, at 5.1 per 100,000; and Asian and Pacific Islanders, at 6.2 per 100,000. Suicide rates among American Indian and Alaskan natives between 15 and 34 years are almost twice the national average for this age range. Young Hispanic females make significantly more suicide attempts than their male or non-Hispanic counterparts.

In the military

In 2008, the rate of suicides in the U.S. Army surpassed the civilian (non-military) rate (19.2 per 100,000), hitting an all-time high of 20.2 suicides per 100,000 people. In that year, at least 128 soldiers committed suicide (with other deaths being investigated as possible suicide cases); suicide deaths numbered 115 and 102 in the two years prior, respectively.

According to the most recent data, roughly five members of the military are unsuccessful in their suicide attempt for every one that is successful. The U.S. Veterans Affairs Department (VA) reported in 2010 that the suicide rate for 17–29 year old male veterans increased by 26% from 2005 to 2007. Despite levelling off in 2010 and 2011, suicide statistics for active-duty troops reached an all-time high in 2012, with 154 suicides already by June 2012. Statistics show that one of the major causes of suicide within these military personnel was substance abuse (drug or alcohol). Between 2005 and 2009 (the most recent data available), the use of drugs or alcohol contributed to over 45% of unsuccessful suicide attempts and 30% of suicide deaths. The Defense Survey of Health-Related Behaviors found that 12% of military personnel had the presence of "dangerous levels" of alcohol or illicit drugs within their bodies. Relationship problems were also a major cause of suicide, with 58% of suicide deaths in 2009 alone, believed to have been caused by such stressful situations. Although causes of high suicide rates among military members are not completely understood, they are exposed to violent combat situations and post-traumatic **stress**, in addition to more typical issues like substance abuse, relationship problems, and financial difficulty.

International

Suicide has become a major social and medical problem around the world, not just in North America. Worldwide suicide rates have increased by 60% since 1960. The **World Health Organization (WHO)** reports that nearly one million people worldwide die annually from suicide, more than the number of people murdered or killed in war. That number of suicides breaks down to 16 deaths per 100,000 people, or one death every 40 seconds. According to **WHO**, more suicides occur in Asia than in any other region of the world, with China, Japan, and India accounting for 40% of the world's suicides. China is also the only country in the world where more women than men take their own lives, with female suicides representing 58% of the total.

Rates among young people have risen even faster, to the point where they are now the age group at highest risk in 35% of the world's countries. Among people 10 to 24 years of age, suicide is the third-leading cause of death in the world, and it is the second-leading cause in persons aged 15 to 44 years. For every 20 attempted tries at suicide, there is one death. In Europe and North America, mental disorders are particularly high in the cause of suicides. All over the world, suicide involves a complex play of biological (genetic), cultural, environmental, psychological, and social factors.

Description

Suicidal behavior is most commonly regarded—and responded to—as a psychiatric or medical emergency, one often committed due to a mental disorder such as bipolar disorder, depression, schizophrenia, or substance abuse. At other times, suicide may be contemplated due to pressures in life, such as financial or legal difficulties, or a troubling interpersonal relationship such as a crumbling marriage. Law enforcement personnel may be involved in preventing an attempted suicide or taking suicidal individuals to a hospital emergency department but not in arresting these persons for breaking the law.

Historical background

Attitudes toward suicide have varied throughout history. The ancient Greeks considered it an offense against the state, which was deprived of contributions by potentially useful citizens. The Romans, by comparison, thought that suicide could be a noble form of death, although they legislated against persons taking their own lives before an impending criminal conviction in order to ensure their families' financial inheritance. Early Christianity, which downplayed the importance of life on Earth, was not critical of suicide until the fourth century, when Algerian philosopher St. Augustine (354–430) condemned it as a sin because it violated the sixth commandment ("Thou shalt not kill."). The view of suicide as a sin prevailed in Western societies for hundreds of years, and many people are still influenced by it, either consciously or unconsciously. For instance, suicide was a felony, and attempted suicide a misdemeanor, in England until 1961.

Austrian neurologist Sigmund Freud (1856–1939) provided the first theory that addressed suicide in terms of a person's inner mental and emotional state. In *Mourning and Melancholia* (1917), he proposed that suicide was the result of turning hostility toward a loved one back on oneself. In *Man against Himself* (1936), American psychiatrist Karl Menninger (1893–1990) extended Freud's contribution to the psychodynamic study of suicide, relating it to such other forms of self-destructive behavior as alcoholism or drug abuse. Some people still refer to such behavior as "slow-motion suicide."

Types of suicidal behavior

Some mental health professionals distinguish five levels of suicidal behavior: completed suicide; suicide attempts, which are potentially fatal; suicide gestures, which involve acting-out behavior that is not necessarily lethal; suicide gambles; and suicidal ideation, or thinking about suicide. An example of a suicide gesture would be cutting one's wrist just deeply enough to draw blood from the skin but not deeply enough to sever veins and arteries. The suicide gamble is a type of suicidal behavior in which the person takes the risk that he or she will be discovered in time and that the discoverer will save them. The suicide of American poet Sylvia Plath (1932–1963) is considered an example of a suicide gamble. Plath gassed herself in the kitchen by turning on her oven without lighting it, but left a note on the door for her children's new nanny, had opened the windows in the children's bedroom to protect them, and had sealed the door to the kitchen with dish towels.

Suicidal ideation, or thinking about suicide, is even more common than suicide gestures or attempted suicide. Suicidal ideation spans a continuum from nonspecific thoughts such as "life is not worth living" to specific ideation. Community surveys indicate that 12–25% of primary- and high-school children have some form of suicidal ideation, whereas 5–10% combine suicidal ideation with a plan or intent to make a suicide attempt. Specific ideation is more closely associated with risk for attempted suicide and frequently occurs in combination with other risk factors.

Risk factors

Some factors increase a person's risk of suicide:

- male gender
- age over 75 years
- family history of suicide or mental illness
- history of suicide attempts
- Caucasian race
- history of abuse
- traumatic experiences after childhood
- recent stressful events, such as separation or divorce, job loss, or death of spouse

- dealing with homosexuality in an unsupportive environment
- lack of a support network, poor relationships with parents or peers, and feelings of social isolation
- chronic medical illness—patients with acquired immune deficiency syndrome (AIDS) have a rate of suicide 20 times that of the general population
- chronic, severe, or intractable pain
- loss of mobility or independence
- access to a firearm—death by firearms accounts for the majority of suicides in the United States
- alcohol or substance abuse—while mood-altering substances do not cause a person to kill himself or herself, they do weaken impulse control
- high blood cholesterol levels
- presence of a psychiatric illness

More than 90% of Americans who commit suicide have a mental illness. Major depression accounts for 60% of suicides, followed by schizophrenia, alcoholism, substance abuse, borderline personality disorder, Huntington's disease, and epilepsy. The lifetime mortality due to suicide in psychiatric patients is 15% for major depression, 20% for bipolar disorder, 18% for alcoholism, 10% for schizophrenia, and 5–10% for borderline and certain other personality disorders. In children and adolescents, the most common triggers of suicidal behavior involve interpersonal conflict or loss, most frequently with parents or romantic attachment figures. **Bullying** by peers has also become a common trigger. Family discord, physical or sexual abuse, and an upcoming legal or disciplinary crisis are also commonly associated with completed and attempted suicides. The most serious suicide attempts involve suicide notes, evidence of planning, and an irreversible method. Most adolescent suicide attempts are of relatively low intent and lethality, and only a minority actually want to die. Usually, children and adolescents who attempt suicide want to escape psychological **pain** or unbearable circumstances, gain attention, influence others, or communicate such strong feelings as rage or love.

Factors that lower the risk of suicide include:

- significant friendship network outside the workplace
- religious faith and practice, especially those that discourage suicide and value life
- stable marriage
- close-knit extended family
- strong interest in or commitment to a project or cause that brings people together, such as community service, environmental concerns, neighborhood associations, animal rescue groups

Ethical issues related to suicide

Several ethical issues related to suicide have emerged as public policy matters in the early twenty-first century. The most controversial of these are the notion of a "right to suicide" and the question of assisted suicide.

RIGHT TO SUICIDE. The idea that suicide is a right among the elderly or those with terminal illnesses surfaced with the 1991 publication of English-born American journalist Derek Humphry's (1930–) *Final Exit*, a controversial book described by its author as a how-to manual for suicide and assisted suicide. Humphry is the founder of the Euthanasia Research and Guidance Organization (ERGO), known until 2003 as the Hemlock Society. Humphry maintains that people have a right to choose the time, place, and method of their death and that rational suicide is a legitimate and even reasonable choice.

People who are often overlooked in discussions of the right to commit suicide, however, are the relatives and friends who are bereaved by the suicide. It is estimated that each person who commits suicide leaves six survivors to deal with the aftermath. On the basis of this figure, there are at least 4.5 million survivors of suicide in the United States. In addition to the grief that ordinarily accompanies death, survivors of suicide often struggle with feelings of guilt and shame as well. Some people have blamed Humphry and his book for their loved one's decision to commit suicide.

ASSISTED SUICIDE. Questions pertaining to the legalization of assisted suicide for persons suffering from a terminal illness are connected in part to increases in the average lifespan. Physician-assisted suicide (also known as physician-assisted death or PAD) was legalized in the Netherlands in April 2001, and in the states of Oregon, Washington, and Montana. As of 2011, it was also legal in Belgium and Luxembourg and was practiced openly in Switzerland. It is important to distinguish between physician-assisted suicide and euthanasia, or "mercy killing." Assisted suicide, which is called "self-deliverance" in Britain, refers to individuals bringing about their own death with the help of another person. Because the other person is often a physician, the act is often called doctor-assisted suicide.

Euthanasia strictly speaking means that the physician or other person is the one who performs the last act that causes death. For example, if a physician injects a patient with a lethal dose of a pain-killing medication, the physician is performing euthanasia. If the physician leaves the patient with a loaded syringe and the patient injects himself or herself with it, the act is an assisted suicide. Euthanasia is illegal in all 50 states.

Causes and symptoms

Causes

One model that has been used by clinicians to explain why people suffering under the same life stresses respond differently is known as the stress/diathesis model. Diathesis is a medical term for a predisposition that makes some people more vulnerable to thoughts of suicide. In addition to factors at the individual level, factors in the wider society have been identified as contributing to the rising rate of suicide in the United States, including:

- Stresses on the nuclear family, including more frequent divorce and economic hardship.

- Loss of a set of moral values held in common by the entire society.

- Weakening of churches, synagogues, neighborhood associations, and other mid-range social groups outside the family. In the past, these institutions often provided a sense of belonging for people from troubled or emotionally distant families.

- Frequent geographical moves, which makes it difficult for people to make and keep long-term friendships outside their immediate family.

- Sensationalized treatment of suicide in the mass media. A number of research studies have shown that there is a definite risk of "contagion" or copycat suicides from irresponsible reporting, particularly among impressionable adolescents. One group of researchers has estimated that as many as 6% of all suicides in the developed countries are copycat suicides.

- Development of medications that allow relatively painless suicide. For most of human history, the available means of suicide were uncertain, painful, or both.

- Easy availability of lethal methods of suicide, most notably firearms, and so-called suicide magnets such as bridges or tall buildings that do not have suicide barriers and are easy to reach. The Golden Gate Bridge in San Francisco, California, is the most notorious public suicide location in the United States; others include the Aurora Bridge in Seattle, Washington, the Sunshine Skyway Bridge in Florida, and the Duke Ellington Bridge in Washington, DC. Other popular suicide locations elsewhere in the world include the Aokigahara Forest at the base of Mount Fuji in Japan, and Beachy Head in the United Kingdom.

The role of the Internet in the rate of adolescent suicide has been debated. On the one hand, there are websites and chat rooms that foster preoccupation with suicide and offer detailed descriptions of suicide methods. There are even instances of adolescents recruiting other adolescents over the Internet to join them in a suicide pact. For instance, seven young people who had met via the Internet committed group suicide by inhaling carbon monoxide from a charcoal burner inside a locked van. Other websites attack psychiatry and mental health professionals, which may steer some vulnerable young people away from seeking help. On the other hand, there are many supportive websites for teens that offer resources (including peer counseling) and contact information for getting help if they are considering suicide.

Media treatment of suicide

In 1989, the **CDC** sponsored a national workshop to address the connection between sensationalized media treatments of suicide and the rising rate of suicide among American youth. The CDC and the American Association of Suicidology subsequently adopted a set of guidelines for media coverage of suicide intended to reduce the risk of copycat suicides.

The CDC guidelines point out that the following types of reporting may increase the risk of copycat suicides:

• Presenting oversimplified explanations of suicide, when in fact many factors usually contribute to it. One example concerns the suicide of the widow of a man who was killed in the collapse of the World Trade Center on September 11, 2001. Most newspapers that covered the story described her death as due solely to the act of terrorism, even though she had a history of depressive illness.

• Giving excessive, ongoing, or repetitive coverage of the suicide.

• Sensationalizing the suicide by including morbid details or dramatic photographs.

• Giving "how-to" descriptions of the method of suicide.

• Referring to suicide as an effective coping strategy or as a way to achieve temporary fame or other goals.

• Glorifying the act of suicide or the person who commits suicide.

• Focusing on the person's positive traits without mentioning his or her problems.

Symptoms

Potential warning signs of suicidal thinking may include:

• reading a lot of books or articles on death and suicide

• talking a lot about death or suicide or expressing feelings of hopelessness

• stockpiling medications

• refusing to take care of oneself

• sudden interest in guns

• giving away cherished possessions, writing long letters, or making other elaborate farewells

• disrupted sleep patterns

• hurriedly revising a will

• increased intake of alcohol or prescription drugs

Diagnosis

The diagnosis of a suicide attempt is often made when the patient either goes to the emergency room of a hospital to seek help or is taken there by family members or first responders. In many cases, the patient will have written a suicide note, talked about his or her intention, or begun to carry out a plan to kill him- or herself. If the patient is not conscious, the doctor will obtain as much information as possible from family members or first responders.

Treatment

Suicide attempts are treated as a psychiatric emergency by police or other rescue personnel. Treatment in a hospital emergency room includes a complete psychiatric evaluation, a mental status examination, and a detailed assessment of the circumstances surrounding the attempt. The physician will interview the person's relatives or anyone else who accompanied the patient in order to obtain as much information as possible. Some questions that the physician will ask include whether the patient had a detailed plan for suicide; whether he or she had the means of suicide at hand; what the patient hoped to gain by killing him- or herself (freedom from pain, reunion with a dead loved one, solution to financial problems); and whether the patient had any tendencies toward homicide. As a rule, suicide attempts requiring advance planning and the use of violent or highly lethal methods are regarded as the most serious. The patient will be kept under observation while decisions are made about the need for hospitalization.

People who have attempted suicide and who are considered a serious danger to themselves or to others can be legally hospitalized against their will. The doctor bases the decision on the severity of the patient's depression or agitation; the presence of other suicide risk factors, including a history of previous suicide attempts, substance abuse, recent stressful events, and symptoms of psychosis; and the availability of friends, relatives, or other social support. If the attempt is judged to be a nonlethal suicide gesture, and the patient has adequate support outside the hospital, he or she may be released after the psychiatric assessment is completed.

Traditional

People who survive a suicide attempt are usually treated with a combination of antidepressant medications and psychotherapy.

Drugs

In 2003, the Food and Drug Administration (FDA) approved the use of clozapine (Clozaril), an antipsychotic medication, for the treatment of patients with schizophrenia who have attempted suicide.

Treatment of suicide survivors

In addition to the grief that ordinarily accompanies death, survivors of a friend or relative's suicide often struggle with feelings of guilt and shame as well. In spite of a general liberalization of social attitudes since World War II (1939–1945), suicide is still stigmatized in many parts of Europe and the United States. Survivors often benefit from group or individual psychotherapy in order to work through such issues as wondering whether they could have prevented the suicide or whether they are at increased risk of committing suicide themselves. Increasing numbers of clergy as well as mental health professionals are trained in counseling survivors of suicide.

Prognosis

The prognosis for a person who has attempted suicide is generally favorable, although further research needs to be done. Many different studies have followed individuals who attempted suicide to determine how likely they are to die by suicide. These studies have generally found that the likelihood is less than 10%. A doctor who studied 515 people who attempted suicide between 1937 and 1971 found that 94% were still alive at the time of his study or had died of natural causes. In general, individuals who attempt suicide and rate highly on intent to commit suicide and hopelessness may be more likely to commit suicide later. These findings may indicate that suicidal behavior is more likely to be a passing response to an acute crisis than a reflection of a permanent state of mind.

Prevention

One reason that suicide is such a tragedy is that most self-inflicted deaths are potentially preventable. Many suicidal people change their minds if they can be helped through their immediate crisis; Dr. Richard Seiden, from the University of California at Berkeley, a specialist in treating survivors of suicide attempts, puts the high-risk period at 90 days after the crisis. Some potential suicides change their minds during the actual attempt; for example, a number of people who survived jumping off the Golden Gate Bridge told interviewers afterward that

---

KEY TERMS

Assisted suicide—A form of self-inflicted death in which individuals voluntarily bring about their own death with the help of another, usually a physician, relative, or friend. Assisted suicide is sometimes called physician-assisted death (PAD).

Cortisol—A hormone released by the cortex (outer portion) of the adrenal gland when a person is under stress. Such levels are now considered a biological marker of suicide risk.

Diathesis—The medical term for predisposition. The stress/diathesis model is a diagram that is used to explain why some people are at greater risk of suicidal behavior than others.

Euthanasia—The act of putting individuals or animals to death painlessly or allowing them to die by withholding medical services, usually because of an incurable disease.

Frontal cortex—The part of the human brain associated with aggressiveness and impulse control. Abnormalities in this part of the brain are associated with an increased risk of suicide.

Self-deliverance—Another term for assisted suicide, more commonly used in Great Britain than in the United States.

Serotonin—A chemical that occurs in the blood and nervous tissue and functions to transmit signals across the gaps between neurons in the central nervous system. Abnormally low levels of this chemical are associated with depression and an increased risk of suicide.

Suicide gesture—Attempted suicide characterized by a low-lethality method, low level of intent or planning, and little physical damage; sometimes called "pseudocide."

Suicide magnet—A bridge, tall building, or geographic location that acquires a reputation for attracting people who want to commit suicide and attempt it.

---

they regretted their action even as they were falling and that they were grateful they survived.

Efforts and Solutions

Brain research is an important means of suicide prevention. Known biological markers for an increased risk of suicide may be correlated with personality profiles linked to suicidal behavior under stress to help identify

QUESTIONS TO ASK YOUR DOCTOR

- There have been a number of suicides in my family. Does that mean that I am at increased risk of suicide?

- How can I help a depressed friend who says that he or she has nothing to live for?

- How can I tell the difference between an occasional blue spell and the kind of depression that can lead to suicide?

- What would you recommend as good ways to deal with occasional thoughts of suicide?

individuals at risk. Brain imaging studies using positron emission tomography (PET) are being used to detect abnormal patterns of serotonin uptake in specific regions of the brain. Genetic studies are also yielding new information about inherited predispositions to suicide.

Research is ongoing to discover better methods of treating depression and other disorders that may influence a person's decision to commit suicide. Primary care physicians are continually learning how to better identify and intervene when treating suicidal patients. An estimated 67% of all adults and 80% of seniors who complete suicide have seen a physician within a month of their death, placing primary care physicians in a good position to evaluate patients for signs of depression. The good news is that depression in adults in any age group is highly treatable, particularly when antidepressant medications are combined with psychotherapy.

People who are concerned about a friend or relative at risk of self-harm should take the following steps:

- Become educated about warning signs and risk factors.

- Identify physicians and other healthcare professionals who know the person and can provide help.

- Talk openly with the person about his or her feelings—although many people are afraid to ask whether someone is thinking about suicide for fear of angering them or giving them an idea, in many cases honest concern is welcomed by the individual.

- Call the local hospital emergency department or 911 if the person seems to be at immediate risk of suicide.

Resources

BOOKS

American Psychiatric Association. *Diagnostic and Statistical Manual of Mental Disorders*. 4th ed., text rev. Washington, DC: American Psychiatric Association, 2000.

Beers, Mark H., and Robert Berkow, eds. *Merck Manual of Geriatrics*. 3rd ed. Whitehouse Station, NJ: Merck, 2005.

Giddens, Sandra. *Suicide*. New York: Rosen Publishing, 2007.

Goldney, Robert D. *Suicide Prevention*. New York: Oxford University Press, 2008.

Kutcher, Stanley P., and Sonia Chehil. *Suicide Risk Management: A Manual for Health Professionals*. Malden, MA: Blackwell Publishing, 2007.

Paris, Joel. *Half in Love with Death: Managing the Chronically Suicidal Patient*. Mahwah, NJ: Lawrence Erlbaum Associates, 2007.

PERIODICALS

Ajdacic-Gross, V., et al. "Methods of Suicide: International Suicide Patterns Derived from the WHO Mortality Databse." *Bulletin of the World Health Organization* 86 (September 2008): 726–32.

Alao, A.O., M. Soderberg, E.L. Pohl, and A.L. Alao. "Cybersuicide: Review of the Role of the Internet on Suicide." *Cyberpsychology and Behavior* 9 (August 2006): 489–93.

American Academy of Hospice and Palliative Medicine. "Position Statement on Physician-Assisted Death." *Journal of Pain and Palliative Care Pharmacotherapy* 21 (April 2007): 55–57.

Apter, A., and R.A. King. "Management of the Depressed, Suicidal Child or Adolescent." *Child and Adolescent Psychiatric Clinics of North America* 15 (October 2006): 999–1013.

Beyer, J.L. "Managing Depression in Geriatric Populations." *Annals of Clinical Psychiatry* 19 (October/December 2007): 221–38.

Burns, Robert. "Military Suicide Rate Surges to Nearly One Per Day This Year." *The Huffington Post*, June 07, 2012. http://www.huffingtonpost.com/2012/06/07/military-suicide-surges-_n_1578821.htmlAccessed August 19, 2012.

Centers for Disease Control and Prevention (CDC). "Alcohol and Suicide among Racial/Ethnic Populations—17 States, 2005–2006." *Morbidity and Mortality Weekly Report* 58 (June 19, 2009): 637–41.

———. "Increases in Age-Group-Specific Injury Mortality—United States, 1999–2004." *Morbidity and Mortality Weekly Report* 56 (December 14, 2007): 1281–84.

Coryell, William H. "Clinical Assessment of Suicide Risk in Depressive Disorder." *CNS Spectrums* 11, no. 6 (2006): 255–461. http://www.cnsspectrums.com/aspx/articledetail.aspx?articleid=474 (accessed November 13, 2011).

Friend, Tad. "Jumpers: The Fatal Grandeur of the Golden Gate Bridge." *New Yorker* (October 13, 2003). http://www.newyorker.com/archive/2003/10/13/031013fa_fact?currentPage=all (accessed July 20, 2011).

Fu, K.W., et al. "Estimating the Risk for Suicide Following the Suicide Deaths of 3 Asian Entertainment Celebrities: A Meta-Analytic Approach." *Journal of Clinical Psychiatry* 70 (June 2009): 869–78.

Guthmann, Edward, et al. "Lethal Beauty." *San Francisco Chronicle* (October 30, 2005). http://www.sfgate.com/cgi-bin/article.cgi?f=/c/a/2005/10/30/MNG2NFF7KI1.DTL (accessed July 20, 2011).

Jelinek, Pauline, and Kimberly Hefling. "Army Suicide Rates Hit Record High." *Huffington Post* (January 29, 2009). http://www.huffingtonpost.com/2009/01/30/army-suicide-rates-hit-re_n_162484.html (accessed July 20, 2011).

Jokinen, A., et al. "HPA Axis Hyperactivity and Attempted Suicide in Young Adult Mood Disorder Inpatients." *Journal of Affective Disorders* 116 (July 2009): 117–20.

Liu, X., A.L. Gentzler, P. Tepper, et al. "Clinical Features of Depressed Children and Adolescents with Various Forms of Suicidality." *Journal of Clinical Psychiatry* 67 (September 2006): 1442–50.

Voaklander, D.C., et al. "Medical Illness, Medication Use, and Suicide in Seniors: A Population-Based Case Control Study." *Journal of Epidemiology and Community Health* 62 (February 2008): 138–46.

Yip, P.S., et al. "Years of Life Lost from Suicide in China, 1990–2000." *Crisis* 29 (March 2008): 131–36.

WEBSITES

Centers for Disease Control and Prevention. "Deaths: Final Data for 2009." *National Vital Statistics Report* 60, no. 3 (March 16, 2011). http://www.cdc.gov/nchs/data/nvsr/nvsr60/nvsr60_03.pdf (accessed August 19, 2012).

WEBSITES

American Academy of Child and Adolescent Psychiatry. "Teen Suicide." *Facts for Families* 10 (May 2008). http://www.aacap.org/cs/root/facts_for_families/teen_suicide (accessed July 20, 2011).

American Association of Suicidology. "Fact Sheets." http://www.suicidology.org/web/guest/stats-and-tools/fact-sheets (accessed July 20, 2011).

———. "If You Are Considering Suicide." http://www.suicidology.org/web/guest/thinking-about-suicide (accessed July 20, 2011).

American Foundation for Suicide Prevention. "About Suicide: Frequently Asked Questions." http://www.afsp.org/index.cfm?fuseaction=home.viewPage&page_id=052618D2-02D2-04B4-00EDA31CFC336B63 (accessed July 20, 2011).

Andrew, Louise B. "Depression and Suicide." Medscape Reference. May 9, 2011. http://emedicine.medscape.com/article/805459-overview (accessed July 20, 2011).

Centers for Disease Control and Prevention. "National Suicide Statistics: At a Glance." September 30, 2009. http://www.cdc.gov/violenceprevention/suicide/statistics/index.html (accessed July 20, 2011).

National Institute of Mental Health. "Suicide Prevention." July 20, 2011. http://www.nimh.nih.gov/health/topics/suicide-prevention/index.shtml (accessed July 20, 2011).

———. "Suicide in the U.S.: Statistics and Prevention." September 30, 2009. http://www.nimh.nih.gov/health/publications/suicide-in-the-us-statistics-and-prevention/index.shtml (accessed July 20, 2011).

Soreff, Stephen. "Suicide." Medscape Reference. January 11, 2011. http://emedicine.medscape.com/article/288598-overview (accessed July 20, 2011).

U.S. Department of Defense and Veterans Administration. "About Suicide." DoD/VA Suicide Outreach. http://www.suicideoutreach.org/about_suicide (accessed July 20, 2011).

ORGANIZATIONS

American Academy of Child and Adolescent Psychiatry, 3615 Wisconsin Ave. NW, Washington, DC 20016-3007, (202) 966-7300, Fax: (202) 966-2891, http://www.aacap.org

American Association of Suicidology, 5221 Wisconsin Ave. NW, Washington, DC 20015, (202) 237-2280, Fax: (202) 237-2282, http://www.suicidology.org/web/guest/home

American Foundation for Suicide Prevention, 120 Wall St., 29th Fl., New York, NY 20016-3007, (212) 363-3500, (888) 333-2377, Fax: (212) 363-6237, inquiry@afsp.org, http://www.afsp.org

American Psychiatric Association, 1000 Wilson Blvd., Ste. 1825, Arlington, VA 22209, (703) 907-7300, apa@psych.org, http://www.psych.org

Mental Health America, 2000 N Beauregard St., 6th Fl., Alexandria, VA 22311, (703) 684-7722, Fax: (703) 684-5968, (800) 969-6642, http://www1.nmha.org

National Alliance on Mental Illness, 3803 N Fairfax Dr., Ste. 100, Arlington, VA 22203, (703) 524-7600, Fax: (703) 524-9094, http://www.nami.org

National Institute of Mental Health, 6001 Executive Blvd., Rm. 8184, MSC 9663, Bethesda, MD 20892-9663, (301) 443-4513, (866) 615-6464, Fax: (301) 443-4279, nimhinfo@nih.gov, http://www.nimh.nih.gov

National Suicide Prevention Lifeline, (800) 274-TALK (8255), http://www.suicidepreventionlifeline.org

U.S. Department of Veterans Affairs (VA), 810 Vermont Ave. NW, Washington, DC United States 20420, (800) 827-1000; Mental health crisis line: (800) 273-8255 (press 1), http://www.va.gov

Rebecca J. Frey, Ph.D.
David A. Brent, M.D.
William A. Atkins, B.B., B.S., M.B.A.
Andrea Nienstedt, M.A.

Sun protection

Definition

Sun protection describes any number of precautions or products intended to protect skin from the sun's harmful ultraviolet (UV) rays.

Demographics

According to the Center for Disease Control and **Prevention (CDC)**, skin **cancer** is the most common form of cancer in the United States. In 2008 (the most recent statistics available as of 2012), nearly 60,000 people in the United States were diagnosed with skin

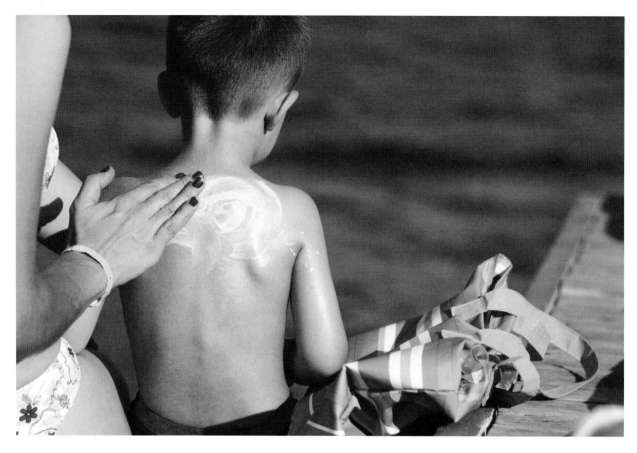

A mother applying sunscreen on her child. Sunscreen should be applied 20-30 minutes before sun exposure. (© iStockphoto. comaydinmutlu)

melanoma (the major form of skin cancer). In the same year, 8,623 people in the United States died from skin melanomas.

Description

Despite the dangers of excessive or unprotected sun exposure, exposure to sunlight is necessary for human survival. The skin absorbs sunlight through UV-B (ultraviolet B) rays and converts it into vitamin D_3 or cholecalciferol. Vitamin D helps the body to properly absorb calcium, among other functions. Though the body's need for sunlight is essential, exposure to sunlight for 10 to 15 minutes, on three occasions per week is enough to satisfy the body's requirements.

The American Academy of Dermatology (AAD) and the U.S. Food and Drug Administration (FDA) have developed a classification system for different skin types and their susceptibility to suntan and sunburn:

- I—extremely sun-sensitive (always burns easily and never tans)
- II—very sun-sensitive (usually burns easily and tans only minimally)
- III—sun-sensitive (sometimes burns and gradually tans to light brown)
- IV—minimally sun-sensitive (burns minimally and always tans to moderate brown)
- V—sun-insensitive (rarely burns and tans well)
- VI—sun-insensitive (never burns and is deeply pigmented)

Tanning

Many Americans, especially a majority of those under 25, believe that tanned skin improves their physical appearance. Tanned skin was not popular in Western civilization until the 1920s, when fashion designer Coco Chanel returned from the French Riviera with a suntan. Tanning can be achieved outside with natural sunlight or indoors with tanning beds or sunlamps, which utilize special light bulbs to create UV rays to darken the skin. Despite the fact that the lighting in tanning beds and sunlamps are known carcinogens, their use remains incredibly popular. Tanning can also cause serious short-term and long-term eye damage. The American Academy of Dermatology (AAD) and the **World Health**

KEY TERMS

Tanning—The usually intentional process of prolonged exposure to UV rays—either from the sun or special light bulbs—in order to darken one's skin.

Sunburn—The inflammation and redness of the skin caused by prolonged exposure to the sun.

Melanoma—A type of skin cancer. Melanoma is the most dangerous of the various types of skin cancer.

Sun Protection Factor (SPF)—A numerical value assigned to sunscreen and sunblock products to communicate the product's ability to protect against UV-B rays. The higher the number, the greater the protection.

Ultraviolet (UV) rays—A term describing the sun's rays and encompassing both UV-A and UV-B rays. In small doses, these rays help the human body create vitamin D, which is needed for many bodily processes. In large doses, these rays can lead to health problems including sunburn, cataracts, blindness, immune system suppression, premature aging, and cancer.

Melanin—A naturally occurring pigment found in human skin, hair, and eyes. Melanin determines skin color and reacts to UV rays to make skin appear tanned.

Organization (WHO) encourage a ban on the use of indoor tanning facilities by minors—in addition to the general health risks posed by tanning, these facilities are generally unregulated and often do not enforce recommended guidelines for progressive tanning schedules and proper eyewear.

Sunburn

Sunburn occurs when skin becomes red and inflamed from overexposure to the sun. Sunburned skin can also blister, and within a few days, the dead skin will peel or flake off. Every year, more than one million Americans suffer from sunburn—of those, one out of every 87 will develop malignant melanoma, which is the most serious type of skin cancer.

Risks

Skin Cancer

Scientists believe that most melanomas are caused by sun exposure from childhood through young adulthood. On average, people will receive 50% to 80% of their lifetime sun exposure before the age of 18. It is believed that roughly 80% of sun exposure occurs incidentally, from day-to-day activities, so proper caution and sun protection are essential, especially during childhood. Though men are more susceptible to skin cancer, studies show they are also less likely to take preventative measures to avoid skin cancer.

Prevention

There are multiple methods of sun protection, and when used properly and consistently they can help avoid the harmful side effects of over exposure to the sun, such as sunburn, eye damage, immune system suppression, premature **aging**, and cancer.

Sunscreen

Sunscreen is one of the most important forms of sun protection. Sunscreen and sunblock come in different types of lotions and gels and are even built into some cosmetic products. Sunscreen and sunblock are labeled to show the degree of protection they offer—labels show a numeric sun protection factor (SPF). The higher the number, the greater the protection. The SPF number only applies to UV-B rays. Though there is currently no system to measure UV-A protection, products labeled "broad-spectrum" offer protection from both UV-A and UV-B rays. SPF 15 is the minimum level of protection most people should use. Sunscreen products are now available with SPF values that approach 100. Individuals with especially fair skin, children, or those at lower or higher altitudes or living closer to the equator should consider products with higher SPF values.

Many sunscreens contain the chemical oxybenzone. Oxybenzone has been shown to cause **allergies**, hormone disruption, and cell damage. The chemical has also been connected to low birth weights in girls whose mothers were in contact with oxybenzone during their pregnancies. As of 2008, the CDC thought that approximately 97% of Americans were contaminated with this ingredient. Sunscreen is not the only product containing oxybenzone; other common products include cosmetics, hair conditioner, and fragrances. In response to the dangers posed by oxybenzone and instances of allergies to sun protection products, companies have developed mineral-based sunscreens and sunscreens that do not contain oxybenzone. These products still provide SPF protection using the recognizable SPF numerical identification.

Babies have particularly thin skin and their bodies are not equipped to process sun in the way that an adult's body is, so infants under six months should be fully covered and kept out of the sun. Most sunscreens are not approved for infants, so it is important to check the label of a sunscreen before applying it to a baby.

To use sunscreen properly, it should be applied daily—including days that are cloudy or cold. Apply sunscreen 15 to 30 minutes before going into the sun. It is important to cover all exposed skin—some commonly forgotten areas include the lips, the ears, the back of the neck, and the feet. Though some sunscreens are labeled "waterproof" or "sweatproof" this additional protection will not last indefinitely, usually these products provide around 80 minutes of protection. It is important to reapply sunscreen every two hours or after the skin has become wet. The amount of sunscreen that is needed varies given a person's size and the amount of their skin that is exposed, but the average amount needed is one ounce. Approximately 25 to 50% of people do not use adequate amounts of sunscreen.

Some medications make an individual particularly susceptible to sun damage or react poorly with sun exposure. It is important to check all medication labels, and if necessary, confer with a physician, before prolonged sun exposure.

Other Forms of Sun Protection

In addition to sunscreen, there are a variety of ways to protect the skin from harmful UV rays. These methods are particularly useful to protect children's delicate skin.

- Wear clothing that covers as much skin as possible. In warm weather, this can be made of lightweight fabrics.

- Avoid being out in the sun when it is at its strongest, "the heat of the day," usually between 11 a.m. and 4 p.m.

- When making outdoor plans, remember that the sun is stronger during the summer, when nearer to the equator, and at high and low altitudes.

- If available (especially for children), wear clothing and swimsuits made from sun-protective fabric.

- Use hats that cover as much of the head and neck as possible.

- Wear sunglasses. Beware, not all sunglasses provide UV protections. Larger sunglasses are more likely to cover the whole eye area, but check sunglass labels to determine the UV protection in the lenses. Labels that read "UV absorption up to 400nm" or "Meets ANSI UV Requirements" will block at least 99% of UV rays. Frames labeled "cosmetic" will probably block around 70% of UV rays, and those with no label will probably offer no UV protection.

- Utilize tents and umbrellas for prolonged outdoor activities.

- Additives are available to use in the washing machine which will add UV protection factor (UPF) to your clothes, without altering the texture or color of the fabric.

Resources

BOOKS

Alic, Margaret. "Tanning." *The Gale Encyclopedia of Medicine.* Ed. Laurie J. Fundukian. 4th ed. Vol. 6. Detroit: Gale, 2011.

Turkington, Carl A., and Ken R. Wells. "Sunburn." *The Gale Encyclopedia of Medicine.* Ed. Laurie J. Fundukian. 4th ed. Vol. 5. Detroit: Gale, 2011.

PERIODICALS

"Mineral sunscreen." *Skin & Allergy News.* July 2012: 34.

"Be sun-savvy and protect your skin from damage: men are more susceptible to skin cancer, but less apt to guard against it. Take precautions, and have your skin checked." *Men's Health Advisor.* 14.7 (2012): 3+.

WEBSITES

American Cancer Society. "How do I protect myself from UV rays?" http://www.cancer.org/Cancer/CancerCauses/SunandUVExposure/SkinCancerPreventionandEarlyDetection/skin-cancer-prevention-and-early-detection-u-v-protectionAccessed August 20, 2012.

Centers for Disease Control and Prevention. "Skin Cancer Statistics." http://www.cdc.gov/cancer/skin/statistics/ Accessed August 20, 2012.

Environmental Working Group. "CDC: Americans Carry Body Burden of Toxic Sunscreen Chemical."http://www.ewg.org/analysis/toxicsunscreen. Accessed August 20, 2012.

National Cancer Institute. "Skin Cancer Home Page."http://www.cancer.gov/cancertopics/types/skin. Accessed August 20, 2012.

Skin Cancer Foundation. "Skin Cancer Facts." http://www.skincancer.org/skin-cancer-information/skin-cancer-facts Accessed August 20, 2012.

ORGANIZATIONS

American Cancer Society, 250 Williams Street NW, Atlanta, GA 30303, (800) 227-2345, http://www.cancer.org

Centers for Disease Control and Prevention, 1600 Clifton Rd., Atlanta, GA 30333, (800) 232-4636, cdcinfo@cdc.gov, http://www.cdc.gov

National Cancer Institute, 6116 Executive Boulevard, Suite 300, Bethesda, MD 20892-8322, (800) 422-6237, http://www.cancer.gov.

Andrea Nienstedt, MA

Swine flu *see* **H1N1 influenza A**

Syphilis

Definition

Syphilis is a sexually transmitted disease (STD) caused by the spirochete bacterium *Treponema pallidum*. The infection is acquired through direct—usually sexual—contact with a syphilis sore. It also can be transmitted from a mother to her child either before or during birth. Untreated syphilis is a systemic, potentially fatal disease that can cause permanent damage to the heart and central nervous system.

Demographics

Syphilis has been a serious public health problem since at least the sixteenth century. Some estimates place the number of worldwide syphilis cases at about 50 million annually. However the incidence of syphilis varies greatly from one region to another and even within small geographical areas.

Overall, the rate of syphilis in the United States has declined 1.6% since 2009, according the Centers for Disease Control and Prevention. In 2010, 45,835 new cases of syphilis were reported in the United States. While this is an increase from the 44,830 cases reported in 2009, it was lower than the 46,292 cases reported in 2008.

Most of the new cases in 2010 occurred among 20- to 24-year–olds, with a total of 2,907 cases reported in that age group, followed by 25- to 29-year-olds (2,455 cases) and 45- to 54-year-olds, 2,056. These figures include only cases of syphilis that were transmitted sexually.

The **CDC** recorded 6,530 cases of syphilis among African Americans, 4,270 among whites, 2,236 among Hispanics, 201 among Asians and Pacific Islanders, and 64 among American Indians and Alaska Natives. The rate of syphilis infection among young African American men increased 134% in a five-year period, including a significant increase among men who have sex with men (MSM).

Syphilis is a problem on a global scale. The **World Health Organization (WHO)** estimates that more than 12 million new cases of syphilis have occurred worldwide since 2009. Four million of those cases occurred in Sub-Saharan Africa, 4 million in South and Southeast Asia, and 3 million in Latin America and the Caribbean.

Syphilis has been closely associated with HIV infection since the late 1980s. Syphilis makes it easier to transmit and acquire HIV. The incidence of syphilis is also high among crack cocaine users.

Description

Although the origin of syphilis remains controversial, evidence suggests that *Treponema* bacteria were brought to Europe from the New World with the return of Christopher Columbus's ships. Syphilis, which is also called *lues* from a Latin word meaning **plague**, was treated with mercury and other dangerous substances until World War I, when more effective treatments based on arsenic or bismuth were introduced. After World War II, penicillin became available to cure syphilis, and the incidence of the disease began to decline.

About 90% of syphilis cases are contracted through sexual contact, usually from people who are unaware that they have the disease. Syphilis is sometimes called the "great imposter," because its symptoms—when present at all—resemble those of various other diseases.

Syphilis is transmitted through direct contact with a syphilis sore, usually through vaginal, anal, or oral sex. Sores usually occur on the external genitals or in the vagina, anus, or rectum, but also can occur on the lips and in the mouth. The chances of contracting syphilis during unprotected sex with a person who has an early stage of the disease are 30–50%. The bacteria also can be transmitted by touching infected sores or using contaminated needles to inject drugs. Babies of infected mothers can be born with congenital syphilis. Transmission through a blood transfusion is very rare because the bacterium cannot survive for more than 24 hours in stored blood, and blood products are screened for the bacteria. Syphilis cannot be spread through toilet seats, doorknobs, swimming pools, hot tubs, bathtubs, shared clothing, or eating utensils. *T. pallidum* is easily killed by heat and drying.

Syphilis has both acute and chronic phases that produce a wide variety of symptoms affecting most of the body's organ systems. The range of symptoms makes it easy to ignore early signs or to confuse it with less serious diseases. Syphilis that is acquired through sexual contact has four stages—primary, secondary, latent, and tertiary. The bacteria can be spread by sexual contact during the first three stages. Although latent syphilis has few external symptoms, the disease continues to progress. Patients with tertiary syphilis cannot infect others.

Syphilis can be transmitted from an infected mother to her fetus through the placenta at any time during pregnancy or through contact with syphilitic ulcers during the birth process. The chances of infection depend on the stage of the mother's disease. Almost all infants born to mothers with untreated primary or secondary syphilis will be infected. If a woman has untreated syphilis acquired within four years of a pregnancy, there is an 80% risk that the newborn will have congenital syphilis. However the infection rate drops to 40% if the mother's disease is in the early-latent stage and to 6–14% if she has late-latent syphilis.

Untreated syphilis can have devastating consequences:

• Syphilis appears to increase a man's risk of developing prostate cancer in later life.

• Cardiovascular syphilis occurs in 10–15% of patients with tertiary syphilis.

• About 8% of those with untreated syphilis develop neurosyphilis 5–35 years after the onset of the primary infection. This central nervous system disease has both physical and psychiatric consequences. It affects men more frequently than women and Caucasians more frequently than blacks.

• General paresis, also called dementia paralytica, results from neurosyphilis and is most common in patients over age 40.

Risk factors

In the United States and Canada, populations at high risk for syphilis include:

• sexually abused children

• sexually active teenagers

• MSM

• women of childbearing age

• prisoners

• abusers of drugs or alcohol

• prostitutes of either sex and their customers

• those infected with another sexually transmitted infection (STI), including HIV/AIDS

Drug abuse can increase the risk of syphilis because of needle sharing and the exchange of sex for drugs. In addition, people abusing drugs or alcohol are more likely to engage in risky sexual practices.

Causes and symptoms

T. pallidum is a thin, spiral- or coil-shaped bacterium that enters the body through mucous membranes or breaks in the skin to cause primary syphilis. The first signs of infection often go unnoticed. After an incubation period of 10–90 days, chancres may develop. These are small blister-like sores about 0.5 in (13 mm) in size. They resemble the ulcers of chlamydia infection, genital **herpes**, or skin tumors. Most chancres are on the genitals, but they also can develop on the breasts or lips or in the mouth. Rectal chancres are common in MSM. Chancres in a woman's vagina or on her cervix are easily overlooked. Chancres are not painful and disappear in three to six weeks without treatment. About 70% of patients with primary syphilis develop swollen lymph nodes near the chancre. The nodes may feel firm or rubbery but are not usually painful.

The disease continues to progress even in the complete absence of symptoms. Secondary syphilis begins between six weeks and six months after infection. Chancres may still be present but are usually healing. Secondary syphilis is a systemic infection marked by the eruption of skin rashes and ulcers in the mucous membranes. The skin rash may resemble other skin disorders such as drug reactions, **rubella**, ringworm, mononucleosis, or pityriasis rosea. Characteristics of a syphilis rash include:

• coppery color

• absence of pain or itching

• occurrence on the palms of the hands and soles of the feet

The skin eruptions may resolve in a few weeks or last as long as a year. Some patients develop condylomata lata—weepy, pinkish or grey patches of flattened skin on moist areas of the body. The skin rashes, mouth and genital ulcers, and condylomata lata are all highly contagious.

About 50% of patients with secondary syphilis develop swollen lymph nodes in the armpits, groin, and neck; about 10% develop inflammations of the eyes, kidney, liver, spleen, bones, joints, or the meninges—membranes covering the brain and spinal cord. Patients also may have flu-like symptoms, including low fever, chills, loss of appetite, headache, runny nose, sore throat, and aching joints.

The latent phase of syphilis is divided into early latency, occurring less than two years after infection, and late latency. During early latency patients are at risk for spontaneous recurrences of the ulcers and skin rashes of secondary syphilis. In late latency, these recurrences are much less common. Late latency can either resolve spontaneously or continue for the remainder of the patient's life.

About 35–40% of untreated syphilis cases progress to the tertiary stage. Tertiary syphilis can be either benign late syphilis or cardiovascular and/or neurosyphilis.

Benign late syphilis begins three to ten years after infection and is characterized by the development of gummas. These are rubbery tumor-like growths that usually involve the skin or long bones but also can develop in the eyes, mucous membranes, throat, liver, or stomach lining. Gummas have become uncommon since the introduction of **antibiotics** for treating syphilis.

Benign late syphilis is usually rapid in onset and responds well to treatment.

Cardiovascular syphilis develops between 10 and 25 years after infection and often occurs along with neurosyphilis. It usually begins as an inflammation of the arteries leading from the heart and causes heart attacks, scarring of the aortic valves, congestive heart failure, or an aortic aneurysm.

There are four types of neurosyphilis:

• Asymptomatic neurosyphilis causes no central nervous system symptoms but can be detected in the spinal fluid.
• Meningovascular neurosyphilis is characterized by changes in the blood vessels of the brain or inflammation of the meninges. It causes headaches, irritability, and visual problems. If the spinal cord is involved, the patient may experience weakness of the shoulder and upper arm muscles.
• Tabes dorsalis is a progressive degeneration of the spinal cord and nerve roots, causing a loss of perception of body position and orientation in space and resulting in loss of muscle reflexes and difficulty walking. Patients may have shooting pains in the legs and periodic episodes of pain in the abdomen, throat, bladder, or rectum. Tabes dorsalis is sometimes called locomotor ataxia.
• General paresis affects the cortex of the brain, with slow, progressive memory loss, inability to concentrate, and loss of interest in self-care. Personality changes may include irresponsible behavior, depression, delusions of grandeur, or complete psychosis.

Syphilis sometimes mimics the symptoms of HIV/AIDS. Conversely, HIV/AIDS appears to increase the severity of syphilis in patients suffering from both diseases and to speed the development or appearance of neurosyphilis. Patients with both syphilis and HIV/AIDS also are more likely to develop lues maligna, a skin condition that sometimes occurs in secondary syphilis and is characterized by areas of ulcerated and dying tissue.

Infants with early congenital syphilis have systemic symptoms that resemble those of secondary syphilis in adults. The central nervous system is affected in 40–60% of children with congenital syphilis. Symptoms include:

• skin rashes
• condylomata lata
• inflammation of the lungs
• persistent runny nose
• swollen lymph nodes
• jaundice

• enlargement of the spleen and liver
• anemia

Symptoms of late congenital syphilis develop after age two and include:

• facial deformities (saddle nose)
• Hutchinson's teeth (abnormal upper incisors)
• saber shins
• dislocated joints
• deafness
• mental retardation
• paralysis
• seizure disorders

Diagnosis

Examination

Diagnosis of syphilis is often delayed:

• The initial chancre may go unnoticed.
• There are wide variations in early symptoms.
• The incubation period varies greatly.
• Patients often do not connect their symptoms with recent sexual contact.

The skin rash of secondary syphilis is sometimes the first symptom to be diagnosed. Women may be diagnosed in the course of a routine gynecological exam. While taking a medical history, the physician will ask about recent sexual contacts to determine whether the patient falls into a high-risk group. Symptoms such as skin rashes or swollen lymph nodes will be noted with respect to the timing of a patient's sexual contacts.

Tests

The definitive diagnosis of syphilis depends on laboratory test results. Various tests also are used as screens for syphilis and for follow-up monitoring after treatment. Because of the long-term risks of untreated syphilis, groups of people are routinely screened for the disease:

• marriage-license applicants
• pregnant women
• children born to infected mothers
• patients with HIV/AIDS
• sexual contacts or partners of patients diagnosed with syphilis

Nontreponemal antigen tests are used as screens for syphilis. They measure the presence of reagin, an antibody formed in reaction to *T. pallidum*. In the venereal disease research laboratory (VDRL) test, a

KEY TERMS

Chancre—An open sore with a firm or hard base that is the initial skin ulcer of primary syphilis.

Condylomata lata—Highly infectious patches of weepy, pink or gray skin in moist areas of the body that occur during secondary syphilis.

Dark field—A microscopy technique in which light is directed at an oblique angle so that organisms appear bright against a dark background.

General paresis—An advanced form of neurosyphilis affecting personality and control of movement and possibly causing convulsions or partial paralysis.

Gumma—A rubbery swelling or tumor that heals slowly and leaves a scar and is a symptom of tertiary syphilis.

Jarisch-Herxheimer reaction—A temporary reaction to penicillin treatment for syphilis that includes fever, chills, and worsening of the skin rash or chancre.

Lues maligna—Areas of ulcerated and dying skin tissue that may occur with secondary syphilis, most frequently in HIV-positive patients.

Meninges—The membranes that cover the brain and spinal cord.

Miasm—In homeopathy, an inherited weakness or predisposition to disease. The syphilitic miasm is considered to be one of the most powerful.

Neurosyphilis—Syphilis of the central nervous system.

Nosode—A homeopathic remedy made from microbes, pus, or other disease material. Syphilinum is a nosode made from a diluted solution of killed *T. pallidum*.

Spirochete—A long, slender, coiled-shape bacterium, such as *T. pallidum* that causes syphilis.

Tabes dorsalis—A progressive deterioration of the spinal cord and spinal nerves that is associated with tertiary syphilis.

Treponema pallidum—The spirochete bacterium that causes syphilis.

sample of the patient's blood serum is mixed with cardiolipin and cholesterol. The formation of clumps indicates a positive reaction. The serum sample can be diluted to determine the concentration of reagin in the patient's blood. The rapid plasma reagin (RPR) test is a kit in which the serum is mixed with cardiolipin on a plastic-coated card that can be examined with the naked eye. Nontreponemal antigen tests require interpretation and sometimes further testing. They can yield both false-negative and false-positive results. False negatives can occur when patients are tested too soon after exposure to syphilis, since it takes about 14–21 days for antibodies to become detectable after infection. False-positive results can be caused by other diseases, including mononucleosis, **malaria**, **leprosy**, rheumatoid arthritis, and lupus. Whereas the overall rate of false positives is 0.8%, the rate of false positives in HIV/AIDS patients is about 4%.

Treponemal antibody tests are used to rule out false-positive results on nontreponemal screening tests. They are more expensive and complicated than nontreponemal tests, but are very specific and sensitive. They measure the presence of antibodies that are specific for *T. pallidum*. These tests include:

- the microhemagglutination-*T. pallidum* (MHA-TP) test, in which sheep red blood cells are coated with *T. pallidum* antigen; the cells clump if the patient's blood contains specific antibodies against the antigen

- the fluorescent treponemal antibody absorption (FTA-ABS) test, in which antibodies in the blood are used to coat *T. pallidum* on a slide and a fluorescein dye causes the coated spirochetes to fluoresce under ultraviolet (UV) light

- the INNO-LIA test—the most accurate antibody test—which uses recombinant and peptide antigens derived from *T. pallidum*

T. pallidum also can be identified in samples of tissue or lymphatic fluid. Slides of fresh samples are examined under microscopic dark-field illumination or slides of dried smears are stained with fluorescein and viewed under UV light.

A high white blood cell count and elevated protein levels in the cerebrospinal fluid (CSF) may suggest neurosyphilis. VDRL or FTA-ABS tests of the CSF are used to diagnose:

- neurosyphilis

- congenital syphilis

- syphilis in HIV/AIDS patients

- patients who are not responding to treatment with penicillin

Patients who test positive for syphilis are tested for HIV infection at the time of diagnosis. All sexual partners of a diagnosed patient must be tested for syphilis.

Treatment

Drugs

Syphilis is treated with antibiotics, either injected intramuscularly (benzathine penicillin G or ceftriaxone) or administered orally (doxycycline, minocycline, tetracycline, or azithromycin). In the vast majority of cases, a single dose of penicillin is sufficient to cure primary and secondary syphilis. Penicillin is less effective in treating later stages, and additional doses may be necessary. Neurosyphilis is treated with a combination of aqueous crystalline penicillin G, benzathine penicillin G, or doxycycline. The levels of penicillin in the patient's body must be kept sufficiently high over a period of days or weeks because *T. pallidum* has a relatively long reproduction time. Follow-up blood tests should be performed every three months to confirm that the patient is completely cured.

Pregnant women with syphilis are treated with tetracycline as early in pregnancy as possible. Infants with proven or suspected congenital syphilis are treated with either aqueous crystalline penicillin G or aqueous procaine penicillin G. Children who acquire syphilis after birth are treated with benzathine penicillin G.

Jarisch-Herxheimer reaction may occur during penicillin treatment for late-primary, secondary, or early-latent syphilis. The patient develops chills, fever, headache, and muscle pains within two to six hours after the penicillin injection and the chancre or rash temporarily worsens. The reaction lasts about one day and is thought to be an allergic reaction to the toxins that are released as massive numbers of spirochetes are destroyed.

Alternative

The historical link between homeopathy and syphilis is Hahnemann's theory of miasms, which labeled the syphilitic miasm as the second-oldest cause of constitutional weakness in humans. Homeopathic practitioners in the United States are banned from claiming that their treatments can cure syphilis. However because of the high incidence of syphilis in HIV/AIDS patients, some alternative practitioners claim that their homeopathic remedies for **AIDS** also are beneficial in treating syphilis. The most frequently suggested remedies are *Medorrhinum, Aurum, Mercurius vivus*, and *Syphilinum*. The use of *Mercurius vivus* reflects the historical use of mercury to treat syphilis. *Syphilinum* is in a class of homeopathic remedies called nosodes, which are made from disease material, such as bacteria, viruses, or pus. *Syphilinum* is made from a dilution of killed *T. pallidum*.

Certain outdated or discredited treatments for syphilis have resurfaced as alternative treatments for HIV/AIDS and **cancer**. Hyperthermia—inducing a fever to treat HIV/AIDS—originated as a treatment for syphilis, in which patients were infected with malaria in an attempt to kill *T. pallidum*. The Hoxsey treatment for cancer, which is no longer legally available in the United States, was developed in the 1920s by Harry Hoxsey and prescribed as a treatment for secondary and tertiary syphilis. The treatment consists of several chemical mixtures applied externally and a formula of nine herbs taken internally. The external formulation contains both arsenic and antimony, which were used to treat syphilis before the advent of antibiotics. The internal herbal formula includes *Phytolacca americana*, or pokeweed, which was used by Native Americans to treat syphilitic chancres, and *Stillingia sylvatica*, or queensroot, which was used in the past to treat syphilis. All of these components are potentially toxic and should not be used to treat syphilis.

Traditional Chinese medicine (TCM) and other alternative approaches emphasize the mental aspects of diseases such as syphilis. Alternative practitioners may recommend mind-body medicine, guided imagery, and affirmations as adjuncts to antibiotic treatment for syphilis.

Home remedies

Although antibiotics are essential for the treatment of syphilis, recovery can be aided by good dietary habits, adequate sleep, exercise, and stress-reduction techniques. Skin rashes and ulcers should be kept clean and dry. Patients must abstain from sexual contact until their disease has been cured. Other people should not be exposed to fluid or discharges from chancres, skin ulcers, rashes, or condylomata lata.

Prognosis

Antibiotics—especially penicillin—cure early-stage syphilis quickly and effectively. Treatment failures do occur, especially in HIV/AIDS patients treated with penicillin. Patients also can be re-infected. Patients should be followed up with blood tests at one, three, six, and 12 months after treatment or until the results are negative. CSF should be tested after one year. Patients with primary and secondary syphilis who remain symptom-free and have negative blood tests for two years after treatment are usually considered cured. Patients with recurrences during the latency period should be tested for re-infection.

In patients with untreated syphilis:

• About 30% undergo spontaneous remission.

• About 30% have lifelong latency.

• About 40% develop potentially fatal tertiary forms of syphilis.

Proper treatment for maternal syphilis during the second and third trimesters of pregnancy reduces the risk of congenital syphilis in the infant from 90% to less than 2%. However nearly 50% of untreated fetuses die shortly before or after birth. Those who survive may appear normal at birth but show signs of infection between three and eight weeks of age.

Prevention

Prevention of syphilis depends on a combination of personal and public health measures. Patients with syphilis do not acquire lasting immunity against the disease, so they can be easily re-infected. The only reliable methods for preventing transmission of syphilis are sexual abstinence or a monogamous relationship between uninfected partners. Condoms reduce the risk of transmission but protect only the covered parts of the genitals. The general public needs to be informed about the transmission and early symptoms of syphilis, and public health facilities must provide for adequate testing and treatment.

U.S. law requires the reporting of all syphilis cases to public health agencies. Sexual contacts of patients diagnosed with syphilis are traced and tested for the disease. This includes all contacts in the past three months for cases of primary syphilis and in the past year for cases of secondary syphilis. Neither patients nor their contacts should have sexual contact until they have been tested and treated. Patients should be informed about the disease and counseled regarding sexual behavior, safe sexual practices, and the importance of completing antibiotic treatment. In addition:

• Sexually active adolescents should be routinely screened for syphilis.

• Pregnant women should be tested for syphilis at the time of their first prenatal visit and again shortly before delivery.

• Many obstetricians and gynecologists recommend the routine screening of non-pregnant women.

• Because of the rising incidence of syphilis worldwide, many public health physicians recommend routine screening of immigrants, refugees, and international adoptees.

Effects on Public Health

The advent of antibiotics and improved public **health education** has made strides in controlling the incidence of syphilis, but this STD is still of concern. The CDC is bringing together healthcare providers,

community leaders, and state and local public health agencies to work together to reduce rates of infection in a Syphilis Elimination Effort (SEE). SEE resources include plans for responses to outbreaks, guidelines for healthcare providers for conducting what can be difficult conversations with patients and their partners, and publications and computer applications that can be used to educate patients and help them finding medical care.

The decline in the number of syphilis cases is in part a result of the CDC's efforts to increase education and public health services, including interventions for high-risk groups such as African Americans and MSM. The incidence of syphilis is often high in urban areas, but some rural locations can have similar rates of infection.

The study of syphilis includes one of the most infamous instances of medical research in history. Between 1932 and 1972, 399 poor African American men were denied treatment for syphilis as part of the Tuskegee Syphilis Study, run by the **United States Public Health Service**. Although the men were told they were being treated for "bad blood," they in fact received no therapeutic treatment at all. In return for their participation, the men received free medical exams, free meals, and burial insurance.

Since the study was brought to public attention in the 1972, it has become a symbol of "racism in medicine, ethical misconduct in human research, the paternalism of physicians, and the government abuse of vulnerable people," according to the final report of the Tuskegee Syphilis Study Legacy Committee. The study continues to affect attitudes among African Americans toward medical studies and even toward routine preventative care.

According to the CDC, several survivors of the men who unwittingly participated in the Tuskegee study are still receiving health benefits from the government, including annual visits from government physicians.

Resources

BOOKS

Holmes, King K., et al., eds. *Sexually Transmitted Diseases.* New York: McGraw-Hill Medical, 2008.

Meredith, Stephanie, et al. *The Global Elimination of Congenital Syphilis: Rationale and Strategy for Action.* Geneva: World Health Organization, 2007.

Parascandola, John. *Sex, Sin, and Science: A History of Syphilis in America.* Westport, CT: Praeger, 2008.

PERIODICALS

Bower, Bruce. "Infectious Voyagers." *Science News* 173, no. 3 (January 19, 2008): 38.

Branger, Judith, et al. "High Incidence of Asymptomatic Syphilis in HIV-Infected MSM Justifies Routine

Screening." *Sexually Transmitted Diseases* 36, no. 2 (February 2009): 84.547–555.

Chesson, Harrell, and Kwame Owusu-Edusei, Jr. "Examining the Impact of Federally-Funded Syphilis Elimination Activities in the USA." *Social Science & Medicine* 67, no. 12 (December 2008): 2059.

WEBSITES

"Syphilis." Sexually Transmitted Diseases Surveillance, 2010, Tables 25, 34, and 35A. (Accessed August 22, 2012) http://www.cdc.gov/std/stats10/tables.htm#syphtables

"Syphilis—CDC Fact Sheet." Sexually Transmitted Diseases. (Accessed August 22, 2012) http://www.cdc.gov/std/Syphilis/STDFact-Syphilis.htm.

"Syphilis." American Social Health Association. (Accessed August 24, 2012) http://www.ashastd.org/std-sti/syphilis.html.

ORGANIZATIONS

American Social Health Association, P.O. Box 13827, Research Triangle Park, NC 27709, (919) 361-8400, (800) 227-8922, Fax: (919) 361-8425, info@ashastd.org, http://www.ashastd.org

National Institute of Allergy and Infectious Diseases (NIAID), Office of Communications and Public Liaison, 6610 Rockledge Drive, Bethesda, MD 20892-66123, (866) 284-4107, http://www3.niaid.nih.gov

U.S. Centers for Disease Control and Prevention (CDC), 1600 Clifton Road, Atlanta, GA 30333, (800) CDC-INFO (232-4636), cdcinfo@cdc.gov, http://www.cdc.gov.

Rebecca J. Frey, Ph.D.
Margaret Alic, Ph.D.
Fran Hodgkins

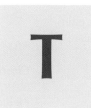

Tetanus

Definition

Tetanus is a rare, but often fatal, disease that affects the central nervous system and causes painful muscular contractions. It begins when tetanus bacteria enter the body, usually through a wound or cut exposed to contaminated soil. Tetanus is easily preventable through **vaccination**.

Description

Tetanus is rare in the United States, with nearly all cases occurring in adults who were not vaccinated as children. It results from infection with a bacterium called *Clostridium tetani*. Spores of the bacterium germinate in the body and produce a neurotoxin that ultimately causes the symptoms, which include convulsive muscle spasms and rigidity that can lead to respiratory paralysis and death. Tetanus is sometimes called "lockjaw" because one of the most common symptoms is spasms that affect the jaw so that it cannot be opened. Sometimes, tetanus affects only the part of the body where the infection began, but in almost all of reported cases, it spreads to the entire body. The incubation period from the time of the injury until the first symptoms appear ranges from two to 50 days. Symptoms usually occur within 5 to 10 days. When symptoms occur early, the chance of death is increased. Tetanus is not contagious.

ORIGINS. Scientists identified *C. tetani* in 1884 as the agent responsible for tetanus. The number of tetanus cases in the United States has steadily decreased since the 1940s, when 500 to 600 cases occurred per year. As of late 2012, about three to four dozen reports of tetanus occur annually in the United States, and all of them are among individuals who lack up-to-date tetanus vaccinations (including regular booster vaccinations).

Neonatal tetanus is a particular problem in developing countries where births may be carried out in non-hygienic conditions. Newborns and their mothers (who have not been properly immunized) are at risk for infection through the cut umbilical cord. Neonatal tetanus is rare in the United States.

Causes and symptoms

CAUSES. Tetanus is caused by a bacterium called *Clostridium tetani*. Its spores (the dormant form) are found in soil, street dust, and animal (or even human) feces. Tetanus spores germinate in the body, producing a highly poisonous neurotoxin in the blood, spreading to the nervous system. The infection is usually transmitted through deep puncture wounds or cuts or scratches that are not cleaned well. Most cases in the United States are associated with such wounds as punctures, lacerations, or abrasions. Many people associate tetanus with rusty nails and other dirty objects, but any wound can be a source. Less-common ways of getting tetanus are intravenous drug use, animal scratches and bites, surgical wounds, dental work, and therapeutic abortion. Cases have also been reported in people with no known wound or medical condition.

SYMPTOMS. The first symptom of tetanus is a stiffened and often locked jaw that prevents the patient from opening his/her mouth or swallowing. This is also called "trismus" and results in a facial expression called a sardonic smile (or risus sardonicus). Stiffness of the neck and other muscles throughout the body and uncontrollable spasms often follow. Sometimes these convulsions are severe enough to cause broken bones. The bacterial toxin (*tetanospasmin*) affects the nerve endings, causing a continuous stimulation of muscles. Other symptoms include:

• irritability

• restlessness

• loss of appetite

• drooling

People who have localized tetanus experience **pain** and tingling only at the wound site and spasms in nearby muscles.

The symptoms of neonatal tetanus typically become noticeable by the baby's third day. At that time, the infant will stop nursing, and his or her body will become increasingly rigid, eventually taking on a characteristic position with the back arched. Convulsions follow. The fatality rate is at least 70%.

Diagnosis

Tetanus is diagnosed by a combination of a physical exam; appearance of muscle spasms, stiffness, and pain indicative of the illness; a review of patient **immunization** history; and patient reports of recent wounds. Early diagnosis and treatment are crucial to recovery from tetanus.

Treatment

Tetanus is a life-threatening disease that requires immediate hospitalization, usually in an intensive care unit (ICU). Treatment can take several weeks and includes **antibiotics** to kill the bacteria and shots of antitoxin to neutralize the toxin. If symptoms have progressed, doctors may prescribe sedatives, morphine, magnesium sulfate, beta blockers, or other medications to help with muscle spasms and to treat respiration and heart issues. In severe cases, patients are placed on an artificial respirator. Recovery can take six weeks or more. After recovery, since the levels of circulating toxin are too low to stimulate natural antibody production, the patient must still be immunized against this disease to prevent reinfection.

PROGNOSIS. About 10–20% of individuals who have tetanus die from the illness. Early diagnosis and treatment improves the prognosis. Neonatal tetanus has a mortality rate of at least 70%.

Prevention

Pre-exposure vaccination

A vaccine is available for tetanus. It is often combined with vaccines for **diphtheria** and/or pertussis. The vaccines are known as DTaP, Tdap, DT, and Td. Specific vaccines are given to individuals at different stages of their lives. For instance, children receive five doses of DTap, four of them by the time they reach 18 months old, and one more between the ages of 4–6. Td is a booster shot for adolescents and adults, and is administered at 10-year intervals.

If a child did not receive the full vaccine regimen, or if an adult never received the vaccine, a doctor should be consulted to arrange the proper vaccine administration.

KEY TERMS

Clostridium—A genus of deadly bacteria that are responsible for tetanus and other serious diseases, including botulism and gas gangrene from war wounds. The bacteria thrive without oxygen.

DTaP—A vaccine that combines diphtheria and tetanus toxoids, and accellular pertussis.

DTP—Diphtheria, tetanus, and whole-cell pertussis vaccine.

Td—Tetanus and diphtheria vaccine.

Toxin—A poisonous substance that flows through the body.

Wound—Any injury that breaks the skin, including cuts, scratches, and puncture wounds.

Side effects of the tetanus vaccine are minor: soreness, redness, or swelling at the site of the injection that appear any time from a few hours to two days after the vaccination and go away in a day or two. Serious allergic or other reactions do occur, but they "are so rare it is hard to tell if they are caused by the vaccine," according to the **Centers for Disease Control and Prevention**. The risk of acquiring tetanus is far higher than the very small risk of having a bad reaction to the vaccine.

Post-exposure care

Keeping wounds and scratches clean is important in preventing infection. Since this organism grows only in the absence of oxygen, wounds must be adequately cleaned of dead tissue and foreign substances. Run cool water over the wound and wash it with a mild soap. Dry it with a clean cloth or sterile gauze. To help prevent infection, apply an antibiotic cream or ointment and cover the wound with a bandage. The longer a wound takes to heal, the greater the chance of infection. If the wound fails to heal, is red or warm, or drains or swells, consult a doctor.

Effects on public health

Tetanus and neonatal tetanus occur rarely in the United States. Neonatal tetanus is, however, a major health concern in developing countries. In 1988, the **World Health Organization (WHO)** put the number of deaths from neonatal tetanus worldwide at 787,000. Unhygienic conditions present during delivery typically were the cause of infections with *C. tetani*. In these cases, medical care was often lacking for those babies who developed neonatal tetanus.

QUESTIONS TO ASK YOUR DOCTOR

- When was my last tetanus shot? Do I need a booster?
- When should my child get the initial tetanus vaccine?
- My child has been sick. Should he still get a tetanus vaccine now?
- My child had a bad reaction to the initial tetanus vaccine. Should she still get the next scheduled tetanus shot?

Costs to society

A 2010 study in the *International Journal of Epidemiology* provided what it called "clear evidence" that a regimen of tetanus immunization had a high impact on the disease. Based on immunization costs of about 60 cents per dose, including full operational costs, and the capability for even weak healthcare systems to disseminate the immunizations, the authors supported vaccinations and related tetanus-elimination goals.

Efforts and solutions

Following WHO's estimation of 787,000 neonatal-tetanus deaths per year, WHO's decision-making body (the World Health Association) along with the United Nations Children's Fund (UNICEF) and the United Nations Population Fund (UNFPA) took action. In 1989, they set a goal of eliminating maternal and neonatal tetanus and established a program called the Maternal and Neonatal Tetanus (MNT) Elimination Initiative. By 2008, the number of deaths had dropped to 59,000. The initiative is still active, especially in the 34 countries that had not eliminated MNT as of February 2012.

Resources

PERIODICALS

Blencowe, Hanna, et al. "Tetanus Toxoid Immunization to Reduce Mortality From Neonatal Tetanus." *International Journal of Epidemiology.* 39, suppl. 1 (2010): i102–109

WEBSITES

"Clostridium." Medical Microbiology Site, Center for Environmental Health and Safety, Southern Illinois University Carbondale.http://www.cehs.siu.edu/fix/medmicro/clost.htm (accessed September 4, 2012).

"Diphtheria, Tetanus, and Pertussis Vaccines: What You Need to Know." Centers for Disease Control and Prevention.

http://www.cdc.gov/vaccines/pubs/vis/downloads/vis-dtap.pdf (accessed September 17, 2012).

"Maternal and Neonatal Tetanus (MNT) Elimination." World Health Organization. http://www.who.int/immunization_monitoring/diseases/MNTE_initiative/en/index.html (accessed September 4, 2012).

"Tetanus." Centers for Disease Control and Prevention. http://www.cdc.gov/nip/publications/pink/tetanus.pdf. (accessed September 4, 2012).

"Tetanus." MedLinePlus, U.S. National Library of Medicine, National Institutes of Health. http://www.nlm.nih.gov/medlineplus/tetanus.html (accessed September 4, 2012).

UNICEF, World Health Organization (WHO), United Nations Population Fund (UNFPA) "Maternal and Neonatal Tetanus Elimination by 2005." http://www.unicef.org/health/files/MNTE_strategy_paper.pdf (accessed September 14, 2012).

ORGANIZATIONS

Centers for Disease Control and Prevention (CDC), 1600 Clifton Road, Atlanta, GA 30333, (800) 232-4636, cdcinfo@cdc.gov, http://www.cdc.gov

United Nations Population Fund (UNFPA), 605 Third Avenue, New York, NY 10158, (212) 297-5000, hq@unfpa.org, http://www.unfpa.org/

World Health Organization, Avenue Appia 20, 1211 Geneva 27, Switzerland, http://www.who.int/.

Lori De Milto
Leslie Mertz, Ph.D.

Tobacco control

Definition

Tobacco control is any effort to reduce or eliminate the use of tobacco, including methods such as the use of public media, banning the use of tobacco in public or private locations, and raising taxes on tobacco products.

Purpose

Smoking increases the risk of coronary **heart disease** by two to four times; of **stroke** by two to four times; of lung **cancer** in men by 23 times; of lung cancer in women by 13 times; and of chronic obstructive lung diseases by 12 to 13 times. The use of tobacco thus is a major contributor to the most serious health problems faced in society as of late 2012. Tobacco control programs are designed to reduce the use of tobacco products and, therefore, reduce the risk of these and other health problems.

Description

The earliest scientific evidence about the harmful effects of tobacco use dates to the middle of the twentieth century (although data existed prior to this time about the risks of smoking). By the 1960s, governmental and professional agencies had begun to take action to make the risks of smoking better known to the general public, with the goal of reducing tobacco use. The key event during this period was the issuance in the United States of the Surgeon General's report *Smoking and Health*, which summarized much of the scientific evidence showing the connection between tobacco use and health problems. A year later, the U.S. Public Health Service (PHS) established the National Clearinghouse for Smoking and Health to promote antismoking efforts (renamed the Office of Smoking and Health of the **Centers for Disease Control and Prevention**), and the British Parliament adopted the first bans on tobacco advertising on television. The next half century saw a protracted and vituperative battle between the tobacco companies and governmental and nongovernmental agencies concerned about the health effects of tobacco use. For almost that entire period, the tobacco companies continued to assert that there was no reputable scientific evidence of the harmful effects of tobacco on human health. Eventually, the tide turned, every tobacco company finally admitted to the extensive existence of such evidence, and most admitted that they had known about the evidence and decided to keep it secret until almost the end of the twentieth century.

Governmental agencies, professional associations, and public health agencies at the international, national, regional, state, and local levels have designed and implemented a large number of campaigns to reduce tobacco use. These campaigns make use of a number of tools, including increasing tobacco taxes, banning advertising in the media, banning smoking in both public and private areas, health warnings on tobacco products, and vigorous educational programs encouraging people to stop smoking or not to begin smoking. Such educational efforts are often focused especially on children and adolescents in an effort to discourage them from ever starting to use tobacco. Perhaps the most comprehensive of all tobacco control initiatives is the Framework Convention on Tobacco Control of the **World Health Organization**, first proposed in 1993 and finally realized in 1998 with the adoption of the Tobacco Free Initiative (TFI). In 2012, the TFI has field offices in six regions, Africa, the Americas, the Eastern Mediterranean, Europe, Southeast Asia, and the Western Pacific, and in a handful of countries where the tobacco epidemic is considered to be "particularly grave," such as Bangladesh, India, Indonesia, and Thailand. **WHO** operatives in these regions work with local health officials to develop campaigns to reduce tobacco use in each location.

A number of organizations concerned with public health issues have joined the battle to combat tobacco use. For example, Action on Smoking and Health (ASH) was founded in England by the Royal College of Physicians in 1971 when it appeared that the government was unlikely to take effective action against the use of tobacco. The ASH movement has since spread to a number of other countries in the world, including Wales, Scotland, Australia, New Zealand, and the United States. Another anti–tobacco organization that started in the United Kingdom is the Smokefree Coalition, a consortium that in 2012 consists of well over a hundred individual health groups, such as Breast Cancer Care, the British Medical Association, the Circulation Foundation, Fatherhood Institute, National Youth Agency, and National Health Service offices in dozens of communities. In the United States, many antismoking groups focus on statewide issues, such as the Arkansas Nonsmokers' Rights Foundation, Tobacco Prevention Program of Santa Barbara (California), Atlanta (Georgia) Coalition against Tobacco, Goshen (Indiana) Community Smoking Awareness, and OOPS (Organization Opposed Public Smoking; Reno, Nevada). Many national associations dealing with specific health problems and their state affiliates are almost always at the forefront of tobacco control programs. These agencies include groups such as the American Lung Association, American Cancer Society, and American Heart Association.

One of the most significant events in the history of the tobacco control movement was the Tobacco Master Settlement Agreement (TMSA), signed in November 1998 between the four largest tobacco companies in the United States and the attorneys general of the 50 states and the District of Columbia. The agreement resolved a large and complex lawsuit originally brought by 46 state attorneys general against Philip Morris, Inc., R. J. Reynolds, Brown & Williamson, and Lorillard who, among them, controlled about 97 percent of the tobacco market in the United States. The suit asked for reparations to the states for the costs of tobacco–related healthcare costs over the years. After years of litigation, the four tobacco companies agreed to pay the states a total of $206 billion over the first 25 years of the agreement, along with a number of other provisions that included:

- a cessation or reduction of certain types of marketing practices, especially those aimed at children and adolescents
- dissolution of certain tobacco advocacy organizations, including the Tobacco Institute and the Council for Tobacco Research
- funding of a new antismoking group known as the American Legacy Foundation, chartered to carry out campaigns against the use of tobacco

In return for these concessions, the tobacco companies were relieved in perpetuity of any future lawsuits against them for health problems resulting from the use of tobacco products. Since the original agreement, tobacco companies have also reached a financial understanding with tobacco growers in 14 states to compensate them for loss of income resulting from the settlement, and 41 additional small tobacco companies have also signed the TMSA, accounting for essentially all tobacco companies in the United States.

Professional publications

Probably the most important single journal in the field of tobacco control is the journal of that name, *Tobacco Control*, published by BMJ Journals. The journal publishes peer–reviewed papers on the nature and consequences of tobacco use worldwide; the effect of tobacco on health, society, the economy, and the environment; efforts to prevent and control the use of tobacco worldwide; education and policies related to tobacco control; the ethics of tobacco use and tobacco control policies; and the activities of the tobacco industry and its supporters. A somewhat more specialized journal is *Tobacco Control and Public Health in Eastern Europe*, which is published in Russian, Ukrainian, and English. In addition, a number of public health journals publish papers on the topic of tobacco control, including the *Journal of Public Health Policy*, the *Journal of Public Health*, and the *Journal of Preventive Medicine*.

Resources

BOOKS

Cairney, Paul, Donley T. Studlar, and Hadii Mamudu. *Global Tobacco Control: Power, Policy, Governance and Transfer.* Houndmills, Basingstoke, Hampshire; New York: Palgrave Macmillan, 2012.

Gupta, Prakash C., et al. *Despair to Hope . . . : Breaking New Grounds in Tobacco Control.* New Delhi: Health for the Millions Trust, 2012.

York, Nancy L., and Suzanne S. Prevost. *Tobacco Control.* Philadelphia: Saunders, 2012.

PERIODICALS

Hackbarth, D. P. "Preventing Adolescent Tobacco Use and Assisting Young People to Quit: Population-, Community-, and Individually Focused Evidence-Based Interventions." *Nursing Clinics of North America* 47. 1. (2012): 119–40.

Nelson, D. E., et al. "News Media Outreach and Newspaper Coverage of Tobacco Control." *Health Promotion Practice* 13. 5. (2012): 642–47.

Sanders, E., et al. "Does the Use of Ingredients Added to Tobacco Increase Cigarette Addictiveness?: A Detailed Analysis." *Inhalation Toxicology* 24. 4. (2012): 227–45.

Schauer, G. L., S. M. Zbikowski, and J. R. Thompson. "Results From an Outreach Program for Health Systems Change in Tobacco Cessation." *Health Promotion Practice* 13. 5. (2012): 657–65.

WEBSITES

Institute for Global Tobacco Control. Johns Hopkins Bloomberg School of Public Health. http://www.jhsph.edu/research/centers-and-institutes/institute-for-global-tobacco-control/ (accessed October 14, 2012).

State of Tobacco Control. American Lung Association. http://www.stateoftobaccocontrol.org/ (accessed October 14, 2012).

Tobacco Control Laws. Campaign for Tobacco-Free Kids. http://www.tobaccocontrollaws.org/ (accessed October 14, 2012).

Tobacco Control State Highlights. Centers for Disease Control and Prevention. http://www.cdc.gov/tobacco/data_statistics/state_data/state_highlights/2010/index.htm (accessed October 14, 2012).

ORGANIZATIONS

American Cancer Society (ACS). International Tobacco Surveillance, 1599 Clifton Rd., N.E., Atlanta, GA 30329-4251, (404) 327-6554, Fax: (404) 327-6450, omar.shafey@cancer.org, www.cancer.org.

World Health Organization. Tobacco Free Initiative (WHO TFI), Avenue Appia 20 1211, Geneva, Switzerland 27, 41 22 791 2126, Fax: 41 22 791 4832, tfi@who.int, www.who.int/tobacco/.

David E. Newton, EdD

Trachoma

Definition

Trachoma, which is also called granular conjunctivitis or Egyptian ophthalmia, is a contagious, chronic inflammation of the mucous membranes of the eyes, caused by *Chlamydia trachomatis*. It is characterized by swelling of the eyelids, sensitivity to light, and eventual scarring of the conjunctivae and corneas of the eyes. Conjunctivitis is an inflammation of the conjunctiva.

Description

Trachoma is the leading cause of blindness in the world. Loss of vision results from recurrent untreated infections, which lead to scarring on the conjunctivae and corneas. As scar tissue accumulates, the conjunctivae and corneas become opaque, resulting in visual impairment. Trachoma is preventable through proper **hygiene** and **sanitation** and is treated with **antibiotics** and sometimes surgery.

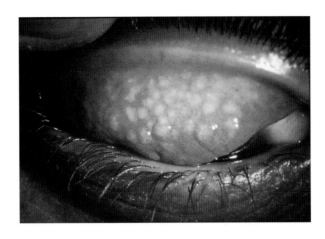

Close up of human eye with growth covering pupil and iris, growth is yellowish and bumpy, outer area of growth is red *(Custom Medical Stock Photo)*

Origin

Trachoma was initially reported by Egyptian, Greek, and Roman physicians in ancient times. A visitor to Egypt in 1745 described the region as "the land of the blind." In 1798, when General Napoleon Bonaparte and the French revolutionary army invaded Egypt, soldiers acquired trachoma and spread the disease to Europe upon their return. By the 1900s, trachoma was prevalent throughout North America and Europe. In the United States, it was endemic in Alabama, Arkansas, Kentucky, Missouri, Oklahoma, Tennessee, Virginia, West Virginia, and neighboring states. As sanitation conditions improved, the prevalence of trachoma in these areas declined radically. However, it continued to be a problem on Native American reservations. In 1937, while working on a Sioux reservation, a physician named Fred Loe, MD, first treated two trachoma patients with sulfonamides. Improvement occurred after five days, and within one month both patients were cured. Shortly thereafter, Dr. Loe treated another 140 patients and realized a 90% cure rate.

Demographics

Nearly 8 million individuals have visual impairment caused by trachoma and more than 500 million are at risk of blindness from it. Trachoma is endemic in more than 50 nations and is most prevalent in portions of Africa, Asia, and the Middle East. In the United States, trachoma is rare, but is found in impoverished regions, such as Appalachia and Native American reservations, where living conditions are crowded and hygiene is poor.

The infection is highly contagious in its early stages, making children more susceptible because of their physical contact with one another. In some urban communities, 60 to 90% of children may have trachoma. Close proximity to children on a daily basis make adult women more susceptible than men.

Causes and symptoms

Trachoma is caused by *C. trachomatis*, a parasitic organism closely related to bacteria. A highly contagious infection, trachoma is transmitted by insects, by hand-to-eye contact, or by the sharing of infected handkerchiefs or towels. The incubation period is about a week. Because close contact facilitates the spread of trachoma, it can easily spread throughout families and community areas.

The early symptoms of trachoma include the development of follicles (small sacs) on the conjunctivae of the upper eyelids, **pain**, swollen eyelids, a discharge, tearing, and sensitivity to light. If the infection is not treated, the follicles develop into large yellow or gray pimples, and small blood vessels develop inside the cornea. In most cases, both eyes are infected.

Repeated infections eventually lead to contraction and turning-in of the eyelids, scarring of the corneas and conjunctivae, eventual blockage of the tear ducts, and blindness.

Diagnosis

Diagnosis is based on a combination of the patient's history (especially for those living or traveling in areas with high rates of trachoma) and examination of the eyes. The doctor will look for the presence of follicles or scarring. He or she will take a small sample of cells from the patient's conjunctivae and examine them, following a procedure called Giemsa staining, to confirm the diagnosis.

Treatment

Treatment of early-stage trachoma consists of four to six weeks of antibiotic treatment with tetracycline, erythromycin, or sulfonamides. Antibiotics should be given without waiting for laboratory test results. Treatment may combine oral medication with antibiotic ointment applied directly to the eyes. A single-dose treatment with azithromycin is an alternative method. Tetracyclines should not be given to pregnant women or children below the age of seven years.

Trachoma treatment may also include a surgical procedure called bilamellar tarsal rotation, which corrects the eyelashes that turn inward. The success rate of the surgery is 80%. If the eyelid does not close properly, a more complex operation is required.

Prognosis

The prognosis for full recovery is excellent if the patient is treated promptly. If the infection has progressed to the stage of follicle development, **prevention** of blindness depends on the severity of the follicles, the presence of additional bacterial infections, and the development of scarring.

Prevention

Vaccines offer temporary protection against trachoma, but there is no permanent **immunization**. Prevention depends upon good hygiene and public health measures:

- Individuals should seek immediate treatment if they show signs of eye infection, and should minimize their contact with others.
- Education should include instruction on handwashing carefully before touching eyes.
- Individuals should seek protection from flies or gnats that settle around the eyes.
- If someone has trachoma (or any eye infection), others should not share towels, pillowcases, etc., and these items should be thoroughly washed.
- If medications are prescribed, the patients should follow the doctor's instructions carefully.

Efforts and solutions

In 1997, the **World Health Organization (WHO)** developed the Alliance for Global Elimination of Trachoma (GET 2020) with an objective of eliminating trachoma by the year 2020. Its efforts incorporate a four-pronged approach using the acronym SAFE:

- **S**urgery to correct the advanced, blinding stage of the disease
- **A**ntibiotics to treat active infection
- **F**acial cleanliness
- **E**nvironmental improvements in the areas of water and sanitation to reduce disease transmission

By 2012, the SAFE strategy was in place in 36 nations. As part of the SAFE strategy, the **WHO** recommends widespread distribution of oral azithromycin in communities afflicted with trachoma. A study reported in *Journal of the American Medical Association (JAMA)* in 2009 found that Ethiopian children experienced reduced mortality when their trachoma was treated with the drug.

Established in 2004, the International Coalition for Trachoma Control (ICTC) is also involved in the worldwide effort to eliminate trachoma and is an advocate for the WHO SAFE strategy. The group collects and disseminates information regarding activities related to trachoma; identifies additional partners in the efforts to control the disease; and heightens awareness of trachoma and strategies underway to address it locally, nationally, and internationally.

Helen Keller International (HKI) also advocates the WHO SAFE strategy. The organization trains surgeons and nurses, provides antibiotic supplies and items needed for surgery, and facilitates the follow-up by patients. HKI provides education to children, instructing them on preventing trachoma and the need to frequently wash their faces. As part of its commitment to eliminate neglected tropical diseases (NTDs), the United Kingdom plays an active role in the quest to eradicate trachoma. In 2012, the United Kingdom announced its support of the International Trachoma Initiative, along with other non-governmental organizations and academic establishments, to perform mapping in more than 30 of the most impoverished nations in the world. The mapping project, led by international charity Sightsavers, serves to identify persons most at risk.

Patients with complications from untreated or repeated infections are treated surgically. Surgery can be used for corneal transplantation or to correct eyelid deformities.

KEY TERMS

Conjunctivitis—Inflammation of the conjunctivae, which are the mucous membranes covering the white part of the eyeball (sclera) and lining the inside of the eyelids.

Cornea—The transparent front part of the eye that allows light to enter.

Ophthalmia—Inflammation of the eye. Usually severe and affecting the conjunctiva. Trachoma is sometimes called Egyptian ophthalmia.

Resources

BOOKS

McPhee, Stephen, and Maxine Papadakis. *Current Medical Diagnosis and Treatment, 2010*, 49th ed. New York: McGraw-Hill Medical, 2009.

PERIODICALS

Burton, Matthew J., and David C. W. Mabey. "The Global Burden of Trachoma: A Review." *PLoS Neglected Tropical Diseases* 3, no. 10 (2009): e460.
Emerson, Paul, et. al. "SAFE Strategy for Blinding Trachoma Addresses Sanitation, The Other Half of MDG7." *The Lancet* 380, no. 9836, 27–28 (2012).

Feibel, Robert M., MD. "Fred Loe, MD, and the History of Trachoma." *Archives of Ophthalmology* 129, no.4 (2011).

Porco, Travis C., PhD, MPH, et.al."Effect of Mass Distribution of Azithromycin for Trachoma Control on Overal Mortality in Ethiopian Children: A Randomized Trial." *The Journal of the American Medical Association (JAMA)* 302(9), 962-968 (2009).

ORGANIZATIONS

Centers for Disease Control and Prevention, 1600 Clifton Road, Atlanta, GA 30333, (800) CDC-INFO (232-4636), cdcinfo@cdc.gov, http://www.cdc.gov.

Helen Keller International, 325 Park Avenue South, 12th Floor, New York, NY 10010, (212) 532-0544, info@hki.org, http://www.hki.org.

International Coalition for Trachoma Control, http://www.trachomacoalition.org.

International Trachoma Initiative, 325 Swanton Way, Decatur, GA 30030, (800) 765-7173, iti@taskforce.org, http://www.trachoma.org.

World Health Organization, Avenue Appia 20, 1211 Geneva, SWITZERLAND 27, 41 22 791-21-11, http://www.who.int.

Rebecca J. Frey, PhD
Rhonda Cloos, RN

Travel health

Definition

Travel is the process of leaving one's home for a journey to another city, town, state, or nation. Maintaining one's health is an important consideration before planning a journey and during the period of travel.

Description

Factors that travelers should take into account when planning a trip include their anticipated health and well being while away from home, potential illness associated with the mode of travel or destination, special precautions, such as vaccines, that may be needed before traveling to certain destinations, items to pack that are essential and may not be available away from home, and warnings that may be in place regarding a destination. Travelers should also be aware of regulations in place regarding the mode of travel.

The United States Bureau of Consular Affairs, a division of the U.S. Department of State, provides a website with updated warnings for travelers. The site contains warnings regarding specific countries.

Health conditions associated with travel

Venous Thromboembolism

Venous thromboembolism (VTE) is a concern for travelers, especially during the journey to their destination. VTE is made up of two conditions: deep vein thrombosis (DVT) and pulmonary embolism (PE). DVT occurs when a deep vein, usually in the legs, is blocked by a clot. The blood clot may form, usually in the legs, due to blood pooling after prolonged sitting in a car, airplane, or other mode of transportation. If the clot breaks loose, it may pass through the vessels into the lung, resulting in a PE, which may be life-threatening.

VTE has been recognized as a problem for airplane travelers as far back as the 1950s. The risk is due to sitting in one position, without movement, for an extended period of time. While studies have shown that the risk for VTE applies to any form of travel in which one stays in the same position for a long period of time, air travel creates higher risk for persons who are less than 5 feet, 3 inches in height. Travelers are two times more likely than non-travelers to develop VTE.

The **Centers for Disease Control and Prevention** lists these risks for VTE on their website, http://www.cdc.gov:

- history of recent major surgery
- paralytic injury to the spinal cord
- victim of multiple trauma
- presence of malignancy
- congestive heart failure, respiratory failure
- hormone replacement therapy, oral contraceptive use
- history of previous VTE
- inherited hypercoagulable medical condition
- acquired hypercoagulable medical condition
- pregnancy
- age of 40 years or more
- obesity
- immobility
- male gender

SIGNS AND SYMPTOMS OF VTE. A person with DVT will show signs such as swelling, redness, **pain**, increased warmth, or feelings of tenderness over the skin in the clot area. These symptoms may be confused with an injury or infection. Some DVTs do not cause symptoms. In these cases, the PE is the first sign that a DVT has occurred.

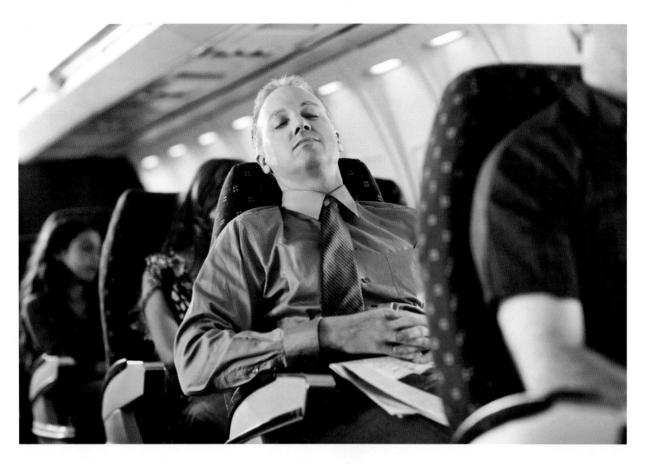

Precautions taken before and during plane travel can cut down on travel-related health problems. *(©iStockphoto.com/ Lifesizeimages)*

Signs of a PE may resemble a heart attack or **stroke**, and may be mild to severe. If a clot has reached the lungs, the most common symptoms are chest pain and shortness of breath. Other signs include feeling dizzy, faint, or having a general sense of malaise.

DIAGNOSIS OF VTE. Imaging tests, such as duplex venous ultrasound, venography, and CT and MRI scans, are required to definitively diagnose DVT. PE is diagnosed via specialized computed tomography (CT) scans or ventilation-perfusion scans.

PREVENTION OF VTE. The American College of Chest Physicians (ACCP) suggests certain measures may help travelers prevent VTE:

• If a flight is eight hours or longer, the traveler should avoid tight clothing around the waist or legs, and should stay hydrated. He or she should also perform frequent contractions of the muscles in the lower legs.

• Those who face extended travel and possess additional risk factors for VTE should take the proscribed precautionary steps and may use below the knee graduated compression stockings, which have been fitted

properly or one preventive dose of low-molecular-weight heparin, administered prior to departure.

• For those traveling long distances, the use of aspirin as a way to prevent VTE is not recommended.

TREATMENT OF VTE. Treatment for DVT without PE usually consists of warfarin (Coumadin) or fondaparinux (Arixta) administered on an outpatient basis. If a patient requires hospitalization, he or she may be given intravenous heparain.

If PE develops, the patient is hospitalized and given anticoagulants.

Travelers' diarrhea

Travelers' diarrhea (TD) is a common condition, experienced by 30 to 70% of travelers, according to the Centers for Disease Control and Prevention. The rate of occurrence depends on the travelers' destinations. The most common cause is poor **hygiene** in restaurants.

In 80 to 90% of cases, the diarrhea is due to bacteria that has been ingested. Because protozoan pathogens take longer to cause symptoms, they account for less than

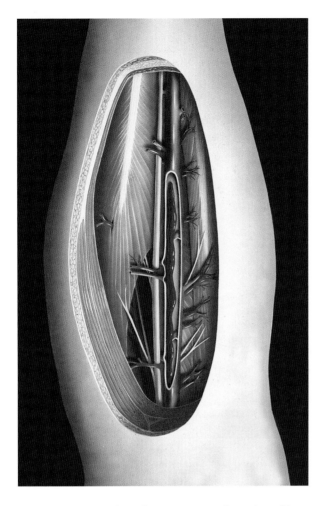

Deep vein thrombosis, which can occur on long plane rides due to lack of circulation. *(Illustration by Electronic Illustrators Group. © 2013 Cengage Learning)*

8% of TD. The most common bacteria pathogens seen in TD are *Escherichia coli, Campylobacter jejuni, Shigella.* and *Salmonella.* The most common protozoan pathogen in TD is *Giardia.*

While males and females are equally at risk, young adults experience TD more commonly than older travelers.

OCCURRENCE OF TD. In terms of TD, the **CDC** divides the world into three grades of risk: low, intermediate, and high.

• Low-risk—United States, Canada, Australia, New Zealand, Japan, and Northern and Western Europe.

• Intermediate-risk—Eastern Europe, South Africa, and some Caribbean islands

• High-risk—Most of Asia, the Middle East, Africa, Mexico, and Central and South America

PREVENTION AND TREATMENT OF TD. Measures that may help prevent TD include use of alcohol-based hand

sanitizers that contain at least 60% alcohol, careful selection of foods and drinks (avoiding items that were washed in nonpotable **water**, or that sat on a buffet for extended periods, or were not well cooked).

Bismuth subsalicylate (BSS) is the main drug used to prevent TD. In the United States, BSS is commonly sold under the trade name Pepto-Bismol. While the use of probiotics has been researched, results are inconclusive.

Antibiotics taken on a prophylactic basis effectively prevent TD. However, this form of prevention is not recommended for most travelers because allergy may develop, as well as antibiotic resistance.

Medications that slow the movement of the colon, or antimotility agents, help to reduce symptoms. These medications are rarely administered to young children.

A major problem associated with TD is the loss of electrolytes. Preventing dehydration is a major concern for young children as well as adults who have a chronic illness. It is important for travelers to take in only rehydrating agents that have been purified. In developing countries, **World Health Organization** ORS (oral rehydrating salts) are often available, and may be added to water that has been boiled or treated.

If the TD has been caused by a parasite, medications used in treatment include metronidazole, tinidazole, and nitazoxanide.

Vaccinations needed for travel

Travel to certain parts of the world may require vaccinations to avoid becoming ill with a disease that is prevalent in the area. Travelers should check the Centers for Disease Control and Prevention website or their local travel clinic well before departure. This is important because some vaccines require several doses, as well as a few weeks or longer to reach optimal effectiveness. Depending on the destination, one or more vaccines from this list may be recommended.

• Measles/Mumps/Rubella (if traveler is not current)—there has been a resurgence of measles in some areas

• Polio

• Avian Influenza A (H5N1)

• Bacille Calmette-Gužrin (BCG)—for the prevention of tuberculosis (TB)

• Hepatitis A

• Hepatitis B

• Rabies

• Cholera

• Diphtheria Tetanus (if traveler is not current with these)

• Meningococcal diseas

• Typhoid

Travelers who are immunodefficient should avoid live vaccines and should discuss this issue with their healthcare provider.

In certain parts of the world, **malaria** is a problem. While a vaccine for malaria is not available, travelers may take preventive measures, such as avoiding mosquito bites through clothing, as well as using insect repellents and considering the use of prophylactic medications (although there are drug resistant strains).

Insect and animal bites

In some areas, insect and tick bites may pose a threat. The CDC recommends using an insect repellent with 30 to 50% DEET. If picaridin is to be used, in 7% or 15% concentrations, it must be applied more often than insect repellents containing DEET.

In areas where mosquitoes and other insects are a problem, travelers should cover themselves by wearing long-sleeved shirts that remain tucked in, as well as long pants and hats. If an area has ticks and fleas, travelers should wear boots and tuck their pants into their socks.

It is important to keep **tetanus** vaccinations current.

Travel while pregnant

The American College of Obstetrics and Gynecology states that it is most safe for a pregnant woman to travel during the second trimester of pregnancy. The organization recommends against traveling overseas during the third trimester due to issues involving access to health care should problems develop such as hypertension, phlebitis, or premature labor. A pregnant woman should discuss travel with her health care provider prior to planning or taking a trip.

If a pregnant women does travel, the issues that should be addressed before departure are:

• intrauterine pregnancy should be confirmed and ectopic pregnancy ruled out

• health insurance coverage for out-of-town services should be investigated

• medical facilities at the destination should be identified and researched

• the need for prenatal care while away should be determined

• the availability of blood that has been screened for HIV and hepatitis B and C in the destination should be determined. The pregnant traveler should be aware of her blood type. Pregnant travelers who are Rh-negative should receive anti-D-immune globulin on a prophylactic basis at approximately 28 weeks' gestation. The immune globulin dose should be repeated following childbirth if the baby is Rh positive.

• risk for influenza should be determined, and the pregnant traveler should discuss influenza vaccine with her physician or healthcare provider

• the presence of TB at the destination should be determined. If risk for TB exists in the region, the pregnant traveler should have a TB skin test before and after traveling.

The most serious risks for pregnant travelers are motor vehicle accidents, **hepatitis** E, and scuba diving (which should be avoided due to the risk of the fetus developing decompression syndrome).

Travel and chronic disease

Travelers who have chronic diseases should discuss with their personal physician or health care provider any special needs or challenges they may experience while traveling. They should request from their physician copies of recent lab tests, EKG tests, or x-rays, depending on the chronic disease that they have. These individuals should, in advance of travel, determine how to obtain medical care at their destination, and what the costs may be if such care becomes necessary.

Persons who take medications on a regular basis should keep these drugs with them at all times. Air travelers should pack medications in their carry-on luggage. They should also carry copies of prescriptions and telephone numbers of their physicians and pharmacies.

Access to water

If a destination's tap water is not chlorinated or if the area's **sanitation** methods are poor, particularly in developing nations, it is important for the traveler to have access to safe **drinking water**. If the tap water is not safe to drink, it also is not safe for making juice, washing produce, using ice, or brushing teeth.

Alternatives when tap water is not safe include bottled water as long as it originates from a source that is trusted. The cap should be completely sealed. If it is not, this may indicate that the bottle was refilled from the tap.

Water may be boiled and cooled. It must be boiled vigorously for one minute and cooled to room temperature without the addition of ice. If the altitude is higher than 6,562 feet (more than 2,000 meters), the water must be boiled for three minutes, or chemical disinfection must be used after the water has been boiled for one minute. Persons must use extreme care with chemical disinfection to avoid a lethal dose. Directions for safely disinfecting water with chemicals may be found at the CDC website. Pregnant women, persons with thyroid conditions, or persons with known hypersensitivity to iodine should not drink water that has been disinfected with iodine. This form of decontamination should not be used continuously for more than a few weeks at a time, according to the CDC.

Resources

BOOKS

Brunette, Gary W., ed. *CDC Health Information for International Travel 2012: The Yellow Book.* New York, NY: Oxford University Press, 2012.

PERIODICALS

Chandra, D., E. Parsini, and D. Mozaffarian. "Meta-analysis: Travel and Risk for Venous Thromboembolism." *Annals of Internal Medicine* 151, no. 3 (2009): 180-190.

Shah, N., H.L. Dupont, and D.J. Ramsey. "Global Etiology of Traveler's Diarrhea." *American Journal of Tropical Medicine* 80, no. 4 (2009): 609-14.

WEBSITES

SafeTravel.dot.gov. http://safetravel.dot.gov/ (accessed September 29, 2012).

Travel Safety. http://www.usa.gov/Topics/Usgresponse/Travel-Safely.shtml (accessed September 29, 2012).

Travel.State.Gov U.S. Department of State. http://travel.state.gov/travel/cis_pa_tw/tw/tw_1764.html (accessed September 29, 2012).

ORGANIZATIONS

Centers for Disease Control and Prevention, 1600 Clifton Road, Atlanta, GA 30333, (800) CDC-INFO (232-4636), cdcinfo@cdc.gov, http://www.cdc.gov.

Rhonda LAST, RN

Tuberculosis

Definition

Tuberculosis (TB) is a chronic, potentially fatal contagious disease that most often affects the lungs but can affect other parts of the body. This **infectious disease** is caused by various strains of mycobacteria but usually by the tubercle bacillus (*Mycobacterium tuberculosis*). It causes small, round swellings (called tubercles) to form on mucous membranes. Tuberculosis is curable and preventable. However, as of 2012, TB is the second most fatal disease in the world, and only HIV/AIDS kills more people annually.

Description

Tuberculosis caused widespread problems in the nineteenth and early twentieth centuries. In 1815, TB caused one in four deaths in England (considered the peak of fatalities in Europe), while it caused one in six deaths in France in 1918. Tuberculosis was commonly called consumption until well into the twentieth century. In 1882, the German microbiologist and physician Heinrich Hermann Robert Koch (1843–1910) isolated the tubercle bacillus (species name *Mycobacterium tuberculosis*) that causes the disease. The tubercle bacillus is transmitted when an infected person coughs or sneezes and another person breathes in the infected droplets. The disease is not spread through kissing or other physical contact.

Before **antibiotics** were discovered in the mid-1900s, the only means of controlling the spread of TB was to isolate patients in sanatoriums or hospitals limited to patients with TB. This practice continues in some countries. The reason for this pattern of treatment was to separate the study of tuberculosis from mainstream medicine. Entire organizations were formed to study not only the disease as it affected individual patients, but also its impact on society. At the beginning of the twentieth century, more than 80% of the **population** in the United States was infected with TB before age 20, and tuberculosis was the single most common cause of death. By 1938, there were more than 700 specialized TB facilities in the United States.

Tuberculosis spread widely in Europe as the result of the industrial revolution in the late nineteenth century when many people moved to towns where they lived in crowded, unsanitary conditions. The disease became widespread somewhat later in the United States.

In the early 1940s, streptomycin was discovered and became the first antibiotic effective against *M. tuberculosis*. For the first time the infection began to be contained. Although other more effective anti-tuberculosis drugs that continue to reduce the number of TB cases have been developed in the past half-century, reports of active TB cases in the United States began to increase in the mid-1980s. This upsurge was in part a result of overcrowding and unsanitary conditions in the poor areas of large cities, prisons, and homeless shelters. Infected visitors and immigrants to the United States also contributed to the resurgence of TB. An additional factor was the **AIDS** epidemic. Individuals with HIV/AIDS are much more likely to develop tuberculosis because of their weakened immune systems than healthy individuals.

The number of reported TB cases in the United States peaked in 1993 and has since declined. New multidrug-resistant strains of TB (MDR TB) have

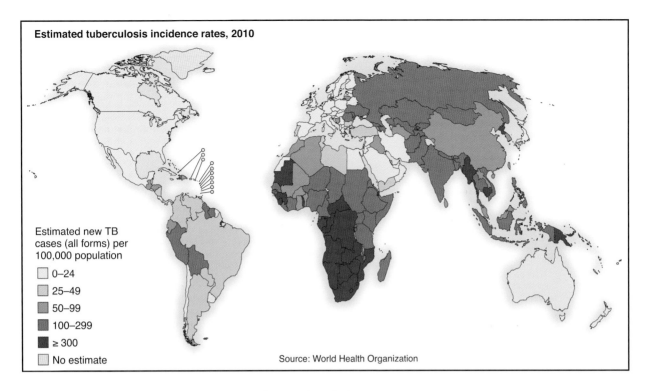

Estimated tuberculosis incidence rates, 2010

Estimated new TB
cases (all forms) per
100,000 population

- 0–24
- 25–49
- 50–99
- 100–299
- ≥ 300
- No estimate

Source: World Health Organization

(Illustration by Electronic Illustrators Group. © 2013 Cengage Learning)

become a major public health concern, with a presence in virtually all countries regularly surveyed by the **World Health Organization (WHO)**. In the mid-2000s, health officials worldwide joined to work at preventing a drug-resistant form of the disease from becoming widespread. By 2007, the **WHO** estimated that 13.7 million chronic, active cases of TB were present around the world.

In 2005, the U.S. **Centers for Disease Control and Prevention (CDC)** reported a record low number of 14,097 cases of active TB in the United States, of which 55% occurred in foreign-born individuals. However, the number of multi-drug resistant strains had increased 13.3% since 2000. The **CDC** estimated that in 2005 about 10 million people in the United States had latent (symptom-free) TB infections.

The WHO estimates that about one-third of the world's population is infected with *M. tuberculosis*. Of those infected, between 5% and 10% will develop active TB. Among individuals who have HIV/AIDS infections, the rate is much higher. The greatest number of active TB infections per capita is found in sub-Saharan Africa where AIDS is epidemic. About one-third of infections occur in Southeast Asia. The WHO estimates that TB caused about 1.6 million deaths worldwide in 2005. Although the rate per capita of active TB is declining worldwide, the absolute number of cases is increasing in many areas because of high population growth.

In 2010, approximately 8.8 million new cases were reported, along with about 1.4 million reported deaths associated with TB, mostly within developing countries of the world. In fact, over 95% of TB deaths occur in low-and middle-income countries. The countries of India and China accounted for about 40% of the world's reported cases of TB in 2010, while Africa reported 24% About 80% of the population in many Asian and African countries test positive for TB, while fewer than 10% do so in the United States. Between 2002 and 2008, the CDC reported that 27 outbreaks of TB involving 398 patients occurred in the United States. Twenty-four of the 27 outbreaks involved U.S.-born patients. One of the major features for nearly all cases was the presence of substance abuse.

The higher rates in developing countries is primarily due to higher rates of HIV infection and its corresponding development of AIDS as compared to developed countries. TB is the leading cause of death for people living with HIV, causing nearly one out of four deaths. However, the WHO reports that the number of people contracting TB is decreasing slowly each year. Its Millennium Development Goal is to reverse the spread of TB by 2015.

Risk factors

People with heightened risks of contracting TB include the elderly, certain racial and ethnic groups, and people with certain lifestyles.

FLORENCE B. SEIBERT (1897–1991)

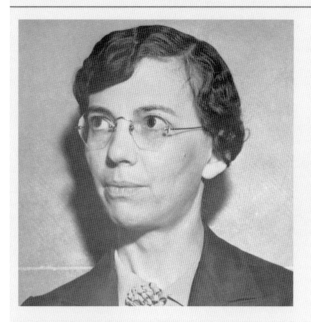

Florence Barbara Seibert was born on October 6, 1897, in Easton, Pennsylvania, the second of three children. She was the daughter of George Peter Seibert, a rug manufacturer and merchant, and Barbara (Memmert) Seibert. At the age of three she contracted polio. Despite her resultant handicaps, she completed high school, with the help of her highly supportive parents, and entered Goucher College in Baltimore, where she studied chemistry and zoology. She graduated in 1918, then worked under the direction of one of her chemistry teachers, Jessie E. Minor, at the Chemistry Laboratory of the Hammersley Paper Mill in Garfield, New Jersey. She and her professor, having responded to the call for women to fill positions vacated by men fighting in World War I, coauthored scientific papers on the chemistry of cellulose and wood pulps.

A biochemist who received her Ph.D. from Yale University in 1923, Florence B. Seibert is best known for her research in the biochemistry of tuberculosis. She developed the protein substance used for the tuberculosis skin test. The substance was adopted as the standard in 1941 by the United States and a year later by the World Health Organization. In addition, in the early 1920s, Seibert discovered that the sudden fevers that sometimes occurred during intravenous injections were caused by bacteria in the distilled water that was used to make the protein solutions. She invented a distillation apparatus that prevented contamination. This research had great practical significance later when intravenous blood transfusions became widely used in surgery. Seibert authored or coauthored more than a hundred scientific papers. Her later research involved the study of bacteria associated with certain cancers. Her many honors include five honorary degrees, induction into the National Women's Hall of Fame in Seneca Falls, New York (1990), the Garvan Gold Medal of the American Chemical Society (1942), and the John Elliot Memorial Award of the American Association of Blood Banks (1962). She died on August 23, 1991.

THE ELDERLY. More than 60% of cases in the United States are diagnosed in people between the ages of 25 and 65 years. About one-quarter of TB cases newly diagnosed occur in people over the age of 65. Many elderly individuals developed TB after acquiring latent TB infection years earlier. As they age, their immune systems can no longer control the disease, and they develop active TB symptoms. In addition, elderly people living in nursing homes and other group facilities are often in close contact with others who may be infected.

RACIAL AND ETHNIC GROUPS. Higher rates of TB are found in the non-white population in the United States, but health researchers have reported that this is related to the socioeconomic status of these groups rather than to race-related biological factors. Individuals of lower socioeconomic status tend to live in more crowded conditions and have less access to health care than higher socioeconomic status individuals. These conditions encourage infection with *M. tuberculosis*.

As of 2012, TB continues to be a major health problem in the United States among certain immigrant groups that come from countries where TB infection is common. California, New York, Texas, and Florida—all states with large immigrant populations—accounted for almost half of all active TB cases. The most common countries of origin for foreign-born persons in the United States with active TB were Mexico, the Philippines, Vietnam, India, and China.

LIFESTYLE FACTORS. The high risk of TB in AIDS patients extends to those infected by HIV who have not yet developed clinical signs of AIDS but whose immune systems are weakened by the virus. People who take drugs that suppress the immune system (for example, transplant patients) are also at higher risk of becoming infected, as are people who have silicosis, a lung disease. Individuals who abuse alcohol, intravenous drug abusers, and the homeless are also at increased risk of contracting TB.

KEY TERMS

Avian influenza—Influenza A virus usually found in birds, but transmitted to humans.

Bacille Calmette-Guérin (BCG)—Vaccine that protects from tuberculosis, derived from weakened live bovine tuberculosis bacillus.

Cholera—Infection of small intestine resulting in watery diarrhea.

Nonpotable—Not safe to drink.

Typhoid—Illness caused by *Salmonelli typhi*. This condition is life-threatening.

Demographics

People infected with TB have a 10% lifetime risk of falling ill with TB. Persons with compromised immune systems, such as people living with HIV, those with malnutrition or diabetes, or people who use tobacco, have a much higher risk of falling ill with TB. In fact, according to the WHO, people infected with HIV and TB are 21 to 34 times more likely to become sick with TB than people without those diseases. In addition, over 20% of TB cases worldwide are attributable to using tobacco products.

Causes and symptoms

The causes and symptoms of tuberculosis involve the way TB is transmitted into the body and its progression once inside. As TB develops inside the body, two common diseases can result: pulmonary tuberculosis and extrapulmonary tuberculosis. In addition, MDR TB has become a major concern in the world. Many similar diseases resemble tuberculosis.

Transmission

Tuberculosis spreads by droplet infection. When a person infected with *M. tuberculosis* exhales, coughs, or sneezes, tiny droplets of fluid containing tubercle bacilli are released into the air. People in close physical contact with the infected person inhale this fine mist. Tuberculosis is not highly contagious compared to some other infectious diseases. Close, frequent, or prolonged contact is needed to spread the disease. Most people do not develop TB even when exposed to a person with active TB. Unlike many other infections, TB is not passed on by contact with a an infected individual's clothing, bed linens, dishes, or cooking utensils. The disease is not spread through kissing or other physical contact. The most important exception is pregnancy. The fetus of an infected mother may contract TB by inhaling or swallowing the bacilli in the amniotic fluid.

Progression

Once a person inhales *M. tuberculosis*, one of four things can happen:

• The person's immune system can kill the bacteria. TB infection does not result, and the person is not contagious.

• The bacteria can become dormant and never grow. Thus, TB symptoms are not seen and the person is not contagious.

• The bacteria can become dormant for a period, then begin to grow. TB symptoms appear a long time after initial infection. The person is not contagious during the dormant period, then becomes contagious when symptoms appear.

• The bacteria multiplies immediately. Active TB symptoms appear, and the person is contagious.

At least 9 out of 10 people infected with *M. tuberculosis* do not develop symptoms of TB, and their chest x-rays remain negative. These people have what is called a latent TB infection. They are not contagious, but they do form a pool of infected individuals who may get sick later and then pass TB on to others. It is thought that more than 90% of cases of active tuberculosis come from this pool. In the United States, there are about 10 million people with latent TB infections. It is impossible to predict which individuals with latent TB infections will develop active TB. An estimated 5% of infected persons get sick within 12 to 24 months of being infected. Another 5% heal initially but, after years or decades, develop active TB either in the lungs or elsewhere in the body. On rare occasions, a previously infected person gets sick again after a later exposure to the tubercle bacillus.

Pulmonary tuberculosis

Pulmonary TB affects the lungs. Its initial symptoms are easily confused with those of other diseases. An infected person may initially feel vaguely unwell or develop a cough that could be blamed on **smoking** or a cold. A small amount of greenish or yellow sputum may be coughed up when the person gets up in the morning. In time, more sputum that is streaked with blood is produced. People who have pulmonary TB do not get a high fever, but they often have a low-grade one. The individual often loses interest in food and may lose weight. Chest pain is sometimes present. If the infection allows air to escape from the lungs into the chest cavity (pneumothorax) or if fluid collects in the pleural space (pleural effusion), the patient may have difficulty breathing. If a young adult develops a pleural effusion, the chance of tubercular infection being the cause is very high.

Before the development of effective TB drugs, many patients became chronically ill with increasingly severe lung symptoms. They lost a great deal of weight and developed a wasted appearance, hence the name consumption. This outcome is uncommon in the twenty-first century where modern treatment methods are available.

Extrapulmonary tuberculosis

Although the lungs are the major site of damage caused by tuberculosis, other organs and tissues in the body may be affected. The usual progression is for the disease to spread from the lungs to locations outside the lungs (extrapulmonary sites). In occasional cases, the first sign of disease appears outside the lungs. The tissues or organs that TB may affect include:

• Bones: TB is particularly likely to attack the spine and the ends of the long bones. Children are especially prone to spinal TB. If not treated, the spinal segments (vertebrae) may collapse and cause paralysis in one or both legs.

• Kidneys: Along with the bones, the kidneys are the most common site of extrapulmonary TB. There may be few symptoms even after part of a kidney is destroyed. TB may also spread to the bladder. In men, it may spread to the prostate gland and nearby structures.

• Female reproductive organs: The ovaries in women may be infected and TB may spread from them to the peritoneum (the membrane lining the abdominal cavity).

• Abdominal cavity: TB peritonitis may cause pain ranging from the vague discomfort of stomach cramps to intense pain that may mimic the symptoms of appendicitis.

• Joints: Tubercular infection of joints causes a form of arthritis that most often affects the hips and knees. The wrist, hand, and elbow joints also may become painful and inflamed.

• Meninges: The meninges are tissues that cover the brain and the spinal cord. Infection of the meninges by the TB bacillus causes TB meningitis, a condition that is most common in young children but is especially dangerous in the elderly. Patients develop headaches, become drowsy and eventually comatose. Permanent brain damage results unless prompt treatment is given. Some patients with TB meningitis develop a tumor-like brain mass called a tuberculoma that causes stroke-like symptoms.

• Skin, intestines, adrenal glands, and blood vessels: All these parts of the body can be infected by *M. tuberculosis*. Infection of the wall of the body's main artery (the aorta), can cause it to rupture with catastrophic results. TB pericarditis occurs when the membrane surrounding the heart (the pericardium) is infected and fills up with fluid that interferes with the heart's ability to pump blood.

• Miliary tuberculosis: Miliary TB is a life-threatening condition that occurs when large numbers of tubercle bacilli spread throughout the body. Huge numbers of tiny tubercular lesions develop that cause marked weakness and weight loss, severe anemia, and gradual wasting of the body.

Multi drug-resistant tuberculosis (MDR TB)

In the twenty-first century, there is increasing concern about strains of *M. tuberculosis* that are resistant to the TB drugs that have brought the disease under control in the past half century. MDR TB is TB that fails to respond to at least two drugs, isoniazid (INH) and rifampin (RIF), which are routinely used to treat TB. In the United States, MDR TB, although rare, is on the rise. The CDC has developed a special group of experts to work with physicians who have patients with MDR TB. There is concern that drug-resistant TB could spread widely and cause a public health crisis. When alternate drug therapy fails to control MDR TB, lung surgery is the preferred treatment option.

Diseases similar to tuberculosis

There are many forms of mycobacteria other than *M. tuberculosis*, the tubercle bacillus. Some cause infections that may closely resemble tuberculosis, but they usually do so only when an infected person's immune system is defective. This occurs, for example, in some HIV-positive people. The most common mycobacteria that infect patients with HIV/AIDS are a group known as *Mycobacterium avium* complex (MAC). People infected by MAC are not contagious, but they may develop a serious lung infection that is highly resistant to antibiotics. MAC infections typically start with the patient coughing up mucus. The infection progresses slowly, but eventually blood is brought up in the sputum, and the patient has trouble breathing. In HIV/AIDS patients, MAC disease can spread throughout the body, with anemia, diarrhea, and stomach pain as common symptoms. Often these patients die unless their immune systems can be strengthened. Other mycobacteria grow in swimming pools and may cause skin infection. Some of them infect wounds and artificial body parts such as breast implants or mechanical heart valves.

Diagnosis

The standard screening test for TB is the tuberculin skin test. This test detects the presence of infection, not of active TB. Tuberculin is an extract prepared from cultures of *M. tuberculosis*. It contains proteins belonging to the bacillus (antigens) to which an infected person has been sensitized. When tuberculin is injected into the skin of an infected person, the area around the injection becomes hard, swollen, and red within one to three days.

Skin tests use a substance called purified protein derivative (PPD) that has a standard chemical composition and is therefore a good measure of the presence of tubercular infection. The PPD test is also called the Mantoux test. The Mantoux PPD skin test is not 100% accurate. It can produce false positive and false negative results. In other words, some people who have a skin reaction are not infected (false positive) and some who do not react are in fact infected (false negative). The PPD test is a highly useful screening test and is required in most states for children wanting to enter school. In addition, anyone who has suspicious findings on a chest x-ray or any condition that makes TB more likely should have a PPD test. People who are in close contact with a TB patient, those who come from a country where TB is common, all healthcare personnel, and persons living or working in institutions, such as prisons, should have a PPD test each year.

To verify the test results, a physician will order a chest x-ray and obtain a sample of sputum or a tissue sample (biopsy) for culture. Three to five sputum samples should be taken early in the morning. Culturing *M. tuberculosis* is useful for diagnosis because the bacillus has certain distinctive characteristics. Unlike many other types of bacteria, mycobacteria can retain certain dyes even when exposed to acid. This acid-fast property is characteristic of the tubercle bacillus.

Body fluids other than sputum can be used for a TB culture. If TB has invaded the brain or spinal cord, culturing a sample of spinal fluid will make the diagnosis. If TB of the kidneys is suspected because of pus or blood in the urine, culture of the urine may reveal a tubercular infection. Infection of the ovaries in women can be detected by inserting a tube with a light on its end (a laparoscope) into the area. Samples also may be taken from the liver or bone marrow to detect the tubercle bacillus.

For most people, a simple skin test is adequate to screen for TB. New advances in the diagnosis of TB use molecular techniques to speed the diagnostic process as well as improve its accuracy. As of 2012, molecular testing is being used more frequently in laboratories around the world. Molecular tests include a polymerase chain reaction to detect mycobacterial DNA in patient specimens; nucleic acid probes to identify mycobacteria in culture; restriction fragment length polymorphism analysis to compare different strains of TB for epidemiological studies; and genetic-based susceptibility testing to identify drug-resistant strains of mycobacteria.

Treatment

Treatment for tuberculosis includes supportive care, drug therapy, and surgery.

Supportive care

In the past, treatment of TB was primarily supportive. Patients were kept in isolation, encouraged to rest, and fed well. If these measures failed, the lung was collapsed surgically so that it could "rest" and heal. Surgical procedures are still used when necessary, but contemporary medicine relies on drug therapy as the mainstay of care. Given an effective combination of drugs, many patients with TB can be treated at home rather than in a sanatorium.

Drug therapy

Most patients with TB recover if given appropriate medication for a sufficient length of time. Three principles govern modern drug treatment of TB:

- Lowering the number of bacilli as quickly as possible. This minimizes the risk of transmitting the disease. When sputum cultures become negative, this has been achieved. Conversely, if the sputum remains positive after five to six months, treatment has failed.
- Preventing the development of drug resistance. For this reason, at least two different drugs and sometimes up to four are always given as initial treatment.
- Long-term treatment to prevent relapse.

Five drugs are most commonly used treat tuberculosis: isoniazid (INH, Laniazid, Nydrazid); rifampin (Rifadin, Rimactane); pyrazinamide (Tebrazid); streptomycin; and ethambutol (Myambutol). The CDC and the American Thoracic Society have developed standard regimens for treating TB in an effort to prevent the spread of drug resistant strains. For lung infections in non-immunocompromised people, the disease is usually treated with a regimen of rifampin and isoniazid (INH) for six months, supplemented in the first two months with pyrazinamide and sometimes ethambutol (or streptomycin in very young children). Because some strains of the disease are highly drug-resistant, cultures are grown from the patient's bacteria and tested with a variety of drugs to determine the most effective treatment, and alternate regimens may be determined to be more appropriate.

Except in cases of MDR TB, prolonged hospitalization is rarely necessary because most patients are no longer infectious after about two weeks of combination treatment. Follow-up involves monitoring side effects and monthly sputum tests. Of the five medications, INH is the most frequently used drug for both treatment and **prevention**. Hospitalization, isolation, and infectious control measures are required for individuals with MDR TB, which is a very serious disease both for the individual and from a public health standpoint. Most states have laws that allow individuals with TB to be hospitalized against their will for non-compliance with treatment.

Surgery

Surgical treatment of TB may be used if drugs fail to control the disease. There are three surgical treatments for pulmonary TB: pneumothorax, in which air is introduced into the chest to collapse the lung; thoracoplasty, in which one or more ribs are removed; and removal of a diseased lung, in whole or in part. Removal is usually required in the case of MDR TB. Individuals can survive with one healthy lung. Extrapulmonary TB may result in the need for other surgeries.

Public health role and response

Several national and international programs have been developed to address the public health concerns with TB. The Stop TB Partnership, which operates through a secretariat hosted by the WHO, in Geneva, Switzerland, created the Global Plan to Stop Tuberculosis. The Plan aims to save 14 million lives between 2006 and 2015, thus reducing the number of deaths and its incidence by 50%. The Partnership is also working to reduce the global incidence of TB to less than one per million people by 2050 and to eliminate TB as a **global public health** problem in that same target year. In addition, the American Thoracic Society has developed a tuberculosis classification system that is used primarily in the U.S. public health program.

Prognosis

Most patients recover from TB if the disease is diagnosed early and given prompt treatment with appropriate medications on a long-term regimen. The relapse rate is less than 4%. The exception is for those with MDR TB. When TB is multi drug-resistant, the prognosis depends largely on the ability to surgically remove all infected tissue. The outcome of surgery depends on where and how widespread the infected area is. Miliary TB is still fatal in many cases but is rarely seen in developed countries.

Prevention

The prevention of TB includes general measures, vaccinations, and prophylactic use of isoniazid.

KEY TERMS

Bacillus Calmette-Guérin (BCG)—A vaccine made from a weakened bacillus similar to the tubercle bacillus that may help prevent serious pulmonary TB and its complications.

Mantoux test—Another name for the PPD test.

Miliary tuberculosis—The form of TB in which the bacillus spreads through all body tissues and organs, producing many thousands of tiny tubercular lesions. It is often fatal unless promptly treated.

Mycobacteria—A group of bacteria that includes *Mycobacterium tuberculosis*, the bacterium that causes tuberculosis, and other forms that cause related illnesses.

Pneumothorax—Air inside the chest cavity that may cause the lung to collapse. It is both a complication of pulmonary tuberculosis and a means of treatment designed to allow an infected lung to rest and heal.

Purified protein derivative (PPD)—An extract of tubercle bacilli that is injected into the skin to find out whether a person presently has or has ever had tuberculosis.

Sputum—Secretions produced in the lung and coughed up. A sign of illness, sputum is routinely used as a specimen for culturing the tubercle bacillus in the laboratory.

Tuberculoma—A tumor-like mass in the brain that sometimes develops as a complication of tuberculosis meningitis.

General measures

General measures such as avoidance of overcrowded and unsanitary conditions are one aspect of prevention. Hospital emergency rooms and similar locations can be treated with ultraviolet light, which has an antibacterial effect. Regular skin testing is required in some jobs and of most children when they enter school and often again when entering college. Although screening does not prevent TB, it allows early treatment of those who are infected, reducing the likelihood that they will spread the disease.

Vaccination

Vaccination is a preventive measure against TB. A vaccine called BCG (Bacillus Calmette-Guérin, named after its French developers) is made from a weakened **mycobacterium** that infects cattle. Vaccination with BCG does not prevent infection by *M. tuberculosis*, but it does strengthen the immune system response and provide partial protection. BCG is used more widely in developing countries than in the United States. The effectiveness of vaccination is still being studied; it is not clear whether the vaccine's effectiveness depends on the population in which it is used or on variations in its formulation.

As of 2007, the first new TB vaccine in 80 years was in clinical trials in South Africa. The new vaccine known as MVA85A (modified vaccinia Ankara 85A), was developed by researchers at Oxford University, England, in response to increasing concern about the rise of MDR TB. This vaccine works with BCG vaccine to increase its effectiveness and produce a very strong immune system response. With phase I clinical trials completed, phase II clinical trials are ongoing in 2012, with a focus on whether the new vaccine actually prevents the disease. In one paper—*A Phase IIa Trial of the New TB Vaccine, MVA85A, in HIV and/or M. Tuberculosis Infected Adults*, published in January 2012 in the *American Journal of Respiratory and Critical Care Medicine*—the South Africa and United Kingdom researchers concluded, "MVA85A was safe and immunogenic in persons with HIV and/or M.tb infection. These results support further evaluation of safety and efficacy of this vaccine for prevention of TB in these target populations." Makers of the vaccine predict that even if clinical trials are successful, the vaccine will not be available on the market until about 2015.

Prophylactic use of isoniazid

INH can be given for the prevention and treatment of TB. INH is effective when given daily over a period of 6 to 12 months to people in high-risk categories. INH appears to be most beneficial to persons under the age of 25 years. Because INH carries the risk of side effects (liver inflammation, nerve damage, changes in mood and behavior) in about one-fifth of people taking the drug, it is important to give it only to persons at special risk. The increase in MDR TB is causing some TB experts to re-evaluate preventative drug treatment.

High-risk groups for whom isoniazid prevention may be justified include:

• close contacts of TB patients, including health care workers

• newly infected patients whose skin test has turned positive in the past two years

• anyone who is HIV-positive with a positive PPD skin test; isoniazid may be given even if the PPD results are negative if there is a risk of exposure to active tuberculosis

• intravenous drug users, even if they are negative for HIV

• persons with positive PPD results and evidence of old disease on their chest x-ray who have never been treated for TB

QUESTIONS TO ASK YOUR DOCTOR

• Should I be worried about tuberculosis?

• How dangerous is tuberculosis?

• Is tuberculosis contagious before symptoms appear?

• What symptoms should I be watching for with regard to TB?

• Should I get tested for TB?

• What should I do if I have a positive test for TB infection?

• If I was exposed to someone with active TB disease, can I give TB to others?

• patients who have an illness or are taking a drug that can suppress the immune system

• persons with positive PPD results who have had intestinal surgery; have diabetes or chronic kidney failure; have any type of cancer; or are more than 10% below their ideal body weight

• people from countries with high rates of TB who have positive PPD results

• people from low-income groups with positive skin test results

• persons with a positive PPD reaction who belong to high-risk ethnic groups (African Americans, Hispanics, Native Americans, Asians, and Pacific Islanders)

• householders who have lived with someone who has been diagnosed with an active TB infection

Resources

BOOKS

Cole, Stewart T., et al., eds.*Tuberculosis and the Tubercle Bacillus.* Washington, DC: ASM Press, 2005.

Magner, Lois N. *A History of Infectious Diseases and the Microbial World (Healing Society: Disease, Medicine, and History).* Westport, CT: Praeger, 2009.

Mayho, Paul, and Richard Coker. *The Tuberculosis Survival Handbook,* 2nd ed. West Palm Beach, FL: Merit Publishing International, 2006.

World Health Organization. *Tuberculosis and Air Travel: Guidelines for Prevention and Control.* 3rd ed. Geneva 27, Switzerland: World Health Organization, 2008.

WEBSITES

Batara, Vandana. *Pediatric Tuberculosis.* Medscape Reference. October 11, 2011. http://emedicine.medscape.com/article/969401-overview (accessed October 13, 2012).

Florence B. Seibert. National Women's Hall of Fame. http://www.greatwomen.org/women-of-the-hall/search-the-hall-results/details/2/138-Seibert (accessed October 13, 2012).

Global Tuberculosis Control 2011. World Health Organization. http://www.who.int/tb/publications/global_report/en/ (accessed October 13, 2012).

Herchline, Thomas E. *Tuberculosis.* Medscape Reference. September 20, 2012. http://emedicine.medscape.com/article/230802-overview (accessed October 13, 2012).

Mitruka, Kiren, John Oeltmann, Kashef Ijaz, and Maryam Haddad. "Tuberculosis Outbreak Investigations in the United States, 2002–2008." *Emerging Infectious Diseases.* March 2011. http://wwwnc.cdc.gov/eid/article/17/3/10-1550_article.htm (accessed October 13, 2012).

Scriba, Thomas J., et al. "A Phase IIa Trial of the New TB Vaccine, MVA85A, in HIV and/or M. Tuberculosis Infected Adults." *American Journal of Respiratory and Critical Care Medicine* 185, no. 7 (April 1, 2012): 769–78. http://ajrccm.atsjournals.org/content/185/7/769.abstract?sid=8f1a92fc-06c0-4106-87cd-1709d3df8d4c (accessed October 13, 2012).

Tuberculosis (TB). Centers for Disease Control and Prevention. September 13, 2012. http://www.cdc.gov/tb/ (accessed October 13, 2012).

Tuberculosis. World Health Organization. Fact sheet No. 104 (March 2012). http://www.who.int/mediacentre/factsheets/fs104/en/index.html (accessed October 13, 2012).

ORGANIZATIONS

American Lung Association, 1301 Pennsylvania Ave., NW, Ste. 800, Washington, D.C. 20004, (202) 785-3355, Fax: (202) 452-1805, info@lung.org, http://www.lung.org/

American Thoracic Society, 25 Broadway, 18th Fl., New York, NY 10004, (212) 315-8600, Fax: (212) 315-6498, atsinfo@thoracic.org, http://www.thoracic.org/

U.S. Centers for Disease Control and Prevention, 1600 Clifton Rd., Atlanta, GA 30333, (800) 232-4636, cdcinfo@cdc.gov, http://www.cdc.gov/

World Health Organization, Avenue Appia 20, Geneva, Switzerland 1211 27, 41 22 791-2111, Fax: 41 22 791-3111, http://www.who.int/en/.

Tish Davidson, AM
Rebecca J. Frey, PhD
Laura Jean Cataldo, RN, EdD
William A. Atkins, BB, BS, MBA

Tularemia

Definition

Tularemia is an illness caused by the bacterium *Francisella tularensis.* It results in fever, rash, and greatly enlarged lymph nodes, and is sometimes called rabbit fever.

Description

Tularemia infects more than 100 wild animals, including rabbits, deer, squirrels, muskrats, beavers, and various birds and insects. Humans can acquire the bacterium directly from contact with the blood or body fluids of these animals, from the bite of an insect (often a tick, fly, or mosquito) that has previously fed on the blood of an infected animal, or from contaminated food or **water**.

Tularemia occurs most often in the summer months. It is most likely to infect people who come into contact with infected animals, including hunters, furriers, butchers, laboratory workers, game wardens, and veterinarians. In the United States, the vast majority of cases of tularemia occur in the southeastern and Rocky Mountain states.

Origins

Tularemia was first described in Japan in 1837, but it was not studied until an outbreak in ground squirrels occurred in Tulare County, California, in 1911. It was subsequently investigated by Dr. Edward Francis. The bacterium that causes the disease, *Francisella tularensis*, was named for the location of the first recognized outbreak and the primary investigator of the outbreak.

Tularemia occurs in the northern hemisphere except in the United Kingdom. In the United States, the number of reported cases of tularemia has declined substantially since the 1950s. Only about 120 cases are reported in the United States each year between 2001 and 2010, although given its rarity and the variety of presenting symptoms, many cases be misdiagnosed and go unreported. In the United States, the majority of reported cases between 2001 and 2010 were in Arkansas and Missouri.

Several outbreaks have occurred in the 2000s in Europe. A large outbreak of tularemia occurred in Kosovo from 1999–2001. The cause was thought to be contaminated food and/or water. At the time, Kosovo was a war zone, and public **hygiene** was compromised. In 2000, substantial outbreaks occurred for the first time in almost 20 years in Sweden and Finland. Transmission was thought to occur through the bite of infected mosquitoes.

Causes and symptoms

Five types of illness may occur, depending on where and how the bacteria enter the body:

- Ulceroglandular/glandular tularemia. 75%–85% of all cases are of this type. This type is often contracted through the bite of an infected tick that has defecated bacteria-laden feces in the area of the bite wound. A tender red bump appears in the area of the original wound. Over a few weeks, the bump develops a punched-out center (ulcer). Nearby lymph nodes grow hugely swollen and very tender. The lymph nodes may drain a thick, pus-like material. Other symptoms include fever, chills, and weakness. In adults, the lymph nodes in the groin are most commonly affected, while in children, the lymph nodes in the neck.

- Oculoglandular tularemia. This type accounts for only 1%–2% of all cases of tularemia. It occurs when a person's contaminated hand rubs his or her eye. The lining of the eyelids and the surface of the white of the eye (conjunctiva) become red and severely painful, with multiple small yellow bumps and pitted sores (ulcers). Lymph nodes around the ears, under the jaw, or in the neck may swell and become painful.

- Oropharyngeal and gastrointestinal tularemia. This type occurs when contaminated meat is undercooked and then eaten, or when water from a contaminated source is drunk. Poor hygiene after skinning and cleaning an animal obtained through hunting can also lead to the bacteria entering through the mouth. Sores in the mouth and throat, as well as abdominal pain, nausea and vomiting, ulcers in the intestine, intestinal bleeding, and diarrhea may all occur.

- Pulmonary tularemia. This rare type of tularemia occurs when a person inhales a spray of infected fluid, or when the bacteria reach the lungs through the blood circulation. A severe pneumonia follows.

- Typhoidal tularemia. This type of tularemia is particularly hard to diagnose, because it occurs without the usual skin manifestations or swelling of lymph glands. Symptoms include continuously high fever, terrible headaches, and confusion. The illness may result in a severely low blood pressure, with signs of poor blood flow to the major organs (shock).

Diagnosis

Samples from the skin lesions can be prepared with special stains, to allow identification of the causative bacteria under the microscope. Other tests are available to demonstrate the presence of antibodies (special immune cells that the body produces in response to the

presence of specific foreign invaders) which increase over time in response to an infection with tularemia. Ordinary blood tests rarely reveal the presence of *F. tularensis*, making diagnosis difficult unless the disease is already suspected.

Treatment

Streptomycin (given as a shot in a muscle) and gentamicin (given either as an injection in a muscle or IV through a needle in the vein) are both used to treat tularemia. Other types of **antibiotics** have been tested, but have often resulted in relatively high rates of relapse (20%). *F. tularensis* is naturally resistant to penicillin and penicillin-related antibiotics. Early treatment is most often successful. Supportive treatment and hospitalization may be necessary if the disease is not treated early.

Prognosis

With early treatment, death rates from tularemia are about 1%. Without treatment, however, the death rate may reach 30%. The **pneumonia** and typhoidal types have the worst prognosis without treatment.

Effects on public health

Tularemia is not a major public health problem as of 2012. However, the **Centers for Disease Control and Prevention (CDC)** do track cases of tularemia. Of more concern is that *F. tularensis* could be used as a weapon of bioterrorism. Transmission is extremely easy. As few as 10–50 bacteria entering the body can cause infection. Although tularemia has not been demonstrated to pass directly from person to person, widespread exposure through contaminated food or water could cause a serious public health threat.

Efforts and solutions

Prevention involves avoiding areas known to harbor ticks and flies, or the appropriate use of insect repellents. Hunters should wear gloves when skinning animals or preparing meat. Others (butchers, game wardens, veterinarians) who work with animals or carcasses should always wear gloves. At one time, a vaccine existed against the disease, but was only given to people at very high risk due to their profession or hobby (veterinarians, laboratory workers, butchers, hunters, game wardens), and as of 2012 was no longer available.

Resources

BOOKS

World Health Organization. *The Vector-Borne Human Infections Of Europe: Their Distribution and Burden on Public Health.* Copenhagen: Denmark, WHO, 2004. 84–86. http://www.euro.who.int/__data/assets/pdf_file/0008/98765/e82481.pdf.

WEBSITES

Centers for Disease Control and Prevention. "Tularemia." http://www.cdc.gov/tularemia (accessed October 19, 2012).

Cleveland, Kerry O. "Tularemia." Medscape Reference. http://emedicine.medscape.com/article/230923-overview (accessed October 19, 2012).

National Center for Biotechnology Information. "Resources for Tularemia." http://www.ncbi.nlm.nih.gov/sites/ga?disorder=Tularemia (accessed October 19, 2012).

ORGANIZATIONS

National Center for Biotechnology Information, 8600 Rockville Pike, Bethesda, MD 20894, (301) 496-2475, http://www.ncbi.nlm.nih.gov

United States Centers for Disease Control and Prevention (CDC), 1600 Clifton Road, Atlanta, GA 30333, (404) 639-3534, (800) CDC-INFO (232-4636), (888) 232-6348, inquiry@cdc.gov, http://www.cdc.gov

World Health Organization, Avenue Appia 20, 1211 Geneva 27, Switzerland, 22 41 791 21 11, Fax: 22 41 791 31 11, info@who.int, http://www.who.int.

Rosalyn Carson-DeWitt, MD
Tish Davidson, AM

Typhoid fever

Definition

Typhoid fever is a severe infection caused by a bacterium, *Salmonella typhi*. *S. typhi* is in the same family of bacteria as the type spread by chicken and eggs, commonly known as **salmonella poisoning** or food poisoning. Unlike the bacteria that cause food poisoning, acquiring the *S. typhi* bacteria does not result in vomiting and diarrhea as the most prominent symptoms in humans. Instead, persistently high fever is the hallmark of *S. typhi* infection.

Description

As of 2012, according to the Mayo Clinic, over 21 million people around the world develop typhoid fever each year, and 200,000 people died of the disease annually. Typhoid fever is passed from person to person through poor **hygiene**, such as incomplete or no hand washing after using the toilet. This allows *S. typhi* to enter the food and **water** supply. The bacteria are ingested and then they are passed into the stool and urine of infected patients. They may continue to be present in the stool of asymptomatic carriers—persons who have recovered from the symptoms of the disease but continue to carry the bacteria. This carrier state occurs in about 3% of all individuals who have recovered from typhoid fever. Persons who are carriers of the disease and who handle food can be the source of epidemic spread of typhoid. One such individual gave her name to the expression "Typhoid Mary," a name given to someone whom others avoid.

One of the largest outbreaks of typhoid fever occurred in 2004–2005 in the Democratic Republic of Congo. In 2004, according to the **World Health Organization (WHO)**, 13,400 cases of typhoid fever were reported in the suburbs of Kimbanseke, Kikimi, Masina, and Ndjili. Between October 1 and December 10, 2004, 615 cases of typhoid fever occurred with peritonitis, along with 134 deaths. The WHO stated that very poor sanitary conditions and a lack of **drinking water** were major causes of the outbreaks. Then, from September 2004 to January 11, 2005, the WHO reported that 42,564 cases and 214 deaths due to typhoid fever occurred in Kinshasa.

Natural disasters are also prime breeding grounds for typhoid fever. The January 2010 earthquake in Haiti displaced hundreds of thousands of people. Human and animal waste accumulated, which caused major diseases, such as typhoid fever, **cholera**, and **shigellosis**, to increase in frequency due to contaminated food and water. The dilapidated health system of Haiti worsened under the stress of these homeless people. Ian Greenwald, the chief medical officer for a Duke University team of doctors working in Haiti, is quoted in *The New York Times* article (February 19, 2010) *Poor Sanitation in Haiti's Camps Adds Disease Risk*: "We're witnessing the setup for the spread of severe diarrheal illnesses in a place where the health system has collapsed and without a functioning sewage system to begin with."

MARY MALLON (1869–1938)

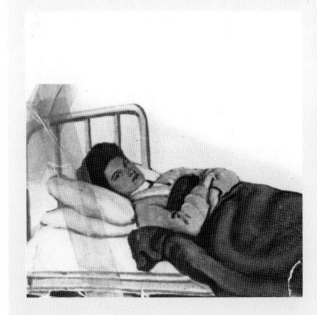

Mallon, Mary (Typhoid Mary), 1914. (© Corbis Corporation. Reproduced by permission)

Mary Mallon was born in Cookstown, Ireland, on September 23, 1869, to Catherine Igo and John Mallon. As a teenager, Mallon left her parents and immigrated to New York to live with an aunt and uncle. Until 1906, when George A. Soper began to study an outbreak of typhoid fever in Long Island, little was known about Mallon.

Soper was called to identify possible causes of an eruption of typhoid fever at a summer house in Oyster Bay. After examining the food and water in a futile attempt to discover contaminants, Soper decided that the disease was probably transmitted by a human carrier. He soon learned that the cook had disappeared and tracked Mallon to her new place of employment, expecting her cooperation in dealing with the matter. Soper eventually turned the case over to the New York City Department of Health. When Mallon was ultimately caught, she refused treatment and was held for three years as a threat to the public. In 1910, a judge granted her release with the stipulation that she not seek employment as a cook, since the disease was transmitted through food. Mallon agreed but, in 1915, an outbreak of typhoid at a hospital was, once again, linked to her. When Soper investigated this incident he learned that employees had nicknamed one of the cooks "Typhoid Mary."

After Mallon was found, she was taken into custody, and spent the rest of her life at Riverside Hospital. Mallon died on November 11, 1938.

Risk factors

Mayo Clinic states that the following are the major risk factors for typhoid fever:

- if a child (although their symptoms are generally milder than are the symptoms of adults)
- if working or traveling to areas where typhoid fever is endemic (such as India, Southeast Asia, Africa, and South America)
- if working as a clinical microbiologist handling *S. typhi* bacteria
- if in close contact with someone who is infected or has recently been infected with typhoid fever
- if having an immune system that is weakened by medications such as corticosteroids or diseases such as human immunodeficiency virus/acquired immune deficiency syndrome (HIV/AIDS)
- if drinking water contaminated by sewage that contains *S. typhi*

Demographics

According to the U.S. **Centers for Disease Control and Prevention (CDC)**, about 400 Americans each year acquire typhoid, most while traveling in developing countries. These areas include Asia, Africa, Latin America, the Caribbean, and Oceania. Although typhoid fever can be found in all those areas, 80% of cases worldwide are found in Bangladesh, China, India, Indonesia, Laos, Nepal, Pakistan, and Vietnam. Around 5% of those Americans who contract the illness abroad become chronic carriers. According to the National Institutes of Health (NIH), a study in the early 2010s found that "the cause of most cases of the disease that did not result from travel abroad could not be accounted for." The NIH stated that about 19% of typhoid cases in the United States (which did not occur while traveling abroad) occurred among groups of people. One of the largest recent outbreaks occurred from orange juice that was contaminated by a food handler. Forty-seven people were sickened from the outbreak in 1998. Typhoid fever is rare in industrialized countries with adequate sewage treatment facilities and clean water supplies.

Causes and symptoms

S. typhi must be ingested to cause disease. Transmission often occurs when a person in the carrier state does not wash hands thoroughly (or not at all) after defecation and serves food to others. This pathway is sometimes called the fecal-oral route of disease transmission. In countries where open sewage is accessible to flies, the insects land on the sewage, pick up the bacteria, and then contaminate food to be eaten by humans. In countries with poor sewage treatment facilities, sewage can contaminate the water supply and typhoid fever can spread by drinking contaminated water.

After being swallowed, the *S. typhi* bacteria enter the digestive tract where they are taken in by cells called mononuclear phagocytes. These phagocytes are cells of the immune system, whose job it is to engulf and kill invading bacteria and viruses. In the case of *S. typhi*, however, the bacteria are able to survive ingestion by the phagocytes, and multiply within these cells. This period of time, during which the bacteria are multiplying within the phagocytes, is the 10- to 14-day incubation period of typhoid fever. When huge numbers of bacteria fill an individual phagocyte, they spill out of the cell and into the bloodstream, where their presence begins to cause symptoms.

The presence of increasingly large numbers of bacteria in the bloodstream (bacteremia) is responsible for an increasingly high fever, which lasts throughout the four to eight weeks of the disease in untreated individuals. Other symptoms of typhoid fever include constipation (at first), nausea, extreme fatigue, headache, joint **pain**, and a rash across the abdomen known as rose spots.

The bacteria move from the bloodstream into certain tissues of the body, including the gallbladder and lymph tissue of the intestine (called Peyer's patches). The tissue's response to this invasion causes symptoms ranging from inflammation of the gallbladder (cholecystitis) to intestinal bleeding to actual perforation of the intestine. Perforation of the intestine refers to an actual hole occurring in the wall of the intestine, with leakage of intestinal contents into the abdominal cavity. This leakage causes severe irritation and inflammation of the lining of the abdominal cavity, which is called peritonitis. Peritonitis is a frequent cause of death from typhoid fever.

Other complications of typhoid fever include liver and spleen enlargement, sometimes so great that the spleen ruptures or bursts; anemia, or low red blood cell count due to blood loss from the intestinal bleeding; joint infections, which are especially common in patients with sickle cell disease and immune system disorders; **pneumonia** caused by a bacterial infection (usually *Streptococcus pneumoniae*), which is able to take hold due to the patient's weakened state; heart infections; and **meningitis** and infections of the brain, which cause mental confusion and even coma. It may take a patient several months to recover fully from untreated typhoid fever.

KEY TERMS

Asymptomatic—A state in which a person experiences no symptoms of a disease.

Bacteremia—Bacteria in the blood.

Carrier—A person who has a particular disease agent present within his or her body, and can pass this agent on to others, but who displays no symptoms of infection.

Epidemic—A large number of cases of the same disease or infection all occurring within a short time period in a specific location.

Incubation period—The time between when an individual becomes infected with a disease-causing agent and when symptoms begin to appear.

Mononuclear phagocyte—A type of cell of the human immune system that ingests bacteria, viruses, and other foreign matter, thus removing potentially harmful substances from the bloodstream. These substances are usually then digested within the phagocyte.

Rose spots—A pinkish rash across the trunk or abdomen that is a classic sign of typhoid fever.

Sickle cell disease—An inherited disorder characterized by a genetic flaw in hemoglobin production. (Hemoglobin is the substance within red blood cells that enables them to transport oxygen.) The hemoglobin that is produced has a kink in its structure that forces the red blood cells to take on a sickle shape, inhibiting their circulation and causing pain. This disorder primarily affects people of African descent.

Diagnosis

In some cases, the doctor may suspect the diagnosis if the patient has already developed the characteristic rose spots, or if he or she has a history of recent travel in areas with poor **sanitation**. The diagnosis is confirmed by a blood culture. Samples of a patient's stool, urine, and bone marrow can also be used to grow *S. typhi* in a laboratory for identification under a microscope. Cultures are the most accurate method of diagnosis. Blood cultures usually become positive in the first week of illness in 80% of patients who have not taken **antibiotics**.

Treatment

Antibiotics are the treatment of choice for typhoid fever. As of the early 2010s, commonly used drugs are ceftriaxone (Rocephin) and cefoperazone (Cefobid). Ciprofloxacin (Cipro, Proquin)) is sometimes given as follow-up therapy. It should be noted, that antibiotic resistance is common in *S. typhi*. Forty-three percent of samples of *S. typhi* collected from patients in the United States were resistant to at least one antibiotic. The choice of antibiotic(s) used to treat typhoid fever is determined by the origin of the disease, sensitivity of cultures of the bacterium to specific antibiotics, and response to treatment.

Carriers of *S. typhi* must be treated even when they do not show any symptoms of the infection, because carriers are responsible for the majority of new cases of typhoid fever. Eliminating the carrier state is a difficult task. It requires treatment with one or even two different medications over a period of four to six weeks. The antibiotics most commonly given are ampicillin (Omnipen, Polycillin, Principen, sometimes given together with probenecid [Benemid]) and amoxicillin (Amoxicot, Amoxil, Dispermox, Moxatag). In the case of a carrier with gallstones, surgery may need to be performed to remove the gallbladder. This measure is necessary because typhoid bacteria are often housed in the gallbladder, where they may survive in spite of antibiotic treatment. In some patients, treatment with rifampin and trimethoprim-sulfamethoxazole is sufficient to eradicate the bacteria from the gallbladder without surgery.

Public health role and response

The U.S. **Centers for Disease Control and Prevention** (**CDC**) recommends that if traveling to a country where typhoid fever is common (generally outside of the United States, Canada, northern Europe, Australia, and New Zealand) or during epidemic outbreaks, then one should consider being vaccinated against typhoid. The CDC recommends that the **vaccination** should be completed at least one to two weeks before the date of departure so that the vaccine has sufficient time to take effect. In addition, the effectiveness of typhoid vaccinations typically last for several years. In addition, **immunization** is not always effective, so some health care providers may recommend taking electrolyte packets along on the trip in case one gets sick. In addition, always drink only boiled or bottled water and eat well-cooked foods while traveling.

The U.S. National Institutes of Health recommend that a health care provider should be summoned if a person has:

• any known exposure to typhoid fever

• been in an endemic area and symptoms of typhoid fever have developed

---

QUESTIONS TO ASK YOUR DOCTOR

- Should I be worried about typhoid fever?
- How dangerous is typhoid fever?
- Is typhoid fever contagious before symptoms appear?
- What symptoms should I be watching for with regard to typhoid?
- If I was exposed to someone with typhoid fever, can I give typhoid to others?
- What types of tests do I need?
- Are treatments available to help me recover from typhoid?
- How long will a full recovery take?
- When can I return to my daily routine?
- What are the possible causes for my symptoms?
- Am I at risk of any long-term complications?

• had typhoid fever and the symptoms return

• developed severe abdominal pain, decreased urine output, or other new symptoms

Prognosis

The prognosis for recovery is good for most patients. In the era before effective antibiotics were discovered, about 12% of all typhoid fever patients died of the infection. As of late 2012, fewer than 1% of patients who receive prompt antibiotic treatment will die. The mortality rate is highest in the very young and very old, and in patients with malnutrition. The most ominous signs are changes in a patient's state of consciousness, including stupor or coma.

Prevention

Hygienic sewage disposal systems in a community, good water treatment facilities, and proper personal hygiene are the most important factors in preventing typhoid fever. Immunizations are available for travelers who expect to visit countries where *S. typhi* is a known public health problem. Some of these immunizations provide only short-term protection (for a few months), while others may be effective for several years. Efforts are being made to develop vaccines that provide a longer period of protection with fewer side effects from the vaccine itself. The most commonly reported side effects are flu-like muscle cramps and abdominal pain.

Resources

BOOKS

Emmeluth, Donald.*Typhoid Fever.* Philadelphia: Chelsea House, 2004.

Ray, Kurt. *Typhoid Fever.* New York: Rosen, 2001.

Shannon, Joyce Brennfleck, editor. *Contagious Diseases Sourcebook: Basic Consumer Health Information about Diseases Spread from Person to Person.* Detroit: Omnigraphics, 2010.

Wilder-Smith, Annelies, Eli Schwartz, and Marc Shaw, editors.*Travel Medicine: Tales Behind the Science.* Amsterdam: Elsevier, 2007.

WEBSITES

Batara, Vandana. *Typhoid Fever.* Centers for Disease Control and Prevention. http://www.cdc.gov/nczved/divisions/dfbmd/diseases/typhoid_fever/ (accessed July 6, 2012).

Diarrhoeal Diseases. World Health Organization. http://www.who.int/vaccine_research/diseases/diarrhoeal/en/index7.html (accessed July 6, 2012).

Romero, Simon. *Poor Sanitation in Haiti's Camps Adds Disease Risk.* The New York Times. http://www.nytimes.com/2010/02/20/world/americas/20haiti.html?_r=1 (accessed July 9, 2012).

Typhoid Fever. Mayo Clinic. http://www.mayoclinic.com/health/typhoid-fever/DS00538 (accessed July 6, 2012).

Typhoid Fever. Medline Plus. http://www.nlm.nih.gov/medlineplus/ency/article/001332.htm (accessed July 6, 2012).

Typhoid Fever. Medscape Reference. http://emedicine.medscape.com/article/231135-overview (accessed July 6, 2012).

Typhoid Fever in Democratic Republic of the Congo. World Health Organization. http://www.who.int/csr/don/2004_12_15/en/ (accessed July 6, 2012).

Typhoid Fever in the Democratic Republic of the Congo—Update. World Health Organization. http://www.who.int/csr/don/2004_12_15/en/ (accessed July 6, 2012).

Typhoid Vaccine—Oral Enteric-Coated Capsule. MedicineNet.com. http://www.medicinenet.com/typhoid_vaccine-oral_enteric-coated_capsule/article.htm (accessed July 6, 2012).

Typhoid Vaccine: What You Need to Know. Centers for Disease Control and Prevention. http://www.cdc.gov/vaccines/Pubs/vis/downloads/vis-typhoid.pdf (accessed July 6, 2012).

ORGANIZATIONS

Centers for Disease Control and Prevention, 1600 Clifton Rd., Atlanta, GA U.S.A. 30333, (800) 232-4636, cdcinfo@cdc.gov, http://www.fda.gov/

National Institute of Allergy and Infectious Diseases, 1301 Pennsylvania Ave., N.W., Ste. 800, Washington, D.C. U.S.A. 20004, 1 (202) 785-3355, Fax: 1 (202) 452-1805, info@lung.org, http://www.lung.org/

World Health Organization, Avenue Appia 20, Geneva, Switzerland 1211 27, 41 22 791-2111, Fax: 41 22 791-3111, cdcinfo@cdc.gov, http://www.who.int/en/.

Rosalyn Carson-DeWitt, MD
Tish Davidson, AM
Paul Checchia, MD
William A. Atkins, BB, BS, MBA

Typhus

Definition

Several different illnesses are called "typhus," all of which are caused by one of the bacteria in the family *Rickettsiae*. Each illness occurs when the bacteria is passed to a human through contact with an infected insect.

Description

The first known description of typhus (probably epidemic typhus) occurred in the late 1480s and early 1490s while Spanish soldiers were fighting during the siege of Granada. Fever, rash, red spots (on their arms, back, and chest), delirium, gangrenous sores, and decaying flesh were some of the common symptoms of typhus during this conflict. At the time, it was called disease gaol, or jail, fever. In 1760, the English government first called it typhus, from the Greek word "typhos." Meaning smoky or hazy, it described the state of mind of those people with the disease. Typhus continued to be a major problem in Europe over the next several centuries, most often due to the crowded and unsanitary living conditions commonly present. In the nineteenth century, many outbreaks occurred around the world. In the 1810s, large numbers of French troops under Napoleon died from typhus, and in the 1830s, hundreds of thousands of Americans and Irish died in several epidemics in both countries.

By the early twentieth century, the cause of epidemic typhus was identified. In 1916 Brazilian physician Henrique da Rocha Lima (1879–1956) discovered its cause while performing typhus research in Germany. Millions of deaths were attributed to typhus in World War I (1914–1918) and World War II (1939–1945). After World War II, the insecticide dichlorodiphenyltrichloroethane (DDT) was used to kill lice, which reduced the number of epidemics and limited their locations to Africa, the Middle East, Eastern Europe, and Asia.

The four main types of typhus are:

- epidemic typhus

- Brill-Zinsser disease

- endemic or murine typhus

- scrub typhus

These four diseases are somewhat similar, but they vary in terms of severity. The specific type of *Rickettsia* that causes the disease varies, as does the specific insect that carries the bacteria.

Epidemic typhus, sometimes called jail fever or louse-borne typhus, is caused by *Rickettsia prowazekii*, which is carried by body lice. When lice feed on a human, they may simultaneously defecate. When a person scratches the bite, the feces that carries the bacteria are scratched into the wound. Body lice are common in areas where there is overcrowding, poor **sanitation**, and poor **hygiene**. As a result, this form of typhus occurs simultaneously in large numbers of individuals living within the same community; that is, in epidemics. Epidemic typhus occurs when cold weather, **poverty**, war, and other disasters result in close living conditions that encourage the maintenance of a **population** of lice living among humans. Some medical historians have reported that the Great **Plague** of Athens in 430 B.C. may have been epidemic typhus. As of late 2012, epidemic typhus is found in the mountainous regions of Africa, South America, and Asia.

Brill-Zinsser disease is a reactivation of an earlier infection with epidemic typhus. It affects people years after they have completely recovered from epidemic typhus. A weakening of a person's immune system (from **aging**, surgery, or illness) can cause the bacteria to gain hold again, causing illness. This disease tends to be extremely mild.

Endemic typhus is carried by fleas. When a flea lands on a human, it may defecate as it feeds. When a person scratches the itchy spot where the flea was feeding, the bacteria-laden feces are scratched into the skin causing infection. The causative bacteria is called *Rickettsia typhi*. Endemic typhus occurs most commonly in warm, coastal regions. In the United States, southern Texas and southern California have the largest number of cases.

Scrub typhus is caused by *Rickettsia tsutsugamushi*. Mites or chiggers carry the bacteria. As the mites feed on humans, they deposit the bacteria. Scrub typhus occurs commonly in the southwest Pacific, Southeast Asia, and Japan. It is a very common cause of illness in people living in or visiting these areas. It occurs more commonly during the wet season.

Risk factors

The risk factors for getting typhus include living in or visiting areas where it is endemic, such as coastal cities where rodent and insect (such as lice, mites, fleas, and ticks) populations are high and in close contact with people, and areas where hygiene is degraded such as within poverty-stricken regions, disaster zones, homeless camps, and other similar places. Typhus is most often contracted during the spring and summer months.

As of 2012, the International Association for Medical Assistance to Travellers identified the following countries as having increased risks for typhus: Bolivia, Burundi, Colombia, Eritrea, Ethiopia, Guatemala, Kenya, Mexico, Peru, Rwanda, and Somalia.

Demographics

Since World War II, large outbreaks of typhus have occurred primarily in three African countries: Burundi, Ethiopia and Rwanda. In Ethiopia, the number of cases reported annually has ranged between 7,000 and 17,000. In 1996, for example, Burundi reported 3,500 cases and that number increased to 20,000 for the period from January to March 1997. In the first two decades of the twenty-first century, the **World Health Organization (WHO)** reported that typhus kills about 0.2 people per million per year.

Causes and symptoms

The four varieties of typhus cause similar types of illnesses, though they vary in severity.

Epidemic typhus causes fever, headache, weakness, and muscle aches. It also causes a rash composed of both spots and bumps. The rash starts on the back, chest, and abdomen, then spreads to the arms and legs. The worst complications involve swelling in the heart muscle (carditis) or brain (**encephalitis**). Without treatment, this type of typhus can be fatal.

Brill-Zinsser disease is quite mild, resulting in about a week-long fever, and a light rash similar to that of the original illness.

Endemic typhus causes about 12 days of high fever, with chills and headache. A light rash may occur.

Scrub typhus causes a wide variety of effects. The main symptoms include fever, headache, muscle aches and pains, cough, abdominal pain, nausea and vomiting, and diarrhea. Some patients experience only these symptoms, while others also develop a rash that can be flat or bumpy. The individual spots develop crusty black scabs. Other patients develop a more serious disease, in which encephalitis, **pneumonia**, and swelling of the liver and spleen (hepatosplenomegaly) occur.

Diagnosis

Numerous tests exist to determine the reactions of a patient's antibodies (immune cells in the blood) to the presence of certain viral and bacterial markers. For instance, a complete blood count (CBC) may show anemia and low platelets. Blood tests for typhus may show: low level of albumin, high level of typhus antibodies, low **sodium** level, moderately high liver enzymes, and mild kidney failure. When the antibodies react in a particular way, it suggests the presence of a rickettsial infection. Many tests require time for processing, so practitioners frequently begin treatment without completing tests, simply on the basis of a patient's symptoms.

Treatment

The **antibiotics** tetracycline or chloramphenicol are used for treatment of each of the forms of typhus. Other antibiotics used for typhus include azithromycin and doxycycline. Tetracycline is taken orally. It is usually not prescribed for children because it can permanently stain their teeth. Besides antibiotics, patients with epidemic typhus may also require oxygen and intravenous fluids. Prompt treatment with one of these antibiotics usually will cure most cases of typhus. Without treatment, typhus can be fatal. The death rate for untreated epidemic typhus varies from 10% for younger people to 40% for older ones.

Public health role and response

Outbreaks of typhus are limited in developed countries like the United States but the disease has the potential to re-emerge. In undeveloped and developing countries, the disease is still responsible for major

QUESTIONS TO ASK YOUR DOCTOR

- Should I be worried about contracting typhus from fleas or lice?
- How dangerous is my form of typhus?
- Is typhus contagious before symptoms appear?
- What symptoms should I watch for with regards to typhus?
- If I was exposed to someone with typhus, can I give it to others?
- What types of tests do I need?
- Are treatments available to help me recover from typhus?
- How long will a full recovery take?
- When can I return to my daily routine?
- What are the possible causes for my symptoms?
- Am I at risk of any long-term complications?

outbreaks. Typhus killed approximately 100,000 people during the civil war in Burundi, which lasted from 1993 to 2005.

The **WHO** published the report *Outbreak Surveillance and Response in Humanitarian Emergencies* in 2012. It states, "Humanitarian emergencies often involve the displacement of large numbers of people. Those affected are frequently settled in temporary locations with high population densities, inadequate food and shelter, unsafe **water**, poor sanitation and lack of infrastructure. These circumstances can increase the risk of transmission of communicable diseases and other conditions, and can thus lead to increased mortality (death). In particular, diseases that have a tendency to become epidemic (referred to as epidemic-prone diseases) can be a major cause of morbidity (sickness) and mortality during emergencies. Rapid detection and prompt response to epidemics among the affected population is a key priority during humanitarian crises." The WHO reports that scrub typhus is one of the most common vector-borne diseases that can occur in humanitarian emergency settings.

Prognosis

The prognosis depends on what types of complications an individual patient experiences. Most patients usually recover well from epidemic typhus with treatment. However, older adults may have as much as a 60% death rate without treatment. Brill-Zinsser disease carries no threat of death. People usually recover uneventfully from endemic typhus, although the elderly, those with other medical problems, or people mistakenly treated with sulfa drugs may have a 1% death rate from the illness. Scrub typhus responds well to appropriate treatment, but untreated patients have a death rate of about 7%.

The relatively high death rate from untreated typhus is one reason there is some concern that its causative organisms might be used in the future as agents of bioterrorism.

Prevention

Prevention for each of these forms of typhus includes avoidance of the insects that carry the causative bacteria. Other preventive measures include good hygiene and the use of insect repellents.

Resources

BOOKS

Beers, Mark H., Robert S. Porter, and Thomas V. Jones, eds. *The Merck Manual of Diagnosis and Therapy*, 18th ed. Whitehouse Station, NJ: Merck Research Laboratories, 2006.

Bynum, William, and Helen Bynum, eds. *Great Discoveries in Medicine*. New York: Thames & Hudson, 2011.

Sartre, Jean-Paul. *Typhus*. London: Seagull Books, 2010.

Shannon, Joyce Brennfleck, ed. *Contagious Diseases Sourcebook: Basic Consumer Health Information about Diseases Spread from Person to Person*. Detroit: Omnigraphics, 2010.

Wilder-Smith, Annelies, Eli Schwartz, and Marc Shaw, eds. *Travel Medicine: Tales Behind the Science*. Amsterdam: Elsevier, 2007.

WEBSITES

David, Patrick. *Typhus*. MedicineNet.com. http://www.medicinenet.com/typhus/article.htm (accessed October 13, 2012).

Typhus. Medline Plus. http://www.nlm.nih.gov/medlineplus/ency/article/001363.htm (accessed October 13, 2012).

Typhus. World Health Organization. May 1997. http://www.who.int/mediacentre/factsheets/fs162/en/index.html (accessed October 13, 2012).

Typhus Fever (Louse-Borne Typhus). International Association for Medical Assistance to Travellers. http://www.iamat.org/disease_details.cfm?id=15 (accessed October 13, 2012).

ORGANIZATIONS

Centers for Disease Control and Prevention, 1600 Clifton Rd., Atlanta, GA 30333, (800) 232-4636, cdcinfo@cdc.gov, http://www.cdc.gov/.

National Institute of Allergy and Infectious Diseases, 1301 Pennsylvania Ave., NW, Ste. 800, Washington, D.C. 20004, (202) 785-3355, Fax: (202) 452-1805, http://www.niaid.nih.gov.

World Health Organization, Avenue Appia 20, Geneva, Switzerland 1211 27, 41 22 791-2111, Fax: 41 22 791-3111, http://www.who.int/en.

Rosalyn Carson-DeWitt, MD
Rebecca J. Frey, PhD
William A. Atkins, BB, BS, MBA

United States Public Health Service (USPHS)

Definition

The United States Public Health Service (USPHS) is the federal agency primarily responsible for public health activities in the United States.

Purpose

The USPHS has three primary objectives: to provide rapid and effective response to public health problems; to provide leadership and excellence in maintaining public health practice; and to advance the knowledge base of public health practices in the United States.

Description

The USPHS was established by the Public Health Service Act of 1944 as the primary agency with the U.S. Department of Health, Education, and Welfare (now the **Department of Health and Human Services**; HHS). The agency has a much longer history, that dates to the establishment of the Marine Hospital Service in 1798, a service that lasted until 1902. The Marine Hospital Service was then renamed the U.S. Public Health and Marine Hospital Service, whose responsibilities were later divided among a number of other federal health agencies, such as the Division of Insular and Foreign Quarantine, the Division of Venereal Diseases, and the Division of Scientific Research. In the 1944 reorgnization act, a number of existing agencies were consolidated under the new USPHS. Today the main health components of the USPHS are the Agency for Healthcare Research and Quality (AHRQ), Agency for Toxic Substances and Disease Registry (ATSDR), **Centers for Disease Control and Prevention (CDC)**, Food and Drug Administration (FDA), Health Resources and Services Administration (HRSA), Indian Health Service (IHS), National Institutes of Health (NIH), and Substance Abuse and Mental Health Services Administration (SAMHSA). The USPHS is under the direction of the Assistant Secretary for Health of the HHS and the Surgeon General of the United States.

A critical part of the USPHS is the USPHS Commissioned Corps, one of the seven "uniformed services" of the U.S. government, which also include the U.S. Army, Navy, Air Force, Marine Corps, Coast Guard, and National Oceanic and Atmospheric Administration Commissioned Corps. The Commissioned Corps consists of more than 6,500 professionals from a wide variety of occupations, such as physicians, dentists, nurses, pharmacists, dietitians, engineers, **environmental health** officers, mental health specialists, optometrists, physician assistants, therapists of all kinds, and veterinarians. The many responsibilities of the Commissioned Corps include: providing service to otherwise underserved populations, such as the urban poor, minority groups, and Native Americans; identifying potential health hazards and developing programs to protect against those hazards; combating the spread of infectious diseases; conducting research on public health problems; monitoring the safety of foods, drugs, commercial products, and other materials used by Americans in their everyday lives; working with nongovernmental agencies and foreign governments to promote good public health policies and practices. Some examples of the programs in which members of the Commissioned Corps have been involved in recent years include the terrorist attacks of September 2001, hurricanes Katrina and Rita in 2005, the 2010 earthquake in Haiti, the Deepwater Horizon oil spill in the Gulf of Mexico in 2010, and the 2011 tsunami and earthquake in Japan, and hurricane Sandy in 2012.

A new component of the Commissioned Corps created within the 2010 Affordable Care Act is the Ready Reserve Corps, a unit roughly comparable to reserve units that exist in other uniformed services. The Ready Reserve Corps will consist of trained professionals in the fields listed who will be available for service in case of emergencies or special needs. They will serve in the corps as volunteers, although they will also be subject to call–up in times of national emergency.

Professional Publications

The various agencies of the USPHS each publish and distribute a very wide selection of print and electronic materials describing the work they do and reporting on their accomplishments. The print and electronic resources of the USPHS itself are somewhat limited and consist primarily of collected articles about the agency's work on the media page of its website and of videos illustrating the work of the typical member of the Commissioned Corps.

Resources

BOOKS

Patel, Kant, and Mark E. Rushefsky. *The Politics of Public Health in the United States.* Armonk, NY: M. E. Sharpe, 2005.

U.S. Public Health Service Commissioned Corps. Rockville, MD: U.S. Public Health Service, U.S. Department of Health & Human Services, 2006.

Williams, Ralph C. *The United States Public Health Service, 1798–1950.* Washington, DC: Commissioned Officers Association of the U.S. Public Health Service, 1951.

PERIODICALS

Flower, Louis, et al. "U.S. Public Health Service Commissioned Corps Pharmacists: Making a Difference in Advancing the Nation's Health." *Journal of the American Pharmacists Association* 49. 3. (2009): 446–452.

Kleinman, D. V., D. J. Hickey, and J. A. Lipton. "Promoting the Public's Oral Health: The Department of Health and Human Services, U.S. Public Health Service, and the U.S. Public Health Service Commissioned Corps." *The Journal of the American College of Dentists* 70. 2. (2003): 16–21.

"You, Too, Can Have a Great Career in the U.S. Public Health Service." *Journal of Environmental Health* 72. 6. (2010): 59–61.

WEBSITES

Commissioned Officers Association of the USPHS Inc. http://www.coausphs.org/ (accessed October 14, 2012).

U.S. Public Health Service. The Social Welfare History Project. http://www.socialwelfarehistory.com/organizations/u-s-public-health-service/ (accessed October 14, 2012).

ORGANIZATIONS

U.S. Public Health Service (USPHS), 5600 Fishers Lane, Rockville, MD 20857, (301) 427-3280, Fax: (301) 427-3431, http://www.usphs.gov/main/contact.aspx, www.usphs.gov/.

David E. Newton, EdD

V

Vaccination

Definition

Vaccination is the injection of a weakened or dead microbe in a person to stimulate the immune system against the microbe and prevent disease.

Purpose

The first vaccine was developed in 1796 by English physician Edward Jenner. Jenner took a few drops of the fluid seeping from a pustule of a woman who was infected with cowpox, and injected it into a healthy young boy. Six weeks later, Jenner injected the boy with fluid from a **smallpox** pustule, and the boy did not develop smallpox, a devastating disease that killed over a million people each year in Europe. Survivors were often left blind, deeply scarred, and deformed. By the start of the twentieth century, vaccines for smallpox, **rabies**, **diphtheria**, **typhoid fever**, and **plague** had been developed. Vaccines are available against more than 20 infectious diseases, including **polio**, **influenza**, **pneumonia**, **whooping cough** (pertussis), **rubella**, **meningitis**, and **hepatitis** B.

Vaccines are medicines that contain weakened or dead bacteria or viruses. When a person is given a vaccine, his or her immune system responds by producing proteins called antibodies. When the person is later exposed to live bacteria or viruses of the same kind that were in the vaccine, the antibodies destroy those organisms and prevent them from making the person sick. Vaccines usually stimulate the cellular immune system as well. In other words, the person becomes immune to the disease that the organisms normally cause. The process of building up immunity by being given a vaccine is called **immunization**.

Vaccines are used in several ways. Some, such as the rabies vaccine, normally are given only when a person is likely to have been exposed to the virus that causes the disease, as through a bite from a wild animal. Others are given to travelers planning to visit countries where certain diseases are common, as in the case of typhoid fever or **yellow fever**. Vaccines such as the influenza vaccine, or the "flu shot," are given mainly to specific groups of people who are at high risk of developing influenza or its complications. There are also vaccines that are given to almost everyone, such as the ones that prevent diphtheria, **tetanus**, polio, or **measles**.

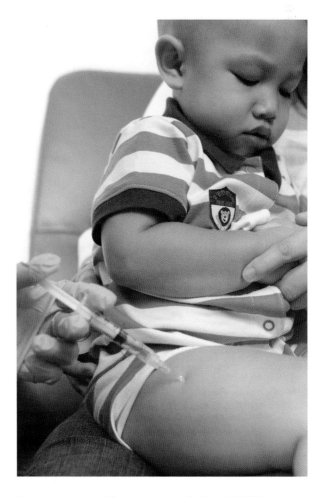

A young boy receiving a vaccine injection. *(CDC/Amanda Mills)*

KEY TERMS

Anthrax—An infectious disease caused by a type of bacterium. The disease can be passed from animals to people and usually is fatal. Symptoms include sores on the skin.

Antibodies—Proteins that are normally produced by specialized white blood cells after stimulation by a foreign substance (antigen) and that act specifically against the antigen in an immune response.

Antigen—Any foreign substance, usually a protein, that stimulates the body's immune system to produce antibodies.

Bacteria—Tiny, single-celled forms of life that cause many diseases and infections.

Chickenpox—A mild disease common in childhood that is caused by a poxvirus; infection can have serious results in adults.

Cholera—An infection of the small intestine caused by a type of bacterium. The disease is spread by drinking water or eating seafood or other foods that have been contaminated with the feces of infected people. It occurs in parts of Asia, Africa, Latin America, India, and the Middle East. Symptoms include watery diarrhea and exhaustion, and it is often fatal to young children and the elderly.

Cowpox—A mild disease in cows that is caused by a poxvirus.

Diphtheria—A serious, infectious disease that produces a toxin (poison) and an inflammation in the membrane lining of the throat, nose, trachea, and other tissues.

Encephalitis—Inflammation of the brain, usually caused by a virus. The inflammation may interfere with normal brain function and may cause seizures, sleepiness, confusion, personality changes, weakness in one or more parts of the body, and even coma.

Feces—The solid aste that is left after food is digested. Feces form in the intestines and pass out of the body through the anus. Also called stool.

Guillain-Barré syndrome (GBS)—A disease of the nerves with symptoms that include sudden numbness and weakness in the arms and legs, sometimes leading to paralysis. The disease is serious and requires medical treatment, but most people recover completely.

H1N1 (Swine Flu)—A disease that was originally found in pigs and can be passed from animal to human or human to human. Symptoms of H1N1 include fever, cough, chills, fatigue, headache, and body aches.

Human papillomavirus (HPV)—The most common sexually transmitted virus, HPV causes genital warts and cervical cancer.

Immune system—The body's natural defenses against disease and infection.

Immunization—Administering a vaccine that stimulates the body to create antibodies to a specific disease (immunity) without causing symptoms of the disease.

Infectious disease—Any disease caused by invasion of a pathogen that subsequently grows and multiplies in the body.

Children routinely are given a series of vaccinations that begin at birth. Given according to a specific schedule, these vaccinations protect against hepatitis B, diphtheria, tetanus, whooping cough, measles, **mumps**, rubella (German measles), varicella (chickenpox), polio, pneumococcus and *Haemophilus influenzae* type b (Hib disease, a major cause of spinal meningitis) and, in some states, hepatitis A. This series of vaccinations is recommended by the American Academy of Family Physicians, the American Academy of Pediatrics, and the **Centers for Disease Control and Prevention (CDC)**. It is required in all states before children can enter school. All states will make exceptions for children who have medical conditions, such as **cancer**, that prevent them

from having vaccinations, and some states also will make exceptions for children whose parents object for religious or other reasons.

Additional vaccines are available for preventing **rotavirus** infection (given to infants), **anthrax**, **cholera**, Japanese **encephalitis**, meningococcal meningitis, plague, **tuberculosis**, typhoid fever, H1N1 (swine flu), yellow fever, chickenpox, human papillomavirus, and zoster (**shingles**).

Description

Most vaccines are given as injections, but a few are given by mouth or as a nasal spray.

KEY TERMS (continued)

Inflammation—Pain, redness, swelling, and heat that usually develop in response to injury or illness.

Influenza—A disease caused by viruses that infect the respiratory tract.

Measles—An acute and highly contagious viral disease marked by distinct red spots followed by a rash that occurs primarily in children.

Meningitis—Inflammation of tissues that surround the brain and spinal cord.

Microbe—A microorganism, especially a bacterium, that causes disease.

Mumps—An acute and highly contagious viral illness that usually occurs in childhood.

Pathogen—A disease-causing microorganism.

Plague—A highly infectious disease that can be fatal if not treated promptly. The bacteria that cause plague mainly infect rats, mice, squirrels, and other wild rodents. The disease is passed to people through fleas. Infected people can then spread the disease to other people.

Rabies—A rare but serious disease caused by a virus carried in saliva. It is transmitted when an infected animal bites a person.

Rubella—A contagious viral disease that is milder than typical measles but is damaging to the fetus when it occurs early in pregnancy. Also called German measles.

Seizure—A sudden attack, spasm, or convulsion.

Smallpox—A highly contagious viral disease characterized by fever, weakness, and skin eruption with pustules that form scabs that slough off, leaving scars.

Tuberculosis—An infectious disease that usually affects the lungs but may also affect other parts of the body. Symptoms include fever, weight loss, and coughing up blood.

Typhoid fever—An infectious disease caused by a type of bacterium and characterized by a lingering fever, diarrhea, feelings of exhaustion and depression, and rose-colored spots on the chest and abdomen. The disease is spread through poor sanitation.

Virus—A tiny, disease-causing particle that can reproduce only in living cells.

Whooping cough—An infectious disease, also called pertussis, especially afflicting children, that is caused by a bacterium and is marked by a convulsive, spasmodic cough, sometimes followed by a shrill intake of breath.

Yellow fever—An infectious disease caused by a virus. The disease, which is spread by mosquitoes, is most common in Central and South America and Central Africa. Symptoms include high fever, jaundice (yellow eyes and skin) and dark-colored vomit, a sign of internal bleeding. Yellow fever can be fatal.

Zoster—A viral disease, also known as shingles or zona, that is characterized by a painful rash and can afflict anyone who has had chickenpox.

Some vaccines are combined in one injection, such as the measles-mumps-rubella (MMR) or diphtheria-tetanus-pertussis (DTaP) combinations.

Recommended dosage

The recommended dosage depends on the type of vaccine and may be different for different patients. Dosage is standardized for each specific type and usually varies based on age. The healthcare professional who gives the vaccine will determine the proper dose.

A vaccination health record helps parents and health care providers keep track of a child's vaccinations. The record should be started when the child has his or her first vaccination and should be updated with each additional vaccination. While most physicians follow the recommended vaccination schedule, parents should understand that some flexibility is allowed, such as if the child is sick at the time the vaccination is due. Slight departures will not prevent the child from developing immunity, as long as all the vaccinations are given at approximately the right times. The child's physician is the best person to decide when each vaccination should be given.

Anyone planning a trip to another country should check to find out what vaccinations are needed. Some vaccinations must be given as much as 12 weeks before the trip, so getting this information early is important. Many major hospitals and medical centers have travel

ALBERT BRUCE SABIN (1906–1993)

Albert Bruce Sabin was born on August 26, 1906, in Bialystok, Russia, to Jacob and Tillie Sabin. In order to escape extreme poverty, the Sabins immigrated to the United States and settled in Paterson, New Jersey. Following his graduation from high school in 1923, Sabin was able to attend dentistry school at New York University due to his uncle's generous offer for financing. However, after reading Paul deKruif's *Microbe Hunters* he became intrigued by virology and the idea of curing epidemic diseases. After two years of dentistry school, Sabin decided to switch to medicine, earning his M.D. in 1931. Sabin completed his residency and internship in the United States and then went to London to conduct research.

Sabin returned to the United States in 1935 to resume his research of polio at the Rockefeller Institute.

In 1953, Jonas Salk announced that he had created a dead-virus polio vaccine that was safe, but soon after its administration many people died. Sabin, however, wanted to create a live-virus vaccine, which he felt would be safer. Sabin diluted three strains of the polio virus and tested these on himself, his family, and other volunteers. These live-virus vaccines (given orally) proved safe and effective and soon became the vaccinations of choice around the world. Sabin's published works include *Viruses and Cancer: A Public Lecture in Conversational Style* (1965), *Behavior of Chimpanzee-Avirulent Poliomyelitis Viruses in Experimentally Infected Human Volunteers* (1955), and *Recent Advances in Our Knowledge of Dengue and Sand Fly Fever* (1955). Sabin died of congestive heart failure on March 3, 1993.

clinics that can provide this information. The Traveler's Health Section of the **Centers for Disease Control and Prevention** website also has information on vaccination requirements.

Precautions

Vaccines are not always 100% effective, and there is no way to predict whether a vaccine will fail to provide adequate immunity in any particular person. To be most effective in preventing disease outbreaks, vaccination programs depend on whole communities participating. The more people who are vaccinated, the lower everyone's risk of being exposed to a disease. Even people who do not develop immunity through vaccination are safer when their friends, neighbors, children, and coworkers are immunized. In addition to vaccines, hand washing and proper **hygiene** are the most effective means for preventing the spread of infectious diseases.

Like most medical procedures, vaccination has risks as well as substantial benefits. Anyone who takes a vaccine should make sure he or she is fully informed about both the benefits and the risks. Any questions or concerns should be discussed with a physician or other health care provider. The Centers for Disease Control and Prevention (CDC) offers substantial information on immunizations and vaccinations.

Vaccines may cause problems for people with certain **allergies**.

• Patients who have allergies to antibiotics neomycin or polymyxin B should not take rubella vaccine, measles vaccine, mumps vaccine, or the combined MMR vaccine.

• Patients who have allergies to baker's yeast should not take the hepatitis B vaccine.

• Patients who have allergies to antibiotics, such as gentamicin sulfate, streptomycin sulfate, or other aminoglycosides, should check with their physicians before taking influenza vaccine, as some influenza vaccines contain small amounts of these drugs.

• Patients who have allergies to eggs should not take vaccines grown in the fluids of chick embryos, including those for influenza, measles, and mumps.

In general, anyone who has had an unusual reaction to a vaccine in the past should inform the physician before taking the same kind of vaccine again. The physician also should be told about any allergies to foods, medicines, preservatives, or other substances.

People with certain other medical conditions should be cautious about taking vaccines. Influenza vaccine, for example, may reactivate the rare Guillain-Barré syndrome (GBS) in people who have had it before. This vaccine also may worsen illnesses that involve the lungs, such as bronchitis or pneumonia. Vaccines that cause fever as a side effect may trigger seizures in people who have a history of seizures caused by fever.

Certain vaccines are not recommended for use during pregnancy, but some may be given to women at especially high risk of getting a specific disease such as polio. Vaccines also may be given to pregnant women to prevent medical problems in their babies. For example, vaccinating a pregnant woman with tetanus toxoid can prevent her baby from getting tetanus at birth.

Women should avoid becoming pregnant for three months after taking rubella vaccine, measles vaccine, mumps vaccine, or the combined MMR, as these vaccines could cause problems in the unborn baby.

Women who are breastfeeding should check with their physicians before taking any vaccine.

Side effects

Most side effects from vaccines are minor and easily treated. The most common are **pain**, redness, and swelling at the site of the injection. Some people may develop a fever or a rash. In rare cases, vaccines may cause severe allergic reactions, swelling of the brain, or seizures. Anyone who has an unusual reaction after receiving a vaccine should contact a physician immediately.

Interactions

Vaccines may interact with other medicines and medical treatments. When this happens, the effects of the vaccine or the other medicine may change, or the risk of side effects may be greater. For example, **radiation** therapy and cancer drugs may reduce the effectiveness of many vaccines or may increase the chance of side effects. Anyone who takes a vaccine should let the physician know all other medicines he or she is taking and should ask whether the possible interactions could interfere with the effects of the vaccine or the other medicines.

Resources

BOOKS

Cave, Stephanie, and Deborah Mitchell. *What Your Doctor May Not Tell You About Children's Vaccinations.* New York: Wellness Central, 2010.

Centers for Disease Control and Prevention. *Epidemiology and Prevention of Vaccine-Preventable Diseases.* Atkinson W., S. Wolfe, and J. Hamborsky, eds. 12th ed., second printing. Washington DC: Public Health Foundation, 2012.

Miller, Neil Z. *Vaccine Safety Manual for Concerned Families and Health Practitioners.* 2nd ed. Santa Fe, NM: New Atlantean Press, 2010.

Offit, Paul A. *The Cutter Incident: How America's First Polio Vaccine Led to the Growing Vaccine Crisis.* New Haven: Yale University Press, 2007.

———. *Vaccinated: One Man's Quest to Defeat the World's Deadliest Diseases.* New York: Collins, 2007.

Queijo, Jon. *Breakthrough: How the 10 Greatest Discoveries in Medicine Saved Millions and Changed our View of the World.* Upper Saddle River, NJ: FT Press Science, 2010.

Sears, Robert. *The Vaccine Book: Making the Right Decision for Your Child.* New York: Little, Brown and Company, 2011.

PERIODICALS

Gans, H.A. "The Status of Live Viral Vaccination in Early Life." Vaccine S0264-410X(12)01363-1 (October 2012).

Lavall, K.H., and A.M. Kennedy. "The Role of Attitudes About Vaccine Safety, Efficacy, and Value in Explaining Parents' Reported Vaccination Behavior." Health Education & Behavior 39:5 (October 2012).

WEBSITES

"Immunization." Medline Plus. http://www.nlm.nih.gov/medlineplus/immunization.html (accessed November 11, 2012).

"Vaccines, Blood & Biologics: Vaccines." U.S. Food and Drug Administration. http://www.fda.gov/BiologicsBlood Vaccines/Vaccines/default.htm (accessed November 11, 2012).

"Vaccines and Immunizations." Centers for Disease Control. http://www.cdc.gov/vaccines (accessed November 11, 2012).

ORGANIZATIONS

American Academy of Pediatrics, 141 Northwest Point Boulevard, Elk Grove Village, IL 60007-1098, (847) 434-4000, Fax: (847) 434-8000, http://www.aap.org

Centers for Disease Control and Prevention (CDC), 1600 Clifton Road, Atlanta, GA 30333, (404) 639-3534, (800) CDC-INFO (800-232-4636). TTY: (888) 232-6348, inquiry@cdc.gov, http://www.cdc.gov

National Institute of Allergy and Infectious Diseases, National Institutes of Health, 6610 Rockledge Drive, MSC 6612, Bethesda, MD 20892-6612, (301) 284-4107, (866) 284-4107 or TDD (800)877-8339 (for hearing impaired), Fax: (301) 402-3573, http://www.niaid.nih.gov/Pages/default.aspx

National Vaccine Program Office, 200 Independence Avenue, SW Room 715-H, Washington, DC 20201, (202) 619-0257, http://www.hhs.gov/nvpo/.

Larry I. Lutwick, MD
Monique Laberge, PhD
Tish Davidson, AM
Paul Checchia, MD
Fran Hodgkins

Veterinary medicine

Definition

Veterinary medicine is the field of medicine that addresses the diseases, disorders, and injuries that may affect nonhuman animals. It focuses on the **prevention**, diagnosis, and treatment of such diseases and injuries, along with the transmission of zoonotic diseases from nonhuman animals to humans.

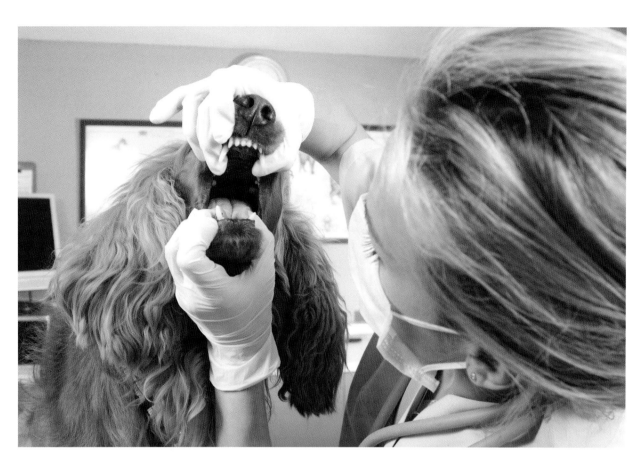

Veterinarian examing a dog. *(Serdar Tibet/Shutterstock.com)*

Purpose

The purpose of veterinary medicine is to provide nonhuman animals with the same type of medical care that is generally available for humans.

Description

The field of veterinary medicine is very similar to that of human medicine, with the major exception of the subject of medical care. As with the human medical profession, veterinary medicine involves the use of workers at various levels of training and expertise, including veterinary physicians (comparable to human medical physicians), veterinary technicians (comparable in many cases to human medical nurses, physicians assistants, nurse practitioners, and similar workers), and veterinary assistants, who may have little or no professional training in the field of veterinary medicine. Veterinary workers with less training than a veterinary physician are sometimes referred to as paraveterinary workers. Veterinary physicians are generally legally certified professionals who have completed undergraduate and graduate training that leads to the degree of doctor of veterinary medicine (DVM), comparable to the degree of

doctor of medicine (MD) in human medicine. Veterinary technicians generally complete at least a two-year college program roughly similar to that of a practical nurse in human medicine. The typical DVM program includes courses such as introduction to veterinary medicine, veterinary anatomy and physiology, cell biology, diagnostic imaging, bacteriology and mycology, parasitology, virology, veterinary surgery, **epidemiology** and public health, endocrine and metabolic diseases, and diseases of farm animals and other animal groups and species.

Veterinary medicine involves the care of all types of animals, including both domestic and wild species. Many veterinarians specialize in the care of special categories of animals, such as small animals (primarily domestic pets, such as dogs, cats, and birds), large animals, farm animals, or wild animals. Specializations are becoming more common also, with many veterinarians choosing to focus on areas such as dentistry, anesthesiology, cardiology, neurology, **nutrition**, and animal behavior. Some veterinarians have also decided to focus on the use of complementary and alternative treatment of animals, such as the use of acupuncture for the treatment of some animal diseases and injuries. The vast majority of veterinary workers are employed in neighborhood clinics, where they

KEY TERMS

Endemic—Characteristic or native to a particular region, species, or population.

One Health—A movement based on the concept of individuals from a wide variety of disciplines to obtain the maximum level of health possible for individuals of all species.

Paraveterinarian—A person who assists a veterinarian in working with nonhuman animals.

Zoonotic disease—A disease that is endemic to animals.

treat their animal clients directly. Some veterinarians are also employed in specialized assignments, however, as at race tracks, in large dairy facilities, or at zoos.

Origins

Abundant evidence indicates that veterinary medicine has been practiced in one form or another from the beginning of recorded history. That is hardly surprising, given the essential role that animals have had as a means of transportation, mechanism for work, source of food, and companion of families since the earliest days of human societies. Some Chinese works of medicine dating to the second millennium B.C., for example, refer to "horse priests" who specialized in the care and treatment of large animals. Many early medical works in China and other countries also included sections on the health and medical problems of nonhuman animals, with suggestions for their treatment and prevention. One authority points out that the first descriptions of acupuncture referred to the use of this procedure on horses rather than animals, since the former were often regarded as more essential to a society than the latter. The world's first formal veterinary school is said to have been founded in Lyon, France, in 1761, and the first degree in veterinary medicine in the United States was granted by Cornell University in 1876.

Demographics

According to a survey by the AVMA, there were 92,547 veterinarians in the United States in 2011, divided almost equally between women (49,353) and men (43,194). In addition to general-practice veterinarians, a number of these individuals were board-certified in a variety of special fields, such as internal medicine (2,257), pathology (1,637), surgery (1,386), preventive medicine (679), radiology (408), emergency and critical care (384), ophthalmology (355), anesthesiology (194), microbiology (216), nutrition (61), behavior (52), clinical pharmacology (48), and sports medicine and rehabilitation (27).

Effects on public health

One area of growing interest among many veterinarians is the concept of One Health, which involves problems posed by zoonotic diseases, diseases that are endemic to nonhuman animals, but that are relatively easily transmitted to humans. Many public health authorities are convinced that zoonotic diseases may be the greatest public health problem among humans in the twenty-first century. Beginning in the mid-twentieth century, a group of veterinarians took the lead in developing mechanisms by which medical experts across all species lines could begin working together to develop a better understanding of the nature of zoonotic diseses, the mechanisms by which they are transmitted across species, and the ways in which veterinarians, physicians, and other health and medical specialists could work together on these issues. Developed originally by members of the veterinary profession, One Health has now become a powerful movement throughout the health and medical profession in the United States and around the world.

Resources

BOOKS

Coston, Bruce R. *The Gift of Pets: Stories Only a Vet Could Tell*. New York: Thomas Dunne Books, 2012.

Division on Earth and Life Studies. *Workforce Needs in Veterinary Medicine*. Washington, DC: National Academies Press, 2012.

Field, Shelly. *Career Opportunities Working with Animals*. New York: Ferguson's, 2012.

Sirois, Margi. *Elsevier's Veterinary Assisting Textbook*. St. Louis: Elsevier/Mosby, 2013.

PERIODICALS

Burns, K. "Task Force Presents Revised Model Practice Act." *Journal of the American Veterinary Medical Association* 240, 1. (2012): 13–4.

Dantas-Torres, F., B.B. Chomel, and D. Otranto. "Ticks and Tick-Borne Diseases: A One Health Perspective." *Trends in Parasitology* 28, 10. (2012): 437–46.

Flatland, B. "Veterinary Laboratory Quality Management—It Takes a Village." *Veterinary Clinical Pathology* 41, 2. (2012): 171–3.

Orand, J.P. "Antimicrobial Resistance and the Standards of the World Organisation for Animal Health." *Revue Scientifique et Technique* 31, 1. (2012): 335–42.

WEBSITES

"Animal and Veterinary." Food and Drug Administration. http://www.fda.gov/AnimalVeterinary/default.htm. (accessed October 31, 2012).

"Careers in Veterinary Medicine." Association of American Veterinary Medicine Colleges. http://www.aavmc.org/students-applicants-and-advisors/careers-in-veterinary-medicine.aspx. (accessed October 31, 2012).

"Preventive Veterinary Medicine." http://www.sciencedirect.com/science/journal/01675877. (accessed October 31, 2012).

"Veterinarians." Occupational Outlook Handbook. http://www.bls.gov/ooh/healthcare/veterinarians.htm. (accessed October 31, 2012).

ORGANIZATIONS

American Veterinary Medical Association (AVMA), 1931 North Meacham Rd., Suite 100, Schaumburg, IL USA 60173–4360, (800) 248–2862, Fax: 1 (847) 925–1329, https://www.avma.org/About/WhoWeAre/Pages/contact.aspx, https://www.avma.org/.

David E. Newton, Ed.D.

Violence

Definition

Violence is the exertion of substantial force, either physical or emotional, with the intent of causing harm to another individual or group of individuals.

Purpose

An individual or group of individuals uses violence on another individual or group of individuals for the purpose of causing serious physical or emotional harm, such as severe injury or death, or feelings of fear, anxiety, or other sense of mental distress.

Description

As youth activist H. Rap Brown once said, "violence is as American as apple pie." He might as easily said, "violence is as natural for humans as breathing," because acts of violence have been a regular part of human life for as long as human history has existed. Indeed, one might argue that the process of civilization is, in some regards, largely an effort to bring under control the violent instincts that seem an inherent part of human life. Violence, therefore, is as old as the human race.

However, discussing violence as a public health issue has a much shorter history, dating back only about to the late 1970s in the United States, and even later in most of the rest of the world. Some historians date the origin of violence as a public health issue in the United States to a 1979 report by the Surgeon General, *Healthy People*, which chronicled the impressive gains made

against **infectious disease** and other traditional health problems in the preceding century. The report then listed 15 areas in which the Surgeon General looked for further progress in the coming years. One of those areas was the prevention of violence. The report noted that as infectious diseases became less significant as the cause of death in the United States, other factors, such as violence, became more important. The nation needed to begin to think of violence, the Surgeon General said, as a problem that could be attacked and solved using the same methods as those used in dealing with other public health problems.

Some two decades later, the **World Health Organization (WHO)** followed the lead of the Surgeon General's report. It placed violence on the agenda of the 1996 World Health Assembly, which eventually adopted a resolution calling violence "a leading worldwide public health proble." Both the **WHO** and a number of public health agencies in countries around the world have since made violence a major focus of their research and policies recommendations. In the United States, for example, a report by the National Research Council and Institute of Medicine resulted in 1983 in the formation of the first public health agency chartered to focus specifically on violence issues, the Division of Injury **Epidemiology** and Control (DIEC) in the **Centers for Disease Control and Prevention (CDC)**.

Defining violence as a public health issue means using familiar and well-tested public health attitudes and methods to attack problems of violence. Those methods include:

- the recognition that homicide, violent crime, and suicide are causes of death, as surely as are heart attacks, obesity, and smoking
- establishing the prevention of homicide, suicide, and other forms of violence as legitimate and essential goals of all public health programs
- conducting research to establish the epidemiological causes of murder, suicide, and other forms of violence
- recognizing violence as a cause of death in the workplace along with other more traditional causes
- discovering and describing homicide and other forms of violence as causes of special concern among certain subgroups within society, such as minorities, the poor, and children
- acknowledging that sexual and physical abuse of children is an essential public health issue, with causes, treatments, and methods of prevention like those used for other types of disease
- recognizing that firearms are a proximate cause of death and other forms of violence and, therefore, a legitimate subject of study by public health authorities

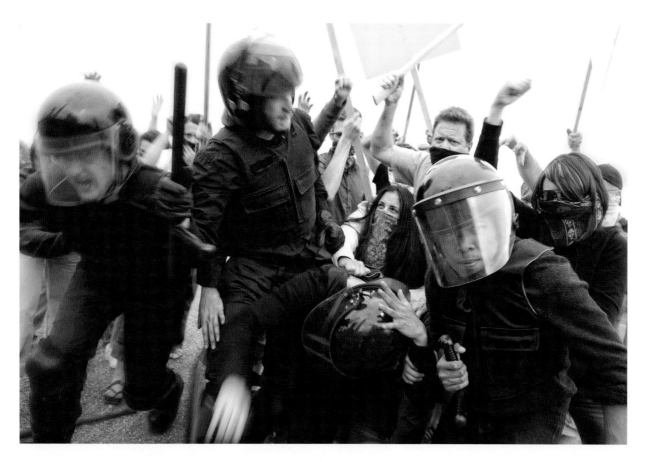

Riot police fight angry mob. (*©iStockphoto.com/inhauscreative*)

The WHO has developed a typology that categorizes various types of violent behavior. At one extreme in that typology is self-directed violence, in which the perpetrator and the victim are the same person. One form of self-directed violence has long been a matter of some interest and concern to health authorities, self-abuse. Only more recently, however, has a more serious form of such violence been included in the panoply of public health challenges, **suicide**. At the other extreme of the WHO typology is group violence, in which many individuals on one side of a dispute commit violence on many individuals on another side of the dispute. This category includes, most obviously, wars and genocide. The WHO also refers to a middle category of violence, interpersonal violence, in which one or a small number of individuals commits violence against another individual or, less commonly, another small group of individuals. The WHO divides this typology along one dimension into physical, sexual, psychological, and deprivation/neglect categories, and the other dimension into individuals against whom violence is committed, such as children, spouses, the elderly, an acquaintance, or a stranger. The WHO suggests that this typology provides a framework within which to study violence and to develop programs for preventing violent acts.

Violence can take many specific forms. For example, one person in a domestic relationship may use physical, sexual, emotional, or some other type of violence in dealing with his or her partner, a phenomenon known as *domestic violence*. Violence in families can also involve the physical, emotional, or sexual abuse of a child, known as *child abuse*. Children and adolescents can also use violence in dealing with their peers, a behavior known as *bullying*. Although the specific actors in these events differ in age, relationship and other characteristics, the acts themselves often have very similar characteristics.

A number of public health agencies have attempted to list a number of acts that can be specifically defined as one form or another of violence. One such list from the government of Newfoundland and Labrador, for example, lists as examples of violence:

• pushing

• pinching

• hair-pulling

• overmedication

• assault

- stabbing
- murder
- forced sexual intercourse
- exhibitionism
- withholding sexual affection
- unfounded allegations of promiscuity and/or infidelity
- name calling
- using silent treatment
- intimidation
- stalking
- threatening to commit suicide
- threats of violence
- threats of abandonment
- verbal aggression
- making fun of religious or spiritual beliefs
- female circumcision
- honor crimes
- cursing
- constant criticism
- expressing distrust
- threats of deportation
- controlling choice of occupation
- denying access to basic needs, such as food and health care
- not paying bills

Demographics

A plethora of data and statistics on all types of violent crimes exists. One of the most useful resources is the U.S. Federal Bureau of Investigation's (FBI) *Uniform Crime Reports*, published annually. Another resource is the Crime and Safety Surveys Program of the National Center for Education Statistics (NECS). The most recent report from the NECS noted that 3.9 percent of all students aged 12 to 18 in U.S. schools in 2009 reported being the target of some type of violent crime. That rate was higher for males than females (4.6 percent compared to 3.2 percent) and highest among Blacks (4.4 percent) compared to Hispanics and Whites (3.9 percent). The most common violent crimes were thefts (2.8 percent of the overall **population**), followed by violent crimes (1.4 percent) and serious violent crimes (0.3 percent), which includes rape, **sexual assault**, robbery, and aggravated assault. Some additional findings of the latest NECS report were that:

- School principals at 85 percent of school surveyed reported at least one violent action during the preceding school year, with a grand total of 1.9 million such events overall for the year (2008–2009).

KEY TERMS

Bullying—A repeated verbal or physical attack by one person on another person, most commonly among children and adolescents.

Collective violence—Violence between two groups of people, as occurs in a war or during genocide.

Domestic violence—Physical, sexual, economic, verbal, or other forms of violence between two people in a close personal relationships, such as a marriage or domestic partnership.

Interpersonal violence—Violence that occurs between two individuals, such as domestic partners, family members, or two unrelated strangers.

Self-directed violence—Suicidal or self-harm acts or thoughts.

Sexual violence—Violence between two or more individuals that involves non-consensual sexual acts with or without physical contact.

Workplace violence—Violence that occurs at the workplace of the perpetrator and/or victim.

- Seven percent of teachers in schools surveyed were threatened with physical attack, 4 percent were actually attacked.

- Four percent of students reported that they feared being physically attacked at school, a significant decrease from 12 percent who reported this feeling in the 1995 NECS survey.

- About 28 percent of students reported being bullied at school, while about 6 percent reported being cyber-bullied. The most common forms of bullying included being the subject of rumors (most common among girls); being pushed, shoved, tripped, or spit on; and being excluded from activities on purpose.

Extensive data are also available on a form of violent behavior that is sometimes not acknowledged as such: suicide. For example, the WHO reports that the three nations in the world with the highest suicide rate for males are Lithuania (61.3 per 100,000 population), Russia (53.9 per 100,000), and Belarus (48.7 per 100,000). The United States reported 17.7 suicides per 100,000 in 2005. The highest rates for females worldwide were from Sri Lanka (22.1 per 100,000), South Korea (16.8 per 100,000), and China (14.8 per 100,000). The comparable rate in the United States was 4.5 per 100,000.

Costs to society

Violence is a large and comprehensive topic, so it is difficult to provide meaningful data on the cost of violence overall to society. However, a number of studies have been done to estimate the cost of certain types of violence to specific nations. In 2003, for example, the **CDC** estimated that domestic violence costs in the United States cost about $5.8 billion annually, although other sources placed that number as high as $12.6 billion. Comparable estimates are available from other nations, such as the United Kingdom (23 billion annually), Canada (CAN$4.2 billion), Australia (A$8.1 billion), and New Zealand (NZ$1.2 billion). In addition to the costs to society, there are additional financial costs for the healthcare of the victims of **domestic abuse**. The CDC has estimated that those costs amounted to about $4.1 billion in 2003.

The financial costs of gun-related violence have also been studied in some detail. According to one frequently-quoted study published in 2000, this form of violence costs Americans about $100 billion annually for medical care, judicial and law enforcement system expenses, security precautions, and reductions in the quality of life. These costs generally extend far beyond those of the immediate victim and his or her family. For example, one study has shown that anywhere from 75 to 93 percent of gunshot victims admitted to a hospital were uninsured, suggesting that their medical costs had to be paid to a considerable extent by the general public. According to one estimate, that fact accounts for a lifetime medical expense to the general public in the United States of $1.1 billion for gunshot victims alone.

Prevention

Violence prevention policies and programs are often classified into one of three general categories: primary, secondary, and tertiary. Primary prevention programs are designed to stop violent acts before they occur. This objective can be accomplished in a number of ways, for example, by changing the attitudes and outlook of potential perpetrators about their victims. Anti-bullying campaigns are often designed with such an objective. Another approach to is remove the mechanism by which violent acts can be carried out, such as increasing the severity of gun possession laws. The likelilhood of success of various primary prevention programs varies widely depending on a host of factors. For example, in the United States in the first decades of the twenty first century, the political climate appears to make it impossible to adjust gun control laws as a primary prevention policy for firearms deaths and injuries.

> ## QUESTIONS TO ASK YOUR DOCTOR
>
> - My son is being bullied on a regular basis at school. What steps can I take to deal with this problem?
> - I know that my neighbor's daughter is being sexually abused at home. What can I do to intervene in this event?
> - I would like to have my children become hunters, but I want them to learn how to use firearms properly. Where I can send them for training in this regard?
> - My husband is constantly being harassed at work by his co-workers. What recourse do we have in such a case?
> - My boss has been making sexual remarks to me lately. I fear that if I complain, I may lose my job. What steps can I take to deal with this problem?

Secondary prevention programs are designed to minimize the results of violent actions once they have occurred. For example, many public health agencies provide recuperative services for rape victims, such as testing for sexually transmitted infections and pregnancy, along with counseling for the victims of rape. Tertiary prevention programs focus on the treatment and recuperation of the victims of violent crime. For example, individuals who have been physically or sexually abused as children may be offered psychological counseling immediately after the event or later in their lives to help them understand the experiences they have been through and to adjust to the violence they have experienced.

Prevention programs can also be classified as universal, targeted (or selective), or indicated programs. Universal programs are those designed for the general population, including anyone who may or may not be at risk for violent behavior. Schools that introduce anti-bullying classes or sessions are making use of universal prevention because some, but not all, students will be subject to this type of violence. Targeted prevention programs are aimed at populations who are known to be at risk for some type of violent behavior or another. For example, a variety of support services are available to low-income single parents who are sometimes overwhelmed with the manifold challenges of holding the family together. Indicated prevention programs are designed for specific individuals who are known to be at risk for specific violent behaviors. For example, some prisons require some or all inmates to participate in violence prevention programs to improve their likelihood of adapting to the post-prison experience.

Resources

BOOKS

Eisler, Barry. *Facing Violence: Preparing for the Unexpected.* Wolfeboro, NH: WMAA Publication Center, 2011.

Hemenway, David. *While We Were Sleeping: Success Stories in Injury and Violence Prevention.* Berkeley: University of California Press, 2009.

Pinker, Steven. *The Better Angels of Our Nature: Why Violence Has Declined.* New York: Penguin Books, 2012.

Wallace, Harvey, and Cliff Robertston. *Family Violence: Legal, Medical, and Social Perspectives*, 6th ed. Upper Saddle River, NJ: Pearson Higher Education, 2010.

PERIODICALS

"ACOG Committee Opinion No. 518: Intimate Partner Violence." *Obstetrics and Gynecology* 119, 2 Pt. 1. (2012): 412–7.

DeVries, K., et al. "Violence against Women Is Strongly Associated with Suicide Attempts: Evidence from the WHO Multi-country Study on Women's Health and Domestic Violence against Women." *Social Science and Medicine* 73, 1. (2011): 79–86.

Fitzpatrick, C., T. Barnett, and L. S. Pagani. "Early Exposure to Media Violence and Later Child Adjustment." *Journal of Development and Behavioral Pediatrics* 33, 4. (2012): 291–7X.

Hall, Ryan C. W., Terri Day, and Richard C. W. Hall. "A Plea for Caution: Violent Video Games, the Supreme Court, and the Role of Science." *Mayo Clinic Proceedings* 86, 4. (2011): 315–21.

WEBSITES

Dahlberg, Linda L., and James A. Mercy. "The History of Violence as a Public Health Issue." http://www.cdc.gov/violenceprevention/pdf/history_violence-a.pdf. (accessed October 3, 2012).

"Futures without Violence." http://www.futureswithout violence.org/. (accessed October 3, 2012).

"Violence." American Psychological Association. http://www.apa.org/topics/violence/index.aspx. (accessed October 3, 2012).

"Violence and Injury Prevention. World Health Organization." http://www.who.int/violence_injury_prevention/violence/en/. (accessed October 3, 2012).

ORGANIZATIONS

Centers for Disease Control and Prevention, 1600 Clifton Rd., N.E., Atlanta, GA USA 30333, 1 (800) 232–4636, cdcinfo@cdc.gov, www.cdc.gov.

David E. Newton, Ed.D.

Visual health

Definition

Visual health is the overall health of the visual system, and the various options available to assist individuals in achieving the best vision possible. Vision is the sense of sight. Total blindness is the inability to tell light from dark, or the total inability to see. Visual impairment or low vision is a severe reduction in vision that cannot be corrected with standard glasses, contact lenses, medicine, or surgery, and reduces a person's ability to function at certain or all tasks. Legal blindness is a severe visual impairment and is not the same as total blindness.

DESCRIPTION. Vision is normally measured using a Snellen chart, which has letters of different sizes that are read, one eye at a time, from a distance of 20 feet. People who have normal vision can read the 20 feet line at 20 feet (the so-called 20/20 line), the 40 feet line at 40 feet, and the 100 feet line at 100 feet. For people who cannot read the 20/20 line, the examiner assigns a ratio based on the smallest line they can read. The first number (numerator) of the ratio is the distance between the chart and the patient, and the second number (denominator) is the distance at which a person with normal vision would be able to read that line. Therefore, a ratio of 20/40 means the patient can see at 20 feet what people with normal vision can see at 40 feet. Legal blindness refers to a best-corrected central vision of 20/200 or worse in the better eye, or a visual acuity of better than 20/200 but with a visual field no greater than 20° (e.g., side vision that is so reduced that it appears as if the person is looking through a tunnel).

When a patient is unable to read any lines on the eye chart, the patient is moved closer until he or she can read the line with the largest letters, which is usually the 200 foot line. The acuity is still measured the same way. A ratio of 5/200 means the person being tested can see at 5 feet what a person with normal vision can see 200 feet.

Eye care professionals measure vision in many ways. Clarity (sharpness) of vision indicates how well a person's central visual status is. The diopter is the unit of measure for refractive errors (inability of the lens to focus an image accurately). Refractive errors, which include nearsightedness (myopia), farsightedness (hyperopia), and astigmatism, indicate the strength of corrective lenses needed. People do not just see straight ahead; the entire area of vision is called the visual field. Some people have good vision (e.g., they can see clearly but have areas of reduced or no vision (blind spots) in parts of their visual field). Others have good vision in the center but poor vision around the edges (peripheral visual field).

Color blindness is the reduced ability to perceive certain colors, usually red and green. It is a hereditary defect and affects very few tasks. "Contrast sensitivity" describes the ability to distinguish one object from another. A person with reduced contrast sensitivity may have problems seeing things in the fog because of the decrease in contrast between the object and the fog.

DEMOGRAPHICS. According to the U.S. Census Bureau report "Americans With Disabilities: 2010," which was issued in July 2012, about 8.1 million people had difficulty seeing, including 2 million who were blind or unable to see. Those numbers compare to 2005 totals of about 7.8 million who had difficulty seeing and about 1.8 million who were blind or unable to see. The 8.1 million total in 2010 represents about 3.3 percent of the overall U.S. **population**. Among those who are 65 years old or older, 9.8 percent had difficulty seeing as of 2010.

Causes and symptoms

Causes

The leading causes of blindness include:

• Macular degeneration, a disease that causes the cells in the macula (a highly sensitized area in the middle of the retina) to die, and gets progressively worse over time.

• Glaucoma, a condition in which the optic nerve is subject to damage—usually, but not always, because of excessively high intraocular pressure (pressure within the eye, also called "IOP"). If untreated, the optic nerve damage results in progressive, permanent vision loss.

• Cataracts, which is a cloudiness of the eye's lens. This can cause blurry vision, difficulty looking at bright lights, and if untreated, vision loss.

• Diabetes mellitus, a set of metabolic diseases characterized by high blood sugar. One complication is diabetic retinopathy, which causes damage to the retina.

Other possible causes include infections and **nutrition** deficiencies.

Infections

Industrialized nations have eliminated most infectious eye diseases through **sanitation**, medication, and public health measures. Viral infections are the main exceptions. Infections that may lead to visual impairment include:

• Herpes simplex keratitis, which is a viral infection of the cornea. Repeated occurrences may lead to corneal scarring.

• Trachoma, a disease caused by an incomplete bacterium *Chlamydia trachomatis* that is transmitted directly from eye to eye, mostly by flies. Standard antibiotics easily treat the disease. If untreated, however, it can lead to blindness. According to the World Health Organization, 6 million people worldwide are blind due to trachoma, and more than 150 million people are in need of treatment.

• River blindness, which is caused by the worm *Onchocerca volvulus*, is found throughout much of the tropics of the Eastern Hemisphere. Transmitted by fly bites, the infection can be treated with a drug called ivermectin (Mectizan). Nevertheless, more than 17 million people worldwide have the disease, and 300,000 of them are blind from it.

Nutrition deficiencies

Vitamin A deficiency is a widespread cause of corneal degeneration in children in developing nations. (Xerophthalmia is a drying of the cornea and conjunctiva, the membrane lining the inside of the eyelids and covering the white part of the eye, which is known as the "sclera.")

Other causes

Exposure of a pregnant woman to certain diseases (e.g., **rubella** or toxoplasmosis) can cause congenital eye problems. Injuries to the eyes can also result in blindness. Very little blindness is due to disease in the brain or the optic nerves. Multiple sclerosis and similar nervous system diseases, brain tumors, diseases of the eye sockets, and head injuries are rare causes of blindness.

Symptoms

People who have low vision have a severe reduction in vision that cannot be corrected with standard glasses, contact lenses, medicine, or surgery, and interferes with their everyday lives. The level of vision reduction varies. People who are completely blind have no vision capabilities.

Diagnosis

A low-vision exam is slightly different from a general exam. Both exams include a case history, visual status, and eye-health evaluation. In a low-vision exam, an eye chart other than a Snellen eye chart may be used. Testing distance will vary. When a patient cannot read the chart at all, the examiner may hold up fingers and ask the patient to count them at various distances. The result is recorded as "counting fingers" at the distance of recognition. If the patient is unable to count fingers at any distance, the examiner will try hand movements, and record the result as "hand movements." If the patient is unable to see hand movements, the examiner will determine whether the patient can detect light from a penlight. Patients who can detect the light, but not its direction, have their vision recorded as "light perception." Patients who can detect its direction have their vision recorded as "light projection." If the patient cannot detect the light at all, the result is recorded as "no light perception."

The doctor will typically also test those activities (e.g., reading or seeing street signs) that are posing difficulties for a person with low vision, and will try different optical and non-optical aids to see whether they help. Finally, the low-vision eye test will check eye health.

Treatment

Vision impairment

Many options, both optical and non-optical, are available for patients with visual impairment. These include:

- telescopes, which a patient may use to read street signs
- hand magnifiers, which can help a patient read labels on items at the store
- stand magnifiers, which can improve a patient's ability to read
- prisms, which help individuals with certain eye diseases by moving the image onto a healthy part of the retina
- closed-circuit television (CCTV), which provides large magnification that a patient may use for such activities as reading
- large-print books and magazines, check-writing guides, large-print dials on the telephone, and other non-optical aids

Glaucoma

If glaucoma is left untreated, optic-nerve damage will result in a progressive loss of vision. Once blindness develops due to glaucoma, it cannot be reversed. With early treatment and monitoring, however, serious vision loss can usually be prevented.

The first line of glaucoma treatment is the use of prescription eyedrops. Several classes of medications are effective at lowering IOP and thus preventing optic nerve damage in chronic and neonatal glaucoma. Patients should discuss the options with their physicians. In addition, patients should inform their doctors of any health conditions they have or any medications they take, including over-the-counter drugs, because these may have an impact on the treatment drugs chosen for the patient. The drugs prescribed to treat glaucoma all have side effects, so patients taking them should be monitored closely, especially for cardiovascular, pulmonary, and behavioral symptoms. Each medication lowers IOP by a different amount, and a combination of medications may be necessary.

A number of laser therapies may be employed to lower eye pressure. These include:

- trabeculoplasty, which opens clogged canals in the trabecular meshwork and allows fluid to flow out of the eye
- laser peripheral iridotomy, which creates a hole in the iris to facilitate fluid outflow
- cyclophotocoagulation, which is directed at the sclera or ciliary tissues and reduces the fluid production

Although studies have shown that marijuana *Cannabis sativa* does lower intraocular pressure in people who have glaucoma, its effects are short in duration, usually only lowering pressure for three or four hours, and is therefore less effective than prescribed glaucoma drugs. In addition, no studies have demonstrated that marijuana effectively treats glaucoma. For these reasons and others, marijuana is not recommended as a treatment for glaucoma.

Cataracts

Cataract surgery falls into two main types: intracapsular and extracapsular. Intracapsular surgery was common before 1980, but it has since been displaced by extracapsular surgery.

Intracapsular surgery is the removal of both the lens and the thin capsule that surround the lens. Removal of the capsule requires a large incision and does not allow comfortable intraocular lens implantation. Thus, people who undergo intracapsular cataract surgery have long recovery periods and have to wear very thick glasses. Extracapsular cataract surgery is the removal of the lens, but the capsule is left in place. Each year in the United States, more than a million cataracts are removed this way. Physicians and researchers continue to improve cataract surgery methods.

Prognosis

For visual impairment, the prognosis generally relates to the severity of the impairment and the ability of the aids to correct it. A good low-vision exam is important, and doctors can alert patients to the latest low-vision aids.

Cataract surgery itself is quite safe and is almost always treated successfully, and about 95% of the time, complications do not occur. If they do, complications include intraocular infection (endophthalmitis), central retinal inflammation (macular edema), post-operative glaucoma, retinal detachment, bleeding under the retina (choroidal hemorrhage), and the occurrence of tiny lens fragments in the back (vitreous) cavity of the eye, all of which can lead to loss of sight.

Cataracts should be removed when they interfere with a person's quality of life.

Prevention

Good **hygiene** (e.g., washing hands frequently) to prevent infection, proper use of contact lenses, and not sharing makeup are just some ways to guard against corneal infections.

EYE EXAMS. Regular eye exams are important to detect silent eye problems (e.g., glaucoma). Performed by an ophthalmologist (M.D. or D.O.) or an optometrist (O.D.), an eye exam can determine whether an individual has any pre-existing or potential vision problems. A child with no symptoms should have an eye exam at age three. Early exams are important because permanent decreases in vision (e.g., amblyopia, also called lazy eye) can occur if not treated early (usually by ages 6–9). With no other symptoms, the second exam should take place before first grade, and according to the American Optometric Association, ensuing eye exams should occur every two years through age 60 and annually after that.

Patients who have risk factors for eye disease should consult their doctors about an appropriate exam schedule. Examples of risk factors include diabetes, a family history of eye disease, or certain ethnic groups (for instance, African Americans are at higher risk for glaucoma). In addition, a person should schedule an eye exam upon notice of any change in vision, eyestrain, blur, flashes of light, a sudden onset of floaters (little dots seeming to float in the air), distortion of objects, double vision, redness, **pain** or discharge. Parents should also watch their children for possible vision problems, and seek eye exams as appropriate. For example, a parent may schedule an eye exam for a child who is having difficulty reading or is rubbing their eyes while reading.

Most exams will include the following procedures:

- information gathering and initial observations

- visual acuity examination, which measures how clearly the patient can see in each eye, with and without any current prescription

- eye movement examination and cover tests, which determine whether the patient can move the eyes to their full extent

- iris and pupil examination, which measure the pupil's response to light (to tell whether it dilates and constricts appropriately), and view the iris for symmetry and physical appearance

- refractive error determination, which examines the refractive error (inability of the lens to focus an image accurately) and obtains a prescription for corrective lenses

---

KEY TERMS

Amblyopia—Decreased visual acuity, usually in one eye, in the absence of any structural abnormality in the eye.

Conjunctiva—The mucous membrane that covers the white part of the eyes (sclera) and lines the eyelids.

Cornea—The clear dome-shaped structure that is part of the front of the eye. It lies in front of the colored part of the eye (iris).

Diabetic retinopathy—Retinal disease caused by the damage that diabetes does to small blood vessels.

Fundus—The inside of an organ. In the eye, the fundus is the back area that can be seen with the ophthalmoscope.

Iris—The colored ring just behind the cornea and in front of the lens that controls the amount of light sent to the retina.

Macula—The central part of the retina where the rods and cones are densest.

Optic nerve—The nerve that carries visual messages from the retina to the brain.

Retina—The light-sensitive layer of the eye.

Sclera—The tough, fibrous, white outer protective covering that surrounds the eye.

Xerophthalmia—A drying of the cornea and conjunctiva.

- ophthalmoscopic examination, which allows the doctor to view the inside back area (fundus) of the eye and examine the retina, blood vessels, optic nerve, and other structures

- slit lamp examination, in which a microscope with an adjustable light source magnifies the external, and some internal, structures of the eyes, and allows the examination of the lid and lid margin, cornea, iris, pupil, conjunctiva, sclera, and lens

- visual field measurement, which maps the patient's field of vision and blindspots

- intraocular pressure (IOP) measurement, which detects the pressure by expelling a puff of air toward the eyeball from a very short distance

PRIMARY AND SECONDARY PREVENTION. Primary **prevention** addresses the causes before they begin. For **trachoma**, for instance, simple sanitation methods can control flies. Likewise, public-health measures can reduce the incidence of many infectious diseases. Sufficient vitamin A, through supplementation when appropriate, will eliminate xerophthalmia. By protecting the eyes against ultraviolet (UV) light through the use of UV coatings on eyewear, individuals may be able to reduce their risk of cataracts, macular degeneration, and some other eye diseases. People should also wear protective glasses or goggles in certain situations, such as when working in certain jobs, playing sports, or even mowing the lawn (due to the potential for an object being thrown by the mower).

Secondary prevention addresses the treatment of established diseases in a timely fashion and before they cause irreversible eye damage. General physical check-ups can also detect systemic diseases such as diabetes or high blood pressure. Control of diabetes is very important in preserving sight.

GENERAL EYE STRUCTURE. Eyes are sphere-shaped. A tough, non-leaky protective sheath (the sclera) covers the entire eye, except for the clear cornea at the front and the optic nerve at the back. Light comes into the eye through the cornea and passes through the lens, which focuses it onto the retina (the innermost surface at the back of the eye). The rods and cones of the retina transform the light energy into electrical messages. The bundle of nerves collectively known as the "optic nerve," transmits those messages to the brain.

The iris, the colored part of the eye shaped like a round picture frame, lies between the dome-shaped cornea and the lens. It controls the amount of light that enters the eye by opening and closing its central hole (pupil) like the diaphragm in a camera. The iris, cornea, and lens are bathed in a liquid called the "aqueous humor," which is somewhat similar to plasma. Nearby ciliary tissues continually produce this liquid, which moves out of the eye through a system of drainage canals (called the "trabecular meshwork") and into the blood-stream. The drainage area is located in front of the iris, in the angle formed between the iris and the point at which the iris appears to meet the inside of the cornea.

Effects on Public Health

About 1 in 28 individuals who are 40 years old or older experience low vision (including blindness). The inability to see clearly can affect an individual's capacity to succeed in school or at work, the overall quality of life, and the ability to live independently. As the U.S. population continues to age, the prevalence of vision loss and vision-related diseases such as glaucoma is expected to rise.

People who have had sight all of their lives find it challenging to adjust to the loss of sight, and this is especially true of older individuals. For instance, a 2012 study in the Journal of the American Medical Association found a correlation between cataract surgery and hip fractures. In this study of about 1.1 million 65-and-older Medicare beneficiaries with cataracts from 2002 through 2009, those who underwent cataract removal had a reduced risk of hip fracture in the year following the surgery, compared to those who did not have the cataract surgery.

Fortunately, preventive measures, including eye exams, can help individuals to receive the vision correction they need in order to see well. Children with good vision can see the blackboard and projected images in class, and therefore usually do better in school than students who cannot see as well. Adult drivers with good vision can read road signs and easily navigate traffic conditions, which may help to reduce the risk of potential accidents. Employees with good vision can avoid dangers in the workplace that they might not otherwise see with poor vision. For these few reasons alone, eye examinations are important to public health.

In addition, eye examinations can discover eye-health problems, such as glaucoma, which can progress to blindness. For instance, a 2010 report of the American Optometric Association reported the results of a year-long, federally funded public-health initiative, called InfactSEE Weeks, that reviewed more than 1,000 comprehensive eye and vision assessments of infants that were conducted in eight states in 2009. According to the report, one in six infants who received exams exhibited an overall cause for concern that necessitated follow-up care. Studies like this one illustrate the need for eye examinations throughout life.

Costs to Society

The financial cost of vision problems is difficult to estimate, but it is large. A 2007 study by Prevent Blindness America noted that among U.S. residents aged 40 or older, the economic cost of four common vision disorders—macular degeneration, cataract, diabetic retinopathy, and glaucoma—combined with that of refractive error, visual impairment, and blindness, totaled $35.4 million for the single year of 2004. That total included $16.2 billion in direct medical costs, $11.2 billion in direct non-medical costs (mainly nursing-home care), and $8 billion in productivity losses.

Another study of the Children's Eye Foundation estimated that the total income loss resulting from blindness was approximately $28 billion per year (in 2007) among the 1.8 million Americans aged 15 and older who are unable to see.

Eye exams are important in identifying many eye problems that, if left unrecognized and untreated, could progress to serious vision loss, possibly even blindness. Eye examinations also determine specific prescriptions for people who have correctable vision problems.

Insurance programs frequently cover at least a portion of the costs for eye examinations.

According to a 2009 study in the Bulletin of the **World Health Organization**, an estimated 158.1 million cases of visual impairment resulted from uncorrected or undercorrected refractive error in 2007. In addition, it estimated global economic productivity loss associated with uncorrected or undercorrected vision at $427.7 billion.

Efforts and Solutions

For those who are blind, a wide range of resources are available to improve the quality of life. Braille and audio and large-print books are increasingly available. Guide dogs provide well-trained eyes and independence. Orientation and mobility training is offered. Special schools for blind children are available, as well as access to disability support through Social Security and private institutions.

Other efforts include initiatives by groups such as Lions Clubs International. Through this organization and its volunteers, 147 million treatments for river blindness have been distributed; nearly 8 million cataract surgeries have been provided; 41 million children in Africa have been vaccinated against **measles**, which causes childhood blindness; eye-health screenings have been provided for millions of individuals every year; and the spread of trachoma in Ethiopia has been lessened by the distribution of 10 million doses of the drug azithromycin annually. Another very active organization is the International Eye Foundation, which is helping to address many vision issues, including river blindness, trachoma, cataract, childhood blindness, and vitamin A deficiency. Many other efforts are under way by governments, agencies, and organizations throughout the United States and around the world to assist those with low vision and to prevent health conditions that lead to low vision.

One global effort to improve access to cataract surgery is VISION2020: the Right to Sight initiative, which is a partnership among the World Health Organization, the International Agency for the Prevention of Blindness, and other agencies working in eye care. The intiative's objective is to provide cataract surgeries at an affordable rate and in an equitable manner to all patients who need them, and to ultimately yield a high success rate in terms of visual outcome and improved quality of life.

Other programs are designed to increase the number of eye examinations performed. One of them is InfantSEE, a public-health program created by Optometry Cares–The AOA Foundation, and The Vision Care Institute, a Johnson & Johnson company. Through the program, which promotes eye and vision care as an integral part of infant wellness and later quality of life, doctors of optometry provide an eye and vision assessment to infants at no charge, regardless of socioeconomic status.

A second AOA program, called Volunteers in Service in Our Nation (VISION USA), provides basic eye health and vision services at no charge to low-income, uninsured individuals and their families. Participating AOA member optometrists donate their services as part of this program.

Additional programs include: EyeCare America, a program of the Foundation of the American Academy of Ophthalmology, which provides eye exams and up to one year of care often at no out-of-pocket cost to those who qualify; VISION USA, coordinated by the American Optometric Association, which provides free eye care to uninsured, low-income Americans; and Sight for Students, a Vision Service Plan program that provides free eye exams and glasses to qualified low-income and uninsured children.

Resources

BOOKS

Domji, Karim, et al. (eds.). *Shields' Textbook of Glaucoma.* 6th ed. Philadelphia, PA: Lippincott Williams & Wilkins, 2010.

Olson, Randall J. et al. *Cataract Surgery From Routine to Complex: A Practical Guide.* 12th ed. Thorofare, NJ: Slack Inc., 2011.

Trope, Graham E. *Glaucoma: A Patient's Guide to the Disease* 4th edition. Toronto: University of Toronto Press, Scholarly Publishing Division, 2011.

PERIODICALS

Baser, Esin F., Goktug Seymenoglu, and Huseyin Mayali. "Trabeculectomy for Advanced Glaucoma." *International Ophthalmology* 31, no. 6 (2011):439–446.

Patalano, Vincent J. III. "The Risks and Benefits of Cataract Surgery." *Digital Journal of Ophthalmology* September 12, 2012. http://www.djo.harvard.edu/site.php?url=/patients/pi/408 (accessed September 11, 2012).

Polack, Sarah, et al. "The Impact of Cataract Surgery on Activities and Time-Use: Results from a Longitudinal Study in Kenya, Bangladesh and the Philippines." PLoS ONE 5, no. 6(2010): e10913. http://www.plosone.org/article/info%3Adoi%2F10.1371%2Fjournal.pone.0010913 (accessed September 11, 2012).

Richman, J., et al. "Relationships in Glaucoma Patients Between Standard Vision Tests, Quality of Life, and Ability to Perform Daily Activities." *Ophthalmic Epidemiology* 17, no. 3 (2010):144–151.

Smith, T.S.T., et al. "Potential Lost Productivity Resulting From the Global Burden of Uncorrected Refractive Error." *Bulletin of the World Health Organization* 87, (2009): 431–437. http://www.who.int/bulletin/volumes/87/08-055673.pdf (accessed September 16, 2012).

Shah, Shaheen P., et al. "Preoperative Visual Acuity Among Cataract Surgery Patients and Countries' State of Development: A Global Study." *Bulletin of the World Health Organization* 89 (2011):749–756. http://www.who.int/bulletin/volumes/89/10/10-080366/en/index.html (accessed September 12, 2012).

Shiuey, Yichieh, and Peter K. Kaiser. "Cataracts." *Digital Journal of Ophthalmology.* http://www.djo.harvard.edu/site.php?url=/patients/pi/407 (accessed September 11, 2012).

Tseng, Victoria L. et al. "Risk of Fractures Following Cataract Surgery in Medicare Beneficiaries." *Journal of the American Medical Association* 308, no. 5(2012):493-501.

WEBSITES

"About Glaucoma." National Glaucoma Research, American Health Assistance Foundation. http://www.ahaf.org/glaucoma/about/ (accessed September 14, 2012).

"Cataract." VISION 2020: A Right to Sight. http://www.vision2020.org/main.cfm?Type=WIBCATARACT&objectid=2572 (accessed September 11, 2012).

"Comprehensive Eye and Vision Examination." American Optometric Association. http://www.aoa.org/x4725.xml (accessed September 13, 2012).

"The Economic Impact of Vision Problems: The Toll of Major Adult Eye Disorders, Visual Impairment, and Blindness on the U.S. Economy." Prevent Blindness America. http://www.preventblindness.org/sites/default/files/national/documents/EI_section2.pdf (accessed September 17, 2012).

"The Eye Exam." A Practical Guide to Clinical Medicine, University of California, San Diego. http://meded.ucsd.edu/clinicalmed/eyes.htm (accessed September 13, 2012).

"Ethnicity and Glaucoma." The Glaucoma Foundation. http://www.glaucomafoundation.org/news_detail.php?id=162 (accessed September 14, 2012).

EyeSmart. "What Are Cataracts?" American Academy of Ophthalmology.http://www.geteyesmart.org/eyesmart/diseases/cataracts.cfm (accessed September 11, 2012).

"Facts About Cataract." National Eye Institute, National Institutes of Health. http://www.nei.nih.gov/health/cataract/cataract_facts.asp (accessed September 11, 2012).

"Facts About Glaucoma." National Eye Institute, National Institutes of Health. http://www.nei.nih.gov/health/glaucoma/glaucoma_facts.asp (accessed September 14, 2012).

Gibson, William E. "Economic Impact of Blindness From Amblyopia." Children's Eye Foundation. http://www.childrenseyefoundation.org/index.php/implementation/economic-impact-of-blindness-from-amblyopia (accessed September 17, 2012).

"Glaucoma Surgery." Glaucoma Research Foundation. http://www.glaucoma.org/treatment/surgery-overview.php (accessed September 14, 2012).

"Glaucoma Treatments." National Glaucoma Research, American Health Assistance Foundation. http://www.ahaf.org/glaucoma/treatment/common/ (accessed September 14, 2012).

"IEF Programs: River Blindness." International Eye Foundation. http://www.iefusa.org/riverblind.shtml (accessed September 17, 2012).

"Is Vision Loss Making It Difficult to Cope?" VisionAware, American Foundations for the Blind, Reader's Digest Partners for Sight. http://www.visionaware.org/ (accessed September 17, 2012).

"Low Vision." National Eye Institute, National Institutes of Health. http://www.nei.nih.gov/health/lowvision/index.asp (accessed September 17, 2012).

"Low Vision." Research to Prevent Blindness. http://www.rpbusa.org/rpb/eye_info/low_vision/ (accessed September 17, 2012).

"Marijuana for Glaucoma: Patients Beware." *Eye to Eye*, The Glaucoma Foundation Newsletter (summer 2010). http://www.glaucomafoundation.org/UserFiles/File/TGF_Summer_10_Web.pdf (accessed September 14, 2012).

"Medical Marijuana." Glaucoma Research Foundation. http://www.glaucoma.org/treatment/medical-marijuana.php (accessed September 14, 2012).

MedlinePlus. "Cataract Removal." U.S. National Library of Medicine, National Institutes of Health. http://www.nlm.nih.gov/medlineplus/ency/article/002957.htm (accessed September 11, 2012).

———. "Standard Ophthalmic Exam." U.S. National Library of Medicine. http://www.nlm.nih.gov/medlineplus/ency/article/003434.htm (accessed September 13, 2012).

"New AOA Report Reveals High Number of Infants with Untreated Eye and Vision Problems." InfantSEE. http://www.infantsee.org/documents/Announcement-2009-IS-CDC-project-results.pdf (accessed September 13, 2012).

"Prevent Blindness, Saving Sight for Millions of People Around the World." Lions Club International. http://www.lionsclubs.org/EN/our-work/sight-programs/index.php (accessed September 17, 2012).

Sight for Students. Vision Service Plan. http://www.sightforstudents.org/ (accessed September 13, 2012).

"Signs of a Vision Problem." Children's Eye Foundation. http://www.childrenseyefoundation.org/index.php/for-parents/signs-of-a-vision-problem (accessed September 17, 2012).

"Types of Glaucoma." Glaucoma Research Foundation. http://www.glaucoma.org/glaucoma/types-of-glaucoma.php (accessed September 14, 2012).

U.S. Census Bureau. "Americans With Disabilities: Household Economic Studies." U.S. Department of Commerce Economics and Statistics Administration. http://www.census.gov/prod/2012pubs/p70-131.pdf (accessed September 17, 2012).

"Vision." HealthyPeople.gov, U.S. Department of Health and Human Services. http://www.healthypeople.gov/2020/topicsobjectives2020/overview.aspx?topicid=42 (accessed September 17, 2012).

"Vision Loss from Eye Diseases Will Increase as Americans Age." National Eye Institute, National Institutes of Health. http://www.nei.nih.gov/news/pressreleases/041204.asp (accessed September 17, 2012).

VISION USA. Optometry Cares, The American Optometric Association Foundation. http://www.optometryscharity.org/vision-usa/ (accessed September 13, 2012).

"Water-Related Diseases: Trachoma." World Health Organization. http://www.who.int/water_sanitation_health/diseases/trachoma/en/index.html (accessed September 17, 2012).

ORGANIZATIONS

American Academy of Ophthalmology (AAO), 655 Beach St., San Francisco, CA 94109, (415) 561-8500, http://www.aao.org.

American Foundation for the Blind, 2 Penn Plaza, Suite 1102, New York, NY 10121, (212) 502-7600, (888) 545-8331, afbinfo@afb.net, http://www.afb.org/.

American Society of Cataract and Refractive Surgery, 4000 Legato Road, Suite 700, Fairfax, VA 22033, (703) 591-2220, http://www.ascrs.org.

Center for Sight and Hearing, 8038 MacIntosh Lane, Rockford, IL 61107, (815) 332-6800, (800) 545-0080, http://www.centerforsighthearing.org/.

Children's Eye Foundation, 1631 Lancaster Drive, Suite 200, Grapevine, TX 76051, (817) 310-2641, info@childrenseyefoundation.org, http://www.childrenseyefoundation.org.

Glaucoma Foundation., 80 Maiden Lane, Suite 1206, New York, NY 10038, (212) 285-0080, info@glaucomafoundation.org, http://www.glaucomafoundation.org.

Glaucoma Research Foundation, 251 Post Street, Suite 600, San Francisco, CA 94108, (415) 986-3162, http://www.glaucoma.org/.

Guide Dogs for the Blind, National Office, P.O. Box 151200, San Rafael, CA 94915-1200, (800) 295-4050, http://www.guidedogs.com.

International Eye Foundation, 10801 Connecticut Avenue, Kensington, MD 20895, (240) 290-0263, ief@iefusa.org, http://www.iefusa.org/.

Lighthouse International, 111 East 59th Street, New York, NY 10022, (212) 821-9200, (800) 829-0500, info@lighthouse.org, http://www.lighthouse.org.

Lions Clubs International, 300 West 22nd Street, Oak Brook, IL 60523, (630) 571-5466, foundation@aoa.org, http://www.lionsclubs.org/EN/index.php.

National Eye Health Education Program, National Eye Institute, 31 Center Dr., MSC 2510, Bethesda, MD 20892-2510, (301) 496-5248, 2020@nei.nih.gov, http://www.nei.nih.gov.

National Eye Institute., 31 Center Dr., MSC 2510, Bethesda, MD 20892-2510, (301) 496-5248, http://www.nei.nih.gov.

National Federation of the Blind, 200 East Wells Street, Baltimore, MD 21230, (410) 659-9314, nfb@nfb.org, http://www.nfb.org.

National Glaucoma Research, American Health Assistance Foundation., 22512 Gateway Center Drive, Clarksburg, MD 20871, (800) 285-0080, info@ahaf.org, http://www.ahaf.org/glaucoma/.

Optometric Glaucoma Society, 3241 South Michigan Avenue, Chicago, IL 60616, (312) 949-7303, mchaglas@ico.edu, http://www.optometricglaucomasociety.org.

Prevent Blindness America, 211 West Wacker Drive, Suite 1700, Chicago, IL 60606, (800) 331-2020, http://www.preventblindness.org.

Research to Prevent Blindness, 645 Madison Ave., Floor 21, New York, NY 10022-1010, (212) 752-4333, (800) 621-0026, inforequest@rpbusa.org, http://www.rpbusa.org.

J. Ricker Polsdorfer, M.D.
Lorraine Lica, Ph.D.
Teresa G. Odle
Mary Bekker
Bonny McClain
Patience Paradox
Laura Jean Cataldo, RN, Ed.D.
Leslie Mertz, Ph.D.

▌Vitamins

Definition

Vitamins are organic compounds found in plants and animals that are necessary in small quantities for life and health. Thirteen different vitamins have been identified as necessary for humans. The body can make small quantities of two of these vitamins, vitamins D and K. All other vitamins must be obtained either from food or from dietary supplements.

Purpose

Each of the 13 vitamins has specific functions, and taken together vitamins play a role in almost every function in the body. They help convert food to energy, and are involved processes as diverse as blood clotting, vision, reproduction, and transmission of nerve impulses.

Description

For centuries before vitamins were formally discovered, people knew that eating certain foods prevented certain diseases. For example, the ancient Egyptians knew that eating liver (later shown to be high in vitamin A) prevented night blindness. Sailors on long voyages often developed a serious disease called **scurvy**. James Lind, a Scottish surgeon who sailed with the British navy conducted the first controlled experiment on vitamins in 1753. He supplemented the regular diet of four groups of sailors with four different foods. The group that received oranges and lemons as supplements did not develop scurvy, while the other three groups did. Although Lind did not know why citrus fruit was essential to health (it is high in vitamin C, and scurvy is caused by vitamin C deficiency), he recognized that it contained some substance that the sailors needed.

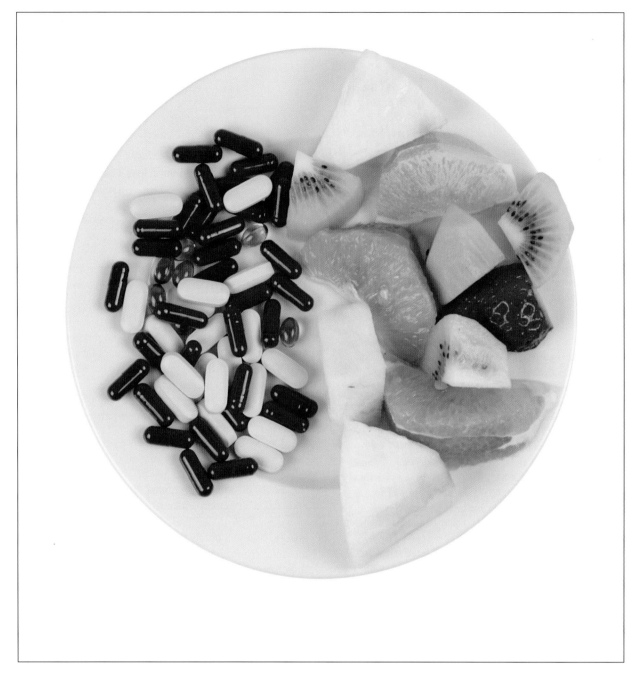

Natural and artificial sources of vitamins. *(Radu Razvan/Shutterstock.com)*

Water-soluble vitamins

Humans need nine water-soluble vitamins. These vitamins dissolve in water and are not stored in the body for long periods. Most excess water-soluble vitamins are removed by the kidneys and leave the body in urine. A list of the water-soluble vitamins and a very brief description of their importance to health are included in this essay. For details on how these vitamins function, see the specific entries for each vitamin. In general, B vitamins tend to be involved in reactions that convert nutrients to energy and

reactions that synthesize new molecules. There are gaps in the numbering of the B-complex vitamins, because compounds originally named as vitamins, such as B4 (adenine), were renamed after further research showed that they did not meet the definition of a vitamin.

- Vitamin B_1 (thiamin): needed to convert carbohydrates to energy

- Vitamin B_2 (riboflavin): helps break down proteins, fats, and carbohydrates and make other vitamins and minerals available to the body

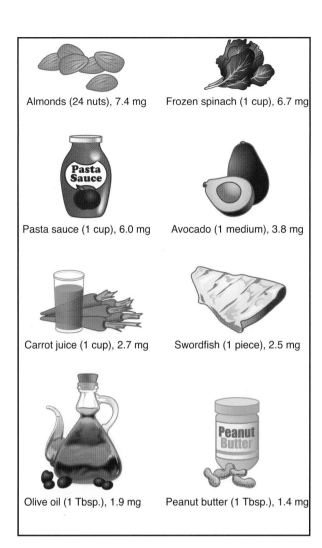

Almonds (24 nuts), 7.4 mg

Frozen spinach (1 cup), 6.7 mg

Pasta sauce (1 cup), 6.0 mg

Avocado (1 medium), 3.8 mg

Carrot juice (1 cup), 2.7 mg

Swordfish (1 piece), 2.5 mg

Olive oil (1 Tbsp.), 1.9 mg

Peanut butter (1 Tbsp.), 1.4 mg

Good food sources for vitamin E. *(Illustration by Electronic Illustrators Group. © 2013 Cengage Learning)*

- Vitamin B_3 (niacin): helps the body process fats and proteins
- Vitamin B_5 (pantothenic acid): helps regulate the chemical reactions that produce energy
- Vitamin B_6 (pyridoxine): involved in the transmission of nerve impulses, formation and functioning of red blood cells, and creation of new cells
- Vitamin B_{12} (cobalamin): necessary for healthy red blood cells, creating new deoxyribose nucleic acid (DNA), and in maintaining nerve cells
- Vitamin C (ascorbic acid): helps form cartilage and connective tissue; as an antioxidant protects cells from free radical damage
- Vitamin H (biotin): joins with enzymes that regulate the breakdown of foods and their use in the body
- Folic acid (folate): helps make new cells; important in development of the fetal nervous system

Fat-soluble vitamins

Humans need four fat-soluble vitamins. Unlike water-soluble vitamins, fat-soluble vitamins can be stored in the body. High levels of these vitamins can cause health problems. Below is a list of the water-soluble vitamins and a very brief description of their importance to health. In general the fat-soluble vitamins have antioxidant activity that helps protect cells from damage. For details on how these vitamins function, see the specific entries for each vitamin.

- Vitamin A (retinol): needed for vision, a healthy immune system, development of the fetus, tissue repair; as an antioxidant protects cells from free radical damage
- Vitamin D (calciferol): involved in building bones, muscle contraction, and nerve impulse transmission.
- Vitamin E: (tocopherol) acts as an antioxidant to protect the body against damage caused by free radicals
- Vitamin K: needed for blood clotting

Vitamin supplements

Before the twentieth century, all vitamins had to come from food. Often individuals on limited diets with little variety developed vitamin deficiency diseases. The period from the 1920s to the 1940s was a time of active research on vitamins. Out of this research came a **food fortification** program in the United States that continues today. Beginning in the late 1930s, the addition of vitamins to common foods, such as flour, milk, and breakfast cereal, substantially reduced vitamin deficiency diseases. Commercially manufactured vitamin supplements also began to appear, and taking a daily multivitamin supplement became popular. By 2007, more than 100 million Americans regularly took some form of vitamin supplement.

Vitamin supplements come as tablets, capsules, and elixirs (liquids). Supplements can contain a single vitamin, a group of related vitamins that work together in the body (e.g., B-complex vitamins), or a mixture of vitamins and minerals (e.g., vitamin D and calcium that work together to build bones). Vitamins are also added to foods that can then be labeled "fortified" or "enriched." Many so-called functional foods, or nutraceuticals, have added vitamins, minerals, and herbs.

In the United States, the Food and Drug Administration (FDA) regulates dietary supplements under the 1994 Dietary Supplement Health and Education Act (DSHEA). Under DSHEA, supplements are subject to the same regulation as food, which is much less rigorous than the regulation of prescription or over-the-counter drugs. Vitamin manufacturers do not have to prove that their products are safe or effective before they can be sold to the public. By contrast, manufacturers of conventional

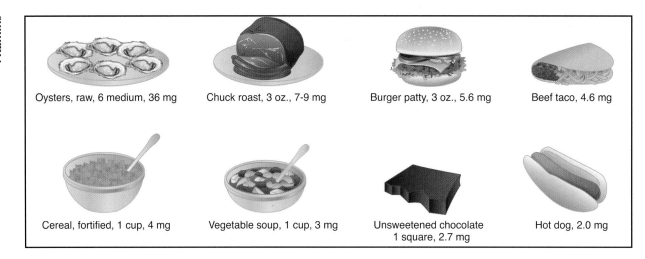

Food sources containing zinc. *(Illustration by Electronic Illustrators Group. © 2013 Cengage Learning)*

prescription and over-the-counter drugs must prove both safety and effectiveness in extensive humans before their product can be marketed.

In 2007, ConsumerLab, an independent testing company in New York, evaluated 21 brands of multivitamins. They found that only 10 of these multivitamins contained all the vitamins and minerals in the quantities listed on the label. In addition, some brands contained contaminants, including lead. To get the most out of vitamin supplements, consumers should

• read the label carefully to understand exactly what is in the supplement

• avoid megadoses of vitamins. The daily value (DV) given on the label should be around 100% for each vitamin

• look for "USP" on the label to verify the supplement meets the strength and purity standards of the U.S. Pharmacopeia, a testing organization

• check the expiration date

• stick with well-known brands

Vitamin requirements

The United States Institute of Medicine (IOM) of the National Academy of Sciences has developed values called Dietary Reference Intakes (DRIs) for most vitamins and minerals. The DRIs consist of three sets of values. The Recommended Dietary Allowance (RDA) defines the average daily amount of the nutrient needed to meet the health needs of 97–98% of the population. The Adequate Intake (AI) is an estimate set when there is not enough information to determine an RDA. The Tolerable Upper Intake Level (UL) is the average maximum amount that can be taken daily without risking negative side effects. The DRIs are calculated for

children, adult men, adult women, pregnant women, and breastfeeding women.

Experts agree that vitamin supplements are not a substitute for nutrients from food. Most healthy people in developed countries who eat a varied diet high in fruits, vegetables, and whole grains get enough vitamins and do not need a vitamin supplement, although many take a daily multivitamin as "insurance." However, some groups do tend to need either general supplement with a multivitamin or supplement with specific vitamins to prevent vitamin deficiency diseases. People in these groups should discuss their vitamin requirements with their healthcare provider. They include:

• the elderly, especially those on restricted diets

• vegans, because they eat no animal products

• breastfed babies of vegan mothers

• people with lactose intolerance or those who do not eat dairy products

• people with alcoholism

• people who have had part of their stomachs or intestines surgically removed

• pregnant women or those who could become pregnant

• people with diseases that interfere with vitamin metabolism

• people taking drugs that interfere with vitamin metabolism

Vitamin excess

Although vitamins play an undeniable role in maintaining health, large doses of vitamins in healthy individuals can cause adverse effects. Almost all vitamin excess (hypervitaminosis) occurs because of supplementation; it is almost impossible to get too many vitamins from food. Although great deal of advertising, especially

KEY TERMS

B-complex vitamins—a group of water-soluble vitamins that often work together in the body. These include thiamine (B_1), riboflavin (B_2), niacin (B_3), pantothenic acid (B_5), pyridoxine (B_6), biotin (B_7 or vitamin H), folate/folic acid (B_9), and cobalamin (B_{12}).

Dietary supplement—a product, such as a vitamin, mineral, herb, amino acid, or enzyme, that is intended to be consumed in addition to an individual's diet with the expectation that it will improve health

Free radical—a molecule with an unpaired electron that has a strong tendency to react with other molecules in DNA (genetic material), proteins, and lipids (fats), resulting in damage to cells. Free radicals are neutralized by antioxidants.

Functional Food—also called nutraceuticals, these products are marketed as having health benefits or disease-preventing qualities beyond their basic supply of energy and nutrients. Often these health benefits come in the form of added herbs, minerals, vitamins, etc.

Mineral—an inorganic substance found in the earth that is necessary in small quantities for the body to maintain a health. Examples include zinc, copper, iron.

on the Internet, suggests that megadoses of certain vitamins can improve athletic performance, prevent and treat chronic disease, delay **aging**, and increase longevity, there is little or no evidence from independent, well-controlled human clinical trials to support these claims. One exception is high dose niacin, which has been used to treat high blood cholesterol levels. Although niacin is very safe at normal doses, the levels needed to lower serum cholesterol, it has been associated with liver damage and, commonly, severe facial flushing. Otherwise, excess water-soluble vitamins are removed from the body in urine. Although large doses of water-soluble vitamins rarely cause health problems, they cannot be used by the body and are a waste of money. Fat-soluble vitamins that are stored in the body can build up to very high levels and cause serious health concerns. People interested in more information about the effects of large doses of vitamins should talk to a healthcare provider.

Precautions

Both too little and too much of any of the 13 human vitamins may cause health consequences. See entries on specific vitamins for more detailed information about potential health concerns.

Interactions

The interactions among various vitamins, enzymes, coenzymes, drugs, and herbal supplements are complex and incompletely understood. See entries on specific vitamins for more detailed information about their interactions.

Complications

Vitamins acquired by eating fruits and vegetables promote health. No complications are expected from vitamins in food. Vitamin supplements may cause hypervitaminosis or interact with other supplements, prescription drugs, over-the-counter drugs, and herbal supplements in ways that cause undesirable side effects. See entries on specific vitamins for more detailed information about potential complications.

Parental concerns

Parents should encourage their children to eat a healthy and varied diet high in fruits, vegetables, and whole grains to meet their vitamin needs.

Most vitamin poisonings and deaths occur in children under age 6 as the result of accidental intake of excessive vitamin supplements. Parents should treat vitamin supplements as they would any drug and store them out of the reach of children.

Resources

BOOKS

Bruning, Nancy Pauling. *The Real Vitamin and Mineral Book: The Definitive Guide to Designing Your Personal Supplement Program.* 4th ed. New York: Avery Publishing Group, 2007.

Gaby, Alan R., ed. *A–Z Guide to Drug-Herb-Vitamin Interactions, Revised and Expanded 2nd Edition: Improve Your Health and Avoid Side Effects When Using Common Medications and Natural Supplements Together.* New York: Three Rivers Press, 2006.

Lieberman, Shari, and Nancy Bruning. *The Real Vitamin and Mineral Book: The Definitive Guide to Designing Your Personal Supplement Program.* 4th ed. New York: Avery, 2007.

Rucker, Robert B., ed. *Handbook of Vitamins.* Boca Raton, FL: Taylor & Francis, 2007.

PERIODICALS

Guyton, J.R., and H.E. Bays. "Safety Considerations with Niacin Therapy." *American Journal of Cardiolology* (March 19, 2007): S22–31.

WEBSITES

American Academy of Family Physicians. "Vitamins and Minerals: How to Get What You Need." FamilyDoctor .org. http://familydoctor.org/familydoctor/en/prevention-wellness/food-nutrition/nutrients/vitamins-and-minerals-how-to-get-what-you-need.html (accessed October 2, 2012).

Mayo Clinic Staff. "Supplements: Nutrition in a Pill?" MayoClinic.com. http://www.mayoclinic.com/health/supplements/NU00198 (accessed October 2, 2012).

MedlinePlus. "Vitamins." U.S. National Library of Medicine, National Institutes of Health. http://www.nlm.nih.gov/medlineplus/vitamins.html (accessed October 2, 2012).

Nemours Foundation. "Vitamins and Minerals." KidsHealth.org. http://kidshealth.org/teen/food_fitness/nutrition/vitamins_minerals.html (accessed October 2, 2012).

U.S. Department of Agriculture, National Agricultural Library. "DRI Tables." Food and Nutrition Information Center. http://fnic.nal.usda.gov/dietary-guidance/dietary-reference-intakes/dri-tables (accessed August 16, 2012).

U.S. Department of Agriculture and U.S. Department of Health and Human Services. *Dietary Guidelines for Americans, 2010.* 7th ed. Washington, DC: U.S. Government Printing Office, December 2010. http://health.gov/dietaryguidelines (accessed September 27, 2012).

ORGANIZATIONS

Academy of Nutrition and Dietetics, 120 South Riverside Plz., Ste. 2000, Chicago, IL 60606-6995, (312) 899-0040, (800) 877-1600, amacmunn@eatright.org, http://www.eatright.org.

British Nutrition Foundation, High Holborn House, 52-54 High Holborn, London, United Kingdom WC1V 6RQ, 44 20 7404 6504, Fax: 44 20 7404 6747, postbox@nutrition.org.uk, http://www.nutrition.org.uk.

Dietitians of Canada, 480 University Ave., Ste. 604, Toronto, Ontario, Canada M5G 1V2, (416) 596-0857, Fax: (416) 596-0603, centralinfo@dietitians.ca, http://www.dietitians.ca.

Institute of Medicine, National Academy of Sciences, 500 Fifth St. NW, Washington, DC 20001, (202) 334-2352, iomwww@nas.edu, http://www.iom.edu.

Office of Dietary Supplements, National Institutes of Health, 6100 Executive Blvd., Rm. 3B01, MSC 7517, Bethesda, MD 20892-7517, (301) 435-2920, Fax: (301) 480-1845, ods@nih.gov, http://ods.od.nih.gov.

U.S. Department of Agriculture, 1400 Independence Ave. SW, Washington, DC 20250, (202) 720-2791, http://www.usda.gov.

U.S. Food and Drug Administration, 10903 New Hampshire Ave., Silver Spring, MD 20993-0002, (888) INFO-FDA (463-6332), http://www.fda.gov.

Tish Davidson, A.M.

∎ Vulnerable populations

Definition

Vulnerable populations, also known as populations at risk or special-needs populations, is a term used in public health, medical ethics, and clinical research to refer to persons whose conditions or situations do not allow them to protect their own interests, either as recipients of health care or as participants in medical research. People who are considered vulnerable do not meet the basic criteria for informed participation in the health care system or in research: namely to be of sound mind; old enough and otherwise able to make personal decisions; and able on social and economic grounds to choose among various healthcare provision or treatment options.

The phrase is also used in disaster management to refer to persons who require special care or assistance in the event of a disaster. As defined by the Pennsylvania Department of Public Health, vulnerable populations are "groups whose needs are not addressed by traditional service providers or who feel they cannot comfortably or safely access and use the standard resources offered in disaster preparedness, relief, and recovery." The English word *vulnerable* comes from the Latin word *vulnus*, which means "wound" or "injury."

Description

There are a number of different groups included in the category of vulnerable populations. In fact, one reason why some public health officials and policy makers are dissatisfied with the phrase is the range of different conditions that have been defined as vulnerable, some of which are longer-lasting or more resistant to medical treatment or social interventions than others. Some analysts have classified vulnerable populations into three categories, according to whether their vulnerabilities are primarily physical, mental, or social.

• Physical: Vulnerable populations in this category include children; the frail elderly; pregnant women; people who are blind, deaf, or otherwise physically disabled; those with such chronic diseases as emphysema and other respiratory diseases, diabetes, hypertension, dyslipidemia, HIV infection, and heart disease. Of those over 65, 87% have one chronic illness; 67% have two or more such illnesses.

• Mental: This category includes those with such serious mental disorders as schizophrenia, bipolar disorder, major depression, as well as a history of suicide attempts. Persons with a history of alcoholism or substance abuse are often included in this category, as are those with such developmental disorders as autism or mental retardation.

- Social: Vulnerable populations in this category include recent legal immigrants, illegal immigrants, refugees, homeless persons, migrant workers, persons who are not proficient in speaking or reading English, Native Americans, former prisoners, persons living in violent or abusive households, and those without access to computers or the Internet. This last group is sometimes referred to as being on the downside of the digital divide.

Some observers make a distinction between vulnerable individuals and vulnerable communities. Vulnerable individuals can often be helped by their social support network of family, friends, churches or other community groups, or by so-called safety-net providers. That is, healthcare providers who accept patients without regard to their ability to pay. Vulnerable communities, on the other hand, are often sources of additional emotional and economic **stress** rather than support to the people who live in them; high crime rates, pollution, few opportunities for employment, easy access to street drugs, substandard housing, loose or nonexistent family ties, fragmented neighborhoods, and other problems place additional burdens on individuals who may be personally vulnerable.

Another finding of recent research is that vulnerability tends to be compounded over the course of a person's life. Such early difficulties as poor parenting, **child abuse**, low educational achievement, and poor **nutrition** increase the likelihood of physical and social vulnerabilities in later life (teenage pregnancy, drug and alcohol abuse, **sexually transmitted diseases**, imprisonment, homelessness, and chronic illnesses). In short, vulnerability is the result of a complex set of conditions that include a person's geographic location (inner city, isolated rural area, Native American reservation, migration from place to place, etc.); socioeconomic status (SES); and personal limitations (physical and mental impairments, **birth defects**, or persistent illness). All these factors can interact in numerous ways to increase an individual's vulnerability.

Demographics

The demographics of vulnerable populations vary according to the specific **population**. Some statistics for the United States are as follows:

- Number of people with chronic medical conditions: 141 million as of 2010, estimated to rise to 171 million (37% of the population) by 2030. Eighty-three percent of healthcare spending goes to 48% of this vulnerable population.

- One in 5 American adults has multiple risk factors for unmet healthcare needs. The three most significant risk factors are low income, lack of health insurance, and the lack of a regular source of health care.

- The true number of homeless people is difficult to estimate because many are transients, but the Department of Housing and Urban Development estimates the number of homeless in the United States at 650,000.

- About 46% of Americans will be diagnosed with a mental disorder at some point in life. Anxiety disorders are the most common, followed by depression and conduct disorders.

- There are an estimated 3 million migrant and seasonal farm workers in the United States as of 2012.

- 2.3 million persons are imprisoned in the United States as of 2012; 67% of those who serve their term reoffend within three years of release.

- The Department of Homeland Security (DHS) estimates the number of illegal immigrants at 11.5 million as of 2012.

- Between 2% and 3% of children and adults in the United States are considered to be mentally retarded. The majority of these (about 80%) have only mild retardation. About 25% of all cases of mental retardation result from genetic disorders.

- About 1.2 million Americans are living with HIV infection as of 2012.

- There are 310 Native American and Alaskan Native reservations as of 2012, with a total of 1 million persons living on them. Another 1.5 million Native Americans live elsewhere than on reservations.

- As of 2012, there are an estimated 410,000 children in foster care in the United States.

- As of 2010, it was reported that 30% of Americans either do not have broadband access or do not use the Internet at all.

- Less than 1% of the United States population lives in isolated or "frontier" rural areas (defined as areas with six or fewer people per square mile); however, these areas cover 45% of the total U.S. land mass. About 18% of people in frontier rural areas are below the poverty line.

The statistics are only "snapshots" of some of the groups that can be considered vulnerable populations. The demographics of vulnerability are further complicated by two important factors: overlap and flux. Overlap refers to the fact that many vulnerable people fall into two or more categories of vulnerability, such as mental illness and substance abuse (sometimes called dual diagnosis patients), or mental retardation and chronic illness. Flux refers to the fact that vulnerability is not always a static or fixed condition; people can move out of certain vulnerable populations by personal choice and lifestyle changes. For example, dropouts can return to school and finish their education; people can move away from isolated rural areas; some people are able to break out of the cycle of drug or alcohol **addiction**, or give up risky sexual behaviors; and some immigrants can improve their mastery of English and assimilate. Conversely, people who are not presently vulnerable may become so at some point in the future as a result of an accident or severe illness.

Effects on public health

The effects of vulnerable populations on public health are varied and complex. Different disciplines within the field of public health tend to focus on different categories of vulnerable populations:

- Epidemiology: Epidemiologists are often concerned with vulnerable populations at risk for high rates of contagious illness, such as the homeless, illegal immigrants, migrant workers, alcoholics and substance abusers, and men who have sex with men.

- Public policy: Public health workers in this field typically focus on vulnerable populations that suffer from health disparities related to unequal access to health care. These include the poor and/or uninsured, the uneducated, those who are not proficient in English, those who live in isolated rural areas, and the frail elderly who may lack transportation. Other public health experts in this field are concerned with research into the causes and interconnections of the social and individual factors that lead to vulnerability.

- Clinical research: Vulnerable populations are of particular concern to those tasked with protecting the rights of human subjects in medical or mental health research. The Office for Human Research Protections (OHRP) of the Department of Health and Human Services (HHS) has detailed regulations for investigators in protecting subjects recruited from vulnerable populations, particularly children, prisoners, and persons who are HIV-positive. On the other hand, many researchers are interested in carrying out studies specifically intended to benefit vulnerable patients, such as trials of new medications for HIV infection, schizophrenia, major depression, and bipolar disorder. With regard to children as subjects, most drugs approved by the Food and Drug Administration (FDA) are evaluated in clinical trials of adults. In many cases, it is helpful to conduct clinical trials in order to determine appropriate dosages of such drugs for children.

- Disaster preparedness. Public health officials concerned with sheltering or evacuating members of vulnerable populations in an emergency concentrate their efforts on those who would be difficult to evacuate quickly (those with mobility impairments, lack of transportation, blind or deaf, developmentally disabled); those who cannot be safely housed in public shelters (persons with contagious illnesses or those who require hospital inpatient care; persons actively abusing drugs or alcohol; those with serious mental illness); and those who are hard to reach with emergency warnings because of language barriers, lack of Internet or telephone access, or distrust of "the system" (illegal immigrants, homeless persons, those who are not proficient in English, former prisoners, etc.).

Costs to society

The costs to society for vulnerable populations are high, particularly in terms of the ever-rising costs of health care. Members of vulnerable populations consume a large proportion of the nation's healthcare resources, particularly those with chronic medical conditions. According to a study done at Johns Hopkins University, 72% of all healthcare spending for the uninsured pays for the care of 31% of patients with chronic conditions, and 83% of Medicaid spending is for 40% of noninstitutionalized beneficiaries with chronic conditions. With reference to substance abusers alone, the estimated annual cost of this vulnerable population in the United States is $200 billion.

In addition to the direct costs of health care, vulnerable people who remain in the workforce are costly to their employers as well in terms of decreased productivity. In terms of absenteeism (missed work days), almost 1 of 4 patients with coronary artery disease report 20 or more of poor health days per year, as do 22% of patients with diabetes and 21% of patients with depression. A closely related problem is presenteeism, which can be loosely defined as the negative effects of a health issue on the employee's work performance. One study of chemical workers found that such disorders as depression, anxiety, or breathing disorders reduced the workers' ability to function on the job by 17% to 38%. The company that was used for the study reported that it lost an average of $6,721 per employee, or 6.8% of its total labor costs across its entire U.S. workforce.

A less easily measured but very real cost to society is the stigma attached to some vulnerable populations. Study after study has shown that the public tends to be more resentful of the healthcare costs of vulnerable populations whose conditions are considered the

KEY TERMS

Digital divide—A term used to refer to inequality between groups or individuals in terms of access to, use of, or knowledge of information and communication technologies (ICTs).

Dual diagnosis—A term used to describe the condition of a person with a diagnosed mental illness and a co-occurring alcohol or substance use disorder.

Ethics—A system of moral standards or values; also the study of such a system.

Presenteeism—A term used to describe inefficiency or poor quality of work from employees who can come to work but are hampered by physical or mental illness.

Safety-net providers—Healthcare providers who offer services to patients regardless of their ability to pay and who have a patient mix with a substantial share of uninsured, Medicaid, or otherwise vulnerable patients.

Stigma—A mark or characteristic trait of a disease or defect; by extension, a cause for reproach or a stain on one's reputation.

outcome of their own poor behaviors and behavioral choices than of those who are considered vulnerable through no fault of their own. Thus, substance abusers, illegal immigrants, persons with HIV infection and other STDs, single mothers, homeless people, and prisoners are typically accorded less compassion and often less public funding. Conversely, federal and state governments are more likely to provide assistance to those who are not seen as responsible for their vulnerability, such as children, the blind, the mentally retarded, disabled veterans, and the elderly. A very real consequence of stigmatizing some vulnerable populations, however, is that it keeps these populations trapped in their situations and ever more susceptible to chronic physical and mental illness in addition to their original problem—thus compounding the long-term costs of their health care to society at large.

Efforts and solutions

As of 2012, there are a number of efforts under way in different areas of public health to address the needs of vulnerable populations:

• Social-scientific research aimed at guiding public policy. Such private foundations as the Commonwealth Fund and the Robert Wood Johnson Foundation (RWJF) provide grant funding for studies of vulnerability in general as well as analyses of specific vulnerable populations. The Commonwealth Fund's stated purpose is to "promote a high-performing health care system that achieves better access, improved quality, and greater efficiency, particularly for society's most vulnerable." The RWJF is the largest philanthropic organization in the United States devoted exclusively to health care.

• Improving access to health care and treatment. Current efforts in this area range from such federal organizations as the Indian Health Service (IHS) and the Department of Veterans Affairs (VA) to local clinics for immigrants and other vulnerable populations staffed by medical students from urban medical schools. Another initiative of this type is the National Health Service Corps (NHSC), a program started in 1972 that offers scholarships and loan forgiveness to medical, nursing, and physician assistant students in return for three to five years of work in isolated rural areas or underserved inner-city locations after graduation. As of 2012, over 60% of doctors who have received NHSC grants or loans remain in their underserved communities after their term of service. About 10.5 million Americans are served by healthcare professionals in the NHSC program in 2012.

• Clinical studies intended to benefit vulnerable populations. An increasing number of clinical trials registered with the National Institutes of Health are directed toward finding treatments or other interventions to help members of vulnerable populations. As of 2012, there are more than 5,500 trials related to HIV infection alone, while there are 204 clinical trials specifically identified as studies of vulnerable populations, ranging from screening for colorectal cancer among Native Americans and follow-up treatment of former prisoners with chronic health conditions to promoting parenting skills in inner-city families and treatment of depression in Hispanic Americans and African Americans.

Resources

BOOKS

Landesman, Linda Young. *Public Health Management of Disasters: The Practice Guide*, 3rd ed. Washington, DC: American Public Health Association, 2012.

Matherly, Deborah, Jane Mobley, and Beverly G. Ward. *Communication with Vulnerable Populations: A Transportation and Emergency Management Toolkit*. Washington, DC: Transportation Research Board of the National Academies, 2011.

Shi, Leiyu, and Gregory D. Stevens. *Vulnerable Populations in the United States*, 2nd ed. San Francisco, CA: Jossey-Bass, 2010.

Stanford, Carla Caldwell, and Valerie J. Connor. *Ethics for Health Professionals*. Burlington, MA: Jones and Bartlett Learning, 2013.

PERIODICALS

Ganz, D., and L. Sher. "Adolescent Suicide in New York City: Plenty of Room for New Research." *International Journal of Adolescent Medicine and Health* 24 (November 29, 2011): 99–104.

Hill, J.H., et al. "Communication Technology Access, Use, and Preferences among Primary Care Patients: From the Residency Research Network of Texas (RRNeT)." *Journal of the American Board of Family Medicine* 25 (September 2012): 625–634.

Nyamathi, A., et al. "Impact of Nursing Intervention on Decreasing Substances among Homeless Youth." *American Journal on Addictions* 21 (November 2012): 558–565.

Nyberg, B.J., et al. "Saving Lives for a Lifetime: Supporting Orphans and Vulnerable Children Impacted by HIV/AIDS." *Journal of Acquired Immune Deficiency Syndromes* 60 (September 15, 2012): Suppl. 3: S127–S135.

Pathman, D.E., et al. "States' Experiences With Loan Repayment Programs for Health Care Professionals in a Time of State Budget Cuts and NHSC Expansion." *Journal of Rural Health* 28 (September 2012): 408–415.

Simpson, V.L. "Making It Meaningful: Teaching Public Health Nursing through Academic-Community Partnerships in a Baccalaureate Curriculum." *Nursing Education Perspectives* 22 (July-August 2012): 260–263.

Swahn, M.H., et al. "Addressing Injuries in Vulnerable Populations: Research Collaborations and Partnerships." *Western Journal of Emergency Medicine* 13 (August 2012): 215–216.

Witgert, K., and C. Hess. "Including Safety-net Providers in Integrated Delivery Systems: Issues and Options for Policymakers." *Issue Brief (Commonwealth Fund)* 20 (August 2012): 1–18.

WEBSITES

"Caring for Vulnerable Populations." American Hospital Association (AHA). http://www.aha.org/research/cor/caring/index.shtml (accessed October 21, 2012).

"Program Areas: Vulnerable Populations." Robert Wood Johnson Foundation (RWJF). http://www.rwjf.org/en/about-rwjf/program-areas/vulnerable-populations/Programs-and-Grants.html (accessed October 22, 2012).

"Vulnerable Populations." Commonwealth Fund. http://www.commonwealthfund.org/Program-Areas/Delivery-System-Innovation-and-Improvement/Vulnerable-Populations.aspx (accessed October 22, 2012).

"Vulnerable Populations." Office for Human Research Protections (OHRP). http://www.hhs.gov/ohrp/policy/populations/index.html (accessed October 20, 2012).

ORGANIZATIONS

American Hospital Association (AHA), 155 N. Wacker Drive, Chicago, IL United States 60606, (312) 422-3000, (800) 424-4301, http://www.aha.org/about/contactus.shtml, http://www.aha.org/.

Commonwealth Fund, One East 75th Street, New York, NY United States 10021, (212) 606-3800, Fax: (212) 606-3500, info@cmwf.org, http://www.commonwealthfund.org/.

National Health Service Corps (NHSC), [no other contact information], (800) 221-9393, http://nhsc.hrsa.gov/.

Office for Human Research Protections (OHRP), Department of Health and Human Services (HHS), 1101 Wootton Parkway, Suite 200, Rockville, MD United States 20852, (240) 453-6900, (866) 447-4777, Fax: (240) 453-6909, OHRP@hhs.gov, http://www.hhs.gov/ohrp/index.html.

Robert Wood Johnson Foundation, P.O. Box 2316, Route 1 and College Road East, Princeton, NJ United States 08543, (877) 843-RWJF, http://pweb1.rwjf.org/global/contactus.jsp, http://www.rwjf.org/.

Rebecca J. Frey, PhD

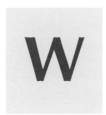

Water

Definition

Water is a chemical compound consisting of two atoms of hydrogen bonded with one atom of oxygen. It is the only substance that can be found in nature in all three forms, solid (ice), liquid (water), and gas (water vapor). Water makes Earth distinctive among all the known planets because Earth alone has sufficient water to support living things. While many living things can survive without oxygen, none can survive without water. Water is truly the stuff of life on Earth.

Description

Nearly three-quarters of the Earth's surface is covered by water, but most of this water is salty ocean water, unsuitable for humans to drink. Most fresh, drinkable water is in the form of ice in glaciers. Only 1% of water is available for humans to drink. Most of it is contained underground in aquifers, but it is also contained in manmade reservoirs, lakes, ponds, and rivers. Not all of this water is potable. Water can be polluted by human activity and contaminated with chemicals, including those from agricultural and manufacturing, and biological materials, including micro-organisms from animal and human waste.

The demands on the world's water supply are increasing as the human **population** of Earth increases. As of 2012, the world's population has topped 7 billion and is expected to double by 2050. Some countries do not have the water resources to support and supply their growing populations because most of the world's water resources are concentrated in nine nations (the United States, Canada, Colombia, Brazil, the Democratic Republic of Congo, Russia, India, China, and Indonesia), according to the World Business Council for Sustainable Development. A considerable amount of water is lost through poorly maintained water systems, evaporation, and poor water-use practices.

Approximately 85% of Americans get their **drinking water** from public drinking water systems. These systems are required to meet safety standards established by the United States **Environmental Protection Agency (EPA)**. The remaining 15% of Americans get their water from private water systems (wells), which are not monitored by the **EPA**. Well owners are responsible for the safety of their own wells.

Public drinking water systems can be divided into two groups: community, which are the water systems that deliver water to homes, and noncommunity, which include nontransient systems, such as those at schools and hospitals, and transient systems, such as those at hotels, campgrounds, and parks. Just 8% of U.S. community water systems provide water to 82% of the U.S. population through large municipal water systems. Because so many people get their drinking water from so few sources, safety and cleanliness are paramount. Contamination can affect thousands, or even millions, of people.

Sources of contaminants that can enter drinking water resources include chemicals and minerals, such as arsenic, radon, and uranium; local land use practices (fertilizer, pesticides, livestock); manufacturing; sewer overflows; and malfunctioning wastewater treatment systems. Regular testing can check for the presence and concentration of more than 90 contaminants, including micro-organisms such as *Salmonella, Cryptosporidium,* and *E. coli,* as well as chemicals, including lead and **sodium**.

Public health monitoring

The United States has been monitoring waterborne disease outbreaks (WBDOs) since 1920. For the past 40 years, three agencies, the EPA, the **Centers for Disease Control and Prevention (CDC)**, and the Council of State and Territorial Epidemiologists have collected data. According to a 2006 report, from 1920 to 2002, at least 1,870 outbreaks were associated with drinking water, an average of 22.5 per year.

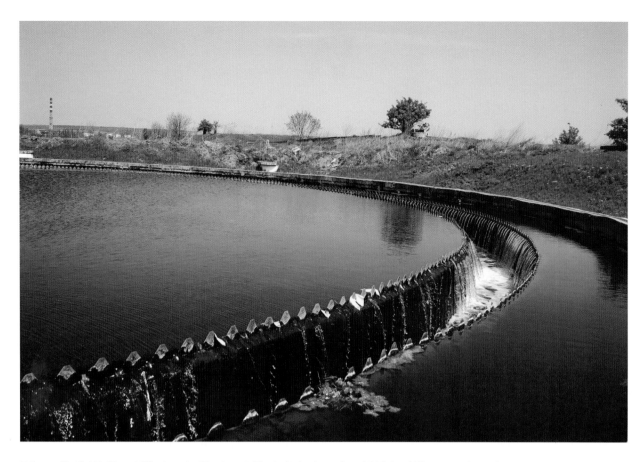

Primary Radial Settler at Wastewater Treatment Plant. *(© Imeleca (Leonid Meleca)/Shutterstock.com)*

The average annual number of WBDOs ranged from a low of 11.1, from 1951 to 1960, to as many as 32.4 from 1971 to 1980. From 1991 to 2002, 207 WBDOs and 433,947 illnesses were reported. Slightly more WBDOs occurred in non-community water systems (42%) than either community (36%) or individual systems (22%).

Since monitoring began, 1,165 Americans have died of WBDOs, most of them in 1940 during an outbreak of **typhoid fever**. However, 54 people died during an outbreak of cryptosporidiosis in Milwaukee, most of them (46) with immune systems compromised by HIV.

Since 1991, reported WBDOs have included:

- acute gastroenteritis, 77 outbreaks, 16,036 cases
- chemical contamination, 33 outbreaks, 577 cases
- giardia, 25 outbreaks, 2,283 cases
- cryptosporidium, 15 outbreaks, 408,371 cases
- norovirus, 12 outbreaks, 3,361 cases
- *E. coli*, 11 outbreaks, 288 cases
- shigella, 9 outbreaks, 663 cases
- campylobacter jejuni, 7 outbreaks, 360 cases
- legionella, 6 outbreaks, 80 cases
- salmonella (non-typhoid), 3 outbreaks, 833 cases
- v. cholera, 2 outbreaks, 114 cases
- hepatitis A, 2 outbreaks, 56 cases

Although public water systems treat water before it arrives at the location where it will be consumed, continued monitoring is essential for protecting the public.

Worldwide public health efforts

Because of its potential to spread disease, the quality of water is of paramount public health concern. According to the **World Health Organization (WHO)**, each year 2 million people die because of diarrheal illnesses related to unsafe water, **sanitation**, and **hygiene**. Most of these people are children under age five. According to current estimates, more than one billion people lack access to an improved water source. An improved water source is one that is safe from outside contamination, especially from fecal matter.

Beginning in 1990, the **WHO** began a global effort to cut in half the number of people in the world who did not have any access to potable water by 2015. Remarkably, that goal was met five years early, in 2010. More than 2 billion people gained access to improved water sources, and 1.8 billion people gained access to improved sanitation facilities between 1990 and 2010 through WHO efforts in cooperation with national governments.

Of those who gained access to improved water sources during that period, almost half lived in China (457 million) and India (522 million). The biggest change has been the increase in the percentage of people with piped water supplies, which rose from 45% in 1990 to 54% in 2010. The percentage of people who rely on surface water has been cut in half, from 6% to only 3, although the remaining amount does include 187 million people.

There is variation between urban and rural areas and between rich and poor populations, and not as much progress has been made in sub-Sarahan Africa and Oceania as in other parts of the world. Much work remains to be done in Kenya, Sudan, Tanzania, Bangladesh, the Democratic Republic of the Congo, Indonesia, Ethiopia, and Nigeria, as well as India and China.

Resources

PERIODICALS

Craun, Michael. "Waterborne outbreaks reported in the United States." *Journal of Water and Health* 04.Suppl 2, 2006. Accessed September 26, 2012.

OTHER

Centers for Disease Control and Prevention (CDC). *Health Studies Branch—Promoting Clean Water for Health.* http://www.cdc.gov/nceh/hsb/cwh/default.htm (accessed September 22, 2012).
WHO/UNICEF Joint Monitoring Programme for Water Supply and Sanitation. *Progress on Drinking Water and Sanitation, 2012 Update.* New York: World Health Organization, 2012.

WEBSITES

World Business Council for Sustainable Development. http://www.wbcsd.org/home.aspx (accessed September 24, 2012).
World Health Organization. *Water, Sanitation, and Health.* http://www.who.int/water_sanitation_health/hygiene/en/ (accessed September 25, 2012).

ORGANIZATIONS

Centers for Disease Control and Prevention, 1600 Clifton Road, Atlanta, GA 30333, (770) 639-3311, cdcinfo@cdc.gov, http:// www.cdc.gov/.
World Health Organization, Avenue Appia 20, 1211 Geneva 27, Switzerland, 41 22 (791) 21 11, Fax: 41 22 (791) 21 11, www.who.int.

Fran Hodgkins

Water fluoridation *see* **Water**

West Nile virus

Definition

West Nile virus spreads to humans through the bite of an infected mosquito. Usually, such bites cause no problems. In some cases, however, individuals may experience illness of varying severity, ranging from mild flu-like symptoms, which are typically described as West Nile fever, to more serious, even life-threatening forms of the illness, which may be called West Nile **encephalitis** or West Nile **meningitis**.

Description

The primary hosts of West Nile virus (WNV) are birds, and scientists have identified the virus in more than 320 species. Some of these birds, such as American crows (*Corvus brachyrhynchos*) and blue jays (*Cyanocitta cristata*), die due to the infection, but most other species survive. The virus can stay alive in birds for several years. When a mosquito bites a bird and draws blood, the virus may pass from the bird to the mosquito, and the mosquito may in turn pass it to birds or to other vertebrates, including humans, that it bites.

WNV is a flavivirus that belongs to the Japanese encephalitis serocomplex, which includes St. Louis encephalitis, Murray Valley encephalitis, and Kunjin virus. Infections generally occur between late summer and early fall in temperate areas, and throughout the year in southern climates. Most people who are infected with the virus experience no symptoms, but in some individuals, the virus can cross the blood-brain barrier and cause severe illness and paralysis.

WNV was originally isolated in a feverish woman living in the West Nile District of Uganda during 1937, although the virus may have been a threat to humans for millennia. According to a research article published in 2003, Alexander the Great may have succumbed to WNV encephalitis in Babylon in 323 BC. The virus was ecologically characterized in Egypt during the 1950s and later linked to severe human meningoencephalitis in elderly patients during a 1957 outbreak in Israel. Since 1937, subsequent outbreaks of WNV have occurred in Africa, Asia, Australia, Western Europe, the Middle East, and tropical islands in the Pacific Ocean.

In the summer of 1999, WNV was first reported in the New York City area and then spread rapidly across the entire continent. The exact pathway of WNV to the United States is unknown, but the transport of infected birds or insects is a suspect. After the virus's arrival in the New York area, the virus spread rapidly across the

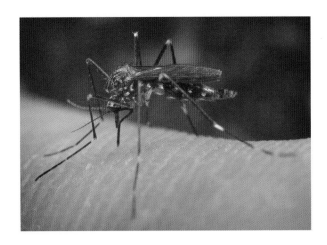

This mosquito, known as Aedes japonicus, was first collected in the U.S. in 1998, and is a major carrier of West Nile Virus. *(CDC/Frank Collins, PhD.)*

United States, as well as north into Canada and south into Mexico. A 2010 study suggested that mosquitoes likely facilitated the spread of the virus west across the United States. In that study, researchers analyzed the DNA gathered from 20 sites in the western United States, and found three large populations of the mosquito species *Culex tarsalis*, which is known to carry the virus and to infect humans. Furthermore, they detected extensive transfer of genes between the populations. This gene transfer, known as gene flow, indicates that the mosquitoes traveled distances consistent with the virus spread.

West Nile virus has claimed the lives of people in the United States. In 2002, a severe U.S. outbreak killed 284 people and caused 2,944 cases of severe brain damage. As of January 2011, the **Centers for Disease Control and Prevention (CDC)** had recorded avian or animal WNV infections in every state except Alaska and Hawaii.

Life cycle and transmission

Like most flaviviruses, the WNV is maintained in a natural host-vector-host cycle, where the primary vector is the mosquito, and the primary hosts are birds. When a mosquito feeds on an infected bird, the virus passes to the insect along with its blood meal. The virus then multiplies rapidly within the mosquito's body and salivary glands over the next few days. When the insect feeds on another animal, including a human, the bite may transmit the virus and cause illness, which may be serious.

Most mosquitoes can become infected with the WNV. However, mosquitoes of the species *Culex pipiens*

in the eastern United States, and *Culex tarsalis* on the West coast are the most common carriers of the virus. *Culex salinarius* is also a concern, because it readily feeds on humans. A **CDC** listing of mosquito species that were positively identified as being infected with West Nile virus from 1999 to 2008 noted 64 species in 10 genera. The genera are: *Aedes, Anopheles, Coquillettidia, Culex, Culiseta, Deinocerites, Mansonia, Orthopodomyia, Psorophora,* and *Uranotaenia.*

Most vertebrates, such as alligators, bats, chipmunks, skunks, squirrels, and rabbits, can also be infected with WNV. Horses, in particular, are commonly infected with WNV. Like humans, the majority of horses suffer either no or mild symptoms, but severe illness and death can and does occur. Relatively few cases exist of dogs and cats becoming infected with WNV. Animals of all species exhibiting fever, weakness, poor coordination, spasms, seizures, and/or personality changes may be infected with WNV.

WNV is not transmitted from person-to-person through casual contact. This includes contact through such means as touch or kissing. In addition, in all situations where standard **infection control** precautions are in force, no reports of patient-to-medical-worker transmission are known. However, one reported case of WNV passing from mother to child via the placenta, and rare incidences of virus transmission through breastfeeding are known. Because of this potential transmission, pregnant mothers should be aware of the presence of WNV in their area and take appropriate precautions. The transmission of WNV has also been evidenced in blood transfusions and in organ transplants, although the current blood supply is now tested for the presence of the WNV. People who are immunocompromised (from disease or from chemotherapy, for example) and people aged 50 and older represent the highest risk group for serious WNV infection. Humans may contract the WNV infection through contact with other infected animals, their blood, or other tissues.

Demographics

In the United States, the CDC monitors and records human WNV infections. In 2011, 712 cases were reported, including 43 fatalities. Infections were reported in 43 states, plus the District of Columbia. The **World Health Organization** also reported West Nile virus infection in several European countries in 2011. From July 2011–August 2011, the countries included Albania (2 cases), Greece (22), Israel (6), Romania (1) and the Russian Federation (11).

Up to 20% of the people who are infected with West Nile virus will experience symptoms. About one in 150 will develop severe illness with symptoms, which may include fever, muscle weakness, coma, paralysis, or others. Among those with severe illness due to West Nile virus, fatality rates range from 3% to 15%. Deaths occur more often in elderly patients.

Causes and symptoms

When a WNV-infected mosquito bites a mosquito, it can transfer the virus to the bird. The virus remains alive and circulates in the bird's bloodstream for several days. If another mosquito again bites a bird while it is carrying the virus, the virus can move into the mosquito with the blood it draws. The virus then moves into the mosquito's salivary glands, and when it bites a human or other animal, it can inject the virus. In some cases, the virus may multiply in the host's body and then cross the blood-brain barrier, which separates the blood from the central nervous system (including the brain and spinal cord). When this occurs, the virus can cause inflammation of brain tissue and interfere with normal operation of the nervous system, causing the described symptoms.

The incubation period for WNV after infection typically ranges between 3 and 14 days. Mild symptoms, also known as West Nile Fever, may last from three days to several weeks. They include:

- eye pain
- fever
- headache
- loss of appetite
- lymphadenopathy (abnormal enlargement of the lymph nodes)
- malaise (nonspecific bodily discomfort)
- myalgia (nonspecific muscular pain/tenderness)
- nausea
- rash (on the neck, torso, and limbs)
- vomiting

In those rare cases where WNV crosses the blood-brain barrier, symptoms may include:

- severe headache
- high fever
- acute muscle weakness
- neck stiffness
- convulsions and tremors
- disorientation and stupor
- paralysis
- coma

People exposed to WNV infection, especially individuals who are immunocompromised or elderly, should contact their health providers immediately if they develop a severe headache accompanied by high fever.

Typically, severe WNV syndromes manifest as one of three syndromes: West Nile encephalitis (inflammation of the brain); West Nile meningitis (inflammation of the meninges of the brain and spinal cord); or West Nile meningoencephalitis (inflammation of both the brain and the meninges). These three syndromes can cause severe brain damage and even death. The majority of these deaths are a result of complication attributable to West Nile meningoencephalitis. Additionally, severe WNV disease can cause acute vision loss due to inflammatory disorders of the eye, such as chorioretinitis, optic neuritis, retinal vasculitis, uveitis, and vitritis. Less frequently, the patient can exhibit acute flaccid paralysis, similar to poliomyelitis (**polio**) or Guillain-Barré syndrome, caused by inflammation of the spinal cord and/or damage to the peripheral nerves. In some severe cases, this acute flaccid paralysis can disrupt muscles that control breathing and result in respiratory failure.

Diagnosis

A proper diagnosis of WNV infection depends heavily upon the symptoms the patient is experiencing, and on thorough laboratory testing that differentiate WNV antibodies from those of similar viruses, because similarities of symptomology between and serological cross-reactivity of WNV and other flaviviruses, may lead to confusion and an incorrect diagnosis. Medical professionals also typically ask patients when and where they have been, as this can also help with diagnosis.

Additionally, health providers should remain constantly aware of the local presence of WNV activity, such as reports of recent animal and/or human cases. Patients with a known susceptibility to WNV (the elderly and immunocompromised) that exhibit symptoms during those time of the year when mosquitoes are present—late spring to early fall in temperate regions, or at any time in warmer climates—should undergo testing for WNV.

Symptomatic WNV infection can be classified as either non-neuroinvasive or neuroinvasive, with each being identified according to certain criteria.

Non-neuroinvasive

The majority of WNV infections are asymptomatic. In approximately 20% of WNV cases, clinically recognizable symptoms can manifest. However, to be clinically classified as non-neuroinvasive West Nile disease, the following must be true:

- no neuroinvasive symptomology
- presence of fever without other recognizable cause
- four-fold or greater increase in serum antibody titer

- virus isolated from and or demonstrated in blood, tissue, cerebrospinal fluid (CSF), or other bodily fluid
- virus-specific immunoglobulin M (IgM antibodies detected in cerebrospinal fluid)

Neuroinvasive

In rare cases (0.7%) of West Nile disease, the virus crosses the blood-brain barrier, causing severe and life-threatening symptoms. Clinical confirmation of neuroinvasive of neuroinvasive disease requires the presence of a fever and at least one of the following:

- acutely altered mental status, such as disorientation, stupor, or coma
- acute central or peripheral neurological difficulties, such as paralysis, nerve palsy, sensory deficits, and abnormal muscle function
- an increased white blood cell concentration in the cerebrospinal fluid coupled with symptoms of meningitis, such as severe headache and neck pain

Treatment

As of 2012, no specific treatment exists for WNV infection. People who have mild symptoms typically recover on their own after a matter of days to weeks. These patients usually recover at home. More severe symptoms may require hospitalization, which includes supportive care to treat the varying symptoms and syndromes associated with the various West Nile diseases. Such care may include the use of intravenous infusions, airway and respiratory management and support, and use of preventive measures against secondary infection.

Prognosis

The West Nile fever offers an excellent prognosis associated with quick recovery and no adverse side-effects. The majority of symptoms will resolve within a few days or weeks of manifestation.

The prognosis is not as positive for patients suffering the more severe syndromes attributable to WNV infection. Symptoms of West Nile encephalitis, West Nile meningitis, and West Nile meningoencephalitis can last for several weeks, and may cause severe and permanent neurological damage. Inflammation can interfere with the brain and central nervous system and result in death, especially among the elderly population. Patients with West Nile poliomyelitis may suffer prolonged muscle weakness and loss of motor control. Long-term rehabilitation is typically required and a full recovery is not assured. If the poliomyelitis affects

---

KEY TERMS

Flavivirus—An arbovirus (a virus transmitted by an insect or other arthropod) that can cause potentially serious diseases, such as dengue, yellow fever, Japanese encaphilitis, and West Nile fever.

Guillain-Barré—A disorder in which the body's immune system attacks part of the peripheral nervous system. Weakness, tingling, and abnormal sensations in the arms and upper body can progress until the muscles become totally disabled and the patient is effectively paralyzed.

Meninges—A series of membranous layers of connective tissue that protect the central nervous system (brain and spinal cord). Damage or infection to the meninges, such as in meningitis, can cause serious neurological damage and even death.

Zoonotic diseases—Diseases caused by infectious agents that can be transmitted between (or are shared by) animals and humans. This can include transmission through the bite of an insect, such as a mosquito.

---

muscles used for breathing, death from respiratory failure may result.

Prevention

Although a vaccine does exist for horses and exotic birds in zoos, no WNV vaccine is available for humans as of 2012. Several pharmaceutical companies, however, have WNV vaccines in various stages of development.

Prevention techniques of WNV typically coincide with avoidance measures against mosquito bites, the primary source of the virus. These include the use of insect repellant on exposed body parts, especially at dawn and dusk when mosquitoes are most active. The CDC recommends one of the following: DEET (N,N-diethyl-m-toluamide or N,N-diethyl-3-methyl-benzamide); picaridin (2-(2-hydroxyethyl)-1-piperidinecarboxylic acid 1-methylpropyl ester); oil of lemon eucalyptus or PMD (para-Menthane-3,8-diol), which is the synthesized version of the oil; or IR3535 (3-[N-Butyl-N-acetyl]-aminopropionic acid, ethyl ester). Other avoidance measures include wearing loose-fitting clothes over the limbs and torso while outdoors, using mosquito coils and/or citronella candles outdoors, limiting outdoor activities during peak biting periods and/or in areas with high mosquito density, and using window and door screens that will keep mosquitoes out of living spaces.

While camping, knockdown spray or bed netting with pyrethrum is suggested. Major cities in the United States have instituted mosquito eradication programs, which involve the use of pesticides to kill mosquito larvae or adults in areas suspected of the presence of infected mosquitoes.

The *Culex pipiens* mosquito is the primary vector of WNV transmission and is also commonly live and feed in urban areas. Special precautions should be taken to reduce exposure to these potentially infected insects. Screen doors and enclosed porches can help keep mosquitoes from coming into the house. It should be noted that studies have shown that mosquito control devices such as "bug zappers" and CO2-baited traps do not significantly reduce the risk of being bitten.

Removing potential mosquito breeding areas from near the home and from the neighborhood can further reduce the risk of bites. Any container that can collect half an inch of standing water can become a potential breeding site in as little as five days. The removal of old tires, empty plant pots, and empty trashcans, as well at the regular cleaning of water sources, such as ponds or birdbaths, can have a substantial impact on mosquito populations. Other recommended strategies for reducing mosquitoes include draining standing water from clogged eaves or other potential but not readily obvious areas, maintaining a proper cover over and **chlorination** of swimming pools and hot tubs.

As of August 2012, reported West Nile cases in the United States were at the highest numbers since 2004, likely due to extreme heat and early summer weather. The hardest hit area was Dallas and its surrounding county, resulting in insecticide spraying efforts after more than 400 cases were reported and almost 20 deaths occured.

Resources

BOOKS

U.S. General Accounting Office. *West Nile Virus Outbreak: Lessons for Public Health Preparedness: Report to Congressional Requesters.* Memphis: Books LLC, 2011.

PERIODICALS

LaDeau, S. L., Marm Kilpatrick, and Marra, P. P. "West Nile Virus Emergence and Large-scale Declines of North American Bird Populations." *Nature* 447 (7 June 2007): 710–713.

Marr J.S., and C.H. Calisher. "Alexander the Great and West Nile Virus Encephalitis." [serial online] December 2003. http://wwwnc.cdc.gov/eid/article/9/12/03-0288.htm. (accessed August 1, 2012).

Venkatesan M., and J.L. Rasgon. "Population Genetic Data Suggest a Role for Mosquito-Mediated Dispersal of West Nile Virus Across the Western United States." *Molecular Ecology* 19, no. 8 (April 2010): 1573–1584.

OTHER

West Nile Virus World Health Organization. http://www.who.int/mediacentre/factsheets/fs354/en/index.html (accessed August 2, 2012).

West Nile Virus U.S. National Library of Medicine. http://ncbi.nlm.nih.gov/pubmedhealth/PMH0004457/ (accessed August 6, 2012).

West Nile Virus: Fight the Bite! Centers for Disease Control and Prevention Division of Vector-Borne Infectious Diseases. http://www.cdc.gov/ncidod/dvbid/westnile/ (accessed August 2, 2012).

West Nile Virus Maps U.S. Geological Survey. http://diseasemaps.usgs.gov/wnv_us_human.html (accessed August 6, 2012).

West Nile Virus Infection (WNV) World Health Organization. http://www.who.int/csr/don/2011_08_16/en/index.html (accessed August 6, 2012).

Wetlands and West Nile Virus U.S. Environmental Protection Agency. http://www.epa.gov/owow/wetlands/pdf/West-Nile.pdf (accessed August 6, 2012).

ORGANIZATIONS

Centers for Disease Control and Prevention (CDC), 1600 Clifton Road, Atlanta, GA 30333, (800) 232-4636, cdcinfo@cdc.gov, http://www.cdc.gov.

National Institute of Allergies and Infectious Diseases, 6610 Rockledge Drive, MSC 6612, Bethesda, MD 20892-6612, (301) 496-5717, (866) 284-4107, ocpostoffice@niaid.nih.gov, http://www.niaid.nih.gov.

World Health Organization, Avenue Appia 20, 1211 Geneva 27, Switzerland 41 22 791 21 11, http://www.who.int.

Jason Fryer
Monique Laberge, PhD
Leslie Mertz, PhD

Whooping cough

Definition

Whooping cough, also known as pertussis, is a highly contagious disease that causes spasms (paroxysms) of uncontrollable coughing, followed by a sharp, high-pitched intake of air that creates the characteristic "whoop" of the disease's name.

Demographics

Pertussis was once one of the most deadly of all infectious childhood diseases in the United States and most other parts of the world. In 1923, 9,269 deaths from the disease were recorded in the United States, the largest number ever. In the period between 1934 and 1943, an average of more than 200,000 new cases of pertussis were being reported annually in the United States, with an average of just over 4,000 deaths per year from the disease. Since the 1940s, the rate of morbidity and mortality from the disease has continued to decrease to very low levels. In 1950, the U.S. **Centers for Disease Control and Prevention (CDC)** reported 120,718 new cases of pertussis in the United States, a number that gradually fell to 14,809 in 1960, 4,249 in 1970, and 1,730 in 1980. Since that time, the number of new cases of pertussis remained at less than 10,000 per year until 2003, when the rate began to climb to a high of 25,616 new cases in 2005. It fell again to a total of 16,858 new cases in 2009. The cause for this resurgence of the disease in the twenty-first century is not known for certain, although some experts believe that doubts about the safety of pertussis vaccines may be partially responsible for fewer children being vaccinated and, hence, at greater risk for the disease.

Pertussis occurs equally in males and females. Whites make up the large majority at over 85% of cases diagnosed. People under the age of 20 years make up over 75% of cases, most of these being reported in children under the age of 1 or between the ages of 10 and 19. Because the whooping cough **vaccination** does not provide lifelong immunity and immunity is no longer evident after 12 years, people must be revaccinated in order to be protected.

Description

Whooping cough is caused by a bacterium called *Bordatella pertussis*. *B. pertussis* causes its most severe symptoms by attaching itself to cells in the respiratory tract that have cilia. Cilia are small, hair-like projections that beat continuously, and serve to constantly sweep the respiratory tract clean of such debris as mucus, bacteria, viruses, and dead cells. When *B. pertussis* interferes with this normal janitorial function, mucus and cellular debris accumulate and cause constant irritation to the respiratory tract, triggering coughing and increasing further mucus production.

Whooping cough is a disease that exists throughout the world. While people of any age can contract whooping cough, children under the age of two are at the highest risk for the disease and for serious complications and death. Apparently, exposure to *B. pertussis* bacteria earlier in life gives a person some immunity against infection with it later on. Subsequent infections resemble the **common cold**.

Causes and symptoms

Whooping cough has four somewhat overlapping stages: incubation, catarrhal, paroxysmal, and convalescent.

An individual usually acquires *B. pertussis* by inhaling droplets infected with the bacteria coughed into the air by someone with the infection. Incubation is the symptomless period of 7 to 14 days after breathing in the *B. pertussis* bacteria and during which the bacteria multiply and penetrate the lining tissues of the entire respiratory tract.

The catarrhal stage is often mistaken for an exceedingly heavy cold. The patient has teary eyes, sneezing, fatigue, a poor appetite, and an extremely runny nose (rhinorrhea). This stage lasts about 10 to 14 days.

The paroxysmal stage, lasting two to four weeks, begins with the development of the characteristic whooping cough. Spasms of uncontrollable coughing, the "whooping" sound of the sharp inspiration of air, and vomiting are all hallmarks of this stage. The whoop is believed to occur due to inflammation and mucus, which narrow the breathing tubes, causing the patient to struggle to get air into his or her lungs and the effort results in intense exhaustion. The paroxysms (spasms) can be induced by activity, feeding, crying, or even overhearing someone else cough.

The mucus produced during the paroxysmal stage is thicker and more difficult to clear than the more watery mucus of the catarrhal stage, and the patient becomes increasingly exhausted attempting to clear the respiratory tract through coughing. Severely ill children may have great difficulty maintaining the normal level of oxygen in their system and may appear somewhat blue (cyanotic) after a paroxysm of coughing due to the low oxygen content of their blood. Such children may experience swelling and degeneration of the brain (encephalopathy), which is believed to be caused both by lack of oxygen to the brain during paroxysms and by bleeding into the brain caused by increased pressure during coughing. Seizures may result from decreased oxygen to the brain. Some children have such greatly increased abdominal pressure during coughing that hernias result. (Hernias are the abnormal protrusion of a loop of intestine through a weak area of muscle.) Another complicating factor during this phase is the development of **pneumonia** from infection with another bacterial agent that takes hold due to the patient's already-weakened condition.

If the patient survives the paroxysmal stage, recovery occurs gradually during the convalescent stage, usually taking about three to four weeks. However, spasms of coughing may continue to occur over a period of months, especially when a patient contracts a cold or other respiratory infection.

Diagnosis

Examination

Diagnosis based just on the patient's symptoms is not particularly accurate, as the catarrhal stage may

KEY TERMS

Bordatella pertussis—A bacterium that causes whooping cough by attaching itself to cells in the respiratory tract.

Cilia—Tiny, hair-like projections from a cell. In the respiratory tract, cilia beat constantly in order to move mucus and debris up and out of the respiratory tree, in order to protect the lung from infection or irritation by foreign bodies.

Encephalopathy—Swelling and degeneration of the brain.

Lymphocytes—A type of white blood cell.

Nasopharynx—The breathing tube continuous with the nose.

Rhinorrhea—A name for the common cold.

appear to be a heavy cold, a case of **influenza**, or a simple bronchitis. Other viruses and **tuberculosis** infections can cause symptoms similar to those found during the paroxysmal stage. The presence of a pertussis-like cough along with an increase of certain specific white blood cells (lymphocytes) is suggestive of whooping cough. However, cough can occur from other pertussis-like viruses.

Tests

The most accurate method of diagnosis is to culture (grow on a laboratory plate) the organisms obtained from swabbing mucus out of the nasopharynx (the breathing tube continuous with the nose). *B. pertussis* can then be identified by examining the culture under a microscope.

Treatment

Drugs

Treatment with the antibiotic erythromycin is helpful only at very early stages of whooping cough, during incubation and early in the catarrhal stage. After the cilia and the cells bearing those cilia are damaged, the process cannot be reversed. Such a patient will experience the full progression of whooping cough symptoms that only improve when the old, damaged lining cells of the respiratory tract are replaced over time with new, healthy, cilia-bearing cells. However, treatment with erythromycin is still recommended to decrease the likelihood of *B. pertussis* spreading. In fact, all members of the household where a patient with whooping cough lives should be treated with erythromycin to prevent the spread of *B. pertussis* throughout the community.

Home remedies

The only other treatment is supportive and involves careful monitoring of fluids to prevent dehydration; rest in a quiet, dark room to decrease paroxysms; and suctioning of mucus. Patients should be hospitalized if at risk for complication, such as infants from birth to six months of age.

Prognosis

Just under 1% of all cases of whooping cough cause death. Children who die of whooping cough usually have one or more of the following three conditions present:

• severe pneumonia, perhaps with accompanying encephalopathy

• extreme weight loss, weakness, and metabolic abnormalities due to persistent vomiting during paroxysms of coughing

• other pre-existing conditions, so that the patient is already in a relatively weak, vulnerable state (such conditions may include low birth weight, poor nutrition, infection with the measles virus, presence of other respiratory or gastrointestinal infections or diseases)

Prevention

The mainstay of **prevention** lies in programs similar to the mass **immunization** program in the United States, which begins immunization inoculations when infants are two months old. The pertussis vaccine, most often given as one immunization together with **diphtheria** and **tetanus** (DTP or DTaP), has greatly reduced the incidence of whooping cough.

There has been some concern about serious neurologic side effects from the vaccine itself. This concern has led many parents in England, Japan, and Sweden to avoid immunizing their children, which in turn has led to major epidemics of disease in those countries. However, several carefully constructed research studies have disproved the idea that the pertussis vaccine is the cause of neurologic damage. Furthermore, a newer formulation of the pertussis vaccine is available. Unlike the old whole cell pertussis vaccine, which is composed of the entire bacterial cell that has been deactivated (and therefore unable to cause infection), the newer acellular pertussis vaccine does not use a whole cell of the bacteria. Instead, it is made up of between two and five chemical components of the *B. pertussis* bacterium. The acellular pertussis vaccine appears to greatly reduce the risk of unpleasant reactions to the vaccine, including high fever and discomfort following vaccination.

Resources

BOOKS

Kitta, Andrea. *Vaccinations and Public Concern in History: Legend, Rumor, and Risk Perception.* New York: Routledge, 2012.

Long, Sarah S. *Principles and Practice of Pediatric Infectious Disease.* Edinburgh: Churchill Livingstone, 2012.

Stratton, Kathleen R., ed. *Adverse Effects of Vaccines: Evidence and Causality.* Washington, DC: National Academies Press, 2012.

Wertheim, Heiman F.L., Peter Horby, and John P. Woodall. *Atlas of Human Infectious Diseases.* Hoboken, NJ: John Wiley & Sons, 2012.

PERIODICALS

Bugenske, E., et al. "Middle School Vaccination Requirements and Adolescent Vaccination Coverage." *Pediatrics* 129, 6. (2012): 1056–63.

Clark, Thomas A., Nancy E. Messonnier, and Stephen C. Hadler. "Pertussis Control: Time for Something New?" *Trends in Microbiology* 20, 5. (2012): 211–13.

Girard, D.Z. "Recommended or Mandatory Pertussis Vaccination Policy in Developed Countries: Does the Choice Matter?" *Public Health* 126, 2. (2012): 129–34.

Libster, R., and K.M. Edwards. "How Can We Best Prevent Pertussis in Infants?" *Clinical Infectious Diseases* 54, 1. (2012): 85–87.

OTHER

Bocka, Joseph J. "Pertussis." Medscape Reference. http://emedicine.medscape.com/article/967268-overview. (accessed on November 2, 2012).

"DTaP Immunization (Vaccine)." Medline Plus. http://www.nlm.nih.gov/medlineplus/ency/article/002021.htm. (accessed on November 2, 2012).

"Pertussis (Whooping Cough) Vaccination." Centers for Disease Control and Prevention. http://www.cdc.gov/vaccines/vpd-vac/pertussis/default.htm. (accessed on November 2, 2012).

"Whooping Cough." Medline Plus. http://www.nlm.nih.gov/medlineplus/whoopingcough.html. (accessed on November 2, 2012).

ORGANIZATIONS

American Academy of Family Physicians, P.O. Box 11210, Shawnee Mission, KS 66207, (913) 906-6000, (800) 274-2237, Fax: (913) 906-6075, http://familydoctor.org/familydoctor/en/about/contact-us.html, http://familydoctor.org.

American Academy of Pediatrics, 141 Northwest Point Blvd., Elk Grove Village, IL 60007-1098, (847) 434-4000, Fax: (847) 434-8000, http://www2.aap.org/visit/contact.htm, http://www.aap.org.

Centers for Disease Control and Prevention (CDC), 1600 Clifton Rd., Atlanta, GA 30333, (404) 639-3534, (800) CDC-INFO (800-232-4636), TTY: (888) 232-6348, inquiry@cdc.gov, http://www.cdc.gov.

National Institute of Allergy and Infectious Diseases Office of Communications and Government Relations, 6610 Rockledge Dr., MSC 6612, Bethesda, MD 20892-6612, (301) 496-5717, (866) 284-4107, or TDD: (800) 877-8339 (for hearing impaired), Fax: (301) 402-3573, ocpostoffice@niaid.nih.gov, http://www3.niaid.nih.gov.

World Health Organization, Avenue Appia 20, 1211 Geneva 27, Switzerland, +22 41 791 21 11, Fax: +22 41 791 31 11, info@who.int, http://www.who.int.

Rosalyn Carson-DeWitt, MD
Tish Davidson, AM
Paul Checchia, MD

Women's health

Description

Women's health is an aspect of public health that has grown in importance over the last several decades due to the increasing recognition that women's bodies respond differently to medications than men's bodies do, and that a healthy woman is the heart of a healthy family.

Demographics

According to the 2010 U.S. Census, 156,964,212 Americans are female, accounting for 50.8% of the total **population**. Of the United States's female population, 22,864,357, or 14.56%, are between the ages of 45 and 54. The number of women over the age of 60 is 31,645,448, or 20%), including more than 44,000 women over 100.

With more than half the nation's population being female, healthcare providers have identified areas of particular interest to women.

From 1980 through 2007, **life expectancy** at birth in the United States increased from 77 years to 80 years for women, according to the **Centers for Disease Control and Prevention**. Women have had longer life expectancy at birth in all decennial periods since 1900, with white females having the longest life expectancy.

Health concerns

Women have some of the same health concerns as men. Like men, women struggle with weight issues. Approximately 60% of adult women in the United States are considered overweight, and one-third of those are considered obese. Weight concerns contribute to other health issues, including **heart disease** and diabetes. Approximately 13 million women live with heart disease (including hypertension), and 8% have diabetes.

GEORGE PAPANICOLAOU (1883–1962)

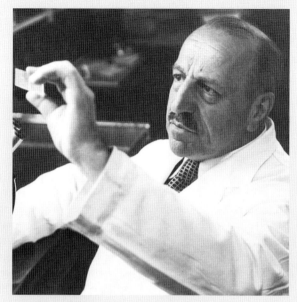

(© Bettmann/CORBIS)

The son of a physician, George Nicholas undertook the study of medicine and received his M. D. from the University of Athens in 1904. After postgraduate work in biology at the Universities of Jena, Freiburg, and Munich, from which he received his doctorate in 1910, he returned to Greece and married Mary Mavroyeni, the daughter of a high-ranking military officer. Papanicolaou decided to forgo the practice of medicine in favor of an academic career, in which his wife served as his lifelong associate. En route to Paris, Papanicolaou stopped for a visit at the Oceanographic Institute of Monaco and accepted an unexpected offer to join its staff. He worked for one year as a physiologist and then returned to Greece following the death of his mother. After serving for two years as second lieutenant in the medical corps of the Greek army during the Balkan War, he immigrated to the United States.

In 1913 Papanicolaou was appointed assistant in the pathology department of New York Hospital, and in 1914 he became assistant in anatomy at Cornell Medical College. Until 1961 he conducted all of his scientific research, devoted almost exclusively to the physiology of reproduction and exfoliative cytology, at these two affiliated institutions, each of which named a laboratory in his honor. He was designated professor emeritus of clinical anatomy at Cornell in 1951. In November 1961 Papanicolaou moved to Florida and became director of the Miami Cancer Institute, but died three months later of an acute myocardial infarction. The institute was renamed the Papanicolaou Cancer Research Institute in November 1962. An indefatigable worker, Papanicolaou is said never to have taken a vacation. Papanicolaou is best known for his development of the technique eponymically termed the Papanicolaou smear, or "Pap test," for the cytologic diagnosis of cancer, especially cancer of the uterus, which is second only to the breast as the site of origin of fatal cancers in American women.

Papanicolaou was invited by Charles R. Stockard, chairman of the Cornell Medical School department of anatomy, to join him in his work in experimental genetics. In 1917 he began a study of the vaginal discharge of the guinea pig, with the hope of finding an indicator of the time of ovulation. He would thus be able to obtain ova at specific stages of development. He sought traces of blood, as seen during estrus in certain other species, such as the cow and bitch, and in the menstrual discharge of primates and women. In the course of his daily examination of the guinea pig vaginal fluid, obtained through a small nasal speculum, Papanicolaou saw no blood. He noted instead a diversity in the forms of the epithelial cells in a sequence of cytologic patterns recurring in a fifteen- to sixteen-day cycle, which he was able to correlate with the cyclic morphologic changes in the uterus and ovary. Papanicolaou thus established the technique that became the standard for studying the sexual (estrous) cycle in other laboratory animals, especially the mouse and rat, and for measuring the effect of the sex hormones.

In 1923 Papanicolaou extended his studies to human beings in an effort to learn whether comparable vaginal changes occur in woman in association with the menstrual cycle. His first observation of distinctive cells in the vaginal fluid of a woman with cervical cancer gave Papanicolaou what he later described as "one of the most thrilling experiences of my scientific career" and soon led to a redirection of his work.

His early reports on cancer detection, however, which appeared from 1928, failed to arouse the interest of clinicians. Cytologic examination of the vaginal fluid seemed an unnecessary addition to the proven procedures for uterine cancer diagnosis-cervical biopsy and endometrial curettage. In 1939, while collaborating with the gynecologist Herbert Traut, Papanicolaou began to concentrate his studies on human beings. Their research culminated in the publication of Diagnosis of Uterine Cancer by the Vaginal Smear. This monograph encompassed a variety of physiologic and pathologic states, including the menstrual cycle, puerperium, abortion, ectopic pregnancy, prepuberty, menopause, amenorrhea, endometrial hyperplasia, vaginal and cervical infections, and 179 cases of uterine cancer (127 cervical and 52 corporeal). The work was instrumental in gaining clinical acceptance of the smear as a means of cancer diagnosis, for superficial lesions could thus be detected in their incipient, preinvasive phase, before the appearance of any symptoms.

The Papanicolaou smear soon achieved wide application as a routine screening technique. The death rate from cancer of the uterus among women aged 35 to 44 who were insured under industrial policies by the Metropolitan Life Insurance Company was almost halved in the decade from 1951 to 1961, decreasing from 16 to 8.2 per 100,000, while the corresponding reduction in the death rate from cancer of all sites was from 74 to 66.

Cancer

Cancer is also a major concern for women. Most people diagnosed with breast cancer are women. About one in eight women will develop invasive breast cancer, while a man's risk of developing breast cancer is 1 in 1,000. Among women, breast cancer is the second most commonly diagnosed cancer, exceeded only by skin cancer. More than 43% of newly diagnosed cases occurred in women age 65 and older. According to the National Cancer Institute, about 124 women out of every 100,000 are diagnosed with breast cancer each year. The incidence is slightly higher for white women than for women of color (127 per 100,000 versus 121 for black women and 94.5 for Asian/Pacific Islanders). The median age for breast cancer diagnosis is 61. In 2011, there were 2.6 million breast cancer survivors in the United States.

Heart disease

Although cancer is an alarming diagnosis, more women actually die from heart disease—more than one-third of women each year. Heart disease is an umbrella term for disorders affecting the heart and blood vessels. It includes heart attacks, arrhythmias (irregular heart beats), coronary artery disease, and conditions and infections that involve the heart's muscle, rhythm, or valves.

Like men, women's risk factors for heart disease include **obesity** and high blood pressure, although women face additional risk factors. Depression and mental state affects women's hearts more than men's hearts. **Smoking** is also a greater contributor to heart disease in women than it is in men. Metabolic syndrome (a combination of high triglycerides, high blood pressure, high blood sugar, and abdominal fat) also has a greater impact in women than in men. In addition, the changing levels of estrogen that occur after a woman goes through menopause can increase her chances of developing blockages in the small arteries of the heart, a type of heart disease called "small vessel heart disease."

Reproductive health

Women's health also include **reproductive health**, including care during pregnancy. Women under the age of 20 and over the age of 35 are generally considered to be at high risk for complications of pregnancy, as are women who are over- or underweight. Among the risks they face are gestational diabetes and preeclampsia, a syndrome that causes high blood pressure, too much protein in the urine, and possible damage to the kidneys and other organs.

Several other complications of pregnancy can occur:

- Ectopic pregnancy, which occurs when the fertilized egg settles in the fallopian tube instead of the uterus; the egg cannot develop, and surgery or medication must be used to remove the tissue

- Hyperemesis gravidarum, which is nausea and vomiting that last far beyond the time of "morning sickness," and can lead to weight loss and dehydration

- Placenta previa, which occurs when the placenta develops over the cervix within the uterus, can lead to bleeding and possible risk to the fetus

- Miscarriage, the unexpected, natural loss of a pregnancy, which occurs in 10 to 15% of pregnancies, usually before the twentieth week. A woman may have a miscarriage without even realizing she was pregnant, and so the total number of miscarried pregnancies may be even higher, as much as 40%. Most miscarriages involve chromosomal disorders in the fetus that would make its survival unlikely. However, drug use, smoking, and alcohol and caffeine can increase the risk of miscarriage.

Mental health

The health of the mind is just as important as the health of the body. **Stress** and anxiety can be part of normal life, but when they do not go away, that may be a sign that there is something more occurring.

Depression is common but serious. Signs of depression include loss of enjoyment in things that used to give pleasure; feelings of hopelessness; pessimism; restlessness; increases or decreases in sleeping and eating; difficulty making decisions and concentrating; and fatigue. A woman who has recently given birth may experience post-partum depression. Fortunately, depression can be treated with medication and talk therapy.

Post-traumatic Stress Disorder (PTSD) can occur in a woman who has lived through a traumatic event. Such an event can be an abusive relationship, a natural disaster, or war. PTSD, like depression, can be treated.

Anxiety disorders include obsessive-compulsive disorder, social phobias, and panic disorder. It is natural to feel anxious at certain times, but when the anxiety interferes with daily life, it is time to speak to a doctor.

Eating disorders include anorexia, bulimia, and binge eating. They are not just about food, but also about body image. These disorders can damage the body and the teeth, especially among those who force themselves to vomit repeatedly. An estimated 10 million

Americans (female and male) struggle with eating disorders, with the peak onset in girls beginning between ages 11 and 13.

Osteoporosis

Osteoporosis is another health issue that women need to be aware of, especially as they get older. It is estimated that half of women over age 50 will break a bone due to osteoporosis, which is a loss of bone mass and the structural deterioration of bone tissue.

Osteoporois affects more than 40 million American women. White and Asian women are at greater risk for the disease, as are women who tend to be small-framed and thin-boned to begin with. The use of cigarettes and certain long-term medications, such as glucocorticoids, can increase the risk of developing the disease, as can anorexia nervosa, an eating disorder.

Staying healthy

To give herself the best chance of staying healthy and to avoid such health problems as heart disease, cancer, and osteroporosis, a woman should do the following:

- Exercise regularly. Get 30 to 60 minutes of exercise several days a week.
- Maintain a healthy weight, and eat more whole grains, fruits, and vegetables and fewer processed foods.
- Avoid smoking tobacco and using illegal drugs.
- Consume alcohol wisely, limiting intake to one drink per day.
- Make sure to consume enough calcium. Women under 50 need 1,000 mg of calcium every day, while women over 51 need 1,200 mg per day. It is found in dairy products or other calcium-rich foods, such as salmon, spinach, and fortified juices or cereals.
- Drink plenty of water.

Public health concerns

Women's health is an integral part of public health. On a global scale, more than 200 million women want to plan their families, but lack access to contraceptives. For many years, hundreds of thousands of women died annually due to complications from pregnancy and childbirth, but that number declined in 2008 to 342,900, according to a study by the University of Queensland that was reported in 2012 in the British medical journal *The Lancet*. Researchers say that this is evidence that public health efforts in the realm of women's health are working. However, in an ironic twist, the number of women in some developed nations, including the United States, who die due to such complications has increased.

The work of state and local public health agencies and organizations, such as the Harvard University School of Public Health, is not done. Politics and religion come between many women and their access to safe medical care.

Resources

PERIODICALS

Centers for Disease Control. *Summary Health Statistics for U.S. Adults: National Health Interview Survey, 2010.* http://www.cdc.gov/nchs/data/series/sr_10/sr10_252.pdf (accessed September 25, 2012).

Health Resources and Services Administration, U.S. Department of Health and Human Services. *Women's Health USA 2010.* http://www.hrsa.gov/ourstories/healthusa2010/ (accessed September 20, 2012).

Langer, Ana. "Finally, Fewer Women Around the World Are Dying from Childbirth. Now to Continue the Trend." *Huffington Post*, April 15, 2010. http://www.huffingtonpost.com/dr-ana-langer/finally-less-women-around_b_538968.html (accessed September 25, 2012).

Office on Women's Health, U.S. Department of Health and Human Services. *Lifetime of Good Health: Your Guide to Staying Healthy.* http://www.womenshealth.gov/publications/our-publications/lifetime-good-health/LifetimeGoodHealth-English.pdf (accessed September 24, 2012).

WEBSITES

Heart Disease. Mayo Clinic. http://www.mayoclinic.com/health/heart-disease/HB00040 (accessed January 10, 2013).

Osteoporosis Overview. NIH Osteoporosis and Related Bone Diseases National Resource Center. http://www.niams.nih.gov/Health_Info/Bone/Osteoporosis/overview.asp#c (accessed September 21, 2012).

Population by Age and Sex, 2000 and 2010, Age and Sex Composition: 2010 2010 Census Briefs, U.S. Census Bureau. http://www.census.gov/prod/cen2010/briefs/c2010br-03.pdf (accessed January 10, 2010).

Surveillance Epidemiology and End Results, National Cancer Institute http://seer.cancer.gov/statfacts/html/breast.html (accessed September 21, 2012).

Women and Heart Disease Fact Sheet, National Coalition for Women with Heart Disease. http://www.womenheart.org/resources/cvdfactsheet.cfm (accessed September 23, 2012).

ORGANIZATIONS

CDC/ATSDR Office of Women's Health Centers for Disease Control and Prevention, 4770 Buford Highway, MS E-89, Atlanta, GA 1 (770) 488-8190, Fax: 1 (770) 488-8280, owh@cdc.gov.

National Eating Disorders Association, 165 West 46th Street, Suite 402, New York, NY 10036, (212) 575-6200, Fax: (212) 575-1650, http://www.nationaleatingdisorders.org/.

Fran Hodgkins

Workplace safety

Definition

Workplace safety refers to all those policies, practices, rules, and regulations designed to protect workers from physical, chemical, biological, and other hazards associated with their jobs and the physical locations in which they work. It also includes efforts by employers, unions, and workers themselves to maintain the highest level of good health possible for employees, their families, and the general community. Workplace safety is also often referred to as "occupational safety and health."

Purpose

The purposes of workplace safety programs are to identify possible hazards faced by workers in their place of employment, to develop programs and other systems to protect workers from those hazards, and to provide an environment that will maximize the physical and mental health of employees.

Description

Employees in virtually every occupation face some type of hazard or another to their physical or mental well-being. Construction workers are at risk for falls or injuries from falling objects. Workers in a refinery are exposed to chemical fumes and are at risk for fires and explosions. Farm workers handle fertilizers and pesticides that may cause respiratory or other bodily damage. Office workers may have to deal with boredom, frustration, **stress**, or other emotional issues.

Machines are a major source of injury in a variety of occupations because of their moving parts. An employee can easily become entangled in gears, sprockets, or rotating shafts, causing loss of a finger, hand, arm, or other body part. Presses and other machines that crush objects can also trap an employee's hand or arm. Objects with knife-like or other sharp edges can also sever body

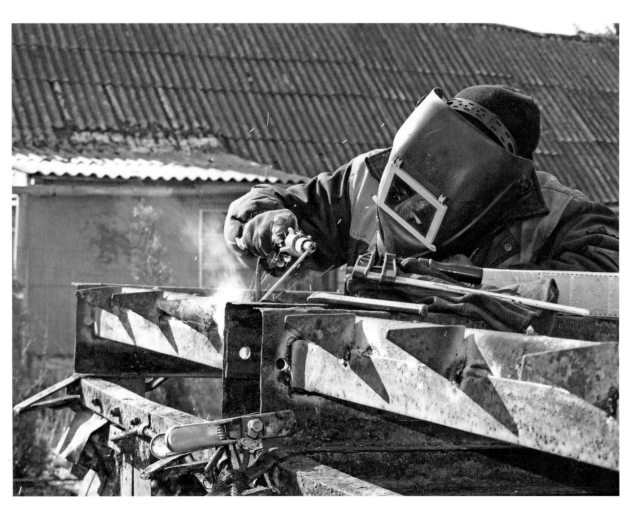

A man properly working with arc welder. (© Grandpa/Shutterstock.com)

HAMILTON, ALICE (1869–1970)

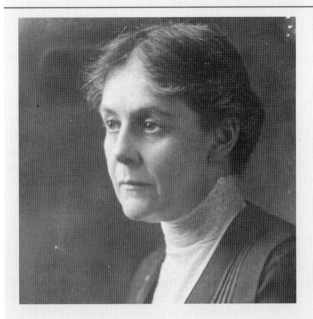

(Library of Congress)

Alice Hamilton was born on February 27, 1869, in New York City, the second of five children born to Montgomery Hamilton, a wholesale grocer, and Gertrude (Pond) Hamilton. She earned a medical degree from the University of Michigan in 1893, without having completed an undergraduate degree and taking surprisingly few science courses. Realizing that she wanted to pursue research rather than medical practice, Hamilton went on to do further studies both in the United States and abroad: from 1895–1896 at Leipzig and Munich; 1896–1897 at Johns Hopkins; and 1902 in Paris at the Pasteur Institute. In 1897 she accepted a post as professor of pathology at the Women's Medical College at Northwestern University in Chicago.

In Chicago Hamilton became a resident of Hull House, the pioneering settlement designed to give care and advice to the poor of Chicago. Under the influence of Jane Addams, the founder of Hull House, Hamilton saw the effects of poverty up close, leading her to a lifelong career focused on industrial medicine.

Alice Hamilton was a pioneer in correcting the medical problems caused by industrialization, awakening the country in the early twentieth century to the dangers of industrial poisons and hazardous working conditions. Through her untiring efforts, toxic substances in the lead, mining, painting, pottery, and rayon industries were exposed and legislation was passed to protect workers. She was also a champion of worker's compensation laws and was instrumental in bringing about this type of legislation in the state of Illinois. A medical doctor and researcher, she was the first woman of faculty status at Harvard University and was a consultant on governmental commissions, both domestic and foreign.

parts. Leaks or breaks in hoses, pipes, liquid reservoirs, or other devices that contain fluids may increase the likelihood of slips and falls that result in broken bones, sprains, or strains.

Inhalation of dust and powders can cause a number of chronic respiratory problems, such as:

• asbestosis

• byssinosis (also known as "brown lung disease")

• pneumoconiosis (also known as "coal worker's pneumoconiosis" or "black lung disease"

• silicosis

• chronic beryllium disease

• chronic pleural disease

• mesothelioma

• hypersensitivy pneumonitis

• occupational lung cancer

Respiratory diseases such as these are a particular hazard in resource recovery occupations, such as coal and metal mining, where naturally occurring materials are broken apart, and small particles, dusts, and powders released in the process are inhaled by workers. Once those particles are inhaled, they tend to become lodged in the lungs, where they accumulate, blocking air passages and causing inflammation of tissues that may result in chronic respiratory disorders, such **asbestosis** (caused by particles of the mineral asbestos), silicosis (caused by small particles of silicon dioxide, or sand), and chronic beryllium disease (caused by small particles of beryllium metal or its ore).

Other possible hazardous present in the workplace include:

• heat from hot machinery, escaping steam, furnaces, molten materials, and other sources that may cause severe burns, heat stroke, exhaustion, cramps, dehydration, dizziness, or other effects, or that scorch clothing or fog safety glasses

• cold, which can produce numbness, frostbite, hypothermia, or other effects that incapacitate a person or reduce work efficiency and effectiveness

• electric shock, which can cause burns, falls, incapacitation, or even death

- chemical exposure to a range of materials, including acids and bases, heavy metals, poisonous compounds, solvents, and flammable and explosive materials, all of which can cause internal distress if swallowed, burns and scarring if in contact with the skin, and respiratory distress if inhaled, any of which can be fatal in the most extreme cases
- fumes and gases that may be annoying or even life-threatening, such oxides of nitrogen, sulfur dioxide, and carbon monoxide
- noise, the effects of which can range from the annoying to they physical damage, as when exposure to very loud sounds may actually cause damage to the eardrum that can result in permanent hearing loss
- high-intensity light or other forms of electromagnetic radiation, such as ultraviolet or infrared radiation, x-rays, or gamma radiation, all of which can damage the eyes, skin, or other parts of the body
- exposure to illegal and unhealthy practices of fellow workers, including smoking, drinking, substance abuse, and careless work behaviors that pose a risk not only to the person doing such behaviors, but also to co-workers in the surrounding environment
- biological agents, including viruses, bacteria, fungi, parasites, and other pathogens that can cause a host of infections
- psychological and social factors, such as stress, violence, burnout, bullying, harassment, and repetitive stress injuries, such as carpal tunnel syndrome.

An additional safety hazard in many occupations is posed by confined spaces. A confined space is a region with one or only a few openings that is not designed for long-term occupancy by employees, with poor ventilation and possibly contaminated air. Examples of confined spaces are storage tanks, compartments of ships, process vessels, pits, silos, vats, degreasing tanks, reaction vessels, boilers, ventilation and exhaust ducts, sewers, tunnels, underground utility vaults, and pipelines. Employees are often required to enter confined spaces for the purpose of service or cleaning such areas and face the risk of becoming trapped inside them. According to the U.S. Bureau of Labor Statistics (BLS), an average of about 92 people in the United States die each year after becoming trapped in a confined space.

Demographics

State, national, and international government and labor organizations collect and maintain extensive databases on the number, causes, and circumstances of workplace injuries and deaths. In the United States, the relevant agency for these data is the U.S. Department of Labor of the Bureau of Labor Statistics. Data announced

by BLS for 2011 indicate that the number of workplace fatalities in the United States has decreased slowly over the past two decades from a high of 6,632 in 1995 to a low of 4,551 in 2010. The most common cause of fatal incidents in 2011 was some type of transportation event, such as an on-road vehicle accident (41 percent of all deaths), followed by **violence** caused by other humans or nonhuman animals (17 percent of all deaths); contact with objects or equipment (15 percent); falls, trips, and slips (14 percent); exposure to harmful substances (9 percent); and fires and explosions (3 percent). Ninety-two percent of all fatalities were male, although males constituted only 57 percent of the work force at the time. The rate of fatalities for each gender was nearly the same for all causes with the exceptions of homicides in the workplace, which accounted for 21 percent of all female deaths and 9 percent of all male deaths, and contact with objects and other equipment, which accounted for 16 percent of all male deaths and 9 percent of all female fatalities. By far the largest age group among 2011 fatalities was workers over the age of 65, with a fatality rate of 10.8 deaths per 100,000 workers. The fatality rate among other age groups was much lower at 4.3 per 100,000 among those 55 to 64 and dropping to a low of 2.3 per 100,000 among those 25 to 34.

The largest number of fatalities in terms of occupation occurred in the transportation and warehousing industry, accounting for a total of 733 deaths in 2011, followed by construction (721 deaths); agriculture, forestry, fishing, and hunting (557 deaths); government (495 deaths); and professional and building services (424 deaths). The highest rate of mortalities in 2011, however, occurred within the agriculture, forestry, fishing, and hunting field (24.4 deaths per 100,000 workers), followed by mining (15.8 deaths per 100,000); transportation and warehousing (15 deaths per 100,000); and construction (8.9 deaths per 100,000). The safest occupations in the United States in 2011 were education and health services, with a death rate of 0.8 per 100,000 workers, and financial services (1.1 deaths per 100,000).

Among specific occupations, the highest death rate per 100,000 workers in the United States in 2011 was the fishing industry, with a rate of 121.2 deaths per 100,000, followed by logging workers (102.4 deaths per 100,000), airline pilots and engineers (57 deaths per 100,000), and refuse and recyclable metal collectors (41.2 deaths per 100,000).

The pattern of nonfatal injuries among American workers in 2011 was somewhat different than the pattern for fatalities. Overall, the rate of nonfatal injuries across all occupations was 3.8 injuries per 100,000 workers, with the highest rates among occupations for nursing and

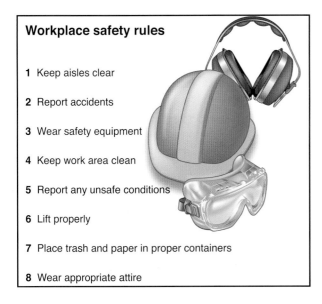

Workplace safety rules

1 Keep aisles clear

2 Report accidents

3 Wear safety equipment

4 Keep work area clean

5 Report any unsafe conditions

6 Lift properly

7 Place trash and paper in proper containers

8 Wear appropriate attire

(Illustration by Electronic Illustrators Group. © 2013 Cengage Learning)

health care facilities employees (13.1 per 100,000); justice, public order, and safety (10.3 per 100,000); construction (8.7 per 100,000); and air transporation (7.3 per 100,000).

Origins

Prior to the twentieth century, workplace safety was a matter of little or no concern to governmental agencies or the general public in the United States or any other country of the world. Certain jobs, such as those in mining and manufacturing, were simply regarded as hazardous, and workers just accepted the risk involved in going to work each day in such jobs. The fatality rate among U.S. coal miners in the last decade of the nineteenth century, for example, was in excess of 325 per 100,000 workers, more than 100 times the comparable rate today. The death rate among railroad workers at the time was somewhat less than that, about 267 deaths per 100,000 workers, about 140 times the rate at the time. Public attitudes began to change during the early part of the twentieth century with the rise of the progressive movement in the United States. For the first time, social reformers began to demand that business and industry accept some measure of responsibility for providing their workers with safe and healthful working conditions. One of the first actions by the U.S. government was the creation of the Bureau of Mines in 1910 following a series of disastrous mine accidents resulting in hundreds of deaths and injuries. In the same year, New York adopted the first workmen's compensation law, a law allowing employees to sue employers for damages resulting from accidents that occurred in

the workplace. Within a decade, largely through the efforts of the new workers unions that were being formed across the country, 44 other states had adopted similar legislation.

In 1971, the U.S. Congress established the first federal agency with specific responsibility for overseeing the safety and health of U.S. workers, the Occupational Safety and Health Administration (OSHA) in the Department of Labor. Under provisions of its original enabling legislation, as well as numerous later bills, OSHA is responsible for a bewildering variety of potential safety hazards and risks as well as a number of occupations and industries. A short list of some of the topics with which OSHA deals includes agricultural operations, the airline industry, **anthrax**, arsenic, asbestos, biofuels, beryllium, biological agents, cadmium, combustible dust, compressed gas and equipment, demolition, diacetyl, ELF radiation, ergonomics, green jobs, hantavirus, heat illness, isocyanates, logging, meat packing, microwave radiation, nursing homes, oil and gas well drilling, the plastic industry, popcorn, Portland cement, reproductive hazards, sawmills, scaffolding, **tularemia**, and violence in the workplace.

Costs to society

The deaths and injuries resulting from workplace accidents are only two measures of their cost to society. Every death and injury is also related to a number of financial and economic costs, both to the injured person and her or his family, as well as to the employer and to society as a whole. A number of economists have attempted to estimate the total cost in dollars to the United States as a result of workplace injuries and deaths, with results that range widely across the board. A 2012 estimate, for example, placed that cost at more than $250 billion. Other estimates range from about $50 billion upwards. These costs include the obvious direct costs associated with an injury of visits to an emergency department, physician fees, other medical bills, medications, and costs of rehabilitation, for example. However, they also include hidden costs that do not immediately come to mind, such as administrative costs in dealing with the injury, increases in insurance premiums, costs of hiring a substitute for the injured worker, effects on employee morale, loss of products and services, delays in filling orders, potential governmental penalties, and attorney fees associated with possible claims. By some estimates, these indirect costs can amount to as much as four times the direct costs of the injury itself.

Prevention

Government, business, and individual employees have all come to the realization that the financial and

KEY TERMS

Confined space—An area with one or only a few opening that is not designed for long-term occupancy by employees, with poor ventilation and possibly contaminated air.

Hazard—A material or condition that can cause injury if not controlled.

Hazard assessment—An attempt to survey an environment to determine which hazards are present in that environment.

Repetitive stress injury—An injury that occurs as a result of repeating some physical action over and over again many times in sequence.

Risk—The possibility of suffering harm from a hazard.

personal costs of workplace injuries and death are so great that programs of injury prevention are not only worth the time and effort, but are essential in the modern world. A number of businesses have adopted accident prevention programs on their own, but most do so because of federal, state, and local regulations that require them to do so. An injury prevention program has a number of primary elements, including:

• Acceptance of management responsibility: The first step in any injury prevention program is an acceptance by a company that it has a responsibility to reduce injuries in its workplace. One concrete expression of this responsibility is the provision for workers of all safety technology available and appropriate for the industry, such as safeguards on machinery, adequate rest times, sufficient safety equipment (safety glasses and gloves, for example), and adequate first aid facilities and equipment.

• Communication with employees: Businesses need to make employees aware of safety issues within the workplace and, preferably, to involve them in the injury-prevention program. For this reason, most businesses today now have safety committees that consist of both managers and employees, to carry out company policies on injury-prevention efforts.

• Hazard assessment and control: One essential step in any injury-prevention program involves a review of the workplace to identify potential risks and hazards to employees and than to develop specific mechanisms for reducing them.

• Accident investigation: Even under the best of circumstances, accidents will occur. A good injury

prevention program will include, therefore, a specific mechanism for investigating the conditions and circumstances surrounding accidents in the workplace to determine what changes are needed to reduce future risks from the same hazard.

• Safety and health recording systems: In some industries, it may be necessary to keep ongoing records of employee exposure to certain types of hazards, such as levels of radiation or exposures to harmful chemicals. These records ensure that employees are not exposed to levels of hazards greater than those recommended by regulatory agencies.

• Safety and health training: Management and unions can work together to provide classes and other training sessions to make employees more aware of the hazards present in the workplace, the steps needed to avoid accidents, and the proper ways to use safety equipment provided by the company.

Resources

BOOKS

American Industrial Hygiene Association; American National Standards Institute. *Occupational Health and Safety Management Systems.* Falls Church, VA: American Industrial Hygiene Association, 2012.

English, Paul F. *Safety Performance in a Lean Environment: A Guide to Building Safety into a Process.* Boca Raton, FL: CRC Press, 2012.

Reese, Charles D. *Accident/incident Prevention Techniques.* Boca Raton, FL: Taylor & Francis, 2012.

Wilborn, Steven L., et al. *Employment Law: Cases and Materials.* New Providence, NJ: LexisNexis, 2012.

PERIODICALS

Kongsvik, T., J. Fenstad, and C. Wendelborg. "Between a Rock and a Hard Place: Accident and Near-miss Reporting on Offshore Service Vessels." *Safety Science* 50, 9. (2012): 1839–46.

Lortie, M. "Analysis of the Circumstances of Accidents and Impact of Transformations on the Accidents in a Beverage Delivery Company." *Safety Science* 50, 9. (2012): 1792–1800.

Saleh, J.H., and C.C. Pendley. "From Learning from Accidents to Teaching about Accident Causation and Prevention: Multidisciplinary Education and Safety Literacy for All Engineering Students." *Reliability Engineering and System Safety* 99. (2012): 105–13.

Smith, E.L. "How Are Nurses at Risk?" *Work* 41, 0. (2012): 1911–9.

WEBSITES

"Cal/OSHA Guide." State of California. Department of Industrial Relations. http://www.dir.ca.gov/dosh/dosh_publications/iipp.html (accessed November 3, 2012).

"Injuries, Illnesses, and Fatalities." U.S. Bureau of Labor Statistics. http://www.bls.gov/iif/oshsum.htm (accessed November 3, 2012).

"Occupational Safety and Health." http://ohsonline.com/Home.aspx (accessed November 3, 2012).

"Workplace Safety and Health." Centers for Disease Control and Prevention. http://www.cdc.gov/workplace/ (accessed November 3, 2012).

ORGANIZATIONS

U.S. Department of Labor. Occupational Safety & Health Administration (OSHA), 200 Constitution Ave., Washington, DC USA 20210, (800) 321–6742, http://www.osha.gov/ecor_form.html, http://www.osha.gov/index.html.

David E. Newton, Ed.D.

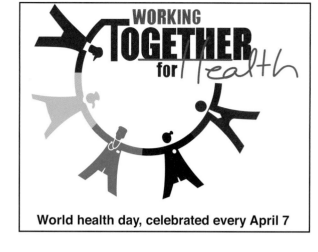

World health day, celebrated every April 7

(Illustration by Electronic Illustrators Group. © 2013 Cengage Learning)

World Health Organization (WHO)

Definition

The World Health Organization (WHO) is the directing and coordinating agency for health within the United Nations (UN).

Purpose

The WHO is responsible for establishing health policies for the UN, providing leadership on health issues worldwide, setting the international health research agenda, monitoring and assessing health trends throughout the world, and providing assistance to individual countries and regions where that may be necessary.

Description

During conferences on the drafting of the United Nations charter after the end of World War II, specific mention was made of the important role of health in the future activities of any international organization created by the charter. By July 22, 1946, all 61 original members of the United Nations had signed a charter for such an organization, which came to be known as the World Health Organization. The WHO officially came into existence when its constitution came into force on April 7, 1948, a day that was proclaimed, and continues to be celebrated annually, as World Health Day.

As of 2012, 194 nations are members of the WHO, with two associate members (Puerto Rico and Tokelau). The organization is run by the World Health Assembly, which meets annually and appoints a Director General and sets general policy for the agency. This policy is carried out by an Executive Board consisting of 34 members with technical expertise in some area of health. The WHO operates regional offices in six parts of the world: Africa, the Americas, Europe, the Eastern Mediterranean, Southeast Asia, and the Western Pacific, and in 147 individual countries. The organization's 2012–13 budget amounted to nearly $4 billion, about a quarter of which comes from contributions from member countries and the rest from donations from other entities. The largest donor to the WHO has traditionally been the United States, followed by Japan, the United Kingdom, Germany, and France.

Each WHO annual budget identifies a number of health priorities to be funded by the agency in the coming year. For fiscal year 2012–13, those priorities were as follows:

- reducing the health, social, and economic burdens associated with communicable diseases
- combating the spread of HIV/AIDS, malaria, and tuberculosis
- preventing and reducing the impact of noncommunicable diseases, mental disorders, violence, and injuries
- reducing morbidity and mortality and improving health during pregnancy, childhood, and adolescence, and improving sexual and reproductive health for individuals at all age levels
- reducing the health consequences of natural and manmade disasters
- preventing or reducing the risks posed by tobacco, alcohol, illegal drugs, unsafe sex, unhealthy diets, and physical inactivity
- working to enhance programs that reduce or eliminate disparity of health care because of income, gender, or human rights factors

- working to reduce environmental threats to good health

- improving nutrition, food safety, and food security

- improving health services for all people through better governance, financing, staffing, and management procedures

- ensuring improved quality, access to, and use of medical equipment

- improving partnerships among WHO and individual nations, as set forth in the Eleventh General Programme of Work

- developing and sustaining WHO as a flexible, learning organization that is able to carry out its mission and goals

This very ambitious agenda means that WHO has developed a number of specific programs for carrying out these and earlier goals and objectives. Some of the organization's current programs include the African Programme for Onchocerciasis, avian **influenza**, child growth standards, Global Alliance against Chronic Respiratory Diseases, humanitarian health action, Initiative for Vaccine Research, Intergovernmental Forum on Chemical Safety, **malaria**, medical devices, Partners for Parasite Control, Polio Eradication Initiative, sexual and **reproductive health**, Tobacco Free Initiative, and the United Nations Road Safety Collaboration. An especially important function of the agency is the collection, analysis, and distribution of data on global health issues. These statistical reports are available on the WHO website.

Professional publications

The WHO library contains a vast collection of books, articles, reports, bibliographies, data sets, and other publications. The organization publishes seven major journals: *Bulletin of the World Health Organization*, *Weekly Epidemiological Record*, *Pan American Journal of Public Health*, *Eastern Mediterranean Health Journal*, *WHO South-East Asia Journal of Public Health*, *Western Pacific Surveillance and Response*, and *WHO Drug Information*. Among the most important regular WHO reports are *The World Health Report*, *World Health Statistics*, *International Travel and Health*, *International Health Regulations*, *The International Classification of Diseases*, and *International Pharmacopoeia*.

Resources

BOOKS

Burci, Gian Luca, and Claude–Henri Vignes. *World Health Organization*. The Hague, Netherlands: Kluwer Law International, 2004.

Chorev, Nitsan. *The World Health Organization between North and South*. Ithaca, NY: Cornell University Press, 2012.

Sayward, Amy L. *The Birth of Development: How the World Bank, Food and Agriculture Organization, and World Health Organization Changed the World, 1945–1965*. Kent, OH: Kent State University Press, 2006.

PERIODICALS

Banerji, Debabar. "The World Health Organization and Public Health Research and Practice in Tuberculosis in India." *International Journal of Health Services* 42. 2. (2012): 341–57.

Chorev, Nitsan. "Restructuring Neoliberalism at the World Health Organization." *Review of International Political Economy* 3. (2012): 1–40.

Sinimole, K. R. "Evaluation of the Efficiency of National Health Systems of the Members of World Health Organization." *Leadership in Health Services* 25. 2. (2012): 139–50

WEBSITES

Leveraging the World Health Organization's Core Strengths. Global Health Policy Center. http://csis.org/files/publication/110502_Reeves_LeveragingWHO_Web.pdf (accessed October 14, 2012).

World Health Organization. New York Times Topics. http://topics.nytimes.com/topics/reference/timestopics/organizations/w/world_health_organization/index.html (accessed October 14, 2012).

World Health Organization. USA Today. http://content.usatoday.com/topics/topic/Organizations/International+Agencies,+Alliances,+Cartels/World+Health+Organization (accessed October 14, 2012).

ORGANIZATIONS

World Health Organization (WHO), Avenue Appia 20, 1211 Geneva 27, Switzerland, 41 22 791 21 11, Fax: 41 22 791 31 11, http://www.who.int/about/contact_form/en/index.html, http://www.who.int/en/.

David E. Newton, EdD

Y-Z

Yellow fever

Definition

Yellow fever, also known as sylvatic fever and viral hemorrhagic fever or VHF, is a severe **infectious disease** caused by a type of virus called a flavivirus. This flavivirus can cause outbreaks of epidemic proportions throughout Africa and tropical America. It is endemic in 33 countries in Africa and 11 countries in South America.

Description

The first written evidence of a yellow fever epidemic occurred in the Yucatan (Mexico) in 1648. Since that time, much has been learned about the transmission patterns of this illness. It is thought that the disease originated in Africa and spread to the Americas in the seventeenth and eighteenth centuries through trading ships. The flavivirus that causes yellow fever was first identified in West Africa, in 1928, and the first vaccine (17D) to fight against the disease was produced by South African-born American microbiologist Max Theiler (1899–1972) at the Rockefeller Institute in New York City in 1937. Based on work from American pathologist and physician Ernest Goodpasture (1886–1960), Theiler used chicken eggs to culture the virus. He won a Nobel Prize in 1951 for his work. Over 400 million doses of vaccine 17D have been used throughout the years.

Many common illnesses in the United States (including the **common cold**, many viral causes of diarrhea, and **influenza**) are spread by direct passage of the causative virus between human beings. Yellow fever, however, cannot be passed directly from one infected human to another. Instead, the virus responsible for yellow fever requires an intermediate vector. A vector is an organism that can carry a particular disease-causing agent (such as a virus or bacteria) without actually developing the disease. In the case of yellow fever, a mosquito is the vector that carries the virus from one host to another.

A host is an animal that can be infected with a particular disease. The hosts of yellow fever include both humans and monkeys. The cycle of yellow fever transmission begins when a tree-hole breeding mosquito bites an infected monkey. This mosquito acquires the virus and can pass the virus to any number of other monkeys that it may bite. This form of yellow fever is known as sylvatic yellow fever, and usually affects humans only incidentally. When an infected mosquito bites a human, the human may acquire the virus. In the case of South American yellow fever, the infected human may return to the city, where an urban mosquito (*Aedes aegypti*) serves as a viral vector, spreading the infection rapidly by biting humans. This form of the disease is known as urban yellow fever or epidemic yellow fever.

Yellow fever epidemics also may occur after flooding caused by earthquakes and other **natural disasters**. They result from a combination of new habitats available for the vectors of the disease and changes in human behavior (spending more time outdoors and neglecting **sanitation** precautions).

Cases of yellow fever are uncommon in the United States and Canada, as of 2012. The last reported case of a U.S. citizen dying of yellow fever concerned a man who contracted yellow fever after visiting Venezuela in 1999. The man had not been vaccinated against yellow fever. The last epidemic in the United States occurred in New Orleans, Louisiana, in 1905.

Risk factors

The major risk factor for contracting yellow fever is residing in or traveling to an area where mosquitoes carry the virus. These areas include South America and sub-Saharan Africa. To provide protection from yellow fever, a **vaccination** is recommended for anyone traveling to affected areas at least 10 to 14 days before the departure date.

WILBUR AUGUSTUS SAWYER (1879–1951)

Wilbur Augustus Sawyer was born in Appleton, Wisconsin, on August 7, 1879, to Minnie Edmea (Birge) and Wesley Caleb Sawyer. The Sawyers moved to Oshkosh, Wisconsin, and finally to Stockton, California, in 1888. Sawyer spent two years at the University of California and then entered Harvard College where he earned his A.B. degree in 1902. In 1906, Sawyer graduated from Harvard Medical School and began a private practice, which lasted until he started his internship at Massachusetts General Hospital. Sawyer returned to California in 1908 in order to obtain a position at the University of California as a medical examiner. He then worked with California State Board of Health from 1910 until 1918. In 1911, Sawyer married Margaret Henderson. The couple had three children.

Sawyer's first publication (1913) dealt with his research of poliomyelitis. His discovery, in 1915, that examination of the individual's stool could lead to detection of the disease was later regarded as very significant. In 1918 and 1919, Sawyer worked to control venereal disease while employed by the Army Medical Corps. In 1926 and 1927, while director of the West African Yellow Fever Commission, Sawyer succeeded in isolating the yellow fever virus. He would ultimately return to the United States, where he and Wray Lloyd would devise an immunization against yellow fever (1931).

In 1944, Sawyer became director of health for the United Nations Relief and Rehabilitation Administration, a position he held for three years. He retired to Berkeley, California where he died on November 12, 1951. The company he built with his brother still thrives today.

Demographics

Anyone can get yellow fever; however, older people are more at risk than younger ones. Yellow fever is found most commonly in men between the ages of 15 and 45 years who work outdoors and live in fever-endemic areas. Race has not been shown to be a factor in contraction or transmission. Between 1970 and 2002, only nine cases of yellow fever were reported in travelers from the United States and Europe. All cases were found in unimmunized travelers who had visited South America or Africa. Seven of the cases were fatal.

According to the **World Health Organization (WHO)**, as of 2011, about 200,000 cases of yellow fever occur annually around the world (mostly in tropical endemic areas of Africa and the Americas), with approximately 30,000 deaths caused by the disease. Thirty-three countries are at risk of yellow fever in Africa and in the Americas; several Caribbean islands and nine South American countries (including Bolivia, Brazil, Columbia, Ecuador, and Peru) are also at risk. Up to 50% of severely affected persons without treatment die from yellow fever. The number of yellow fever cases has increased over the past several decades primarily due to fewer people becoming immune to it and fewer immunizations, along with environmental factors, such as urbanization, deforestation, global climate change, and **population** movements into areas more prone to the virus. The vaccine for yellow fever protects humans for 30 to 35 years. About 95% of people vaccinated are immune to the disease within one week of the vaccination.

Causes and symptoms

Once a mosquito passes the yellow fever virus to a human, the chance of disease developing ranges from 5–20%. Infection may be fought off by the host's immune system or may be so mild that it is never identified.

In human hosts who develop the disease yellow fever, there are five distinct stages through which the infection evolves. These have been termed the periods of incubation, invasion, remission, intoxication, and convalescence.

Yellow fever's incubation period (the amount of time between the introduction of the virus into the host and the development of symptoms) is three to six days. During this time, there are generally no symptoms identifiable to the host.

The period of invasion lasts two to five days, and begins with an abrupt onset of symptoms, including fever and chills, intense headache and lower backache, muscle aches, nausea, and extreme exhaustion. The patient's tongue shows a characteristic white, furry coating in the center, surrounded by a swollen, reddened margin. While most other infections that cause a high fever also cause an increased heart rate, yellow fever results in an unusual finding, called Faget's sign. This is the simultaneous occurrence of a high fever with a slowed heart rate. Throughout the period of invasion, there are live viruses circulating in the patient's bloodstream. Therefore, a mosquito can bite an ill patient, acquire the virus, and continue passing it on to others.

The next phase is the period of remission. The fever falls, and symptoms decrease in severity for several hours to several days. In some patients, this signals the end of the disease, while in others, this is the calm before the storm.

The period of intoxication represents the most severe and potentially fatal phase of the illness. During this time, lasting three to nine days, a type of degeneration of the internal organs (specifically the kidneys, liver, and heart) occurs. This fatty degeneration results in what is considered the classic triad of yellow fever symptoms: jaundice, black vomit, and the dumping of protein into the urine. Jaundice causes the whites of the patient's eyes and the patient's skin to take on a distinctive yellow color. This is due to liver damage and the accumulation of a substance called bilirubin, which is normally processed by a healthy liver. The liver damage also results in a tendency to bleed and the patient's vomit appears black due to the presence of blood. Protein, which is normally kept out of the urine by healthy, intact kidneys, appears in the urine due to disruption of the kidney's healthy functioning.

Patients who survive the period of intoxication enter a relatively short period of convalescence. They recover with no long-term effects related to the yellow fever infection. Surviving an infection with the yellow fever virus results in lifelong immunity against repeated infection by the virus.

The course of yellow fever is complicated in some patients by secondary bacterial infections.

Diagnosis

Diagnosis for yellow fever includes examination, testing, and procedures.

Examination

A diagnosis of yellow fever may be suspected during a physical examination when the classic triad of symptoms are present. These include:

- a sudden onset of fever, chills, intense headaches and lower backaches, muscle aches, nausea, and exhaustion
- Faget's sign—simultaneous occurrence of a high fever and decreased heart rate
- a white furry coating in the center of the tongue surround by a swollen, red margin

Tests

Diagnosis of yellow fever depends on the examination of blood by various techniques in order to demonstrate either yellow fever viral antigens (the part of the virus that stimulates the patient's immune system to respond) or specific antibodies (specific cells produced by the patient's immune system that are directed against the yellow fever virus). The most rapid method of diagnosis, as of 2012, was capture enzyme immunoassay.

Procedures

Typically, the only procedure required for diagnosis is a blood draw so that the blood can be evaluated for signs of yellow fever.

Treatment

Treatment for yellow fever includes traditional approaches, along with the use of drugs.

Traditional

As of 2012, the only treatments for yellow fever are given to relieve its symptoms. Fevers and **pain** should be relieved with acetaminophen, not aspirin or ibuprofen, both of which could increase the already-present risk of bleeding. Dehydration (due to fluid loss, both from fever and bleeding) needs to be carefully avoided. This can be accomplished by increasing fluids. The risk of bleeding into the stomach can be decreased through the administration of antacids and other medications. Hemorrhage (heavy bleeding) may require blood transfusions. Kidney failure may require dialysis (a process that allows the work of the kidneys in clearing the blood of potentially toxic substances to be taken over by a machine, outside of the body).

Drugs

There are no antiviral treatments available as of 2012 to combat the yellow fever virus. Nonclinical research has yielded limited results.

Researchers have found that ribavirin (Virazole, Rebetol), a drug that is given by mouth to treat **hepatitis** C, is successful in reducing mortality from yellow fever in hamsters, but only if given within 120 hours of infection. Another drug, Interferon-alpha has also been found to reduce mortality in monkeys with yellow fever but only when administered within 24 hours of infection.

Public health role and response

The **World Health Organization** (**WHO**) recommends routine childhood vaccination to prevent yellow fever in endemic countries where epidemics are possible. Quick detection of yellow fever and fast response of governments through emergency vaccination campaigns are important in controlling outbreaks. WHO recommends that at-risk countries maintain at least one national laboratory where blood tests for yellow fever can be performed.

The organization Secretariat for the International Coordinating Group (ICG) for Yellow Fever Vaccine Provision provides an emergency stockpile of yellow fever vaccines whenever outbreaks occur in any country of the world. WHO also leads the Yellow Fever Initiative (YFI), which is a preventive vaccination effort for at-risk countries, especially 12 participating African countries where the disease is most likely to occur. The YFI recommends "including yellow fever vaccines in routine

KEY TERMS

Antibody—A protein normally produced by the immune system to fight infection or rid the body of foreign material. The material that stimulates the production of antibodies is called an antigen. Specific antibodies are produced in response to each different antigen and can only inactivate that particular antigen.

Antigen—Any foreign substance, usually a protein, that stimulates the body's immune system to produce antibodies.

Bilirubin—A reddish-yellow bile pigment made by the liver.

Dialysis—The cleansing of the blood through use of a special machine that filters the blood. The process is performed when the kidneys are unable to filter blood properly.

Epidemic—A situation in which the number of cases of a particular disease exceeds the endemic or average number of cases. Infections of such diseases often spread through a population of people in a relatively short period of time.

Faget's sign—The simultaneous occurrence of a high fever with a slowed heart rate.

Flavivirus—The species to which the virus that causes yellow fever belongs.

Hemorrhage—Abnormal and obsessive bleeding.

Host—The organism (such as a monkey or human) in which another organism (such as a virus or bacteria) is living.

Jaundice—The yellowing of the skin and whites of the eyes caused by an increased level of bilirubin in the blood.

Sylvatic—Pertaining to or living in the woods or forested areas. The form of yellow fever transmitted by mosquitoes to rainforest monkeys is called sylvatic yellow fever.

Vector—A carrier organism (such as a fly or mosquito) that serves to deliver a virus (or other agent of infection) to a host.

QUESTIONS TO ASK YOUR DOCTOR

- Should I be worried about contracting yellow fever?
- Should I receive a yellow fever vaccination?
- What symptoms should I watch for with regard to yellow fever?
- What are my treatment options and the risks associated with treatment?
- How long will I be taking medication for yellow fever? What are the potential side effects of my medication?
- Does my yellow fever medication interact with my medicines or supplements?
- When can I resume my normal activities? When can I return to work?
- What can I do to reduce my risk for having yellow fever again?
- How often will I need to follow-up with my doctor?
- What community support and other resources are available to help me?

Prognosis

Five to 10 percent of all diagnosed cases of yellow fever are fatal. Jaundice occurring during a yellow fever infection is an extremely grave predictor as 20–50% of these patients die of the infection. Death may occur due to massive bleeding (hemorrhage), often following a lapse into a comatose (unconscious) state.

Prevention

A very safe and very effective yellow fever vaccine exists. The Arilvax vaccine is made from a live attenuated (weakened) form of the yellow fever virus, strain 17D. In the United States, the vaccine is given only at Yellow Fever Vaccination Centers authorized by the U.S. Public Health Service. About 95% of vaccine recipients acquire long-term immunity to the yellow fever virus. Careful measures to decrease mosquito populations in both urban areas and jungle areas where humans are working, along with programs to vaccinate all people living in such areas, are necessary to avoid massive yellow fever outbreaks.

Individuals planning to travel in countries where yellow fever is endemic may obtain up-to-date

infant immunizations (starting at age 9 months), implementing mass vaccination campaigns in high-risk areas for people in all age groups aged 9 months and older, and maintaining surveillance and outbreak response capacity."

information on yellow fever vaccination from the U.S. **Centers for Disease Control and Prevention (CDC)**.

Resources

BOOKS

Crosby, Molly Caldwell. *The American Plague: The Untold Story of Yellow Fever, the Epidemic That Shaped Our History.* New York: Berkley Books, 2006.

Shannon, Joyce Brennfleck, editor. *Contagious Diseases Sourcebook: Basic Consumer Health Information about Diseases Spread from Person to Person.* Detroit: Omnigraphics, 2010.

Shmaefsky, Brian R. *Yellow Fever.* New York: Chelsea House, 2010.

Wilder-Smith, Annelies, Eli Schwartz, and Marc Shaw, editors. *Travel Medicine: Tales Behind the Science.* Amsterdam: Elsevier, 2007.

WEBSITES

Busowski, Mary T. *Yellow Fever.* Medscape Reference. http://emedicine.medscape.com/article/232244-overview (accessed October 9, 2012).

Country List: Yellow Fever Vaccination Requirements and Recommendations; and Malaria Situation. World Health Organization. http://www.who.int/ith/ITH2010country list.pdf (accessed October 9, 2012).

Dugdale, David, and Jatin M. Vyas. *Yellow Fever.* Medline-Plus. http://www.nlm.nih.gov/medlineplus/ency/article/001365.htm (accessed October 9, 2012).

Yellow Fever. Fact Sheet No. 100. World Health Organization. http://www.who.int/mediacentre/factsheets/fs100/en/ (accessed October 9, 2012).

Yellow Fever. Mayo Clinic. http://www.mayoclinic.com/health/yellow-fever/DS01011 (accessed October 9, 2012).

Yellow Fever Vaccine. Medline Plus. http://www.nlm.nih.gov/medlineplus/druginfo/meds/a607030.html (accessed October 9, 2012).

ORGANIZATIONS

Centers for Disease Control and Prevention, 1600 Clifton Rd., Atlanta, GA 30333, (800) 232-4636, cdcinfo@cdc.gov, http://www.cdc.gov.

National Institute of Allergy and Infectious Diseases, 6610 Rockledge Dr., MSC 6612, Bethesda, MD 20892, (301) 496-5717, (866) 284-4107, Fax: (301) 402-3573, http://www.niaid.nih.gov.

World Health Organization, Avenue Appia 20, Geneva, Switzerland 1211 27, 41 22 791-2111, Fax: 41 22 791-3111, http://www.who.int/en/.

Rosalyn Carson-DeWitt, MD
Tish Davidson, AM
Paul Checchia, MD
William A. Atkins, BB, BS, MBA

Zoonosis

Definition

Zoonosis, also called zoonotic disease, refers to diseases or infections that can be naturally passed (transmitted) from vertebrate animals, whether wild or domesticated, to humans, and vice versa. According to the **World Health Organization (WHO)**, more than 250 distinct zoonoses have been medically described.

Description

Bacteria, fungi, **parasites**, viruses, and other disease-causing organisms cause zoonosis. The following are examples of zoonosis caused by:

- bacteria: leptospirosis (scientific name *Leptopiras spp*), which is transmitted by direct contact with an infected animal or indirect contact with urine-infected food, soil, or water
- fungi: aspergillosis (*Aspergillus fumigatus*, which is transmitted by the inhalation of fungal spores
- parasites: raccoon roundworm (*Baylisascaris procyonis*), which is transmitted by the ingestion of eggs
- viruses: rabies (no scientific name), which is transmitted by a bite wound

In the twenty-first century, zoonoses continue to be significant public health threats around the world, affecting hundreds of thousands of people annually especially in developing countries. However, most zoonoses can be prevented.

Many modern diseases are known to have started as zoonotic diseases when humans first began to record history. Biblical references to a **plague** are thought to have been caused by bacterial zoonosis transmitted from fleas to humans. The Plague of Athens, in 430 BC is thought to have been caused by one of the bacteria in the family Rickettsiae. History continues to hold the secret as to when many diseases were first transported from other animals to humans. Medical science is quite confident, however, that many long-known diseases, such as **influenza** (flu), **smallpox**, and **measles**, had their beginnings as zoonotic diseases. In addition, even though with much less certainty, the **common cold** may have first been a problem in other animals before becoming a problem for humans. Other diseases that were virtually unknown within humans in the twentieth century, such as **West Nile virus**, are causing serious problems with people in the twenty-first century.

Although many diseases are species specific, meaning that they can only occur in one animal species, many other diseases can be spread between different animal species. These are infectious diseases caused by bacteria, viruses, or other disease-causing organisms that can live as well in humans as in other animals.

There are different methods of transmission for different diseases. In some cases, zoonotic diseases are transferred by direct contact with infected animals, much as being near an infected human can cause the spread of an **infectious disease**. Other diseases are spread by **drinking water** that contains the eggs of parasites. The eggs enter the **water** supply from the feces of infected animals. Others are spread by eating the flesh of infected animals. Tapeworms are spread this way. Insect vectors spread other diseases. An insect, such as a flea or tick, feeds on an infected animal, and then feeds on a human. In the process, the insect transfers the infecting organism.

The **Centers for Disease Control and Prevention (CDC)**, headquartered in Atlanta, Georgia, has said that most **emerging diseases** around the world are zoonotic. The director of the CDC has stated that 11 of the last 12 emerging infections in the world with serious health consequences have probably arisen from animal "1"s. Wild animal trade occurs across countries and many people take in wild animals as domestic pets. However, many pet shops and food markets are not properly testing for diseases and parasites that can cause harm to humans and other animals.

Some zoonotic diseases are well known, such as plague (rats) and **Lyme disease** (deer ticks). Others are not as well known. For example, elephants may develop **tuberculosis** and spread it to humans.

Risk factors

According to the **WHO**, the largest risk for the transmission of zoonotic disease "occurs at the human-animal interface through direct or indirect human exposure to animals, their products, and/or their environments." The WHO adds, "More than 60% of the newly identified infectious agents that have affected people over the past few decades have been caused by pathogens originating from animals or animal products. Seventy percent of these zoonotic infections originate from wildlife."

Many zoonoses continue to occur in several developing countries of the world. These continue to be transmitted to humans through bites from infected mammals (**rabies**), food (such as **brucellosis** and tuberculosis), and insects (Rift Valley Fever), along with environmental contamination (echinococcosis/hydatidosis).

Demographics

Human health has been adversely effected by zoonoses. One particular major outbreak involved the Nipah virus and **severe acute respiratory syndrome (SARS)** coronavirus (CoV). Such outbreaks are becoming more complex due to changing circumstances.

A 2010 paper "Public Health Threat of New, Reemerging, and Neglected Zoonoses in the Industrialized World" in the CDC publication *Emerging Infectious Diseases* discusses how zoonoses are changing in the face of these changing circumstances:

- changes in agriculture, such as containment of large numbers of animals or close proximity of several different species, can promote the spread of disease between animals

- increased movement of people, animals, and products across the globe allows introduction of disease and disease carriers to more populations despite measures to control spread of disease

- movement of people into natural habitats for housing or tourism puts them in circumstances where they may be exposed to new types of zoonoses

- changes in climate may promote opportunity for mutation or variation of pathogens as well as the vectors they use to spread disease

Causes and symptoms

The following is a partial list of animals and the diseases that they may carry. Not all animal carriers are listed, nor are all the diseases that the various species may carry.

- Bats are important rabies carriers and also carry other viral diseases that can affect humans.

- Cats may carry the causative organisms for plague, anthrax, cowpox, tapeworm, and many bacterial infections.

- Dogs may carry plague, tapeworm, rabies, Rocky Mountain Spotted Fever, and Lyme disease.

- Horses may carry anthrax, rabies, and *Salmonella* infections.

- Cattle may carry the organisms that cause anthrax, European tick-borne encephalitis, rabies, tapeworm, *Salmonella* infections, and many bacterial and viral diseases.

- Pigs are best known for carrying tapeworm, but may also carry a large number of other infections including anthrax, influenza, and rabies.

- Sheep and goats may carry rabies, European tick-borne encephalitis, *Salmonella* infections, and many bacterial and viral diseases.

- Rabbits may carry plague and Q-Fever.

- Birds may carry *Campylobacteriosis*, *Chlamydia psittaci*, *Pasteurella multocida*, *Histoplasma capsulatum*, *Salmonellosis*, and others.

Zoonotic diseases may be spread in different ways. Tapeworms can often spread to humans when people eat the infected meat of cattle and swine. Other diseases are transferred by insect vectors, often blood-feeding insects that carry the cause of the disease from one animal to another.

Diagnosis

Diagnosis of the disease is made by identifying the infecting organism. Each disease has established symptoms and tests. Identifying the carrier may be easy or may be more difficult when the cause is a common infection. For example, tapeworms are usually species specific. Cattle, pigs, and fish all carry different species of tapeworms, although all can be transmitted to humans who eat undercooked meat containing live tapeworm eggs. Once the tapeworm has been identified, it is easy to tell from which species the tapeworm came.

Other zoonotic infections may be more difficult to identify. Sometimes the infection is common among both humans and animals, and it is impossible to tell the difference. Snakes may carry the bacteria *Escherichia coli* and *Proteus vulgaris*, but since these bacteria are already common among humans, it would be difficult to trace infections back to snakes.

Increased trade between nations and changes in animal habitats has introduced new zoonotic diseases. These may be found in animals transported from one nation to another, bringing with them new diseases. In some cases, changes in the environment lead to changes in the migratory habits of animal species, bringing new infections.

Treatment

The treatment of zoonotic infections depends on the specific disease. Many are treated with prescription drugs such as **antibiotics**. For instance, Lyme disease is caused by the bacterium *Borrelia burgdorferi*. The bacterium gets inside a tick from infected deer, mice, or other animals. The tick can then attach itself onto the skin of a human. The infected tick feeds on a person's blood, which then infects the human. Lyme disease is treated with antibiotics.

Public health role and response

The Global Early Warning System for Major Animal Diseases, including Zoonoses (GLEWS) is an early warning system for outbreaks of animal diseases. The

---

KEY TERMS

Anthrax—A disease of warm blooded animals, particularly cattle and sheep, transmissible to humans. The disease causes severe skin and lung damage.

Bovine spongiform encephalopathy—Also known as Mad Cow disease, a progressive, fatal disease of the nervous system of domestic animals that is transmitted by eating infected food.

Lyme disease—An acute disease that is usually marked by skin rash, fever, fatigue, and chills. Left untreated, it may cause heart and nervous system damage.

Q-Fever—A disease marked by high fever, chills, and muscle pain. It is seen in North America, Europe, and parts of Africa. It may be spread by drinking raw milk or by tick bites.

Zoonotic—A disease that can be spread from animals to humans.

World Health Organization (WHO), the Food and Agricultural Organization of the United Nations (FAO), and the World Organization for Animal Health (OIE) created GLEWS. It is used to help alert the international community in the **prevention** and control of threats from animal diseases, including zoonoses.

Prognosis

The prognosis for zoonoses is dependent on the particular organism. However, for the most part, the prognosis for fully recovering from such a disease is good if treatment is promptly given with appropriate medicine.

Prevention

Prevention of zoonotic infections may take different forms, depending on the nature of the carrier and the infection.

Some zoonotic infections can be avoided by immunizing the animals that carry the disease. Pets and other domestic animals should have rabies vaccinations, and wild animals are immunized with an oral vaccine that is encased in suitable bait. In some places, the bait is dropped by airplane over the range of the potential rabies carrier. When the animals eat the bait, they also ingest the oral vaccine, thereby protecting them from rabies and reducing the risk of spread of the disease. This method

QUESTIONS TO ASK YOUR DOCTOR

- Should I be worried about zoonotic disease?
- What are the possible causes for my symptoms?
- What symptoms should I be watching for with regards to this zoonotic disease?
- If I was exposed to someone with a zoonotic disease, can I give it to others?
- What types of tests do I need?
- Are treatments available to help me recover from zoonotic disease? What are the risks associated with treatment?
- How long will a full recovery take?
- When can I return to my daily routine?
- Am I at risk of any long-term complications?

has been used to protect foxes, coyotes, and other wild animals.

Zoonotic diseases that are passed by eating the meat of infected animals can often be prevented by proper cooking of the infected meat. Tapeworm **infestations** can be prevented by cooking, and *Salmonella* infections from chickens and eggs can be prevented by ensuring that both the meat and the eggs are fully cooked.

For other zoonotic diseases, programs are in place to eliminate the host, or the vector, that spreads the disease. Plague is prevented by elimination of rats—a common "1" of the infection—and of fleas that carry the disease from rats to humans. Efforts around the world to control bovine spongiform encephalitis, better known as Mad Cow disease, have focused on the destruction of infected cattle to prevent spread of the disease. Regulations on the makeup of the cattle feed to ensure safety and prevent the disease have helped curb its spread.

Other means of prevention simply rely on care. People living in areas where Lyme disease is common are warned to take precautions against the bite of the deer tick, which transfers the disease. These precautions include not walking in tall grass, not walking bare legged, and wearing light-colored clothing so that the presence of the dark ticks can be readily seen.

Resources

BOOKS

Link, Kurt. *Understanding New, Resurgent, and Resistant Diseases: How Man and Globalization Create and Spread Illness.* Westport, CT: Praeger, 2007.

Palmer, S. R., et al., eds. *Oxford Textbook of Zoonoses: Biology, Clinical Practice, and Public Health Control.* Oxford: Oxford University Press, 2011.

Shannon, Joyce Brennfleck, ed. *Contagious Diseases "1"book: Basic Consumer Health Information about Diseases Spread from Person to Person.* Detroit: Omnigraphics, 2010.

Wilder-Smith, Annelies, Eli Schwartz, and Marc Shaw, eds. *Travel Medicine: Tales Behind the Science.* Amsterdam: Elsevier, 2007.

PERIODICALS

Cutler, Sally J., Anthony R. Fooks, and Wim H.M. van der Poel. "Public Health Threat of New, Reemerging, and Neglected Zoonoses in the Industrialized World." *Emerging Infectious Diseases* 16, no. 1 (January 2010): DOI 10.3201/eid1601.081467.

WEBSITES

Outbreak Alerts: Global Early Warning System for Major Animal Diseases, including Zoonoses (GLEWS). World Health Organization. http://www.who.int/zoonoses/outbreaks/en/ (accessed July 6, 2012).

Zoonoses. World Health Organization. http://www.who.int/foodsafety/zoonoses/en/ (accessed October 13, 2012).

Zoonoses and Veterinary Public Health (VPH). World Health Organization. http://www.who.int/zoonoses/en/ (accessed October 13, 2012).

ORGANIZATIONS

Centers for Disease Control and Prevention, 1600 Clifton Rd., Atlanta, GA 30333, (800) 232-4636, cdcinfo@cdc.gov, http://www.cdc.gov/.

National Institute of Allergy and Infectious Diseases, 1301 Pennsylvania Ave., NW, Ste. 800, Washington, DC 20004, (202) 785-3355, Fax: (202) 452-1805, http://www.niaid.nih.gov.

World Health Organization, Avenue Appia 20, Geneva, Switzerland 1211 27, 41 22 791-2111, Fax: 41 22 791-3111, http://www.who.int/en/.

Samuel D. Uretsky, PharmD
Teresa G. Odle
William A. Atkins, BB, BS, MBA

ORGANIZATIONS

The following is an alphabetical compilation of relevant organizations listed in the *Resources* sections of the main body entries. Although the list is comprehensive, it is by no means exhaustive. It is a starting point for gathering further information. Many of the organizations listed have links to additional related websites. E-mail addresses and web addresses listed were provided by the associations; Gale, Cengage Learning is not responsible for the accuracy of the addresses or the contents of the websites.

A

AARP
601 E St., N.W.
Washington, DC 20049
Toll free: (888) 687–2277
E-mail: member@aarp.org
Web site: http://www.aarp.org/

Academy of General Dentistry
211 E. Chicago Ave., Suite 900
Chicago, IL 60611
Web site: http://www.knowyourteeth
.com/aboutagd/

**Academy of Nutrition and Dietetics
[formerly the American Dietetic
Association]**
120 South Riverside Plaza, Suite 2000
Chicago, IL 60606-6995
Phone: (312) 899-0040
Toll free: (800) 877-1600
Web site: http://www.eatright.org/

Academy of Nutrition and Dietetics
120 South Riverside Plaza., Ste. 2000
Chicago, IL 60606-6995
Phone: (312) 899-0040
Toll free: (800) 877-1600
E-mail: amacmunn@eatright.org
Web site: http://www.eatright.org

Academy of Nutrition and Dietetics
120 South Riverside Plz., Ste. 2000
Chicago, IL 60606-6995
Phone: (312) 899-0040
Toll free: (800) 877-1600
E-mail: amacmunn@eatright.org
Web site: http://www.eatright.org

**Academy of Correctional Health
Professionals**
P.O. Box 11583
Chicago, IL 60611
Toll free: (877) 549–2247
Fax: 1 (773) 880–2424
E-mail: academy@correctionalhealth.org
Web site: http://www.correctionalhealth
.org/index.asp

Act Against Bullying
PO Box 57962
London, W4 2TG
Phone: 44 020 8995 9500
E-mail: info@actagainstbullying.org
Web site: http://www.actagainstbullying
.org/index.htm

Administration on Aging
One Massachusetts Ave., N.W.
Washington, DC 20001
Phone: 1 (202) 619-0724
Fax: 1 (202) 357-3555
E-mail: aoainfo@aoa.hhs.gov
Web site: http://www.aoa.gov/

Adult Congenital Heart Association
6757 Greene St., Suite 335
Philadelphia, PA 19119-3508
Phone: (215) 849-1260
Toll free: (888) 921-2242
Fax: (215) 849-1261
E-mail: info@achaheart.org
Web site: http://www.achaheart.org

**African Women's Health Center,
Brigham and Women's Hospital**
75 Francis St.
Boston, MA 02115
Phone: 1 (617) 732-5500
Web site: http://www.brighamand
womens.org/Departments_and
_Services/obgyn/services/african
womenscenter/default.aspx

**Agency for Healthcare Research and
Quality (AHRQ)**
540 Gaither Road, Suite 2000
Rockville, MD 20850
Phone: (301) 427-1104
Web site: http://www.ahrq.gov/

**Agency for Toxic Substances and
Disease Registry, Centers for
Disease Control and
Prevention**
4770 Buford Hwy N.E.
Atlanta, GA 30341
Toll free: (800) 232-4636
Web site: http://www.atsdr.cdc.gov/

Agricultural Research Service
Jamie L. Whitten, Bldg. 1400
Independence Avenue, SW
Washington, DC 20250
Phone: (301) 504-1637
Web site: http://www.ars.usda.gov

AIDS.GOV
200 Independence Ave., S.W., Rm 443H
Washington, DC 20201
Toll free: (800) 448-0440
E-mail: contact aids.gov.
Web site: http://www.aids.gov

Al-Anon/Alateen
1600 Corporate Landing Pkwy.
Virginia Beach, VA 23454
Phone: 1 (757) 563-1600
Fax: 1 (757) 563-1655
Toll free: (800) 877-1600
E-mail: wso@al-anon.org
Web site: http://www.al-anon.alateen.org/

Alcoholics Anonymous
475 Riverside Dr. at West 120th St.
New York City, NY 10115
Phone: 1 (212) 870-3400
Web site: http://www.aa.org/

**Alexander Graham Bell Association
for the Deaf and Hard of Hearing**
3417 Volta Place NW
Washington, DC 20007
Phone: (202) 337-5220
Web site: http://nc.agbell.org/

**Allergy and Asthma Foundation of
America**
8201 Corporate Drive, Suite 1000
Landover, Maryland 20785
Toll free: (800) 727-8462
E-mail: Info@aafa.org
Web site: aafa.org

**Allergy and Asthma Network:
Mothers of Asthmatics (AANMA)**
2751 Prosperity Ave., Suite 150
Fairfax, VA 22031
Toll free: (800) 878-4403
Fax: (703) 573-7794
Web site: http://www.aanma.org

Alliance for Healthy Cities
Kanda–surugadai 2–1–19–1112,
    Chiyoda–ku
Tokyo, 101–0062
Phone: 3 5577 6780
Fax: 3 5577 6780
E-mail: alliance.ith@tmd.ac.jp
Web site: http://www.alliance-healthy
    cities.com/

**Alliance for the Prudent Use of
    Antibiotics (APUA)**
200 Harrison Avenue, Posner 3
    (Business)
Boston, MA 02111
Phone: (617) 636-0966
Fax: (617) 636-0458
E-mail: apua@tufts.edu
Web site: http://www.tufts.edu/med
    /apua/

America's Clean Water Foundation
750 First St. NE, Ste. 1030
Washington, DC 20002
Phone: (202) 898-0908
Fax: (202) 898-0977
E-mail: webmasteracwf@acwf.org
Web site: http://agripollute.nstl.gov.cn
    /MirrorResources/6492/index.html

**American Academy of Allergy,
    Asthma & Immunology (AAAAI)**
555 East Wells Street
Milwaukee, WI 53202-3823
Phone: (414) 272-6071
Web site: http://www.aaaai.org/

**American Academy of Child and
    Adolescent Psychiatry (AACAP)**
3615 Wisconsin Avenue, NW
Washington, DC 20016-3007
Phone: (202) 966-7300
Fax: (202) 966-2891
Web site: http://www.aacap.org

**American Academy of Dermatology
    (AAD)**
PO Box 4014
Schaumburg, IL 60168
Toll free: (866) 503-7546
E-mail: MRC@aad.org
Web site: http://www.aad.org

**American Academy of
    Environmental Engineers (AAEE)**
130 Holiday Ct., Suite 100
Annapolis, MD 21401
Phone: (410) 266-3311
Fax: (410) 266-7653
E-mail: info@aaee.net
Web site: www.aaee.net

**American Academy of Environmental
    Medicine**
6505 E Central Ave., No. 296
Wichita, KS 67206
Phone: (316) 684-5500

Fax: (316) 684-5709
E-mail: administrator@aaemonline.org
Web site: http://aaemonline.org

**American Academy of Experts in
    Traumatic Stress**
203 Deer Rd.
Ronkonkoma, NY 11779
Phone: (631) 543-2217
Fax: (631) 543-6977
E-mail: info@aaets.org
Web site: http://www.aaets.org

**American Academy of Family
    Physicians**
P.O. Box 11210
Shawnee Mission, KS 66207
Phone: (913) 906–6000
Toll free: (800) 274-2237
Fax: (913) 906–6075
E-mail: http://familydoctor.org/
    familydoctor/en/about/contact-us
    .html
Web site: http://familydoctor.org

**American Academy of Neurology
    (AAN)**
201 Chicago Avenue South
Minneapolis, MN 55415
Toll free: (800) 879-1960
Web site: http://www.aan.com/

**American Academy of
    Ophthalmology (AAO)**
655 Beach St.
San Francisco, CA 94109
Phone: (415) 561-8500
Web site: http://www.aao.org

**American Academy of Orthopaedic
    Surgeons (AAOS)**
6300 North River Road
Rosemont, IL 60018-4262
Phone: (847) 823-7186
Fax: (847) 823-8125
Web site: http://orthoinfo.aaos.org

**American Academy of Pediatrics
    (AAP)**
141 Northwest Point Blvd.
Elk Grove, IL 60007-1098
Phone: (847) 434-8000
Web site: http://www.aap.org

American Academy of Peridontology
737 N. Michigan Avenue, Suite 800.
Chicago, IL 60611-6660
Phone: (312) 787-5518
Web site: http://www.perio.org/

**American Academy of Sleep
    Medicine**
2510 N Frontage Rd.
Darien, IL 60561
Phone: (630) 737-9700
Fax: (630) 737-9790
E-mail: inquiries@assmnet.org
Web site: http://www.aasmnet.org

**American Association of
    Naturopathic Physicians**
4435 Wisconsin Ave., NW, Suite 403
Washington, DC 20016
Phone: (202) 237-8150
Fax: (202) 237-8152
Toll free: (866) 538-2267
E-mail: member.services@
    naturopathic.org
Web site: http://naturopathic.org/

**American Association of Poison
    Control Centers (AAPCC)**
Toll free: (800) 222-1222
E-mail: info@aapcc.org
Web site: http://www.aapcc.org/dnn
    /Home.aspx

American Association of Suicidology
5221 Wisconsin Ave. NW
Washington, DC 20015
Phone: (202) 237-2280
Fax: (202) 237-2282
Web site: http://www.suicidology.org
    /web/guest/home

**American Associations of Poison
    Control Centers**
515 King St., Ste. 510
Alexandria, VA 22314
Phone: (703) 894-1858
Fax: (703) 683-2812
Web site: http:// info@aapcc.org

**American Biological Safety
    Association**
1200 Allanson Rd.
Mundelein, IL 60060
Phone: (847) 949-1517
Toll free: (866) 425-1385
Fax: (847) 566-4580
E-mail: info@absa.org
Web site: http://www.absa.org

**American Board of Industrial
    Hygiene**
6015 W St. Joseph, Suite 102
Lansing, MI 48917
Phone: (517) 321-2638
Fax: (517) 321-4624
Web site: http://www.abih.org

American Botanical Council
6200 Manor Rd.
Austin, TX 78723
Phone: (512) 926-4900
Fax: (512) 926-2345
E-mail: abc@herbalgram.org
Web site: http://cms.herbalgram.org

American Burn Association
311 S Wacker Dr., Ste. 4150
Chicago, IL 60606
Phone: (312) 642-9260
Fax: (312) 642-9130
E-mail: info@ameriburn.org
Web site: http://www.ameriburn.org

American Cancer Society
250 Williams Street NW
Atlanta, GA 30303
Toll free: (800) 227-2345
Web site: https://www.cancer.org/

American Cancer Society (ACS),
International Tobacco Surveillance
1599 Clifton Rd., N.E.
Atlanta, GA 30329-4251
Phone: (404) 327-6554
Fax: (404) 327-6450
E-mail: omar.shafey@cancer.org
Web site: www.cancer.org

American Chronic Pain Association
P.O. Box 850
Rocklin, CA 95677
Fax: (916) 632–3208
Toll free: (800) 533–3231
E-mail: APA@pacbell.net
Web site: http://www.theacpa.org

American College of Allergy, Asthma,
and Immunology
85 W Algonquin Rd., Ste. 550
Arlington Heights, IL 60005
Web site: http://allergy.mcg.edu

American College of Emergency
Physicians (ACEP)
1125 Executive Cir.
Irving, TX 75038-2522
Phone: (972) 550-0911
Toll free: (800) 798-1822
Fax: (972) 580-2816
Web site: http://www.acep.org

American College of Epidemiology
(ACE)
1500 Sunday Drive, Suite 102
Raleigh, NC 27607
Phone: (919) 861-5573
Fax: (919) 787-4916
E-mail: info@acepidemiology.org
Web site: http://acepidemiology.org/

American College of Gastroenterology
(ACG)
6400 Goldsboro Rd., Suite 200
Bethesda, MD 20817
Phone: (301)263-9000
E-mail: info@acg.gi.org
Web site: http://www.acg.gi.org/

American College of Hyperbaric
Medicine
6737 W. Washington St., Ste. 3265
West Allis, WI 53214
Phone: (414) 918-9300
Fax: (414) 918-9301
E-mail: admin@achm.org
Web site: http://www.achm.org

American College of Medical
Toxicology (ACMT)
10645 N. Tatum Blvd., Suite 200-111
Phoenix, AZ 85028

Phone: (623) 533-6340
Fax: (623) 533-6520
E-mail: info@acmt.net
Web site: http://www.acmt.net/

American College of Nutrition
300 S. Duncan Ave., Ste. 225
Clearwater, FL 33755
Phone: (727) 446-6086
Fax: (727) 446-6202
E-mail: office@AmericanCollegeof
Nutrition.org
Web site: http://www.americancollege
ofnutrition.org

American College of Obstetricians
and Gynecologists (ACOG)
409 12th St., S.W., P.O. Box 96920
Washington, DC 20090-6920
Phone: 202-638-5577
E-mail: resources@acog.org
Web site: http://www.acog.org/

American College of Sports
Medicine
401 West Michigan Street
Indianapolis, IN 46206-3233
Phone: (317) 637-9200
Fax: (317) 634-7817
Web site: http://www.acsm.org

American College of Toxicology
(ACTOX)
9650 Rockville Pike, #3408
Bethesda, MD 20814
Phone: (301) 634-7840
Fax: (301) 634-7852
Web site: http://www.actox.org/

American Congress of Obstetricians
and Gynecologists (ACOG)
P.O. Box 70620
Washington, DC 20024-9998
Phone: (202) 638-5577
Toll free: (800) 673-8444
Web site: http://www.acog.org/

American Contact Dermatitis Society
2323 North State Street #30
Bunnell, FL 32110
Phone: (386) 437-4405
Fax: (386) 437-4427
E-mail: info@contactderm.org
Web site: http://www.contactderm.org

American Council on Exercise
4851 Paramount Drive
San Diego, CA 92123
Phone: (858) 279-8227
Toll free: (888) 825-3636
Fax: (858) 576-6564
E-mail: support@acefitness.org
Web site: http://www.acefitness.org

American Council on Science and
Health
1995 Broadway, Ste. 202
New York, NY 10023

Phone: (212) 362-7044
Toll free: (866) 905-2694
Fax: (212) 362-4919
E-mail: acsh@acsh.org
Web site: http://www.acsh.org

American Dental Association
211 E. Chicago Avenue
Chicago, IL 60611-2678
Phone: (312) 440-2500
Web site: http://www.ada.org

American Diabetes Association
1701 North Beauregard St.
Alexandria, VA 22311
Toll free: (800) DIABETES
(342-2383)
E-mail: askADA@diabetes.org
Web site: http://www.diabetes.org

American Dietetic Association
120 South Riverside Plaza,
Suite 2000
Chicago, IL 60606-6995
Toll free: (800) 877-1600
Web site: http://www.eatright.org

American Fertility Organization
315 Madison Avenue, Suite 901
New York, NY 10017
Toll free: (888) 917-3777
Web site: http://www.theafa.org/

American Foundation for Suicide
Prevention
120 Wall St., 29th Fl.
New York, NY 20016-3007
Phone: (212) 363-3500
Toll free: (888) 333-2377
Fax: (212) 363-6237
E-mail: inquiry@afsp.org
Web site: http://www.afsp.org

American Foundation for the Blind
2 Penn Plaza, Suite 1102
New York, NY 10121
Phone: (212) 502-7600
Toll free: (888) 545-8331
E-mail: afbinfo@afb.net
Web site: http://www.afb.org/

American Heart Association
7272 Greenville Ave.
Dallas, TX 75231
Toll free: (800) 242-8721
Web site: http://www.heart.org

American Hospital Association
(AHA)
155 N. Wacker Drive
Chicago, IL 60606
Phone: (312) 422-3000
Toll free: (800) 424-4301
E-mail: http://www.aha.org/about
/contactus.shtml
Web site: http://www.aha.org/

American Industrial Hygiene Association
3141 Fairview Park Drive, Suite 777
Falls Church, VA 22042
Phone: (703) 849-8888
Fax: (703) 207-3561
E-mail: infonet@aiha.org
Web site: http://www.aiha.org

American Institute of Homeopathy
801 N. Fairfax St., Suite 306
Alexandria, VA 22314
Toll free: (888) 445-9988
Web site: http://www.homeopathy
usa.org

American Institute of Stress
124 Park Avenue
Yonkers, NY 10703
Phone: (914) 963-1200
E-mail: stress125@optonline.net
Web site: http://www.stress.org

American Kidney Fund
11921 Rockville Pike, Ste. 300
Rockville, MD 20852
Toll free: (800) 638-8299
Web site: http://www.kidneyfund.org

American Legion
700 N Pennsylvania St.
Indianapolis, IN 46206
Toll free: (800) 433-3318
Web site: http://www.legion.org

American Liver Foundation (ALF)
39 Broadway, Suite 2700
New York, NY 10006
Phone: (212) 668-1000
Fax: (212) 483-8179
E-mail: http://www.liverfoundation.org
/contact/
Web site: http://www.liverfoundation
.org/

American Lung Association
1301 Pennsylvania Ave., NW,
Ste. 800
Washington, DC 20004
Phone: (202) 785-3355
Fax: (202) 452-1805
Toll free:
E-mail: info@lung.org
Web site: http://www.lung.org/

American Lyme Disease Foundation
P. O. Box 466
Lyme, CT 06371
E-mail: inquire@adlf.com
Web site: http://www.aldf.com

American Medical Association
515 N. State St.
Chicago, IL 60654
Toll free: (800) 621-8335
Web site: http://www.ama-assn.org

American Mosquito Control Association
15000 Commerce Pkwy., Ste. C
Mount Laurel, NJ 08054
Phone: (856) 439-9222
Fax: (856) 439-0525
E-mail: amca@mosquito.org
Web site: http://www.mosquito.org

American Pain Society
4700 W. Lake Ave.
Glenview, IL 60025
Phone: (847) 375-4715
Fax: (866) 574-2654
E-mail: info@ampainsoc.org
Web site: http://www.ampainsoc.org/

American Physical Therapy Association
1111 North Fairfax Street
Alexandria, VA 22314-1488
Phone: (703) 684-APTA (2782).
TDD: (703) 683-6748
Toll free: (800) 999-APTA (2782
Fax: (703) 683-6748
Web site: http://www.apta.org

American Physical Therapy Association
1111 North Fairfax Street
Alexandria, VA 22314-1488
Phone: (703) 684-APTA (2782).
TDD: (703) 683-6748
Toll free: (800) 999-APTA (2782
Fax: (703) 683-6748
Web site: http://www.apta.org

American Pregnancy Association
1425 Greenway Drive, Suite 440
Irving, TX 75038
Phone: (972) 550-0140
E-mail: Questions@American
Pregnancy.org
Web site: http://www.american
pregnancy.org

American Psychiatric Association
1000 Wilson Blvd, Ste. 1825
Arlington, VA 22209-3901
Phone: (703) 907-7300
Toll free: (888) 357-7924
E-mail: apa@psych.org
Web site: http://www.psych.org

American Public Health Association (APHA)
800 I Street, NW
Washington, DC 20001-3710
Phone: (202) 777-APHA
Fax: (202) 777-2534
Web site: http://apha.org/

American Red Cross
2025 E Street
Washington, DC 20006
Phone: (202) 303-4498

Toll free: (800) RED-CROSS
(733-2767)
Web site: http://www.redcross.org/

American School Health Association (ASHA)
4340 East West Hwy., Suite 403
Bethedsa, MD 20814
Phone: 1 (301) 652-8072
Fax: (301) 652-8077
E-mail: info@ashaweb.org
Web site: http://www.ashaweb.org/

American Society for Metabolic and Bariatric Surgery
100 SW 75th Street, Ste. 201
Gainesville, FL 32607
Phone: (352) 331-4900
Toll free:
Fax: (352) 331-4975
E-mail: info@asmbs.org
Web site: http://www.asbs.org

American Society for Nutrition
9650 Rockville Pike
Bethesda, MD 20814
Phone: (301) 634-7050
Fax: (301) 634-7894
Web site: http://www.nutrition.org

American Society for Reproductive Medicine
1209 Montgomery Hwy.
Birmingham, AL 35216-2809
Phone: (205) 978-5000
E-mail: asrm@asrm.org
Web site: http://www.asrm.org

American Society of Cataract and Refractive Surgery
4000 Legato Road, Suite 700
Fairfax, VA 22033
Phone: (703) 591-2220
Web site: http://www.ascrs.org

American Society of Clinical Oncology
2318 Mill Road, Suite 800
Alexandria, Virginia 22314
Phone: (571) 483-1300
Web site: http://www.asco.org

American Society of Plastic Surgeons
444 E Algonquin Rd.
Arlington Heights, IL 60005
Phone: (847) 228-9900
Web site: http://www.plasticsurgery.org

American Sociological Association (ASA)
1430 K St., N.W., Suite 600
Washington, DC 20005
Phone: (202) 383-9005
Fax: (202) 638-0882
E-mail: http://www.asanet.org/contactus
.cfm
Web site: http://www.asanet.org/

American Stroke Association (ASA)
7272 Greenville Avenue
Dallas, TX 75231
Toll free: (888) 478-7653
E-mail: strokeinfo@heart.org
Web site: http://www.strokeassociation
.org/

American Thoracic Society
25 Broadway, 18th Fl.
New York, NY 10004
Phone: (212) 315-8600
Fax: (212) 315-6498
E-mail: atsinfo@thoracic.org
Web site: http://www.thoracic.org/

American Veterinary Medical Association (AVMA)
1931 North Meacham Rd., Suite 100
Schaumburg, IL 60173–4360
Toll free: (800) 248-2862
Fax: (847) 925-1329
Web site: http://www.avma.org

Americans for Nonsmokers' Rights
2530 San Pablo Avenue, Suite J
Berkeley, CA 94702
Phone: (510) 841-3032
Web site: http://www.no-smoke.org/
index.php

Amnesty International
1 Easton Street
London, WC1X 0DW
Phone: 44 20 74135500
Fax: 44 20 79561157
Web site: http://www.amnesty.org

Anxiety Disorders Association of America
8701 Georgia Ave., Ste. 412
Silver Spring, MD 20910
Phone: (240) 485-1001
Web site: http://www.adaa.org

APEC Emerging Infections Network
1107 NE 45th St., Ste. 400,
Box 354809
Seattle, WA 98195
E-mail: apecein@u.washington.edu
Web site: http://depts.washington.edu

Armed Forces Health Surveillance Center (AFHSC)
11800 Tech Road, Suite 220
Silver Spring, MD 20904
Phone: (301) 319-3240
Fax: (301) 319-7620
E-mail: AFHSC.Web@amedd.army.mil
Web site: http://www.afhsc.mil/home

Arthritis Foundation
PO Box 7669
Atlanta, GA 30357-0669
Toll free: (800) 283-7800
Web site: http://www.arthritis.org

Ask Me 3, National Patient Safety Foundation (NPSF)
268 Summer Street, 6th floor
Boston, MA 02210
Phone: 1 (617) 391-9900
Fax: 1 (617) 391-9999
E-mail: http://www.npsf.org/contact-us/
Web site: http://www.npsf.org/for-
healthcare-professionals/programs
/ask-me-3/

Association for Professionals in Infection Control and Epidemiology (APIC)
1275 K St., N.W., Suite 1000
Washington, DC 20005–4006
Phone: 1 (202) 789-1890
Fax: 1 (202) 789-1899
E-mail: http://www.apic.org/About-
APIC/Contact-Us/Form
Web site: http://www.apic.org/

Association of Black Cardiologists
5355 Hunter Road
Atlanta, GA 30349
Phone: (404) 201-6600
Toll free: (800) 753-9222
Fax: (404) 201-6601
E-mail: abcardio@abcardio.org
Web site: http://www.abcardio.org

Association of Occupational and Environmental Clinics (AOEC)
1010 Vermont Ave., NW #513
Washington, DC 20005
Phone: (202) 347-4976
Toll free: (888) 347-AOEC
Fax: (202) 347-4950
E-mail: aoec@aoec.org
Web site: http://www.aoec.org/

Association of Public Health Nurses (APHN)
PO Box 7440
Oklahoma City, OK 73153
Phone: (405) 271-9444, X56531
E-mail: askaphn@phnurse.org
Web site: http://www.phnurse.org/

Association of Reproductive Health Professionals - East
1901 L St., N.W., Suite 300
Washington, DC 20036
Phone: 1 (202) 466–3825
E-mail: ARHP@arhp.org
Web site: http://www.arhp.org/

Association of Schools of Public Health (ASPH)
1900 M Street NW, Suite 710
Washington, DC 20036
Phone: (202) 296-1099
Fax: (202) 296-1252
E-mail: info@asph.org
Web site: http://www.asph.org/

Association of State and Territorial Health Officers (ASTHO)
2231 Crystal Dr., Suite 450
Arlington, VA 22202
Phone: (202) 371-9090
Fax: (571) 527-3189
Web site: http://www.astho.org/

Asthma and Allergy Foundation of America
1233 20th Street, NW, Suite 402
Washington, DC 20036
Toll free: (800) 7-ASTHMA or
(800) 727-8462
E-mail: info@aafa.org
Web site: http://www.aafa.org

Autism Research Institute/Autism Resource Center
4182 Adams Avenue
San Diego, CA 92116
Phone: English: (866) 366-3361;
Spanish: (877) 644-1184 ext. 5
Fax: (619) 563-6840
Web site: http://www.autism.com

Autism Society of America
4340 East–West Hwy, Suite 350
Bethesda, MD
Phone: (301) 657-0881
Toll free: (800) 3-AUTISM [(800)
328-8476]
Web site: http://www.autismsource.org

Autism Speaks
1 East 33rd Street, 4th Floor
New York, NY 10016
Phone: (212) 252-8584
Fax: (212) 252-8676
E-mail: contactus@autismspeaks.org
Web site: http://www.autismspeaks.org

B

Better Hearing Institute
1444 I St. NW, Ste. 700
Washington, DC 20005
Phone: (202) 449-1100
Fax: (202) 216-9646
E-mail: mail@betterhearing.org
Web site: http://www.betterhearing.org

Bill & Melinda Gates Foundation
500 Fifth Ave. N
Seattle, WA 98102
Phone: (206) 709-3100
E-mail: info@gatesfoundation.org
Web site: http://www.gates
foundation.org

Brain Aneurysm Foundation (BAF)
269 Hanover Street, Building 3
Hanover, MA 02339
Phone: (781) 826-5556
Toll free: (888) 272-4602

E-mail: office@bafound.org
Web site: http://www.bafound.org/

**Brain Injury Association
of America**
1608 Spring Hill Rd., Suite 110
Vienna, VA 22182
Phone: (703) 761-0750
Fax: (703) 761-0755
Toll free: (800) 444-6443
E-mail: braininjuryinfo@biausa.org
Web site: http://www.biausa.org

**Brendan B. McGinnis Congenital
CMV Foundation**
P.O. Box 1718
Wheat Ridge, CO 8003401718
E-mail: mcginnis@cmvfoundation.org
Web site: http://cmvfoundation.org/

British Nutrition Foundation
High Holborn House, 52-54 High
Holborn
London, WC1V 6RQ
Phone: 020 7404 6504
Fax: 020 7404 6747
E-mail: postbox@britishnutrition.org.uk
Web site: http://www.britishnutrition
.org.uk

C

**Canadian Association of
Naturopathic Doctors**
20 Holly St., Ste. 200
Toronto, M4S 3B1
Phone: (416) 496-8633
Fax: (416) 496-8634
Toll free: (800) 551-4381
Web site: http://www.cand.ca

Canadian Diabetes Association
National Life Building, 1400–522
University Ave.
Toronto, M5G 2R5
Toll free: (800) 226-8464
E-mail: info@diabetes.ca
Web site: http://www.diabetes.ca

Canadian Pain Society
1143 Wentworth St. West, Suite 202
Oshawa, L1J 8P7
Phone: (905) 404–9545
Fax: (905) 404–3727
E-mail: http://www.canadianpainsociety
.ca/en/contact.html
Web site: http://www.canadianpain
society.ca

CARE International Secretariat
Chemin de Balexert 7–9
Chatelaine, 1219
Phone: 41 22 795 10 20
Fax: 41 22 795 10 29
Toll free: (800) 521-CARE (2273)

Web site: http://www.care-
international.org

Carter Center (The)
One Copenhill, 453 Freedom Parkway
Atlanta, GA 30307
Phone: (404) 420-5100
Toll free: (800) 550-3560
E-mail: carterweb@emory.edu
Web site: http://www.cartercenter.org/

**Center for Emerging and Neglected
Diseases (CEND)**
University of California, Berkeley,
444A Li Ka Shing Center
Berkeley, CA 94720-3370
Phone: (510) 664-4867
E-mail: cend@berkeley.edu
Web site: http://globalhealth.berkeley
.edu/cend/index.html

**Center for Environmental Research
and Children's Health (University
of California at Berkeley)**
1995 University Ave., Ste. 265
Berkeley, CA 94720-7392
Phone: (510) 643-9598
Fax: (510) 642-9083
E-mail: cerch@berkeley.edu
Web site: http://cerch.org

Center for Evidence-Based Policy
Oregon Health and Science University,
3455 SW US Veterans Hospital
Road, Mailstop SN-4N
Portland, OR 97239-2941
Phone: (503) 494-2182
Fax: (503) 494-3807
E-mail: centerebp@ohsu.edu
Web site: http://www.ohsu.edu/xd/
research/centers-institutes/evidence-
based-policy-center/index.cfm/

**Center for Food Safety and Applied
Nutrition (CFSAN), U.S. Food and
Drug Administration**
5100 Paint Branch Pkwy.
College Park, MD 20740
Toll free: (888) SAFEFOOD
(723-3366)
E-mail: consumer@fda.gov
Web site: http://www.fda.gov/Food
/default.htm

Center for Food Safety
660 Pennsylvania Ave. SE, Ste. 302
Washington, DC 20003
Phone: (202) 547-9359
Fax: (202) 547-9429
E-mail: office@centerforfoodsafety.org
Web site: http://www.centerforfood
safety.org

**Center for Hearing and
Communications**
50 Broadway, Sixth Floor
New York City, NY 10004

Phone: (917) 305-7700
Web site: http://www.chchearing.org/

**Center for Infectious Disease
Dynamics (CIDD)**
The Pennsylvania State University, 208
Mueller Lab
University Park, PA 16802
E-mail: http://www.cidd.psu.edu
/contact-info
Web site: http://www.cidd.psu.edu/

**Center for Internet Addiction
Recovery**
P.O. Box 72
Bradford, PA 16701
Phone: (814) 451-2405
Fax: (814) 368-9560
Web site: http://www.netaddiction.com

**Center for Nutrition Policy and
Promotion (CNPP), U.S.
Department of Agriculture
(USDA)**
3101 Park Center Drive, 10th Floor
Alexandria, VA 22302-1594
Phone: (703) 305-7600
Fax: (703) 305-3300
Web site: http://www.cnpp.usda.gov/

Center for Reproductive Rights
120 Wall St.
New York City, NY 10005
Phone: 1 (917) 637-3600
Fax: (917) 637-3666
Web site: http://reproductiverights.org/

Center for Rural Affairs
145 Main Street, P.O. Box 136
Lyons, NE 60606
Phone: (402) 687-2100
E-mail: info@crfa.org
Web site: www.cfra.org

Center for Sight and Hearing
8038 MacIntosh Lane
Rockford, IL 61107
Phone: (815) 332-6800
Toll free: (800) 545-0080
Web site: http://www.centerforsight
hearing.org/

**Center for the Study of Bioterrorism
and Emergency Infections-Saint
Louis University**
3545 Lafayette, Ste. 300
St. Louis, MO 63104
Web site: http://bioterrorism.slu.edu

**Centers for Disease Control and
Prevention (CDC)**
1600 Clifton Rd.
Atlanta, GA 30333
Phone: (404) 639–3534
Toll free: (800) CDC–INFO (800–232–
4636). TTY: (888) 232–6348
E-mail: inquiry@cdc.gov
Web site: http://www.cdc.gov

Centers for Disease Control and Prevention (CDC), Bacterial Diseases Branch
Foothills Campus
Fort Collins, CO 80521
Toll free: (800) CDC-INFO (232-4636)
E-mail: cdcinfo@cdc.gov
Web site: http://www.cdc.gov/

Centers for Disease Control and Prevention (CDC), National Center on Birth Defects and Developmental Disabilities (NCBDDD)
1600 Clifton Road, MS E-87
Atlanta, GA 30333
Toll free: (800) CDC-INFO (232-4636)
E-mail: cdcinfo@cdc.gov
Web site: http://www.cdc.gov/

Centers for Disease Control and Prevention—Bioterrorism Preparedness & Response Program (CDC)
1600 Clifton Rd.
Atlanta, GA 30333
Phone: (404) 639-3534
Toll free: (888) 246-2675
E-mail: cdcresponse@ ashastd.org
Web site: http://www.bt.cdc.gov

Centers for Disease Control and Prevention, Public Inquiries/MASO
Mailstop F07, 1600 Clifton Road
Atlanta, GA 30333
Toll free: (800) 311-3435
Web site: http://www.cdc.gov

Centers for Disease Control Malaria Hotline
Phone: (770) 332-4555

Centers for Disease Control Travelers Hotline
Phone: (770) 332-4559

Centers for Medicare 3000
Toll free: (877) 267-2323
Web site: https://www.cms.gov/

Central Institute for the Deaf
825 South Taylor Avenue
St. Louis, MO 63110
Phone: (314) 977-0132
Toll free: (877) 444-4574
Web site: http://www.cid.edu/home
.aspx

Centre for Addiction and Mental Health
33 Russell St.
Toronto, M5S 2S1
Phone: (416) 535-8501
Toll free: (800) 463-6273
Web site: http://www.camh.net

Chagas Disease Foundation (The)
1191 DaAndra Drive

Watkinsville, GA 30677
Phone: (641) 715-3900 ext.46250#
E-mail: chagasfoundation@gmail.com
Web site: http://www.chagasfound.org/

Charity Navigator
139 Harristown Rd., Ste. 201
Glen Rock, NJ 07452
Phone: (201) 818-1288
Fax: (201) 818-4694
E-mail: info@charitynavigator.org
Web site: http://www.charitynavigator
.org

Chartered Institute of Environmental Health
Chadwick Court, 15 Hatfields
London, SE1 8DJ
Phone: (0) 20 7928 6006
Fax: (0) 20 7827 5862
E-mail: https://forms.cieh.org/ciehorg
/forms/ciehform.aspx?ekfrm=154
Web site: http://www.cieh.org/

Chemical Safety and Hazard Investigation Board (CSB)
2175 K Street NW
Washington, DC 20037
Phone: (202) 261-7600
Fax: (202) 261-7650
E-mail: http://www.csb.gov/service
/contact.aspx
Web site: http://www.csb.gov/

Chicago Electrical Trauma Research Institute
4047 W 40th St.
Chicago, IL 80532
Phone: (773) 904-0347
Toll free: (800) 516-8709
E-mail: info@cetri.org
Web site: http://www.cetri.org/

Children & Nature Network
7 Avenida Vista Grande B-7, no. 502
Santa Fe, NM 87508
E-mail: info@childrenandnature.org
Web site: http://www.cnaturenet.org

Children's Eye Foundation
1631 Lancaster Drive, Suite 200
Grapevine, TX 76051
Phone: (817) 310-2641
E-mail: info@childrenseyefoundation
.org
Web site: http://www.
childrenseyefoundation.org

Children's Hemiplegia and Stroke Association CHASA)
4101 W. Green Oaks, Suite 305,
no. 149
Arlington, TX 76016
Web site: http://www.chasa.org/

Coalition for Evidence-Based Policy
1725 I Street, NW, Suite 300
Washington, DC 20006

Phone: (202) 349-1130
Fax: (202) 349-3915
E-mail: jbaron@coalition4evidence.org
Web site: http://coalition4evidence.org
/wordpress/

Cochrane Collaboration, United States Cochrane Center
Center for Clinical Trials, Johns
Hopkins Bloomberg School of
Public Health, 615 N. Wolfe Street,
Mail RM W5010
Baltimore, MD 21205
Phone: (410) 502-4419
Fax: (410) 502-4621
E-mail: uscc@jhsph.edu
Web site: http://www.cochrane.org/
Web site: United States home page:
http://us.cochrane.org/

Collaborative on Health and the Environment (CHE)
P.O. Box 316
Bolinas, CA 94924
Phone: 415-868-0970
Fax: 415-868-2230
E-mail: info@Healthand
Environment.org
Web site: http://www.healthand
environment.org/index.php

Commonwealth Fund
One East 75th Street
New York, NY 10021
Phone: (212) 606-3800
Fax: (212) 606-3500
E-mail: info@cmwf.org
Web site: http://www.commonwealth
fund.org/

Congenital CMV Foundation
12801 Crossroads Parkway South,
Suite 200
City of Industry, CA 91746
Web site: http://www.congenitalcmv.org

Consumer Product Safety Commission
4330 East West Hwy.
Bethesda, MD 20814
Phone: (301) 504-7923
Web site: http://www.cpsc.gov/

Convention on Biological Diversity
413 Saint-Jacques St., Ste. 800
Montreal, H2Y 1N9
Phone: 1 (514) 288-2220
Fax: 1 (514) 288-6588
E-mail: bch@cbd.int
Web site: http://bch.cbd.int

Council of State and Territorial Epidemiologists (CSTE)
2872 Woodcock Blvd. Suite 303
Atlanta, GA 30341
Phone: (770) 458-3811
Fax: (770) 458-8516
Web site: http://www.cste.org/dnn/

Council on Education for Public Health (CEPH)
1010 Wayne Avenue, Suite 220
Silver Spring, MD 20910
Phone: (202) 789-1060
Fax: (202) 789-1895
Web site: http://www.ceph.org/

Creutzfeldt-Jakob Disease Foundation
3632 W Market St.
Akron, OH 44333
Toll free: (800) 659-1991
E-mail: help@cjdfoundation.org
Web site: http://www.cjdfoundation.org

D

Department of Health (UK), Customer Service Centre
Richmond House, 79 Whitehall
London, SW1A 2NS
Phone: 020 7210 4850
Fax: 020 7210 5952
E-mail: http://www.info.doh.gov.uk/
contactus.nsf/memo?openform
Web site: http://www.dh.gov.uk/en

Dietitians of Canada
480 University Ave., Ste. 604
Toronto, M5G 1V2
Phone: (416) 596-0857
Fax: (416) 596-0603
E-mail: centralinfo@dietitians.ca
Web site: http://www.dietitians.ca

Divers Alert Network
6 W Colony Place
Durham, NC 27705
Phone: (919) 684-2948
Fax: (919) 490-6630
Toll free: (800) 446-2671
Web site: http://www.
diversalertnetwork.org

Division of Aging and Seniors, Health Canada, Public Health Agency of Canada
1015 Arlington Street
Winnipeg, R3E 3R2
Phone: (204) 789-2000
E-mail: ph-sp-info@phac-aspc.gc.ca
Web site: http://www.phac-aspc.gc.ca/
seniors-aines/

Division of Toxicology and Environmental Medicine
4770 Buford Hwy NE
Atlanta, GA 30341
Toll free: (800) CDC-INFO
E-mail: cdcinfo@cdc.gov
Web site: http://www.atsdr.cdc.gov/

Donate Life America
701 E. Bird St., 16th Floor

Richmond, VA 23219
Phone: (804) 377-3580
Web site: http://www.donatelife.net

E

Earth Day Network
1616 P St. NW, Ste. 340
Washington, DC 20036
Phone: (202) 518-0044
E-mail: buchanan@earthday.org
Web site: http://www.earthday.org

Environmental Defense Fund
1875 Connecticut Ave. NW, Ste. 600.
Washington, DC 20009
Toll free: (800) 684-3322
Web site: http://www.edf.org/

Environmental Protection Agency (EPA)
Ariel Rios Building, 1200 Pennsylvania Avenue, N.W.
Washington, DC 20460
Phone: (202) 272-0167
Web site: http://www.epa.gov/

Environmental Research Foundation
PO Box 160
New Brunswick, NJ 08908
Phone: 1 (732) 828-9995
E-mail: erf@rachel.org
Web site: http://www.rachel.org/

Environmental Working Group (The)
1436 U Street NW, Suite 100
Washington, DC 20009
Phone: 1 (202) 667-6982
Web site: http://www.ewg.org

EuroGentest
Gasthuisberg O&N, Herestraat 49, Box 602
Leuven, 3000
Web site: http://www.eurogentest.org

European Bioinformatics Institute
Wellcome Trust Genome Campus, Hinxton
Cambridge, CB10 1SD
Phone: 44 (0)1223 494 444
Fax: 44 (0)1223 494 468
Web site: http://www.ebi.ac.uk

European Cities Against Drugs
Hantverkargatan 3D, City Hall, S-105-35
Stockholm
Phone: 46-8-5082-9362
Fax: 46-8-5082-9436
E-mail: ecad@ecad.net
Web site: http://www.ecad.net

European Commission, Directorate General for Health and Consumers
B-1049
Brussels

Phone: 011 32 (2) 299-11-11
Web site: http://ec.europa.eu/dgs/
health_consumer/index_en.htm

European Food Safety Authority
Via Carlo Magno 1A
Parma, 43126
Phone: 0521 036111
Fax: 0521 036110
Web site: http://www.efsa.europa.eu

European Society of Cardiology
The European Heart House, 2035 Route des Colles, B.P. 179-Les Templiers
Sophia-Antipolis, 06903
Phone: 33 4.9294 7600
Fax: 33 4 9294 7601
E-mail: http://www.escardio.org/Pages
/contactus.aspx
Web site: http://www.escardio.org

Exxon Valdez Oil Spill Trustee Council
4230 University Dr., Ste. 230
Anchorage, AK 99508-4650
Phone: (907) 278-8012
Fax: (907) 276-7178
Toll free: (800) 478-7745
Web site: http://www.evostc.state.ak.us

F

Federal Bureau of Investigation
J. Edgar Hoover Building, 935 Pennsylvania Avenue NW
Washington, DC 20535-0001
Phone: (202) 324-3000
Web site: http://www.fbi.gov

Federal Communications Commission
445 12th Street, SW
Washington, DC 20554
Phone: 1 (202) 418-1440
Fax: 1 (866) 418-0232
Toll free: (888) CALL FCC (225-5322)
E-mail: fccinfo@fcc.gov
Web site: http://www.fcc.gov

Federal Emergency Management Agency (FEMA), U.S. Department of Homeland Security
500 C St. SW
Washington, DC 20472
Phone: (206) 646-2500
Toll free: (800) 621-FEMA (3362)
Web site: http://www.fema.gov

Fetal Alcohol Syndrome (FAS) World Canada
250 Scarborough Golf Club Rd.
Toronto, M1J 3G8
Phone: (416) 264-8000
Fax: (416) 264-8222
E-mail: info@fasworld.com
Web site: http://www.fasworld.com

Food Allergy and Anaphylaxis Network (FAAN)
11781 Lee Jackson Hwy., Ste. 160
Fairfax, VA 22033
Toll free: (800) 929-4040
Fax: (703) 691-2713
E-mail: faan@foodallergy.org
Web site: http://www.foodallergy.org

Food and Agriculture Organization of the United Nations (FAO Headquarters)
Viale delle Terme di Caracalla
Rome, 00153
Phone: 39 06 570 53625
Fax: 39 06 5705 3699
E-mail: AGN-Director@fao.org
(Nutrition and Consumer Protection)
Web site: http://www.fao.org

Food and Drug Administration (FDA)
10903 New Hampshire Ave.
Silver Spring, MD 20993
Toll free: (888) INFO-FDA
Web site: http://www.fda.gov/

Food and Nutrition Information Center, National Agricultural Library
10301 Baltimore Ave., Rm. 105
Beltsville, MD 20705
Phone: (301) 504-5414
Fax: (301) 504-6409
E-mail: fnic@ars.usda.gov
Web site: http://fnic.nal.usda.gov

Food Safety and Inspection Service (FSIS), U.S. Department of Agriculture (USDA)
1400 Independence Ave. SW
Washington, DC 20250-3700
Toll free: (888) 674-6854 (USDA Meat and Poultry Consumer Hotline)
E-mail: MPHotline.fsis@usda.gov
Web site: http://www.fsis.usda.gov

Food Standards Agency
Aviation House, 125 Kingsway
London, WC2B 6NH
Web site: http://www.food.gov.uk

Foundation for Health in Aging
40 Fulton Street, 18th Floor
New York, NY 10038
Phone: (212) 308-1414
Web site: http://www.healthinaging
.org

G

Gay and Lesbian Medical Association
1326 18th Street NW, Suite 22
Washington, DC 20036

Phone: (202) 600-8037
E-mail: info@glma.org
Web site: http://www.glma.org

Glaucoma Foundation
80 Maiden Lane, Suite 1206
New York, NY 10038
Phone: (212) 285-0080
E-mail: info@glaucomafoundation.org
Web site: http://www.glaucoma
foundation.org

Glaucoma Research Foundation
251 Post Street, Suite 600
San Francisco, CA 94108
Phone: (415) 986-3162
Web site: http://www.glaucoma.org/

Global Alliance Against Chronic Respiratory Diseases, World Health Organization
20 Avenue Appia
Geneva 1211 27
E-mail: gard@who.int
Web site: http://www.who.int/gard/en

Global Fund to Fight AIDS, Tuberculosis, and Malaria
Geneva Secretariat, Chemin de Blandonnet 8, 1214 Vernier
Geneva
Phone: 41 58 791-1700
Fax: 41 58 791-1701
E-mail: info@theglobalfund.org
Web site: http://www.theglobalfund
.org/en

GMHC [formerly Gay Men's Health Crisis]
446 West 33rd Street
New York, NY 10001-2601
Phone: (212) 367-1000
Toll free: (800) 243-7692
E-mail: http://www.gmhc.org/about-us
/contact-us
Web site: http://www.gmhc.org/

Guide Dogs for the Blind, National Office
P.O. Box 151200
San Rafael, CA 94915-1200
Toll free: (800) 295-4050
Web site: http://ww.guidedogs.com

Guttmacher Institute
125 Maiden Lane, 7th Floor
New York, NY 10038
Phone: (212) 248-1111
Web site: http://www.guttmacher.org

H

Hazelden Foundation
PO Box 11
Center City, MN 55012-0011

Phone: (651) 213-4200
Toll free: (800) 257-7810
E-mail: info@hazelden.org
Web site: http://www.hazelden.org

Health Physics Society
1313 Dolley Madison Blvd., Ste. 402
McLean, VA 22101
Phone: (703) 790-1745
Fax: (703) 790-2672
E-mail: hps@burkinc.com
Web site: www.hps.org

Health Resources and Services Administration, U.S. Department of Health and Human Services
5600 Fishers Lane
Rockville, MD 20857
Toll free: (888) 275–4772
E-mail: ask@hrsa.gov
Web site: http://www.hrsa.gov/

Hearing Loss Association of America
7910 Woodmont Avenue, Suite 1200
Bethesda, MD 20814
Phone: (301) 657-2248
Web site: http://www.hearingloss.org/

Heart Foundation
80 William St., Level 3
Sydney, 2011
Phone: 02 9219 2444
Toll free: 300 36 27 87
E-mail: http://www.heartfoundation.
org.au/about-us/contact-us/Pages
/contact-form.aspx
Web site: http://www.heartfoundation
.org.au

Helen Keller International
325 Park Avenue South, 12th Floor
New York, NY 10010
Phone: (212) 532-0544
E-mail: info@hki.org
Web site: http://www.hki.org

Henry J. Kaiser Family Foundation
2400 Sand Hill Road
Menlo Park, CA 94025
Phone: (650) 854-9400
Fax: (650) 854-4800
Web site: http://www.kff.org/

Human Factors and Ergonomics Society
PO Box 1369
Santa Monica, CA 90406-1369
Phone: (310) 394-1811
Fax: (310) 394-2410
E-mail: info@hfes.org
Web site: www.hfes.org

Human Rights Watch
350 Fifth Avenue, 34th Floor
New York, NY 10118
Phone: (212) 290 4700
Fax: (212) 736 1300
Web site: http://www.hrw.org

I

Immunization Action Coalition (IAC)
1573 Selby Avenue, Suite 234
Saint Paul, MN 55104
Phone: (651) 647-9009
Fax: (651) 647-9131
E-mail: admin@immunize.org
Web site: http://www.immunize.org

**Infectious Diseases Society of
America (IDSA)**
1300 Wilson Blvd., Ste. 300
Arlington, VA 22209
Phone: (703) 299-0200
Fax: (703) 299-0204
E-mail: info@idsociety.org
Web site: http://www.idsociety.org

**Information Centres Service.
Strategic Communications
Division. Department of Public
Information. United Nations**
New York, NY 10017
E-mail: dpi_dis_unit@un.org
Web site: http://www.un.org/en/

Institute for Altitude Medicine
PO Box 1229
Telluride, CO 81435
Phone: (970) 728-6767
E-mail: info@altitudemedicine.org
Web site: http://www.altitudemedicine
.org

Institute for Health Policy Solutions
1444 "Eye" St., N.W., Suite 900
Washington, DC 20005
Phone: (202) 789-1491
Fax: (202) 789-1879
E-mail: pshrestha@ihps.org
Web site: http://www.ihps.org/

Institute of Food Technologies
525 W. Van Buren, Ste. 1000
Chicago, IL 60607
Phone: (312) 782-8424
Fax: (312) 792-8348
E-mail: info@ift.org
Web site: http://www.ift.org

**Institute of Medicine, National
Academy of Sciences**
500 Fifth St. NW
Washington, DC 20001
Phone: (202) 334-2352
E-mail: iomwww@nas.edu
Web site: http://www.iom.edu

**International Agency for Research
on Cancer**
150 Cours Albert Thomas, CEDEX 08
Lyons, 69372
Phone: 33 0 4 72 73 8485
Fax: 33 0 4 72 73 8575
Web site: http://www.iarc.fr

International AIDS Society (IAS)
Ave. Louis Casaï 71, P. O. Box 28
Geneva, CH - 1216 Cointrin
Phone: (0) 22-7 100 800
Fax: (0) 22-7 100 899
E-mail: info@iasociety.org
Web site: http://www.iasociety.org

**International Association of Wildland
Fires**
1418 Washburn St.
Missoula, MT 59801
Phone: (406) 531-8264
Toll free: (888) 440-4293
E-mail: iawf@iawfonline.org
Web site: http://www.iawfonline.org

**International Atomic Energy Agency
(IAEA)**
Vienna International Center,
PO Box 100
Vienna, A-1400
Phone: ? 2600-0
Fax: ? 2600-7
E-mail: Official.Mail@iaea.org
Web site: http://www.iaea.org

**International Centre for Genetic
Engineering and Biotechnology
Biosafety**
Padriciano 99
Trieste, 34149
Phone: 39 (040) 3757320
Fax: 39 (040) 226555
E-mail: biosafe@icgeb.org
Web site: www.icgeb.org

**International Coalition for Trachoma
Control**
Web site: http://www.
trachomacoalition.org

**International Committee of the Red
Cross**
19 Avenue de la Paix
Geneva 1202
Phone: 41 22 734 60 01
Fax: 41 22 733 20 57
E-mail: webmaster@icrc.org
Web site: http://www.icrc.org

**International Council for the Control
of Iodine Deficiency Disorders**
PO Box 51030, 375 des Epinettes
Ottawa, K1E 3E0
Web site: http://www.iccidd.org

International Eye Foundation
10801 Connecticut Avenue
Kensington, MD 20895
Phone: (240) 290-0263
E-mail: ief@iefusa.org
Web site: http://www.iefusa.org/

**International Federation of Red
Cross and Red Crescent Societies**
PO Box 372
Geneva 1211

Phone: 41 22 730 42 22
Fax: 41 22 733 03 95
Web site: http://www.ifrc.org

**International Food Information
Council Foundation**
1100 Connecticut Ave., NW Ste. 430
Washington, DC 20036
Phone: (202) 296-6540
E-mail: info@foodinsight.org
Web site: http://www.foodinsight.org

International Leptospirosis Society
Faculty of Medicine, Nursing and
Health Sciences, Monash
University3800
Phone: 3 9905 4301
Fax: 3 9905 4302
E-mail: enquiries@med.monash.edu.au
Web site: http://www.med.monash.edu.
au/microbiology/staff/adler/ils.html

International Manganese Institute
17 rue Duphot
Paris
Phone: (0) 145 63 06 34
Fax: (0) 1 42 89 42 92
Web site: http://www.manganese.org

**International Occupational Hygiene
Association**
5/6 Melbourne Business Court,
Pride Park
Derby, DE24 8LZ
Phone: (332) 298 101
Fax: (332) 298 099
E-mail: admin@ioha.net
Web site: http://www.ioha.net

International Rescue Committee
122 E 42nd St.
New York, NY 10168-1289
Phone: (212) 551-3000
Fax: (212) 551-3179
Web site: http://www.rescue.org

**International Society for Infectious
Diseases (ISID)**
9 Babcock Street, 3rd Floor
Brookline, MA 02446
Phone: (617) 277-0551
Fax: (617) 278-9113
E-mail: info@isid.org
Web site: http://www.isid.org/index
.shtml

**International Society for Traumatic
Stress Studies**
111 Deer Lake Rd., Ste. 100
Deerfield, IL 60015
Phone: (847) 480-9028
Fax: (847) 480-9282
Web site: http://www.istss.org

**International Society of Explosives
Engineers (ISEE)**
30325 Bainbridge Rd.
Cleveland, OH 44139

Phone: (440) 349-4400
Fax: (440) 349-3788
Web site: http://www.isee.org

International Society of Exposure Science Secretariat
c/o JSI Research and Training Institute, 44 Farnsworth St.
Boston, MA 02201
Phone: (617) 482-9485
Fax: (617) 482-0617
Web site: http://isesweb.org

International Solid Waste Association
Auerspergstrasse 15, Top 41
Vienna, 1080
Phone: 43 1 (253) 6001
Fax: 43 1 (253) 6001 99
E-mail: iswa@iswa.org
Web site: http://www.iswa.org

International Trachoma Initiative
325 Swanton Way
Decatur, GA 30030
Toll free: (800) 765-7173
E-mail: iti@taskforce.org
Web site: http://www.trachoma.org

International Union for Conservation of Nature
Rue Mauverney 28
Gland, 1196
Phone: 41 (999) 0000
Fax: 41 (999) 0002
Web site: http://www.iucn.org

International Union of Geodesy and Geophysics
Hertzstrasse 16
Karlsruhe, 76187
Phone: 49 (721) 6084-4494
Fax: 49 (721) 711-73
E-mail: secretariat@iugg.org
Web site: http://www.iugg.org

J

Juvenile Diabetes Research Foundation International
26 Broadway, 14th Fl.
New York, NY 10004
Toll free: (800) 533-CURE (2873)
Fax: (212) 785-9595
E-mail: info@jdrg.org
Web site: http://www.jdrf.org

L

La Leche League International
957 N Plum Grove Rd
Schaumburg, IL 60173
Phone: (847) 519-7730
Toll free: (800) LA-LECHE (525-3243)

Fax: (847) 969-0460
Web site: http://www.llli.org

Leukemia and Lymphoma Society
1311 Mamaroneck Avenue, Suite 310
White Plains, New York 10605
Phone: (914) 949-5213
Web site: http://www.lls.org

Lighthouse International
111 East 59th Street
New York, NY 10022
Phone: (212) 821-9200
Toll free: (800) 829-0500
E-mail: info@lighthouse.org
Web site: http://www.lighthouse.org

Lions Clubs International
300 West 22nd Street
Oak Brook, IL 60523
Phone: (630) 571-5466
E-mail: foundation@aoa.org
Web site: http://www.lionsclubs.org /EN/index.php

Lyme Disease Network of NJ.
43 Winton Road
East Brunswick, NJ 08816
Web site: http://www.lymenet.org

M

March of Dimes Birth Defects Foundation
1275 Mamaroneck Ave.
White Plains, NY 10605
Phone: (914) 997-4488
Web site: http://www.modimes.org

Men Can Stop Rape
1003 K Street NW, Suite 200
Washington, DC 20001
Phone: (202) 265-6530
Toll free: (800) 656-4673
E-mail: info@mencanstoprape.org
Web site: http://www.mencanstoprape .org/

Men's Health Network
PO Box 75972
Washington, DC 20013
Phone: (202) 543-6462
E-mail: info@menshealthnetwork.org
Web site: http://www.menshealth network.org

Meningitis Research Foundation
Midland Way
Thornbury, BS25 2BS
Phone: 01454 281811
Fax: 01454 281094
E-mail: info@meningitis.org
Web site: http://www.meningitis.org

Mental Health America
2000 N Beauregard St., 6th Fl.

Alexandria, VA 22311
Phone: (703) 684-7722
Fax: (703) 684-5968
Toll free: (800) 969-6642
Web site: http://www1.nmha.org

Mine Safety and Health Administration
4015 Wilson Blvd.
Arlington, VA 22203
Toll free: (877) 778-6055
E-mail: MSHAhelpdesk@dol.gov
Web site: http://www.msha.gov

Mothers Against Drunk Driving
511 E. John Carpenter Freeway, Suite 700
Irving, TX 75062
Phone: (877) 275-6233
Web site: http://www.madd.org/

N

National Abortion Federation
1660 L Street, NW, Suite 450
Washington, DC 20036
Phone: (202) 667-5881
E-mail: naf@prochoice.org
Web site: http://www.prochoice.org

National Agriculture Center, U.S. Environmental Protection Agency
901 N 5th St.
Kansas City, KS 66101
Toll free: (888) 663-2155
Fax: (913) 551-7270
E-mail: agcenter@epa.gov
Web site: http://www.epa.gov /agriculture/agctr.html

National Alliance on Mental Illness
3803 N. Fairfax Dr., Ste. 100
Arlington, VA 22203
Phone: (703) 524-7600
Fax: (703) 524-9094
Toll free: (800) 950-6264
Web site: http://www.nami.org

National Association of Anorexia Nervosa & Associated Disorders
800 E. Diehl Rd. #160
Naperville, IL 60563
Phone: (630) 577-1333
Phone: (630) 577-1330 (helpline)
E-mail: anadhelp@anad.org
Web site: http://www.anad.org

National Association of Community Health Centers (NACHC)
7501 Wisconsin Ave., Suite 1100W
Bethesda, MD 20814
Phone: (301) 347-0400
E-mail: http://www.nachc.com/contact-us .cfm
Web site: http://www.nachc.com/

**National Association of Community
Health Centers (NACHC)**
7501 Wisconsin, Ave., Suite 1100W
Bethesda, MD 20814
Phone: (301) 347-0400
E-mail: http://www.nachc.com/contact-us
.cfm
Web site: http://www.nachc.com/

**National Association of County and
City Health Officials (NACCHO)**
1100 17th St., N.W., 17th floor
Washington, DC 20036
Phone: 1 (202) 783-5550
Fax: 1 (202) 783-1583
E-mail: info@naccho.org
Web site: www.naccho.org/

**National Association of Emergency
Medical Technicians (NAEMT)**
PO Box 1400
Clinton, MS 39060–1400
Phone: (601) 924-7744
Toll free: (800) 34-NAEMT
Fax: (601) 924-7325
E-mail: info@naemt.org
Web site: http://www.naemt.org/

**National Association of Local Boards
of Health (NALBOH)**
1840 East Gypsy Lane Rd.
Bowling Green, OH 43402
Phone: (419) 353-7714
Fax: (419) 352-6278
E-mail: http://www.nalboh.org/Staff.htm
Web site: http://www.nalboh.org/

National Association of the Deaf
8630 Fenton Street, Suite 820
Silver Spring, MD 20910
Phone: (301) 587-1788
Web site: http://www.nad.org/

National Cancer Institute (NCI)
6116 Executive Blvd., Ste. 300
Bethesda, MD 20892-8322
Toll free: (800) 422-6237
E-mail: http://www.cancer.gov/global
/contact/email-us
Web site: http://www.cancer.gov

**National Center for Biotechnology
Information**
National Library of Medicine Building
38A
Bethesda, MD 20894
Phone: 1 (301) 496-2475
E-mail: info@ncbi.nlm.nih.gov
Web site: http://www.ncbi.nlm.nih.gov

**National Center for Emerging and
Zoonotic Infectious Diseases,
Centers for Disease Control and
Prevention**
1600 Clifton Rd.
Atlanta, GA 30333
Toll free: (800) 232-4635

E-mail: cdcinfo@cdc.gov
Web site: http://www.cdc.gov/ncezid/

**National Center for Environmental
Health, Centers for Disease
Control and Prevention**
1600 Clifton Rd., N.E.
Atlanta, GA 30333
Toll free: 1 (800) 232-4636
E-mail: cdcinfo@cdc.gov
Web site: www.cdc.gov/nceh/

**National Center for Farmworker
Health, Inc.**
1770 FM 967
Buda, TX 78610
Phone: 1 (512) 312-2700
Toll free: (800) 531-5120
Fax: 1 (512) 312-2600
E-mail: info@ncfh.org
Web site: http://www.ncfh.org/

National Center for Policy Analysis
12770 Coit Rd., Suite 800
Dallas, TX 75251-1339
Phone: (972) 386-6272
Fax: (972) 386-0924
Web site: http://www.ncpa.org

**National Center for Post Traumatic
Stress Disorder (PTSD), U.S.
Department of Veterans Affairs**
810 Vermont Ave. NW
Washington, DC 20420
Phone: (802) 296-6300
E-mail: ncptsd@va.gov
Web site: http://www.ncptsd.va.gov

**National Center on Addiction and
Substance Abuse at Columbia
University**
633 Third Avenue, 19th Floor
New York, NY 10017-6706
Phone: (212) 841-5200
Web site: http://www.casa
columbia.org

National Child Abuse Hotline
Toll free: (800) 4-A-CHILD
(422-4453)
Web site: http://answers.usa.gov

**National Children's Leukemia
Foundation**
7316 Avenue U
Brooklyn, New York 11234
Phone: (800) 448-4673
Web site: http://www.leukemia
foundation.org

**National Clearinghouse for Alcohol
and Drug Information**
P.O. Box 2345
Rockville, MD 20847-2345
Toll free: (877) SAMHSA-7
Fax: (240) 221-4292,
Web site: http://ncadi.samhsa.gov

**National Coalition Against Domestic
Violence**
One Broadway, Suite B210
Denver, CO 80203
Phone: (303) 839-1852
Fax: (303) 831-9251
E-mail: mainoffice@ncadv.org
Web site: http://www.ncadv.org/

**National Coalition for Cancer
Survivorship**
1010 Wayne Avenue, Suite 770
Silver Spring, MD 20910
Toll free: (877) 622-7937
Web site: http://www.canceradvocacy
.org/

**National Community Development
Association (NCDA)**
522 21st St., N.W., #120
Washington, DC 20006
Phone: (202) 293-7587
Fax: (202) 887-5546
E-mail: ncda@ncdaonline.org
Web site: http://www.ncdaonline.org/

**National Comprehensive Cancer
Network**
275 Commerce Drive, Suite 300
Fort Washington, Pennsylvania
19034
Phone: (215) 690-0300
Web site: http://www.nccn.org

**National Council for Community
Behavioral Healthcare**
1701 K St. NW, Ste. 400
Washington, DC 20006
Phone: (202) 684-7457
Fax: (202) 386-9391
E-mail: communications@thenational
council.org
Web site: http://www.TheNational
Council.org

National Council on Aging (NCOA)
1901 L Street NW, 4th Floor
Washington, DC 20036
Phone: (202) (301) 479-1200
Web site: http://www.ncoa.org/

**National Council on Alcohol and
Drug Dependence**
244 East 58th Street 4th Floor
New York, NY 10022
Phone: (212) 269-7797
Toll free: 24-hour help line: (800)
NCA-CALL
Fax: (212) 269-7510
E-mail: national@mcadd.org
Web site: http://www.ncadd.org

**National Council on Child Abuse
TTY (866) 569-1162**
Fax: (703) 738-4929
E-mail: info@niddk.nih.gov
Web site: http://digestive.niddk.nih.gov

National Domestic Violence Hotline
Toll free: (800) 799-SAFE (7233)
Web site: http://answers.usa.gov

National Earthquake Information Center
PO Box 25046, DFC, MS 967
Denver, CO 80225
Phone: (303) 273-8500
Fax: (303) 273-8450
E-mail: sedas@neis.cr.usgs.gov
Web site: http://www.neic.usgs.gov

National Eating Disorders Association
165 West 46th Street, Suite 402
New York, NY 10036
Phone: 1 (212) 575-6200
Fax: 1 (212) 575-1650
Web site: http://www.nationaleating
disorders.org/

National Environmental Education Foundation
4301 Connecticut Ave., Ste. 160
Washington, DC 20008
Phone: (202) 833-2933
Fax: (202) 261-6464
Web site: http://www.outdoor
foundation.org

National Environmental Health Association (NEHA)
720 S. Colorado Blvd., Suite 1000-N
Denver, CO 80246
Phone: (303) 756-9090
Toll free: (866) 956-2258
Fax: (303) 691-9490
E-mail: staff@neha.org
Web site: www.neha.org

National Eye Health Education Program, National Eye Institute
31 Center Dr., MSC 2510
Bethesda, MD 20892-2510
Phone: (301) 496-5248
E-mail: 2020@nei.nih.gov
Web site: http://www.nei.nih.gov

National Eye Institute
31 Center Dr., MSC 2510
Bethesda, MD 20892-2510
Phone: (301) 496-5248
Web site: http://www.nei.nih.gov

National Federation of the Blind
200 East Wells Street
Baltimore, MD 21230
Phone: (410) 659-9314
E-mail: nfb@nfb.org
Web site: http://www.nfb.org

National Foundation for Infectious Diseases (NFID)
4733 Bethesda Avenue, Suite 750
Bethesda, MD 20814
Phone: (301) 656-0003
Web site: http://www.nfid.org

National Glaucoma Research, American Health Assistance Foundation
22512 Gateway Center Drive
Clarksburg, MD 20871
Toll free: (800) 285-0080
E-mail: info@ahaf.org
Web site: http://www.ahaf.org
/glaucoma/

National Health Information Center. Office of Disease Prevention and Health Promotion. U.S. Department of Health and Human Services
P. O. Box 1133
Washington, DC 20013-1133
Phone: (847) 434-4000
Web site: http://www.health.gov/nhic/

National Health Service Corps (NHSC)
[no other contact information]
Toll free: (800) 221-9393
Web site: http://nhsc.hrsa.gov/

National Hearing Conservation Association
3030 W 81st Ave.
Westminster, CO 80031
Phone: (303) 224-9022
Fax: (303) 458-0002
E-mail: nhcaoffice@hearingconservation
.org
Web site: http://www.hearingconservation
.org

National Heart Lung and Blood Institute Health Information Center
PO Box 30105
Bethesda, MD 20824-0105
Phone: (301) 592-8573;
    TTY: (240) 629-3255
Fax: (240) 629-3246
E-mail: nhlbiinfo@nhlbi.nih.gov
Web site: http://www.nhlbi.nih.gov

National Highway Traffic Safety Administration
1200 New Jersey Avenue, SE
Washington, DC 20590
Phone: 1 (202) 366-9742
Fax: 1 (202) 366-6916
E-mail: Lori.Millen@dot.gob
Web site: www.distraction.gov

National Human Genome Research Institute (NHGRI)
Building 31, Room 4B09, 31 Center
Drive, MSC 2152, 9000
Rockville Pike
Bethesda, MD 20892-2152
Phone: (301) 402-0911
Fax: (301) 402-2218
Web site: http://www.genome.gov/

National Hurricane Center
11691 SW 17th St.
Miami, FL 33165
Phone: (305) 229-4404
E-mail: NHC.Public.Affairs@noaa.gov
Web site: http://www.nhc.noaa.gov

National Institute of Allergies and Infectious Diseases
6610 Rockledge Dr., MSC 6612
Bethesda, MD 20892-6612
Phone: (301) 496-5717
Fax: (301) 402-3573
Toll free: (866) 284-4107
E-mail: ocpostoffice@niaid.nih.gov
Web site: http://www.niaid.nih.gov

National Institute of Arthritis and Musculoskeletal and Skin Diseases (NIAMS)Information Clearinghouse
1 AMS Circle
Bethesda, MD 20892-3675
Phone: (301) 495-4484
Toll free: (877) 22-NIAMS (226-4267);
    TTY: (301) 565–2966
E-mail: NIAMSinfo@mail.nih.gov
Web site: http://www.niams.nih.gov

National Institute of Child Health and Human Development (NICHD)
P.O. Box 3006
Rockville, MD 30847
Toll free: (800) 370-2943,
    TTY: (800) 320-6942
Fax: (866) 760-5947
E-mail: NICHDInformationResource
Center@mail.nih.gov
Web site: http://www.nichd.nih.gov

National Institute of Dental and Craniofacial Research
31 Center Drive, MSC 2190,
    Building 31, Room 5B55
Bethesda, MD 20892-2190
Toll free: (866) 232-4528
E-mail: nidcrinfo@mail.nih.gov
Web site: http://www.nidcr.nih.gov/

National Institute of Diabetes and Digestive and Kidney Diseases
Office of Communications & Public
    Liaison, NIDDK, NIH Building 31,
    Rm. 9A06, 31 Center Dr.,
    MSC 2560
Bethesda, MD 20892-2560
Phone: (301) 496-3583
Web site: http://www2.niddk.nih.gov

National Institute of Environmental Health Science
PO Box 12233, MD K3-16
Research Triangle Park, NC 27709
Phone: (919) 541-1919
Fax: (919) 541-4395
Web site: http://www.niehs.nih.gov

National Institute of Mental Health
6001 Executive Blvd., Rm. 8184,
 MSC 9663
Bethesda, MD 20892-9663
Phone: (301) 443-4513
Toll free: (866) 615-6464
E-mail: nimhinfo@nih.gov
Web site: http:// www.nimh.nih.gov

National Institute of Neurological
 Disorders and Stroke (NINDS)
P.O. Box 5801
Bethesda, MD 20828
Phone: (301) 496-5751.
 TTY: (301) 468-5981
Toll free: (800) 352-9424
Web site: http://www.ninds.nih.gov

National Institute of Occupational
 Safety and Health, Centers for
 Disease Control and Prevention
1600 Clifton Rd.
Atlanta, GA 30333
Toll free: (800) 232-4636
E-mail: cdcinfo@cdc.gov
Web site: http://www.cdc.gov/niosh/

National Institute on Aging (NAI)
Bldg. 31, Rm. 5C27, 31 Center Dr.,
 MSC 2292
Bethesda, MD 20892
Phone: (301) 496-1752
Toll free: (800) 222-2225
Fax: (301) 496-1072
E-mail: niaic@nia.nih.gov
Web site: http://www.nia.nih.gov/

National Institute on Alcohol Abuse
 and Alcoholism (NIAAA)
5635 Fishers Lane, MSC 9304
Bethesda, MD 20892-9304
Phone: (301) 443-3860
Web site: http://www.niaaa.nih.gov

National Institute on Deafness and
 Other Communication Disorders
 (NIDCD)
31 Center Drive, MSC 2320
Bethesda, MD 20892-2320
Toll free: (800) 241-1044
Fax: (301) 770-8977
E-mail: nidcdinfo@nidcd.nih.gov
Web site: http://www.nidcd.nih.gov/
 index.asp

National Institute on Drug Abuse
 (NIDA)
6001 Executive Boulevard, Room 5213
Bethesda, Maryland 20892-9561
Phone: 1 (301) 443-1124
E-mail: information@nida.nih.gov
Web site: www.drugabuse.gov

National Institutes of Health
9000 Rockville Pike
Bethesda, MD 20892
Phone: (301) 496-4000

E-mail: NIHinfo@od.nih.gov
Web site: nih.gov

National Kidney Disease Education
 Program
3 Kidney Information Way
Bethesda, MD 20892
Toll free: (866) 4-KIDNEY (454-3639)
Fax: (301) 402-8182
E-mail: nkdep@info.niddk.nih.gov
Web site: http://www.nkdep.nih.gov

National Kidney Foundation
30 East 33rd St.
New York, NY 10016
Phone: (212) 889-2210
Toll free: (800) 622-9010
Fax: (212) 689-9261
Web site: http://www.kidney.org

National Law Center on
 Homelessness and Poverty
1411 K Street NW, Suite 1400
Washington, DC 20005
Phone: (202) 638-2535
Toll free: (202) 628-2737
Web site: http://www.nlchp.org/

National Lead Information Center
 (The)
422 S. Clinton Ave.
Rochester, NY 14620
Toll free: (800) 424-5323
Fax: (585) 232-3111
Web site: http://www.epa.gov/lead/
 pubs/nlic.htm

National Library of Medicine
Web site: http://www.nlm.nih.gov/
 medlineplus/medicaid.html

National Living Donor Assistance
 Center
2461 S. Clark Street, Suite 640
Arlington, VA 22202
Phone: (703) 414-1600
E-mail: NLDCA@livingdonor
 assistance.org
Web site: http://www.livingdonor
 assistance.org

National Meningitis Association
PO Box 725165
Atlanta, GA 31139
Phone: 1 (866) FONE-NMA (366-3662)
Fax: 1 (877) 703-6096
Web site: http://www.nmaus.org

National Necrotizing Fasciitis
 Foundation
2731 Porter SW
Grand Rapids, MI 49509
E-mail: nnfffeb@aol.com
Web site: http://www.nnff.org

National Network for Immunization
 Information
301 University Blvd.

Galveston, TX 77555-0350
Phone: (409) 772-0199
Fax: (409) 772-5208
E-mail: nnii@i4ph.org
Web site: http://www.
 immunizationinfo.org

National Oceanic and Atmospheric
 Administration
1401 Constitution Ave. NW, Rm. 5128
Washington, DC 20230
Web site: http://www.noaa.gov

National Office for Marine Biotoxins
 and Harmful Algal Blooms, Woods
 Hole Oceanographic Institution
Biology Dept., MS No. 32
Woods Hole, MA 02543
Phone: (508) 289-2252
Fax: (508) 457-2180
E-mail: jkleindinst@ whoi.edu
Web site: http://www.redtide
 .whoi.edu/hab

National Office of Public Health
 Genomics
1600 Clifton Rd.
Atlanta, GA 30333
Phone: (770) 488-8510
Toll free: (888) MODIMES (663–4637)
Fax: (770) 488-8355
E-mail: genetics@cdc.gov
Web site: http://www.cdc.gov/genomics

National Organization of State
 Alcohol/Drug Abuse Directors
1025 Connecticut Avenue NW, Suite
 605 Washington, DC 20036
Phone: (202) 293-0090

National Organization on Fetal
 Alcohol Syndrome (NOFAS)
900 17th St., NW, Suite 910
Washington, DC 20006
Phone: (202) 785-4585
Toll free: (800) 66-NOFAS
Fax: (202) 466-6456
Web site: http://www.nofas.org

National Park Conservation
 Association
777 6th St. NW, Ste. 700
Washington, DC 20001
Phone: (202) 223-6722
Toll free: (800) NAT-PARK
 (628-7275)
Fax: (202) 454-3333
E-mail: npca@npca.org
Web site: http://www.npca.org

National Park Foundation
1201 Eye St. NW, Ste. 550B
Washington, DC 20005
Phone: (202) 354-6460
Fax: (202) 371-2066
E-mail: ask-npf@nationalparks.org
Web site: http://www.nationalparks.org

National Pesticide Information Center, Oregon State University
333 Weniger Hall
Corvallis, OR 97331-6502
Toll free: (800) 858-7378
E-mail: npic@ace.orst.edu
Web site: http://npic.orst.edu

National Rural Health Association
1108 K Street NW, 2nd Floor
Washington DC 20005-4094
Phone: (202) 639-0550
Fax: (202) 639-0559
E-mail: dc@NRHArural.org
Web site: www.ruralhealthweb.com

National Safety Council
1121 Spring Lake Dr.
Itasca, IL 60143-3201
Phone: (630) 285-1121
Toll free: (800) 621-7615
E-mail: info@cetri.org
Web site: http://www.nsc.org/Pages
/Home.aspx

National Shingles Foundation
590 Madison Ave., 21st Floor
New York, NY 10022
Phone: (212) 222-3390
Fax: (212) 222-8627
Web site: http://www.vzvfoundation
.org

National Sleep Foundation
1010 North Glebe Rd., Suite 310
Arlington, VA 22201
Phone: (703) 243-1697
E-mail: nsf@sleepfoundation.org
Web site: http://www.sleepfoundation
.org

National Society of Genetic Counselors
401 N. Michigan Ave.
Chicago, IL 60611
Phone: (312) 321–6834
Fax: (312) 673–6972
E-mail: nsgc@nsgc.org
Web site: http://www.nsgc.org

National Solid Waste Management Association
4301 Connecticut Ave. NW, Ste. 300
Washington, DC 20008
Phone: (202) 244-4700
Toll free: (800) 424-2869
Fax: (202) 966-4824
Web site: http://www.environmentalist
severyday.org

National STD and AIDS Hotline
Toll free: (800) 227-8922

National Stroke Association (NSA)
9707 E. Easter Lane, Suite B
Centennial, CO 80112
Toll free: (800) STROKES

E-mail: info@stroke.org
Web site: http://www.stroke.org/site
/PageNavigator/HOME

National Suicide Prevention Lifeline
Toll free: (800) 274-TALK (8255)
Web site: http://www.
suicidepreventionlifeline.org

National Toxicology Program (National Institute of Environmental Health Sciences)
PO Box 12233
Research Triangle Park, NC 27709
Web site: http://ntp.niehs.nih.gov

National Vaccine Injury Compensation Program
Parklawn Building, Room 11C-26
5600 Fishers Lane
Rockville, MD 20857
Toll free: (800) 338-2382
Web site: http://www.hrsa.gov
/vaccinecompensation/index.html

National Vaccine Program Office. U.S. Dep. of Health & Human Services
200 Independence Ave. SW,
Rm. 715-H
Washington, DC 20201
Phone: (202) 690-5566
E-mail: nvpo@hhs.gov
Web site: http://www.hhs.gov/nvpo

National Wildfire Suppression Association
PO Box 330
Lyons, OR 97358
Toll free: (877) 676-6972
Fax: (866) 854-8186
Web site: http://www.nwsa.us

National Wildlife Federation
PO Box 1583
Merrifield, VA 22116-1583
Phone: 1 (703) 438-6000
Toll free: (800) 822-9919
Web site: http://www.nwf.org

Nature Conservancy (The)
4245 North Fairfax Dr., Ste. 100
Arlington, VA 22203-1606
Phone: (703) 841-5300
Toll free: (800) 628-6860
E-mail: member@tnc.org
Web site: http://www.nature.org

Noise Pollution Clearinghouse
P.O. Box 1137
Montpelier, VT 05601–1137
Toll free: (888) 200-8332
E-mail: http://www.nonoise.org/cgi-bin
/info-request.cgi
Web site: http://www.nonoise.org/

O

Obesity Prevention Center, University of Minnesota
1300 S Second St., Ste. 300
Minneapolis, MN 55454
Phone: (612) 625-6200
E-mail: umopc@epi.umn.edu
Web site: http://www.ahc.umn.edu/opc
/home.html

Obesity Society (The)
8757 Georgia Ave., Ste. 1320
Silver Spring, MD 20910
Phone: (301) 563-6526
Fax: (301) 563-6595
Web site: http://www.obesity.org
Web site: http://www.obesity.org
/resources-for/consumer.htm

Occupational Health & Safety Administration, U.S. Department of Labor
200 Constitution Ave.
Washington, DC 20210
Toll free: (800) 321-OSHA (6742)
Web site: http://www.osha.gov

Office for Human Research Protections (OHRP), Department of Health and Human Services (HHS)
1101 Wootton Parkway, Suite 200
Rockville, MD 20852
Phone: (240) 453-6900
Toll free: (866) 447-4777
Fax: (240) 453-6909
E-mail: OHRP@hhs.gov
Web site: http://www.hhs.gov/ohrp
/index.html

Office for Victims of Crime, U.S. Department of Justice
810 7th Street NW, 8th Floor
Washington, DC 20531
Phone: (202) 307-1034
Toll free: (800) 656-5983
Web site: http://www.ojp.usdoj.gov/ovc/

Office of Cancer Clinical Proteomics Research, Center for Strategic Scientific Initiatives, Office of the Director, National Cancer Institute
31 Center Drive, MS 2580
Bethesda, MD 20892-2580
Phone: 1 (301) 451-8883
E-mail: cancer.proteomics@mail.nih.gov
Web site: http://proteomics.cancer.gov

Office of Communications and Public Liaison, National Institute of Diabetes and Digestive and Kidney Diseases (NIDDKD)
31 Center Dr., MSC 2560, Bldg. 31,
Rm. 9A06

Bethesda, MD 20892–2560
Phone: 1 (301) 496-3583
E-mail: http://www2.niddk.nih.gov
/Footer/ContactNIDDK
Web site: http://www2.niddk.nih.gov/

**Office of Dietary Supplements,
National Institutes of Health**
6100 Executive Blvd., Rm. 3B01,
MSC 7517
Bethesda, MD 20892-7517
Phone: (301) 435-2920
Fax: (301) 480-1845
E-mail: ods@nih.gov
Web site: http://ods.od.nih.gov

**Office of Disease Prevention and
Health Promotion, U.S.
Department of Health and
Human Services**
1101 Wootton Pkwy., Suite LL100
Rockville, MD 20852
Phone: 1 (240) 453-8280
Fax: 1 (240) 453-8282
Web site: http://odphp.osophs.dhhs.gov/

**Office of Minority Health and
Health Disparities**
1600 Clifton Road
Atlanta, GA 30333
Toll free: 800-232-4636
Web site: http://www.cdc.gov/omhd/

Office of Minority Health
Post Office Box 37337
Washington, DC 20013-7337
Toll free: 800-444-6472
Web site: http://minorityhealth.hhs.gov/

**Office of Public Health Genomics,
Centers for Disease Control
and Prevention**
1600 Clifton Rd., N.E., MS E61
Atlanta, GA 30333
Phone: 1 (404) 498–0001
E-mail: genomics@cdc.gov
Web site: http://www.cdc.gov/genomics/

**Office of the Special Assistant for
Gulf War Illnesses**
Force Health Protection & Readiness
Policy & Programs Four Skyline
Place, 5113 Leesburg Pike, Ste. 901
Falls Church, VA 22041
Toll free: (800) 497-6261
Web site: http://www.gulflink.osd.mil

**Office of the United Nations High
Commissioner for Human
Rights**
Palais des Nations
Geneva, CH-1211
Phone: 41 22 917 9220
E-mail: InfoDesk@ohchr.org
Web site: http://www.ohchr.org

**Office on Women's Health, U.S.
Department of Health and
Human Services**
200 Independence Ave., S.W.
Washington, DC 20201
Phone: 1 (917) 637-3600
Web site: http://www.womenshealth.gov/

Olweus Bullying Prevention Program
Toll free: (800) 328-9000
E-mail: olweusinfo@hazelden.org
Web site: http://www.olweus.org
/public/index.page

Oncology Nursing Society
125 Enterprise Drive
Pittsburgh, Pennsylvania 25275
Phone: (866) 257-4667
Web site: http://www.ons.org

Optometric Glaucoma Society
3241 South Michigan Avenue
Chicago, IL 60616
Phone: (312) 949-7303
E-mail: mchaglas@ico.edu
Web site: http://www.optometricglaucom
asociety.org

Oral Cancer Foundation
3419 Via Lido # 205
Newport Beach, CA 92663
Toll free: (949) 646-8000
E-mail: info@oralcancerfoundation.org
Web site: http://www.oralcancer
foundation.org/

Outdoor Foundation
1776 Massachusetts Ave. NW, Ste. 450
Washington, DC 20036
Phone: (202) 271-3252
E-mail: info@outdoorfoundation.org
Web site: http://www.outdoor
foundation.org

Overeaters Anonymous
PO Box 44020
Rio Rancho, NM 87174
Phone: (505) 891-2664
Fax: (505) 891-4320
Web site: http://www.oa.org

Oxfam America
226 Causeway St., 5th Fl.
Boston, MA 02114-2206
Phone: (617) 482-121
Fax: (617) 728-2594
Toll free: (800) 77-OXFAM (776-9326)
Web site: http://www.oxfamamerica.org

Oxfam International Secretariat
266 Banbury Rd., Ste. 20
Oxford, OX2 7DL
Phone: 44 865 339 100
Fax: 44 865 339 101
Web site: http://www.oxfam.org

P

Pan American Health Organization
525 23rd St. NW
Washington, DC 20037
Phone: (202) 974-3000
Fax: (202) 974-3663
Web site: www.paho.org

Parents Anonymous
675 W. Foothill Blvd., Suite 220
Claremont, CA 91711-3475
Phone: (909) 621-6184
Fax: (909) 625-6304
Web site: http://www.parents
anonymous.org

**Parents, Families and Friends of
Lesbians and Gays (PFLAG)**
1828 L Street, NW, Suite 660
Washington, DC 20036
Phone: (202) 467-8180
E-mail: info@pflag.org
Web site: http://community.pflag.org

Partnership for a Drug-free America
405 Lexington Avenue, Ste 1601
New York, NY 10174
Phone: (212) 922-1560
Fax: (212) 922-1570
Web site: http://www.drugfree.org

**Partnership for Food Safety
Education**
2345 Crystal Dr., Ste. 800
Arlington, VA 22202
Phone: (202) 220-0651
Fax: (202) 220-0873
E-mail: info@fightbac.org
Web site: http://www.fightbac.org

**Pesticide Action Network North
America**
1611 Telegraph Ave., Ste. 1200
Oakland, CA 94612
Phone: (510) 788-9020
Web site: http://www.panna.org

**Planned Parenthood Federation of
America**
434 West 33rd Street
New York, NY 10001
Phone: (212) 541-7800
Web site: http://www.planned
parenthood.org/

Prevent Blindness America
211 West Wacker Drive, Suite 1700
Chicago, IL 60606
Toll free: (800) 331-2020
Web site: http://www.preventblindness
.org

Prevent Child Abuse America
500 North Michigan Avenue, Suite 200
Chicago, IL 60611-3703

Phone: (312) 663-3520
Toll free: 1-800-CHILDREN
Fax: (312) 939-8962
E-mail: mailbox@preventchildabuse.org
Web site: http://www.preventchild
abuse.org/index.shtml

Prevention Research Center in St. Louis (PRC-StL)
Washington University, 660 S. Euclid
Ave., Campus Box 8109
Saint Louis, MO 63110
Phone: (314) 362-9643
E-mail: prcstl@wustl.edu
Web site: http://prcstl.wustl.edu/Pages
/default.aspx

Project EAT, Eating Among Teens
University of Minnesota, 1300 S.
Second St., Suite 300
Minneapolis, MN 55454
Phone: (612) 624-1818
Web site: http://www.epi.umn.edu
/research/eat/index.shtm

Public Health Accreditation Board (PAHB)
1600 Duke St., Suite 440
Alexandria, VA 22314
Phone: (703) 778-4549
Fax: (703) 778-4556
E-mail: info@phaboard.org
Web site: http://www.phaboard.org/

Public Health Foundation (PHF)
1300 L St., Suite 800
Washington, DC 20005
Phone: (202) 218-4400
Fax: (202) 218-4409
E-mail: info@phf.org
Web site: www.phf.org

Pulmonary Fibrosis Association
811 W Evergreen Avenue, Suite 303
Chicago, IL 60642-2642
Toll free: (888) 733-6741
E-mail: info@pulmonaryfibrosis.org
Web site: http://www.pulmonary
fibrosis.org

R

Rape, Abuse, and Incest National Network
2000 L Street NW, Suite 406
Washington, DC 20036
Phone: (202) 544-1034
Toll free: (800) 656-4673
E-mail: info@rainn.org
Web site: http://www.rainn.org/

Research to Prevent Blindness
645 Madison Ave., Floor 21
New York, NY 10022-1010
Phone: (212) 752-4333

Toll free: (800) 621-0026
E-mail: inforequest@rpbusa.org
Web site: http://www.rpbusa.org

RESOLVE, The National Infertility Association
1760 Old Meadow Rd., Suite 500
McLean, VA 22102
Phone: (703) 556-7172
E-mail: info@resolve.org
Web site: http://www.resolve.org

Robert Wood Johnson Foundation
P.O. Box 2316, Route 1 and
College Road East
Princeton, NJ 08543
Toll free: (877) 843-RWJF
E-mail: http://pweb1.rwjf.org/global
/contactus.jsp
Web site: http://www.rwjf.org/

S

Save the Children (United Kingdom)
1 St. John's Lane
London, EC1M 4AR
Phone: 44 20 7012 6400
E-mail: supporter.care@savethe
children.org.uk
Web site: http://www.savethechildren
.org.uk

Save the Children (United States)
54 Wilton Rd.
Westport, CT 06880
Phone: (203) 221-4030
Toll free: (800) 728-3843
E-mail: twebster@savechildren.org
Web site: http://www.savethechildren.org

Shriners Hospitals for Children
2900 Rocky Point Drive
Tampa, FL 33607
Phone: (813) 281-0300
Web site: http://www.shrinershq.org
/Hospitals/Main

Sierra Club
85 Second St., 2nd Fl.
San Francisco, CA 94105
Phone: (415) 977-5500
Fax: (415) 977-5797
E-mail: information@sierraclub.org
Web site: http://www.sierraclub.org

Sierra Club Canada
412-1 Nicholas St.
Ottawa, K1N 7B7
Phone: 1 (613) 241-4611
Toll free: 1 (888) 810-4204
Web site: http://www.sierraclub.ca

Sight & Hearing Association (The)
1246 University Avenue West,
Suite 226

St. Paul, MN 55104-4125
Phone: (651) 645-2546
Toll free: (800) 992-0424
E-mail: mail@sightandhearing.org
Web site: http://www.sightandhearing
.org/

Skin Cancer Foundation
149 Madison Ave., Ste. 901
New York, NY 10016
Phone: (212) 725-5176
E-mail: http://www.skincancer.org
/contact-us
Web site: http://www.skincancer.org

Society for Public Health Education (SOPHE)
10 G St., N.W., Suite 605
Washington, DC 20002
Phone: (202) 408-9804
Fax: (202) 408-9815
E-mail: info@sophe.org
Web site: www.sophe.org

Society of Environmental Toxicology and Chemistry (Asia/Pacific/Latin and North America)
229 South Baylen St., 2nd Fl.
Pensacola, FL 32502
Phone: (850) 469-1500
Fax: (850) 469-9778
E-mail: setac@setac.org
Web site: http://www.setac.org

Society of Forensic Toxicologists (SOFT)
One MacDonald Center, 1 N.
MacDonald Street, Suite 15
Mesa, AZ 85201
Toll free: (888) 866-SOFT (7638)
E-mail: office@soft-tox.org
Web site: http://soft-tox.org/

STOP COMV—The CMV Action Network
P.O. Box 6221
Sunnyvale, CA 94088-2214
E-mail: email@stopcmv.org
Web site: http://www.stopcmv.org/

STOP Cyberbullying
Phone: (201) 463-8663
E-mail: parry@aftab.com
Web site: http://www.stopcyberbullying
.org/index2.html

STOP Foodborne Illness
3759 N Ravenswood, Ste. 224
Chicago, IL 60613
Phone: (773) 269-6555
Fax: (773) 883-3098
Toll free: (800) 350-STOP
Web site: http://www.
stopfoodborneillness.org

Substance Abuse and Mental Health Services Administration
1 Choke Cherry Rd.

Rockville, MD 20857
Toll free: (877) SAMHSA-7 (726-4727)
Fax: (240) 221-4292
E-mail: SAMHSAInfo@samhsa.hhs.gov
Web site: http://www.samhsa.gov

Superfund, TRI, EPCRA, RMP & Oil Information Center
Ariel Rios Bldg., 1200 Pennsylvania Ave. NW
Washington, DC 20460
Phone: (703) 412-9810
Toll free: (800) 424-9346
Web site: http://www.epa.gov/ superfund

T

Texas Department of Health Bioterrorism Preparedness Program (TDH)
1100 W 49th Street
Austin, TX 78756
Phone: (512) 458-7676
Toll free: (800) 705-8868
Web site: http://www.tdh.state.tx.us /bioterrorism/default.htm

U

U.S. Administration on Aging
1 Massachusetts Avenue NW
Washington, DC 20001
Phone: (202) 619-07240
E-mail: aoainfo@aoa.hhs.gov
Web site: http://www.aoa.gov

U.S. Department of Agriculture
1400 Independence Ave. SW, Rm. 1180
Washington, DC 20250
Phone: (202) 720-2791
Web site: http://www.usda.gov

U.S. Department of Health & Human Services
200 Independence Avenue, S.W.
Washington, DC 20201
Toll free: (877) 696-6775
Web site: www.hhs.gov

U.S. Department of Labor Occupational Safety and Health Administration (OSHA)
200 Constitution Avenue
Washington, DC 20210
Toll free: (800) 321-6742
Web site: http://www.osha.gov/

U.S. Department of Transportation
1200 New Jersey Avenue Southeast
Washington, DC 20590
Phone: 1 (202) 366-4542
Web site: www.dot.gov

U.S. Department of Veterans Affairs
810 Vermont Ave. NW
Washington, DC 20420
Toll free: (877) 222-8387
Web site: http://www.publichealth .va.gov

U.S. National Park Service
1849 C St. NW
Washington, DC 20240
Phone: (202) 208-3818
Web site: http://www.nps.gov

U.S. Public Health Service (USPHS)
5600 Fishers Lane
Rockville, MD 20857
Phone: (301) 427-3280
Fax: (301) 427-3431
E-mail: http://www.usphs.gov/main /contact.aspx
Web site: www.usphs.gov/

Undersea and Hyperbaric Medical Society
21 W Colony Place, Ste. 280
Durham, NC 27705
Phone: (919) 490-5140
Fax: (919) 490-5149
Toll free: (877) 533-UHMS (8467)
E-mail: uhms@uhms@org

UNICEF Headquarters
2 United Nations Plaza
New York, NY 10017
Phone: (212) 326-7000
Fax: (212) 887-7465
Web site: http://www.unicef.org

UNICEF Innocenti Research Centre
Piazza SS. Annunziata, 12 50122
Florence
Phone: 39 055 20330
Fax: 39 055 2033220
Web site: http://www.unicef-irc.org/

United Mine Workers of America (UMWA)
18354 Quantico Gateway Dr., Suite 200
Triangle, VA 22172-1179
Phone: (703) 291-2400
Web site: http://www.umwa.org/

United Nations Environment Programme Global Environment Facility
UNEP-GEF Biosafety Unit DEPI, UNEP
Nairobi
Phone: 254 (20) 7624066
E-mail: unepgef@unep.org
Web site: http://www.unep.org /biosafety

United Nations Foundation
1800 Massachusetts Ave. NW, Ste. 400
Washington, DC 20036
Phone: (202) 887-9040
Fax: (202) 887-9021

E-mail: inquiries@un.org
Web site: http://www.unfoundation.org

United Nations High Commissioner for Refugees
Case Postale 2500
CH-1211Genève 2 Dépôt
Phone: 41 22 739 8111
Fax: 41 22 739 7377
Web site: www.unhcr.org

United Nations Office on Drugs and Crime
PO Box 500
Vienna, A 1400
Phone: 43 (1) 26060
Fax: 43 (1) 263 3389
E-mail: info@unodc.org
Web site: https://www.unodc.org

United Nations Population Fund (UNFPA)
605 Third Avenue
New York, NY 10158
Phone: (212) 297-5000
E-mail: hq@unfpa.org
Web site: http://www.unfpa.org/

United Network for Organ Sharing
P.O. Box 2484
Richmond, VA 23218
Phone: (804) 782-4800
Web site: http://www.unos.org

United States Agency for International Development (USAID)
Office of the Administrator, Ronald Reagan Building, 1300 Pennsylvania Avenue, N.W.
Washington, DC 20523
Phone: (202) 712-4810
Fax: (202) 216-3524
E-mail: http://www.usaid.gov/comment
Web site: http://www.usaid.gov/

United States Consumer Products Safety Commission
4330 East West Highway
Bethesda, MD 20814
Phone: (301) 504-7923; TTY(301) 595-7054
Toll free: (800) 638-2772
Fax: Fax (301) 504-0124 and (301) 504-0025
Web site: http://www.cpsc.gov

United States Department of Agriculture (USDA)
1400 Independence Ave. SW
Washington, DC 20250
Phone: (202) 720-2791
Web site: http://www.usda.gov/wps /portal/usdahome

United States Department of Agriculture Food Safety and Inspection Service
1400 Independence Ave., S.W.

Washington, DC 20250
Phone: (402) 344 5000
Toll free: (800) 233 3935
Fax: (402) 344 5005
Web site: http://www.fsis.usda.gov

**United States Department
of Defense (DOD)**
1400 Defense Pentagon
Washington, DC 20301–1400
Phone: 1 (703) 571–3343
E-mail: http://www.defense.gov
/landing/comment.aspx
Web site: http://www.defense.gov/

**United States Department of Health
and Human Services**
200 Independence Avenue SW
Washington, DC 20201
Web site: http://www.hhs.gov

United States Department of Labor
Frances Perkins Building, 200
Constitution Avenue, N.W.
Washington, DC 20210
Toll free: (866) 487-9243
Web site: www.dol.gov

**United States Department of
Veterans Affairs (DVA)**
810 Vermont Ave., N.W.
Washington, DC 20420
E-mail: http://www.va.gov
/landing2_contact.htm
Web site: http://www.va.gov/

**United States Food and Drug
Administration (FDA)**
10903 New Hampshire Avenue
Silver Spring, MD 20993
Toll free: (888) INFO-FDA
(463-6332)
Web site: http://www.fda.gov

W

Water Environment Federation
601 Wythe St.
Alexandria, VA 22314-1994
Fax: (703) 684-2492

Toll free: (800) 666-0206
Web site: http://www.wef.org

Water Quality Association
4151 Naperville Road
Lisle, IL 60532
Phone: (630) 505-0160
Fax: (630) 505-9637
Web site: http://www.wqa.org

**Weight-Control Information
Network (WIN)**
1 WIN Way
Bethesda, MD 20892-3665
Phone: (202) 828-1025
Toll free: (877) 946-4627
Fax: (202) 828-1028
E-mail: win@http://win.niddk.nih.gov
Web site: http://win.niddk.nih.gov

Women, Infants, and Children
Supplemental Food Programs Division,
Food and Nutrition Service, USDA,
3101 Park Center Dr., Rm. 520
Alexandria, VA 22302
Phone: (202) 305-2746
Fax: (703) 305-2196
Web site: http://www.fns.usda.gov

Workplace Bullying Institute (WBI)
PO Box 29915
Bellingham, WA 98228
Web site: http://www.workplace
bullying.org

World Food Programme (WFP)
Via C. G. Viola 68, Parco dei Medici
Rome 00148
Phone: 06 65131
Fax: 06 6590632
E-mail: http://www.wfp.org/contact
Web site: http://www.wfp.org/

World Health Organization (WHO)
Avenue Appia 20
1211 Geneva 27
Phone: 22 41 791 21 11
Fax: 22 41 791 31 11
E-mail: info@who.int
Web site: http://www.who.int

World Health Organization Europe
Scherfigsvej 8, DK-2100

Copenhagen
Phone: 45 391-1717
E-mail: infohcp@euro.who.int
Web site: http://www.euro.who.int/en/home

**World Health Organization, Tobacco
Free Initiative (WHO TFI)**
Avenue Appia 20 1211
Geneva, 27
Phone: 41 22 791 2126
Fax: 41 22 791 4832
E-mail: tfi@who.int
Web site: www.who.int/tobacco/

World Medical Association
13, ch. Du Levant
Ferney-Voltaire, 01210
Phone: 4 (50) 40 75 75
Fax: 4 (50) 40 59 37
E-mail: wma@wma.net
Web site: http://www.wma.net/en/

**World Organization for Animal
Health (OIE)**
12, rue de Prony
Paris, 75017
E-mail: oie@oie.int
Web site: http://www.oie.int

**World Organization of Volcano
Observatories**
903 Koyukuk Dr.
Fairbanks, AK 99775
Phone: (907) 474-1542
Fax: (907) 474-7290
E-mail: wovo.iavcei@gmail.com
Web site: http://www.wovo.org

**World Recreation Association
of the Deaf**
Post Office Box 3211
Quartz Hill, CA 93586
Phone: (661) 952-7752
Web site: http://www.wrad.org/

Z

Zero Population Growth
1400 16th Street NW, Suite 320
Washington, DC 20036

GLOSSARY

The glossary is an alphabetical compilation of terms and definitions listed in the *Key Terms* sections of the main body entries. Although the list is comprehensive, it is by no means exhaustive.

A

ABLATIVE. Also known as "ablation" and referring to the surgical removal of lesions associated with HPV.

ABSCESS. An area of inflamed and injured body tissue that fills with pus.

ABSTINENCE. Intentional refraining from some or all forms of sexual activity.

ACAMPROSATE. An anti-craving medication used to reduce the craving for alcohol.

ACETYLCHOLINE. A chemical called a neurotransmitter that functions to excite nerve cells.

ACETYLCHOLINESTERASE. An enzyme that breaks down acetylcholine.

ACHALASIA. An esophageal disease of unknown cause, in which the lower sphincter or muscle is unable to relax normally, and leads to the accumulation of material within the esophagus.

ACQUIRED IMMUNE DEFICIENCY SYNDROME (AIDS). HIV infection that has led to certain opportunistic infections, cancers, or a CD4+ T-lymphocyte (helper cell) blood cell count lower than 200/mL.

ACTIVE IMMUNIZATION. Treatment that provides immunity by challenging an individual's own immune system to produce antibodies against a particular organism, in this case the rabies virus.

ACUTE PAIN. Pain in response to injury or another stimulus that resolves when the injury heals or the stimulus is removed.

ACUTE RESPIRATORY DISTRESS SYNDROME. A serious reaction to various forms of injuries to the lung, which is characterized by inflammation of the lung, leading to impaired gas exchange and release of inflammatory mediators causing inflammation and low blood oxygen and frequently resulting in multiple organ failure. This condition is life threatening and often lethal, usually requiring mechanical ventilation and admission to an intensive care unit.

ACUTE RETROVIRAL SYNDROME (ARS). A syndrome that develops in about 30% of HIV patients within a few weeks of infection. ARS is characterized by nausea, vomiting, fever, headache, general tiredness, and muscle cramps.

ACUTE TOXICITY. Health problems that occur shortly after exposure and last a relatively short period of time.

ACYCLOVIR. An antiviral drug that is available in oral, intravenous, and topical forms and that blocks replication of the varicella zoster virus.

ADDICTION. The state of being both physically and psychologically dependent on a substance.

ADDICTIVE PERSONALITY. The concept that addiction is the result of pre-existing character defects.

ADENOSINE. A nucleoside that plays multiple physiological roles in energy transfer and molecular signaling, as a component of RNA, and as an inhibitory neurotransmitter that promotes sleep.

ADIPOSE TISSUE. Fat tissue.

ADJUSTMENT DISORDER. A psychiatric disorder marked by inappropriate or inadequate responses to a change in life circumstances. Depression following retirement from work is an example of adjustment disorder.

AEROBIC EXERCISE. Any exercise that increases the body's oxygen consumption and improves the functioning of the cardiovascular and respiratory systems.

AGGRAVATED SEXUAL ABUSE. Sexual acts forced upon an individual by use of physical force; threats of death, injury, or kidnapping; or substances that render that individual unconscious or impaired.

AIDS DEMENTIA COMPLEX. A type of brain dysfunction caused by HIV infection that causes difficulty thinking, confusion, and loss of muscular coordination.

ALCOHOL USE DISORDERS INVENTORY TEST (AUDIT). A test for alcohol use developed by the World Health Organization (WHO). Its ten questions address three specific areas of drinking over a 12-month period: the amount and frequency of drinking, dependence upon alcohol, and problems that have been encountered due to drinking alcohol.

ALLERGEN. A foreign substance, such as mites in house dust or animal dander which, when inhaled, causes the airways to narrow and produces symptoms of asthma.

ALLERGENIC. Acting as an allergen or inducing an allergic response.

ALLERGIC RHINITIS. Inflammation of the mucous membranes of the nose and eyes in response to an allergen. Hay fever is seasonal allergic rhinitis.

ALPHA-FETOPROTEIN. A substance produced by a fetus' liver that can be found in the amniotic fluid and in the mother's blood. Abnormally high levels of this substance suggests there may be defects in the fetal neural tube, a structure that will include the brain and spinal cord when completely developed. Abnormally low levels suggest the possibility of Down syndrome.

ALVEOLI. The little air sacs clustered at the ends of the bronchioles, in which oxygen-carbon dioxide exchange takes place.

ALZHEIMER'S DISEASE. A condition causing a decline in brain function that interferes with the ability to reason and to perform daily activities.

AMBIENT CONDITIONS. Conditions in the surrounding environment.

AMBLYOPIA. Decreased visual acuity, usually in one eye, in the absence of any structural abnormality in the eye.

AMEBOMA. A mass of tissue that can develop on the wall of the colon in response to amebic infection.

AMINO ACIDS. Complex molecules that form proteins. There are 20 different common types of amino acids that join to form proteins. A diet must include a minimum number of amino acids to keep a person healthy.

AMNESIA. A loss of memory that may be caused by brain injury, such as concussion.

AMPLITUDE. A measure of the amount of energy carried by a wave.

ANAEROBIC. Occurring or growing in the absence of oxygen.

ANAEROBIC BACTERIA. Bacteria that grow and reproduce in an oxygen-free environment, such as the bacterium that causes tetanus.

ANAPHYLAXIS. Severe, potentially fatal hypersensitivity caused by previous exposure to an allergen that can result in blood vessel dilation and a sharp drop in blood pressure, smooth muscle contraction, and difficulty breathing.

ANEMIA. Red blood cell deficiency.

ANENCEPHALY. A birth defect in which the baby is born without a forebrain and with part of the skull and scalp missing. Babies with this defect either are stillborn or die shortly after birth.

ANEURYSM. A pouch-like bulging of a blood vessel. Aneurysms can rupture, leading to stroke.

ANGINA. Chest pain.

ANGIOEDEMA. Severe non-inflammatory swelling of the skin, organs, and brain, possibly accompanied by fever and muscle pain.

ANGIOGRAM. An x-ray image of one or more blood vessels.

ANGIOPLASTY. A surgical operation to clear a narrowed or blocked artery.

ANTHELMINTHIC (ALSO SPELLED ANTHELMINTIC). A type of drug or herbal preparation given to destroy parasitic worms or expel them from the body.

ANTHRAX. A disease of warm blooded animals, particularly cattle and sheep, transmissible to humans. The disease causes severe skin and lung damage.

ANTI-ANDROGEN. A substance that inhibits the body's reception of any of the androgen hormones, such as testosterone.

ANTI-MOTILITY MEDICATIONS. Medications such as loperamide (Imodium), dephenoxylate (Lomotil), or medications containing codeine or narcotics which decrease the ability of the intestine to contract. This can worsen the condition of a patient with dysentery or colitis.

ANTIBIOTIC. A substance, such as a drug, that can stop bacteria from growing, or destroy the bacteria.

ANTIBIOTIC RESISTANCE. The ability of infectious agents to change their biochemistry in such a way as to make an antibiotic no longer effective.

ANTIBODY. Specialized cells of the immune system that can recognize organisms that invade the body (such as bacteria, viruses, and fungi). The antibodies are then able to set off a complex chain of events designed to kill these foreign invaders.

ANTIDEPRESSANTS. A type of medication that is used to treat depression; it is also sometimes used to treat autism.

ANTIDOTE. A medication or remedy for counteracting the effects of a poison.

ANTIEMETIC. A type of drug given to control nausea and vomiting.

ANTIGEN. A foreign protein or particle that causes the body to produce specific antibodies that bind to it.

ANTIGENS. Markers on the outside of such organisms as bacteria and viruses, which allow antibodies to recognize foreign invaders.

ANTIMICROBIAL. A general term for any drug that is effective against disease organisms, including bacteria, viruses, fungi, and parasites. Antibiotics, which are used to treat bacterial infections, are one type of antimicrobial.

ANTIMICROBIAL AGENTS. A general term for drugs that kill or inhibit the growth of microbes.

ANTIOXIDANT. Any substance that reduces the damage caused by oxidation, such as the harm caused by free radicals.

ANTIOXIDANTS. A class of biochemicals that have been found to protect cells from free-radical damage.

ANTISEPTIC AGENT. Any substance that inactivates microorganisms or inhibits their growth on living tissues.

ANTISEPTIC HANDRUBBING. Cleaning the hands with any antiseptic agent that does not require the use of water or a drying cloth.

ANTISEPTIC HANDWASHING. Washing the hands with soap and water, or other detergents containing an antiseptic agent.

ANTITOXIN. An antibody that neutralizes a toxin.

ANXIETY. Worry or tension in response to real or imagined stress, danger, or dreaded situations. Physical reactions, such as fast pulse, sweating, trembling, fatigue, and weakness may accompany anxiety.

APNEA. The transient cessation of breathing.

APPENDICITIS. Condition characterized by the rapid inflammation of the appendix, a part of the intestine.

APPETITE SUPPRESSANT. A drug that reduces appetite.

ARACHNOID MATER. The middle layer of the meninges.

ARRHYTHMIA. Any of a number of conditions in which there is abnormal electrical activity in the heart. Some arrhythmias are minor, while others are

potentially life-threatening. They are also called "cardiac dysrhythmias."

ARTEMINISININS. A family of antimalarial products derived from an ancient Chinese herbal remedy. Two of the most popular varieties are artemether and artesunate, used mainly in Southeast Asia in combination with mefloquine.

ASBESTOS. Asbestos is the commercial name, not a mineralogical term, given to a variety of six naturally occurring fibrous minerals that have been mined for wide use because of their heat resistance and chemical resistance properties. These minerals possess high tensile strength, flexibility, resistance to chemical and thermal degradation, and electrical resistance. These minerals have been used for decades in more than 3,000 types of commercial products, such as insulation and fireproofing materials, automotive brakes, textile products, and cement and wallboard materials. Asbestos has been classified as a known human carcinogen by the U.S. Department of Health and Human Services, the EPA, and the International Agency for Research on Cancer.

ASCITES. The condition that occurs when the liver and kidneys are not functioning properly and a clear, straw-colored fluid is excreted by the membrane that lines the abdominal cavity (peritoneum).

ASCORBIC ACID. Another term for vitamin C, a nutrient found in fresh fruits and vegetables. Good sources of vitamin C in the diet are citrus fruits like oranges, lemons, limes, grapefruits, berries, tomatoes, green peppers, cabbage, broccoli, and spinach.

ASEPTIC. Sterile; containing no microorganisms, especially no bacteria.

ASEPTIC MENINGITIS. A term that is sometimes used for meningitis that is not caused by bacteria.

ASEXUALITY. Lack of interest in sexual activity or lack of sexual attraction to others. It should not be confused with abstinence, which is a behavioral choice.

ASPERGER SYNDROME. Children who have autistic behavior but no problems with language and no clinically significant cognitive delay.

ASPIRATION. A situation in which solids or liquids which should be swallowed into the stomach are instead breathed into the respiratory system.

ASSERTIVE COMMUNITY TREATMENT (ACT). A service-delivery model for providing comprehensive, highly individualized, locally based treatment directly to patients with serious, persistent mental illnesses.

ASSISTED SUICIDE. A form of self-inflicted death in which individuals voluntarily bring about their own death with the help of another, usually a physician, relative, or friend. Assisted suicide is sometimes called physician-assisted death (PAD).

ASTHMA. A lung condition, usually of allergic origin, in which the airways become narrow due to smooth muscle contraction, causing wheezing, coughing, and shortness of breath.

ASTM. ASTM International, previously the American Society for Testing and Materials, develops standards for product quality and safety.

ASYMPTOMATIC. Persons who carry a disease and are usually capable of transmitting the disease but who do not exhibit symptoms of the disease are said to be asymptomatic.

ATHEROSCLEROSIS. A buildup of plaque in the arteries, also called hardening of the arteries.

ATOPIC DERMATITIS. A skin condition resulting from exposure to airborne or food allergens.

ATOPY. Genetic predisposition toward the development of allergies.

ATRESIA. A condition in which a body orifice or passage is abnormally closed or absent. In esophageal atresia, the esophagus is closed before it reaches the stomach.

ATRIAL FIBRILLATION. A disorder of the heartbeat associated with a higher risk of stroke. In this disorder, the upper chambers (atria) of the heart do not completely empty when the heart beats, which can allow blood clots to form.

AUTOMATED EXTERNAL DEFIBRILLATOR (AED). A portable electronic device that automatically diagnoses potentially life-threatening cardiac arrhythmias (ventricular fibrillation and ventricular tachycardia) and is able to treat them through defibrillation.

AUTOSOMAL DISEASE. A disease caused by a gene mutation located on a chromosome other than a sex chromosome.

AUTOSOMAL DOMINANT INHERITANCE. A pattern of inheritance in which a trait will be expressed if the gene is inherited from either parent.

AVIAN CHLAMYDIOSIS. An illness in pet birds and poultry caused by *Chlamydia psittaci*. It is also known as parrot fever in birds.

AVIAN INFLUENZA. Influenza A virus usually found in birds, but transmitted to humans.

B

B CELL. A type of white blood cell produced in the bone marrow that makes antibodies against viruses.

B-COMPLEX VITAMINS. a group of water-soluble vitamins that often work together in the body. These include thiamine (B_1), riboflavin (B_2), niacin (B_3), pantothenic acid (B_5), pyridoxine (B_6), biotin (B_7 or vitamin H), folate/folic acid (B_9), and cobalamin (B_{12}).

BABESIOSIS. A disease caused by protozoa of the genus *Babesia* characterized by a malaria-like fever, anemia, vomiting, muscle pain, and enlargement of the spleen. Babesiosis, like Lyme disease, is carried by a tick.

BACILLE CALMETTE-GUÉRIN (BCG). Vaccine that protects from tuberculosis, derived from weakened live bovine tuberculosis bacillus.

BACILLUS. A rod-shaped bacterium. The organism that causes cholera is a gram-negative bacillus.

BACILLUS CALMETTE-GUÉRIN (BCG). A vaccine made from a weakened bacillus similar to the tubercle bacillus that may help prevent serious pulmonary TB and its complications.

BACTEREMIA. The presence of bacteria in the bloodstream.

BACTERIA. Tiny, one-celled forms of life that cause many diseases and infections.

BACTERICIDAL. A state that prevents growth of bacteria.

BACTERIOPHAGE. A type of virus that can be used to treat bacterial infections. Bacteriophages (or simply phages) work by injecting their own genetic material into bacteria and forcing the bacteria to produce new virus particles rather than a new generation of bacteria.

BACTERIOSTATIC. A substance that kills bacteria.

BARIATRICS. The branch of medicine that deals with the prevention and treatment of obesity and related disorders.

BASE PAIR. A pair of two nitrogen bases, such as adenine and thymine or guanine and cytosine.

BEHAVIORAL THERAPY. Form of psychotherapy used to treat depression, anxiety disorders, phobias, and other forms of psychopathology.

BELL'S PALSY. Facial paralysis or weakness with a sudden onset, caused by swelling or inflammation of the seventh cranial nerve, which controls the facial muscles.

Disseminated Lyme disease sometimes causes Bell's palsy.

BENIGN. Mild, nonmalignant. Recovery is favorable with treatment.

BENZODIAZEPINES. A class of drugs that have a hypnotic and sedative action, used mainly as tranquilizers to control symptoms of anxiety.

BETA-BLOCKER. A drug that blocks some of the effects of fight-or-flight hormone adrenaline (epinephrine and norepinephrine), slowing the heart rate and lowering the blood pressure.

BEVEL. The flat aperture on one side of a needle at the tip.

BILE. A yellow-green fluid secreted by the liver that aids in the digestion of fats.

BILIRUBIN. A reddish-yellow bile pigment made by the liver.

BINGE DRINKING. Consumption of five or more alcoholic drinks in a row on a single occasion.

BINGE-EATING DISORDER. A condition characterized by uncontrolled eating.

BIOACCUMULATION. The absorption and buildup of a toxic substance within the tissues of an organism. Bioaccumulation can move up the food chain when one animal feeds on another contaminated by the toxin and is in turn consumed by a larger predator.

BIODIVERSITY. The extent of the variety of life forms within a given ecosystem. Biodiversity is an important measurement of the health of an ecosystem.

BIOFEEDBACK. A technique in which patients learn to modify certain body functions, such as temperature or pulse rate, with the help of a monitoring machine.

BIOGAS. Gas produced by the decay of organic matter in the absence of oxygen. Sources of biogas include sewage, manure, landfills, swamps, marshes, and animal manure.

BIOHAZARDOUS. Describes biological agents or conditions and materials that pose potential hazards or harms to people and the environment.

BIOMONITORING. A method for detecting the presence and amount of environmental chemicals in the human body, usually obtained from blood or urine samples. It is a more accurate measure of the effects of chemical exposure on human health than simply measuring the levels of chemicals in soil, air, water, or food.

BIOPSY. The surgical removal and microscopic examination of living tissue for diagnostic purposes.

BIOSTATISTICS. The branch of statistics that focuses on the collection and analysis of biological and medical data.

BIOTERRORISM. The intentional use of disease-causing microbes or other biologic agents to intimidate or terrorize a civilian population for political or military reasons.

BIOTINIDASE DEFICIENCY. An inherited metabolic disorder in which biotin (vitamin B_7 is not released from proteins in the diet during digestion, leading to a deficiency of this vitamin.

BIOTOXIN. Any toxin produced by a living organism.

BIOTYPE. A variant strain of a bacterial species with distinctive physiological characteristics.

BIPOLAR DISORDER. Formerly called manic-depressive disorder. A mood disorder characterized by alternating periods of overconfidence and activity (manic highs) and depressive lows.

BLACK DEATH. Also known as The Plague, the Black Death is a bacterial infection that caused millions of deaths in Europe during the 14th century.

BLASTOCYST. A cluster of cells representing multiple cell divisions that have occurred in the Fallopian tube after successful fertilization of an ovum by a sperm. This is the developmental form which must leave the Fallopian tube, enter the uterus, and implant itself in the uterus to achieve actual pregnancy.

BLOOD-BRAIN BARRIER. A specialized, semi-permeable layer of cells around the blood vessels in the brain that controls which substances can leave the circulatory system and enter the brain.

BODY MASS INDEX (BMI). Also known as BMI, the index determines whether a person is at a healthy weight, underweight, overweight, or obese. The BMI can be calculated by converting the person's height into inches. That amount is multiplied by itself and then divided by the person's weight. That number is then multiplied by 703. The metric formula for the BMI is the weight in kilograms divided by the square of height in meters.

BONE MARROW. Spongy material that fills the inner cavities of the bones. The progenitors of all the blood cells are produced in this bone marrow.

BORDATELLA PERTUSSIS. A bacterium that causes whooping cough by attaching itself to cells in the respiratory tract.

BOTULISM. A life-threatening paralytic illness from food contaminated with botulinum toxin from the bacterium *Clostridium botulinum*.

BOVINE SPONGIFORM ENCEPHALOPATHY. Also known as Mad Cow disease, a progressive, fatal disease of the nervous system of domestic animals that is transmitted by eating infected food.

BRAIN STEM. The posterior portion of the brain that connects directly to the spinal cord. It regulates breathing, heart function, and the sleep-wake cycle as well as maintaining consciousness.

BRAXTON HICKS' CONTRACTIONS. Short, fairly painless uterine contractions during pregnancy that may be mistaken for labor pains. They allow the uterus to grow and help circulate blood through the uterine blood vessels.

BRONCHIAL TUBES. The major airways to the lungs and their main branches.

BRONCHITIS. Inflammation of the mucous membrane of the bronchial tubes of the lung that can make it difficult to breathe.

BRONCHOSCOPY. The examination of the bronchi (the main airways of the lungs) using a flexible tube (bronchoscope). Bronchoscopy helps to evaluate and diagnose lung problems, assess blockages, obtain samples of tissue and/or fluid, and/or to help remove a foreign body.

BROWNFIELD. A term used to describe previously used or underused commercial or industrial buildings that are contaminated by sufficiently low levels of pollutants that they can be reused after being cleaned up.

BUBO. A swollen lymph node resulting from an infection. Buboes are characteristic of bubonic plague but may also occur in syphilis, tuberculosis, or gonorrhea. The English word is derived from the Greek word for groin, which is the most common location for buboes to appear.

BULLYCIDE. Suicide attributed to the victim's having been bullied.

BULLYING. A repeated verbal or physical attack by one person on another person, most commonly among children and adolescents.

BURDEN OF DISEASE. A measure of the impact of disease as measured by mortality, morbidity, financial cost, or other measures.

BURNOUT. An emotional condition, marked by fatigue, loss of interest, or frustration, that interferes with job performance. Burnout is usually regarded as the result of prolonged work-related stress.

C

CAGE. A four-question assessment for the presence of alcoholism in both adults and children.

CALCIUM CHANNEL BLOCKER. A drug that blocks the entry of calcium into the muscle cells of small blood vessels (arterioles) and keeps them from narrowing.

CALICIVIRUS. A member of the Caliciviridae family of viruses that includes noroviruses.

CALORIE. A unit of food energy.

CAMPYLOBACTER. A genus of bacteria that is found in almost all raw poultry and that can contaminate food and cause illness.

CANNABINOID. Any one of a class of compounds that stimulate the cannabinoid receptor sites in the human body. In humans, cannabinoid receptors primarily affect the nervous system—including the brain, spinal cord, and peripheral nerves—and the immune system—which helps the body fight disease and infection. Cannabinoids are separated into three classifications: endocannabinoids (which are produced naturally within the body); phytocannabinoids (which are found in plants) including tetrahydrocannabinol (THC), the psychoactive component of cannabis; and synthetic cannabinoids (which are manufactured in a laboratory).

CAPITAL IMPROVEMENTS. Major improvements to an organization, such as addition of facilities and upgraded equipment.

CAPSAICIN. An active ingredient from hot chili peppers that is used in topical ointments to relieve pain. It appears to work by reducing the levels of a chemical substance involved in transmitting pain signals from nerve endings to the brain.

CAPSID. The outer protein coat of a virus.

CAR BED. A type of car seat, most commonly used for infants born prematurely. A car bed allows the child to be securely fastened while lying down as opposed to being in a seated position. As a result of frequently having underdeveloped respiratory systems, many premature babies have serious difficulty breathing in a traditional seated car seat.

CARBOHYDRATE. A class of nutrients that includes sugars, starches, celluloses, and gums, which are a major source of calories from foods.

CARBON MONOXIDE. With the chemical formula CO (where C stands for carbon, and O for oxygen), a colorless, odorless, and tasteless gas that is toxic to humans in higher than normal concentrations.

CARBOXYHEMOGLOBIN (COHB). Hemoglobin that is bound to carbon monoxide instead of oxygen.

CARCINOGEN. A substance that causes or increases the risk of cancer in human or animals.

CARCINOGENIC. Having a tendency to cause cancer.

CARDIAC ARREST. A condition in which the heart stops functioning. Fibrillation can lead to cardiac arrest if not corrected quickly.

CARRIER. An individual who possesses a genetic mutation associated with a recessive disorder, but who usually does not display symptoms of that disease. Carriers can pass the mutation on to their offspring.

CARRIER STATE. The continued presence of an organism (bacteria, virus, or parasite) in the body that does not cause symptoms but is able to be transmitted and infect other persons.

CATECHOLAMINES. Hormones and neurotransmitters including dopamine, epinephrine, and norepinephrine.

CATEGORICALLY NEEDY. A term that describes certain groups of Medicaid recipients who qualify for the basic mandatory package of Medicaid benefits. There are categorically needy groups whom states participating in Medicaid are required to cover, and other groups whom the states have the option to cover.

CATHETERIZATION. Inserting a tube into the bladder so that a patient can urinate without leaving the bed.

CAUSATIVE AGENT. An organism that causes a disease.

CD4. A type of protein molecule in human blood. The HIV virus infects cells with CD4 surface proteins and, as a result, depletes the number of T cells, B cells, natural killer cells, and monocytes in the patient's blood.

CD4 COUNT. A measure of the strength of the immune system. HIV continually kills CD4 cells. Over time, the body can not replace these lost CD4 cells and their number declines. AS this happens, the body becomes more susceptible to infections. A normal CD4 count is 1000. The body starts to get more frequent common infections at around a count of 400. At around a CD4 count of 200, the body becomes susceptible to many unusual infections. It is best to start medications for HIV before the CD4 count drops below 200 to prevent these infections from developing.

CELIAC DISEASE. A condition in children and adults where the body is unable to tolerate wheat protein (gluten).

CENTRAL NERVOUS SYSTEM (CNS). Part of the nervous system consisting of the brain, cranial nerves, and spinal cord. The brain is the center of higher processes, such as thought and emotion, and is responsible for the coordination and control of bodily activities and the interpretation of information from the senses. The cranial nerves and spinal cord link the brain to the peripheral nervous system, that is the nerves present in the rest of body.

CEPHALOSPORINS. A class of beta-lactam antibiotics originally derived from the fungus *Acrimonium*, which was previously called *Cephalosporium*.

CERCARIAE. The free-living form of the schistosome worm that has a tail, swims, and has suckers on its head for penetration into a host.

CEREBRAL EMBOLISM. A blockage of blood flow through a vessel in the brain by a blood clot that formed elsewhere in the body and traveled to the brain.

CEREBRAL THROMBOSIS. A blockage of blood flow through a vessel in the brain by a blood clot that formed in the brain itself.

CEREBROSPINAL FLUID (CSF). Fluid made in chambers within the brain which then flows over the surface of the brain and spinal cord. CSF provides nutrition to cells of the nervous system, as well as providing a cushion for the structures of the central nervous system.

CEREBROSPINAL FLUID ANALYSIS. A analysis that is important in diagnosing diseases of the central nervous system. The fluid within the spine will indicate the presence of viruses, bacteria, and blood. Infections such as encephalitis will be indicated by an increase of cell count and total protein in the fluid.

CERVICAL INTRA-EPITHELIAL NEOPLASIA (CIN). A precancerous condition in which a group of cells grow abnormally on the cervix but do not extend into the deeper layers of this tissue.

CERVIX. Narrow, lower end of the uterus forming the opening to the vagina.

CHANCRE. An open sore with a firm or hard base that is the initial skin ulcer of primary syphilis.

CHELATION THERAPY. The use of such chemicals as BAL (British Anti-Lewisite) or EDTA in conventional medicine to treat heavy metal poisoning. Some practitioners of alternative medicine use these chemicals to remove toxins in general from the body or to treat autism and heart disease.

CHEMOTHERAPY. Treatment with certain anticancer drugs.

CHICKENPOX. A mild disease common in childhood that is caused by a poxvirus; infection can have serious results in adults.

CHILD DEVELOPMENT. The process of physical, intellectual, emotional, and social growth that occurs from infancy through adolescence. Erik Erikson, Margaret Mahler, Sigmund Freud, and Jean Piaget are among the best known child development theorists.

CHILD LABOR TAX LAW. Passed by Congress in 1919, this law put an excise tax on companies that employed children younger than 14 years of age, or those between 14 and 16 years of age who worked more than eight hours per day or more than six days per week. The Supreme Court declared this law unconstitutional in 1922.

CHLAMYDIA. A microorganism that resembles certain types of bacteria and causes several sexually transmitted diseases in humans.

CHLAMYDIA PSITTACI. An organism related to bacteria that infects some types of birds and can be transmitted to humans to cause parrot fever.

CHLAMYDIOSIS, PSITTACOSIS, OR ORNITHOSIS. Other names for parrot fever in humans.

CHLOASMA. A skin discoloration common during pregnancy, also known as the "mask of pregnancy" or melasma, in which blotches of pale brown skin appear on the face. It is usually caused by hormonal changes. The blotches may appear in the forehead, cheeks, and nose, and may merge into one dark mask. It usually fades gradually after pregnancy, but it may become permanent or recur with subsequent pregnancies. Some women may also find that the line running from the top to the bottom of their abdomen darkens. This is called the linea nigra.

CHLORACNE. A skin eruption of blackheads, cysts, and acne-like pustules, most often caused by exposure to toxic chemicals.

CHLOROQUINE. An antimalarial drug that began being used in the 1940s and stopped being used after evidence of quinine resistance appeared in the 1960s. In the early 2000s, it was considered ineffective against falciparum malaria almost everywhere. However, because it is inexpensive, it continued to be still the antimalarial drug most widely in Africa. Native individuals with partial immunity may have better results with chloroquine than travelers with no previous exposure.

CHOLERA. An infection of the small intestine caused by a type of bacterium. The disease is spread by drinking water or eating seafood or other foods that have been contaminated with the feces of infected people. It occurs in parts of Asia, Africa, Latin America, India, and the Middle East. Symptoms include watery diarrhea and exhaustion and are often fatal to young children and the elderly.

CHOLESTEROL. A fat-soluble steroid alcohol (sterol) found in animal fats and oils, and produced in the body from saturated fats. Cholesterol is required to produce vitamin D and various hormones and for the formation of cell membranes. High cholesterol levels contribute to the development of atherosclerosis.

CHRONIC. Disease or condition characterized by slow onset over a long period of time.

CHRONIC OBSTRUCTIVE PULMONARY DISEASE (COPD). Chronic obstructive pulmonary disease (COPD) is a progressive disease that makes it hard to breathe. COPD can cause coughing that produces large amounts of mucus (a slimy substance), wheezing, shortness of breath, chest tightness, and other symptoms. Cigarette smoking is the leading cause of COPD. Most people who have COPD smoke or used to smoke. Long-term exposure to other lung irritants, such as air pollution, chemical fumes, or dust, also may contribute to COPD.

CHRONIC PAIN. Pain that lasts beyond the term of an injury or painful stimulus. The term can also refer to cancer pain, pain from a chronic or degenerative disease, and pain from an unidentified cause.

CHRONIC TOXICITY. Health problems that occur over a long period of time and that last for an extended period.

CILIA. Tiny, hair-like projections from a cell. In the respiratory tract, cilia beat constantly in order to move mucus and debris up and out of the respiratory tree, in order to protect the lung from infection or irritation by foreign bodies.

CIRCADIAN RHYTHM. A 24-hour cycle of physiological or behavioral activities.

CIRCUMCISION. A procedure, usually with religious or cultural significance, in which the prepuce—the skin covering the tip of the male penis or the female clitoris, is cut away.

CIRRHOSIS. Disruption of normal liver function by the formation of scar tissue and nodules in the liver.

CLEFT PALATE. A congenital malformation in which there is an abnormal opening in the roof of the mouth that allows the nasal passages and the mouth to be improperly connected.

CLINDAMYCIN. An antibiotic that can be used instead of penicillin.

CLINICAL NUTRITION. The use of diet and nutritional supplements as a way to enhance health prevent disease.

CLITORIDECTOMY. A procedure in which the clitoris and possibly some of the surrounding labial tissue at the opening of the vagina is removed.

CLITORIS. The small erectile organ at the front of the female vulva that is the site of female sexual pleasure.

CLOSTRIDIUM. A genus of deadly bacteria that are responsible for tetanus and other serious diseases, including botulism and gas gangrene from war wounds. The bacteria thrive without oxygen.

CLOSTRIDIUM PERFRINGENS. A bacterium that is a common food contaminant.

COAGULATION. In water treatment, this refers to adding a chemical to the water to cause particles in the water to clump so that they can be strained out.

COERCION. Use of force to threaten a person to do something against his or her will. In domestic abuse, the abuser uses coercion to gain control over the victim.

COGNITIVE BEHAVIORAL THERAPY. A type of psychotherapy in which people learn to recognize and change negative and self-defeating patterns of thinking and behavior.

COGNITIVE-BEHAVIORAL THERAPY. A type of psychotherapy used to treat anxiety disorders (including PTSD) that emphasizes behavioral change as well as alteration of negative thought patterns.

COINFECTION. Invasion of the body by two viruses at about the same time.

COLIC. Excessive crying in an otherwise healthy infant.

COLITIS. Inflammation of the colon or large bowel, which has several causes. The lining of the colon becomes swollen and ulcers often develop. The ability of the colon to absorb fluids is also affected and diarrhea often results.

COLLECTIVE VIOLENCE. Violence between two groups of people, as occurs in a war or during genocide.

COLONIC HYDROTHERAPY. In alternative medicine, the use of enemas to cleanse the lower bowel in the belief that this process removes toxic wastes from the body.

COLONOSCOPY. A medical procedure that allows a doctor to examine the interior lining of the rectum and colon for abnormalities. It is typically used as a screening test for colon cancer.

COLPOSCOPY. Procedure in which the cervix is examined using a special microscope.

COMMON COLD. A mild illness caused by a upper respiratory viruses. Usual symptoms include nasal congestion, coughing, sneezing, throat irritation, and a low-grade fever.

COMMUNICABLE DISEASE. An infectious, contagious disease transmitted by bacteria or viral organisms.

COMMUNITY. All those individuals within a geographical area with common social, cultural, racial, religious, socioeconomic, and other characteristics.

COMMUNITY COALITION. A group of individuals and/or agencies with common interests in some particular issue, such as a health problem of concern to them all.

COMMUNITY MENTAL HEALTH CLINIC (CMHC). A community-based provider of limited or comprehensive mental health services; usually at least partially publicly funded.

COMMUNITY PARTNERSHIPS. All of those relationships among individuals, groups, and agencies within a community among whom are shared common goals, responsibilities, resources, and accountability for public health policies and practices.

COMORBID. Referring to the presence of one or more diseases or disorders in addition to the patient's primary disorder.

COMORBIDITY. Diagnosis of two or more illnesses at the same time. It is common in behavioral health for adults to have more than one disorder simultaneously.

COMPLIANCE. The degree to which a population obeys public safety standards or obeys the statutes of laws.

COMPROMISED. Lacking adequate resistance to disease.

COMPUTED TOMOGRAPHY. Abbreviated CT, a medical imaging method that uses tomography along with computer processing to generate three-dimensional images from a series of two-dimensional x-ray images.

COMPUTERIZED TOMOGRAPHY (CT) SCAN. A test to examine organs within the body and detect evidence of tumors, blood clots, and accumulation of fluids.

CONCENTRATED ANIMAL FEEDING OPERATION (CAFO). An agricultural operation in which animals are raised in confined situations, with animals, feed, manure, urine, dead animals, and production operations concentrated in a small area.

CONDOM. A thin sheath worn over the penis during sexual intercourse to prevent pregnancy or the transmission of STDs. There are also female condoms.

CONDYLOMATA ACUMINATA (SINGULAR, CONDYLOMA ACUMINATUM). The medical term for infectious warts on the genitals caused by HPV.

CONDYLOMATA LATA. Highly infectious patches of weepy, pink or gray skin in moist areas of the body that occur during secondary syphilis.

CONFINED SPACE. A region with one or only a few opening that is not designed for long-term occupancy by employees, with poor ventilation and possibly contaminated air.

CONGENITAL. A condition that is present at birth.

CONJUGATION. The transfer of genetic material between two bacteria through cell-to-cell contact.

CONJUNCTIVA. The mucous membrane that lines the inside of the eyelid and the exposed surface of the eyeball.

CONJUNCTIVITIS. Inflammation of the conjunctiva, the membrane covering the white part of the eye.

CONSANGUNITY. Relation to a common ancestor; blood relative.

CONSOLIDATION. A condition in which lung tissue becomes firm and solid rather than elastic and air-filled because it has accumulated fluids and tissue debris.

CONTACT DERMATITIS. Skin inflammation resulting from contact with an allergen or other substance.

CONTAGIOUS DISEASE. a highly communicable disease with the ability to spread rapidly from one source to other through contact or proximity.

CONTAMINATION. The process by which an object or body part becomes exposed to an infectious agent such as a virus.

CONTRACEPTION. The use of a device, sexual practice, or chemical intended to prevent conception; birth control. It should not be confused with safe sex.

CONTRIBUTION-BASED ASSISTANCE. Financial or other type of aid to a person or a family for which the individual or family has made some type of contribution, such as payments toward Social Security or Medicare.

COORDINATED SCHOOL HEALTH (CSH). A program developed by the Centers for Disease Control and Prevention for improving student health in the United States.

CORECTIONAL INSTITUTION. A prison or jail.

CORNEA. The clear dome-shaped structure that is part of the front of the eye. It lies in front of the colored part of the eye (iris).

CORONARY ARTERIES. The main arteries that provide blood to the heart. The coronary arteries surround the heart like a crown, coming out of the aorta, arching down over the top of the heart, and dividing into two branches. These are the arteries in which heart disease occurs.

CORONAVIRUS. A genus of viruses that cause respiratory disease and gastroenteritis.

CORTICOSTEROIDS. A group of hormones produced naturally by the adrenal gland or manufactured synthetically. They are often used to treat inflammation. Examples include cortisone and prednisone.

CORTISOL. A hormone produced by the adrenal glands near the kidneys in response to stress.

COWPOX. A mild disease in cows that is caused by a poxvirus.

CREDENTIAL. A document that serves as proof of a person's competence in a specific field. Academic degrees, diplomas, certificates given on completion of an examination, and identification badges are all examples of credentials.

CREUTZFELDT-JAKOB DISEASE. A rare and progressive disease that targets certain brain tissue and causes early dementia and loss of muscle coordination.

CROP ROTATION. The practice of growing a series of different crops with different water and nutrient requirements in the same plot of land in successive seasons. Crop rotation helps to restore nutrients to the soil and reduces the likelihood of crop failure due to plant diseases or pests.

CRYOTHERAPY. The use of liquid nitrogen or other forms of extreme cold to destroy tissue.

CULTURE. A laboratory system for growing bacteria for further study.

CUMULATIVE. Increasing in effects or quantity by successive additions.

CURETTE. A spoon-shaped instrument used to remove tissue from the inner lining of the uterus.

CUSTOMARY LAW. A law that has been established due to the belief among those involved that a practice is legally binding and the evidence of widespread and consistent practice in a particular social setting.

CUTANEOUS. Pertaining to the skin

CYANOSIS. A bluish tinge to the skin that can occur when the blood oxygen level drops too low.

CYBERBULLYING. The use of electronic devices, including computers, cell phones, and other mobile devices, to bully by means of hurtful messages, spreading rumors, or misusing social media.

CYTOKINES. A class of proteins, including interferons and interleukins, that are released by cells as part of the immune response and as mediators of intercellular communication.

D

DARK FIELD. A microscopy technique in which light is directed at an oblique angle so that organisms appear bright against a dark background.

DEBRIDEMENT. The surgical removal of dead tissue.

DECIBEL. A logarithmic unit of measure comparing the intensity of two sounds (or other forms of energy) with each other.

DEET. A slightly yellow oily substance that can be applied to skin or clothing to protect against flea bites, tick bites, and the bites of other insects that can spread disease. The full chemical name of DEET is N,N-Diethyl-meta-toluamide.

DEFICIT. In medicine, the loss or impairment of a function or ability.

DEHYDRATION. The abnormal depletion of body fluids, as from vomiting and diarrhea.

DELAYED HYPERSENSITIVITY REACTIONS. Allergic reactions mediated by T cells that occur hours to days after exposure to the antigen.

DEMOGRAPHIC CHARACTERISTICS. Population measures, such as age, gender, race, and ethnicity.

DEPARTMENT OF HEALTH (UK). The national agency responsible for public health, adult social care, and the National Health Service.

DEPARTMENT OF HEALTH AND HUMAN SERVICE (DHHS). A federal agency that houses the Centers for Medicare and Medicaid Services and distributes funds for Medicaid.

DEPENDENCE. A state in which a person requires a steady concentration of a particular substance to avoid experiencing withdrawal symptoms.

DEPOLARIZATION. A change in a cell's membrane potential, making its electrical charge more positive or less negative. Defibrillation essentially depolarizes a portion of the heart muscle, allowing the heart's natural pacemaker to reestablish normal heart rhythm.

DEPRESSION. A mental condition in which a person feels extremely sad and loses interest in life. A person with depression may also have sleep problems and loss of appetite and may have trouble concentrating and carrying out everyday activities. Severe depression may instigate a suicide attempt.

DERMATOME. An area of skin which is serviced by a single ganglian from the spinal cord.

DERMIS. The basal layer of skin; it contains blood and lymphatic vessels, nerves, glands, and hair follicles.

DESIGNER DRUGS. A class of substances that are specifically created to avoid traditional means of detection, including drug laws and testing. Designer drugs often consist of multiple variations of an original compound or they are created to mimic the effects of other popular illicit drugs.

DETOXIFICATION. A structured program for removing stored toxins from the body.

DEVELOPED NATION. A country with highly-developed socioeconomic status. Citizens of developed nations are not usually subject to the same levels of political instability as citizens of developing nations. Developed nations also have more established municipal infrastructures, better human rights records, as well as increased access to health care and education.

DEVELOPING NATION. A country characterized by a minimal level of socioeconomic development. Citizens of developing nations are often subject to political crisis or instability, low productivity farming, human rights violations, limited infrastructures for things like sanitation and water distribution, limited access to healthcare and education. According to the United Nations (UN), of the least developed nations, 33 are in Africa, 14 in Asia, and Haiti in the Caribbean.

DIABETIC RETINOPATHY. Retinal disease caused by the damage that diabetes does to small blood vessels.

DIALYSIS. A form of treatment for patients with kidneys that do not function properly. The treatment removes toxic wastes from the body that are normally removed by the kidneys.

DIAPHRAGM. A dome-shaped device used to cover the back of a woman's vagina during intercourse in order to prevent pregnancy.

DIATHESIS. The medical term for predisposition. The stress/diathesis model is a diagram that is used to explain why some people are at greater risk of suicidal behavior than others.

DIAZINON. A member of the organophosphate family of pesticides. This chemical causes nerve and reproductive damage.

DIETARY SUPPLEMENT. A product, such as a vitamin, mineral, herb, amino acid, or enzyme, that is intended to be consumed in addition to an individual's diet with the expectation that it will improve health

DIETITIAN. A health care professional who specializes in individual or group nutritional planning, public education in nutrition, or research in food science. To be licensed as a registered dietitian (RD) in the United States, a person must complete a bachelor's degree in a nutrition-related field and pass a state licensing examination. Dietitians are also called nutritionists.

DIGITAL DIVIDE. A term used to refer to inequality between groups or individuals in terms of access to, use of, or knowledge of information and communication technologies (ICTs).

DIOXIN. The name of a family of highly toxic chlorinated chemicals that are known carcinogens as well as environmental pollutants.

DIPHTHERIA. A serious, infectious disease that produces a toxin (poison) and an inflammation in the membrane lining of the throat, nose, trachea, and other tissues.

DIPHTHERIA–TETANUS–PERTUSSIS (DTP). The standard preparation used to immunize children against diphtheria, tetanus, and whooping cough. A so-called "acellular pertussis" vaccine (aP) is usually used since its release in the mid-1990s in a combined vaccine known as DTaP.

DISABILITY-ADJUSTED LIFE-YEARS (DALYS). A term used to describe the health effects of some environmental factor, defined as the sum of the potential years of life lost due to premature death and the equivalent years of healthy life lost by virtue of being in states of poor health or disability.

DISSEMINATED. Scattered or distributed throughout the body. Lyme disease that has progressed beyond the stage of localized EM is said to be disseminated.

DISSEMINATED INTRAVASCULAR COAGULATION (DIC). An abnormal activation of blood clotting mechanisms that occurs in response to various diseases, including plague. Small blood clots form inside the blood vessels, disrupting normal clotting elsewhere in the body and leading to abnormal bleeding in the skin, digestive tract, and other organs.

DISSOCIATION. The splitting off of certain mental processes from conscious awareness. Many PTSD patients have dissociative symptoms.

DISULFIRAM. A medication that has been used since the late 1940s as part of a treatment plan for alcohol abuse. Sold under the trade name Antabuse, it produces changes in the body's metabolism of alcohol that cause headaches, vomiting, and other unpleasant symptoms if the patient drinks even small amounts of alcohol.

DNA. The abbreviation for deoxyribonucleic acid, the molecule in which genetic information is stored.

DNA PROBE. An agent that binds directly to a predefined sequence of nucleic acids.

DOMESTIC VIOLENCE. Physical, sexual, economic, verbal, or other forms of violence between two people in a close personal relationships, such as a marriage or domestic partnership.

DOMINANT INHERITANCE. A pattern of inheritance in which a trait or disease is conferred by one gene or allele. A parent with a disorder caused by a dominant allele has a 50% chance of passing the trait for disease to their offspring.

DOPAMINE. A neurochemical made in the brain that is involved in many brain activities, including movement and emotion.

DOUBLE BURDEN OF DISEASE. The situation in which a country or region has to simultaneously address problems posed by both infectious and non-infectious (degenerative) diseases.

DTAP. A vaccine that combines diphtheria and tetanus toxoids, and accellular pertussis.

DTP. Diphtheria, tetanus, and whole-cell pertussis vaccine.

DUAL DIAGNOSIS. A term used to describe the condition of a person with a diagnosed mental illness and a co-occurring alcohol or substance use disorder.

DURA MATER. The outermost layer of the meninges.

DYSENTERY. Intestinal infection marked by diarrhea containing blood and mucus.

DYSPHAGIA. Difficulty in swallowing.

E

EATING DISORDER. A condition characterized by an abnormal attitude towards food, altered appetite control, and unhealthy eating habits that affect health and the ability to function normally.

EBOLA. The disease caused by the newly described and very deadly Ebola virus found in Africa.

ECHOCARDIOGRAM. An image of the heart created by ultrasound waves.

ECTOPARASITE. A parasite that lives on or just below the exterior surface of an animal.

ECTOPIC PREGNANCY. Pregnancy in which a fertilized egg begins to develop outside the uterus. An ectopic pregnancy can be life-threatening to the woman and must be terminated.

ECZEMA. An inflammatory skin condition characterized by redness, itching, and oozing lesions, which become crusty, scaly, or hardened.

EDWARDS SYNDROME. A genetic disorder caused by an extra copy (trisomy) of chromosome 18. It is characterized by heart abnormalities, kidney malformations, and disorders of other internal organs; few newborns survive past the first week of life. The syndrome is named for John H. Edwards (1928–2007), a British geneticist who first described it in 1960.

EFFERENT NERVES. Nerves that convey impulses away from the central nervous system to the periphery.

EL NIÑO-SOUTHERN OSCILLATION (ENSO). A recurrent weather pattern across the tropical Pacific characterized by alternating wetter-than-normal and drier-than-normal conditions in large portions of Africa, eastern Asia, and South America.

ELECTROCARDIOGRAM. A test that measures the electrical activity of the heart. Also called an ECG or EKG.

ELECTROENCEPHALAGRAM (EEG). A chart of the brain waves picked up by the electrodes placed on the scalp. Changes in brain wave activity can be an indication of nervous system disorders.

ELECTROLYTES. Salts and minerals that ionize in body fluids. Common human electrolytes include sodium, chloride, potassium, and calcium. Electrolytes control the fluid balance of the body and are important in muscle contraction, energy generation, and almost all major biochemical reactions in the body.

ELECTROMAGNETIC RADIATION (EMR). A type of energy that is both absorbed and emitted by particles. Forms of EMR demonstrate wave-like movement as they travel through space and can be measured along the electromagnetic spectrum based on the frequency of wavelengths of emitted light or energy. Forms of EMR include radio radiation, infrared radiation, light on the visible spectrum, ultraviolet light, X-rays and Gamma rays.

ELECTROPHORESIS. A process used in molecular biology, biochemistry, and clinical chemistry to separate and identify specific proteins as well as DNA and RNA fragments. Polyacrylamide, a compound containing acrylamide, is used in this process.

ELEPHANTIASIS. A condition characterized by the gross enlargement of limbs and/or the genitalia that is also accompanied by a hardening and stretching of the overlying skin. Often a result of an obstruction in the lymphatic system caused by infection with a filarial worm.

ELISA PROTOCOLS. ELISA is an acronym for "enzyme-linked immunosorbent assay;" it is a highly sensitive technique for detecting and measuring antigens or antibodies in a solution.

EMBOLUS. A clot that forms in the heart and travels through the circulatory system to another part of the body.

EMBRYO. An unborn child during the first eight weeks of development following conception (fertilization with sperm). For the rest of pregnancy, the embryo is known as a fetus.

EMERGENCY MANAGEMENT. An overall term for organization and management procedures for critical events that includes response to and recovery from emergencies as well as emergency preparedness.

EMETIC. A medication or substance given to induce vomiting.

EMPOWERMENT. The act of investing individuals with an understanding of their own potential and their own self-worth, while simultaneously providing them with the tools by which to achive their maximum personal potential.

ENAMEL. The hard, white, outer layer of the tooth.

ENCEPHALITIS. An inflammation and swelling of the brain, usually due to infections with bacteria, viruses, or other agents. It may be contracted through contaminated foods or drinks, from insect or tick bites, or by other means.

ENCEPHALOPATHY. Brain disorder characterized by memory impairment and other symptoms.

ENDEMIC. Referring to an infectious disease that is constantly present in a particular country or region, though generally under control.

ENDEMIC AREA. A geographical area where a particular disease is prevalent.

ENDOCARDITIS. An infection of the inner membrane lining of the heart.

ENDOCRINE DISRUPTOR. A foreign chemical that, when introduced into the body, acts on it similarly to a naturally-occurring hormone. In addition to Bisphenol A, other endocrine disruptors include dichlorodiphenyltrichloroethane (DDT)—which is an insecticide now banned in the US, and polychlorinated biphenyl (PCBs)—which are toxic and commonly found in coolants and pesticides.

ENDOCRINE SYSTEM. Glandular body system which dispatches hormones to regulate body functions. The endocrine system includes the thyroid, adrenal glands, and hypothalamus. This system affects other organs including the liver, pancreas, and kidneys and manages hormones like estrogen, testosterone, cortisol, and insulin.

ENDOMETRIUM. The lining of the uterus.

ENDOPARASITE. A parasite that lives within the body of an animal.

ENDORPHINS. A class of peptides in the brain that are produced during exercise and bind to opiate receptors, resulting in pleasant feelings and pain relief.

ENDOSCOPY. Exam using an endoscope (a thin, flexible tube equipped with a lens or miniature camera to view various areas of the gastrointestinal tract). When the procedure is performed to examine certain organs such as the bile ducts or pancreas, the organs are not viewed directly, but rather indirectly through the injection of x ray.

ENFORCEMENT. The degree to which a population is held to the statutes of a particular law.

ENRICHMENT. The addition of vitamins and minerals to improve the nutritional content of a food.

ENTEROTOXIN. A type of harmful protein released by bacteria and other disease agents that affects the tissues lining the intestines.

ENTEROVIRUSES. Viruses that live in the gastrointestinal tract. Coxsackie viruses, viruses that cause hand–foot–mouth disease, are an enterovirus.

ENTITLEMENT. A program that creates a legal obligation by the federal government to any person, business, or government entity that meets the legally defined criteria. Medicaid is an entitlement both for eligible individuals and for the states that decide to participate in it.

ENVIRONMENTAL EPIDEMIOLOGY. The study of the effects of exposure to environmental hazards on human health.

ENZYME. A protein that speeds up a chemical reaction but is not consumed during the process.

EPIDEMIC. An outbreak of disease where the number of cases exceeds the usual (endemic) or typical number of cases.

EPIDEMIC PAROTITIS. The medical name for mumps.

EPIDEMIOLOGY. A field of medical science dealing with the incidence, distribution, and control of disease in a population.

EPIGLOTTITIS. An infection of the epiglottis that causes inflammation and can lead to an obstructed airway and inability to breathe. Epiglottitis can be caused by H. influenzae.

EPINEPHRINE. Adrenalin; a hormone released into the bloodstream in response to stress. Its many effects include stimulating the heart and increasing blood pressure, metabolic rate, and blood glucose concentration.

EPITHELIAL. Referring to the epithelium, the layer of cells forming the epidermis of the skin and the surface layer of mucous membranes.

EPITHELIUM. The layer of cells covering the body's surface and lining the internal organs and various glands.

EPIZOOTIC. An outbreak of a contagious disease among animals.

EQUIVALENT CARE. The concept that a prisoner is legally eligible for a level and health and medical care equivalent to that of a non-incarcerated person.

ERADICATE. To completely do away with something, eliminate it, end its existence.

ERYTHEMA MIGRANS (EM). A red skin rash that is one of the first signs of Lyme disease in about 75% of patients.

ERYTHROGENIC TOXIN. A toxin or agent produced by the scarlet fever-causing bacteria that causes the skin to turn red.

ERYTHROMYCIN. An antibiotic that can be used instead of penicillin.

ESSENTIAL FATTY ACIDS. Sources of fat in the diet, including omega-3 and omega-6 fatty acids.

ESSENTIAL MEDICINES. Drugs that satisfy the health care needs of the majority of the population; they should therefore be available at all times in adequate amounts and in appropriate dosage forms, at a price the community can afford.

ETHANOL. The chemical name for beverage alcohol. It is also sometimes called "ethyl alcohol" or "grain alcohol" to distinguish it from isopropyl or rubbing alcohol.

ETHICS. A set of principles of correct conduct that help individuals and groups decide the moral action to take in a specific situation.

ETIOLOGY. The cause or origin of a disease; also, the scientific study of disease causation.

EUKARYOTE. A single-cell or multicellular organism with a clearly defined nucleus.

EUSTACHIAN TUBE. A thin tube between the middle ear and the pharynx. Its purpose is to equalize pressure on either side of the eardrum.

EUTHANASIA. The act of putting individuals or animals to death painlessly or allowing them to die by withholding medical services, usually because of an incurable disease.

EXANTHEM (PLURAL, EXANTHEMS OR EXANTHEMATA). A skin eruption regarded as a characteristic sign of such diseases as measles, German measles, and scarlet fever.

EXERCISE. Any type of physical activity requiring physical effort, generally carried out for the purpose of maintaining or improving health and fitness.

EXOTOXIN. A poisonous secretion produced by bacilli which is carried in the bloodstream to other parts of the body.

F

FAGET'S SIGN. The simultaneous occurrence of a high fever with a slowed heart rate.

FAIR LABOR STANDARDS ACT (FLSA). Passed in 1938 as part of President Roosevelt's New Deal, FLSA provided regulations for employers to improve conditions of workers. The FLSA included certain statutes that applied specifically to the employment of minors. FLSA continues to be the primary federal law governing child labor in the United States.

FALLOPIAN TUBES. The thin tubes (two fo them) that connect the ovary to the uterus. Ova (eggs) travel from the ovary to the uterus. If the egg has been fertilized, it can implant in the uterus.

FAMCICLOVIR. An oral antiviral drug that blocks the replication of the varicella zoster virus.

FAST. A period of at least 24 hours in which a person eats nothing and drinks only water.

FAT. Molecules composed of fatty acids and glycerol; the slowest utilized source of energy, but the most energy-efficient form of food. Each gram of fat supplies about nine calories, more than twice that supplied by the same amount of protein or carbohydrate.

FEBRILE. Characterized or caused by fever.

FECES. The solid waste that is left after food is digested. Feces form in the intestines and pass out of the body through the anus. Also called stool.

FEDERAL POVERTY LEVEL (FPL). The definition of poverty provided by the federal government, used as the reference point to determine Medicaid eligibility for certain groups of beneficiaries. The FPL is adjusted every year to allow for inflation.

FEEDSTOCK. A chemical that is used in the commercial or industrial preparation of other chemicals.

FERMENTATION. A reaction performed by yeast or bacteria to make alcohol.

FERTILIZATION. The joining of the sperm and the egg; conception.

FETUS. An unborn child from the end of the eights week after fertilization until birth.

FIBROID TUMORS. Non-cancerous (benign) growths in the uterus. Fibroid tumors, which occur in 30–40% of women over age 40, do not need to be removed unless they are causing symptoms that interfere with a woman's normal activities.

FIRST RESPONDER. A generic term for the first medically trained responder to arrive at the scene of an emergency. First responders include police officers, firefighters, emergency medical technicians, and paramedics.

FLACCID. Weak, soft, or floppy.

FLAGELLUM. A tail-like projection extending from the cell walls of certain bacteria. Its name is the Latin word for whip.

FLASHBACK. A temporary reliving of a traumatic event.

FLAVIVIRUS. An arbovirus (a virus transmitted by an insect or other arthropod) that can cause potentially serious diseases, such as dengue, yellow fever, Japanese encaphilitis, and West Nile fever.

FLUORESCENT ANTIBODY TEST (FA TEST). A test in which a fluorescent dye is linked to an antibody for diagnostic purposes.

FLUORIDE. A compound believed to combat cavities in teeth.

FLUORODOSIS. A cosmetic dental problem that can be caused by the presence of too much fluoride in drinking water. Fluorodosis causes brown spots on the teeth but does not weaken them in any way.

FLUOROQUINOLONES. A class of synthetic broad-spectrum antibiotics that contain a fluorine atom in addition to the basic quinolone structure. They work by preventing the DNA in bacteria from unwinding and replicating.

FLY ASH. Fine particles of ash produced from the combustion of solid fuel.

FOOD INSECURITY. A limited or uncertain ability to obtain nutritionally adequate and safe foods in socially acceptable ways.

FOOD SAFETY AND INSPECTION SERVICE (FSIS). The public health agency within the U.S. Department of Agriculture that is responsible for the safety of meat, poultry, and egg products.

FOOD-BORNE ILLNESS. A disease that is transmitted by eating or handling contaminated food.

FOOD-IRRADIATION METHODS. A process using radiant energy to kill microorganisms in food, to extend the amount of time in which food can be sold and eaten safely.

FOODBORNE DISEASE. An illness caused by consuming a food or drink infected with pathogens.

FORCIBLE SODOMY. Forced oral or anal intercourse.

FOREMILK. Thin watery milk found at the beginning of breast feeding.

FORENSIC. Pertaining to matters of interest in a court of law.

FORMULARY. A book containing a list of pharmaceutical substances along with their formulas, uses, and methods of preparation.

FORTIFICATION. The addition of vitamins and minerals to improve the nutritional content of a food.

FOSSIL FUELS. Any type of fuel, such as coal, natural gas, peat, and petroleum, derived from the decomposed remains of prehistoric plants and animals.

FRAGILE X SYNDROME. A genetic condition related to the X chromosome that affects mental, physical and sensory development.

FREE RADICAL. An unstable molecule that causes oxidative damage by stealing electrons from surrounding molecules, thereby disrupting activity in the body's cells.

FREQUENCY. The number of wave fronts that pass a given point in space in some specified period of time, such as one second.

FRONTAL CORTEX. The part of the human brain associated with aggressiveness and impulse control. Abnormalities in this part of the brain are associated with an increased risk of suicide.

FULMINANT. Occurring or flaring up suddenly and with great severity. A potentially fatal complication of amebic dysentery is an inflammation of the colon known as fulminant colitis.

FULMINATING COLITIS. A potentially fatal complication of amebic dysentery marked by sudden and severe inflammation of the intestinal lining, severe bleeding or hemorrhaging, and massive shedding of dead tissue.

FUNCTIONAL FOOD. also called nutraceuticals, these products are marketed as having health benefits or disease-preventing qualities beyond their basic supply of energy and nutrients. Often these health benefits come in the form of added herbs, minerals, vitamins, etc.

FUNDUS. The inside of an organ. In the eye, the fundus is the back area that can be seen with the ophthalmoscope.

FUNGI. A kingdom of saprophytic and parasitic spore–producing organisms that include mushrooms and yeast.

FUNGICIDE. A substance capable of killing or stopping the growth of fungi.

G

GALACTOSEMIA. A rare genetic disorder where an infant cannot metabolize the sugar in breast milk, and therefore cannot breastfeed.

GANGLION. A mass of nerve tissue outside of the central nervous system.

GANGRENE. Death of tissue due to loss of blood supply followed by bacterial invasion and putrefaction.

GAS GANGRENE. A potentially fatal form of gangrene (tissue death) caused by a bacterial infection. Gas gangrene usually occurs at the site of a wound, including a surgical incision.

GASTRIC LAVAGE. A technique for washing poison out of the stomach by instilling water or saline solution through a tube, removing the stomach contents by suction, and repeating the process until the washings are free of poison. The procedure is also called "stomach pumping."

GASTROENTERITIS. An inflammation of the lining of the stomach and intestines, usually caused by a viral or bacterial infection.

GASTROINTESTINAL. Pertaining to the stomach and intestines.

GASTROPLASTY. A surgical procedure used to reduce digestive capacity by shortening the small intestine or shrinking the side of the stomach.

GASTROSCHISIS. A birth defect in which there is an opening in the abdominal wall (usually to the right of the umbilicus) that allows the intestines to protrude through it.

GENE MAPPING. The process of determining the location of genes (or DNA segments) on a chromosome.

GENE TRANSFER. The exchange of genetic material between bacteria during conjugation. It is a common mechanism for developing antimicrobial resistance.

GENERAL PARESIS. An advanced form of neurosyphilis affecting personality and control of movement and possibly causing convulsions or partial paralysis.

GENETIC CLUSTER. A group of viral strains with very similar, yet distinct, nucleic acid sequences.

GENETICALLY MODIFIED (GM OR GMO) FOODS. Food or ingredients derived from genetically modified organisms.

GENOCIDE. The deliberate killing of a racial or ethnic group.

GENOGROUP. Related viruses within a genus; may be further subdivided into genetic clusters.

GENOME. The complete set of genetic information in an organism.

GENOMICS. The study of an organism's complete genome.

GEOGRAPHIC INFORMATION SYSTEM (GIS). Any program or process that makes use of computer technology to capture, store, analyze, interpret, and report geographic data.

GERIATRICS. The field of medicine that deals with the health of elderly people.

GERM. A common term for a microorganism that causes disease.

GHRELIN. A peptide hormone secreted primarily by the stomach that has been implicated in the control of food intake and fat storage.

GINGIVITIS. Inflammation of the gums, seen as painless bleeding during brushing and flossing.

GLOMERULONEPHRITIS. A serious inflammation of the kidneys that can be caused by streptococcal bacteria; a potential complication of untreated scarlet fever.

GLUCOCORTICOSTEROIDS. Also called glucocorticoids, a class of steroid hormones that play important roles in metabolism and the immune system. Synthetic glucocorticosteroids are drugs given to control certain allergic and immune system disorders; they include cortisone, prednisone, aldosterone, and dexamethasone. These drugs suppress the immune response to infection; thus they can increase a person's risk of listeriosis.

GRADUATED DRIVERS LICENSE (GDL). A licensing program for young adults that requires them to complete a probationary period before obtaining a full license. This probationary period usually requires the novice driver to gain so many hours driving under the supervision of a licensed adult. The probationary period also limits the conditions under which a novice driver can drive, such as before a certain time of night, and without any additional passengers. GDLs have been shown to reduce the number of teenage driving accidents and fatalities.

GRAM'S STAIN. A dye staining technique used in laboratory tests to determine the presence and type of bacteria.

GRAM-NEGATIVE. Refers to the property of many bacteria that causes them to not take up color with Gram's stain, a method which is used to identify bacteria. Gram-positive bacteria which take up the stain turn purple, while Gram-negative bacteria which do not take up the stain turn red.

GRANULES. Small packets of reactive chemicals stored within cells.

GRANULOMA. A group of macrophages. This is a mass that forms when macrophages have grouped together to attempt the digestion of a potential threat but are unable to eliminate the threat.

GRAY LITERATURE. A term used by librarians to refer to written material that is not published commercially or is not generally accessible to the public. Gray literature includes such material as conference proceedings, working papers, technical reports, and the like.

GREEN REVOLUTION. A series of agricultural research and development programs from the 1940s through the 1970s that included the development of high-yielding food crops, expansion of irrigation, and distribution of seeds and fertilizers in India and other countries with recurrent famines.

GREENHOUSE EFFECT. The overall warming of Earth's atmosphere as the result of atmospheric pollution by gases.

GREENHOUSE GASES. Any gas (such as carbon dioxide and ozone) that absorbs radiation and contributes to the warming of Earth's atmosphere by reflecting radiation from the surface of Earth.

GRIEF COUNSELING. A form of psychotherapy designed to help people cope with emotional responses to extraordinarily stressful events in their lives, such as the death of a loved one or long-term unemployment.

GUILLAIN-BARRÉ SYNDROME. Progressive and usually reversible paralysis or weakness of multiple muscles usually starting in the lower extremities and often ascending to the muscles involved in respiration. The syndrome is due to inflammation and loss of the myelin covering of the nerve fibers, often associated with an acute infection.

GUINEA WORM EMBRYO. The guinea worm at its earliest life stage prior to or shortly after being expelled from an adult female worm.

GUINEA WORM LARVAE. The guinea worm during its middle life stage as it matures within a water flea. The larvae can only grow to adulthood within a human host.

GUMMA. A rubbery swelling or tumor that heals slowly and leaves a scar and is a symptom of tertiary syphilis.

H

H1N1 (SWINE FLU). A disease that was originally found in pigs and can be passed from animal to human or human to human. Symptoms of H1N1 include fever, cough, chills, fatigue, headache, and body aches.

HALLUCINATION. A false or distorted perception of objects, sounds, or events that seems real. Hallucinations usually result from drugs or mental disorders.

HALOACETIC ACIDS (HAA5). a group of five chemicals that are potentially formed when organic matter in drinking water reacts with chlorine during the chlorination disinfection process. The five Haloacetic acids are: monochloroacetic acid, dichloroacetic acid, thrichloroacetic acid, monobromoacetic acid, and dibromoacetic acid. These chemicals are potentially harmful to human health and are thus regulated by the Environmental Protection Agency (EPA).

HAND WASHING. Any act or set of acts performed to remove dirt, microbes, and other materials from the hands.

HANTAVIRUS. A group of arboviruses that cause hemorrhagic fever (characterized by sudden onset, fever, aching, and bleeding in the internal organs).

HAZARD. In the context of emergency preparedness, a general term for any agent, whether biological, chemical, mechanical, or other, that is likely to cause harm to humans or the environment in the absence of protective measures.

HAZARD ASSESSMENT. An attempt to survey an environment to determine which hazards are present in that environment.

HDL CHOLESTEROL. High-density lipoprotein cholesterol is a component of cholesterol that helps protect against heart disease. HDL is nicknamed "good cholesterol."

HEALTH ASSESSMENT. The process of collecting, analyzing, assessing, and disseminating data and information about health status, risk factors, resource availability, individual concerns, environmental health factors, and any and all other factors impacting public health issues in a community.

HEALTH CARE FINANCING ADMINISTRATION (HCFA). A federal agency that provides guidelines for the Medicaid program.

HELMINTHS. Parasitic worms, such as tapeworms or liver flukes, that can live in the human body.

HEMODIALYSIS. The removal of waste products from the blood stream in patients with kidney failure. Blood is removed from a vein, passed through a dialysis machine, and then put back into a vein.

HEMOGLOBIN (HB). A molecule that normally binds to oxygen in order to carry it to our cells, where it is required for life.

HEMOLYTIC BACTERIA. Bacteria that are able to burst red blood cells.

HEMOLYTIC UREMIC SYNDROME (HUS). Kidney failure, usually in infants and young children, that can be caused by food contaminated with bacteria such as STEC or *Shigella*.

HEMORRHAGE. Bleeding that is massive, uncontrollable, and often life-threatening.

HEMORRHAGIC. A condition resulting in massive, difficult-to-control bleeding.

HEPATITIS. The medical term for inflammation of the liver. It can be caused by toxic substances or alcohol as well as infections.

HERB. In alternative medicine, a plant or plant derivative or extract prescribed for health or healing.

HERPESVIRUS. Any one of a large family of viruses (Herpesviridae) that cause diseases in humans and other animals.

HIGH-RISK HPV TYPE. A member of the HPV family of viruses that is associated with the development of cervical cancer and precancerous growths.

HIGHLY ACTIVE ANTIRETROVIRAL THERAPY (HAART). An individualized combination of three or more antiretroviral drugs used to treat patients with HIV infection. It is sometimes called a drug cocktail.

HISTAMINE. A chemical released by mast cells during an allergic reaction and which has a variety of effects on other cells.

HIVES. A raised, itchy area of skin that is usually a sign of an allergic reaction.

HOMEOPATHY. The use of diluted remedies that have energetic, rather than chemical, properties. They are prescribed according to the axiom that "like cures like."

HORMONE THERAPY. Treatment of cancer by inhibiting the production of hormones such as testosterone and estrogen.

HOST. The organism (such as a monkey or human) in which another organism (such as a virus or bacteria) is living.

HUMAN CHORIONIC GONADOTROPIN (HCG). A hormone produced by the placenta during pregnancy.

HUMAN IMMUNODEFICIENCY VIRUS (HIV). A transmissible retrovirus that causes AIDS in humans. Two forms of HIV are now recognized: HIV-1, which causes most cases of AIDS in Europe, North and South America, and most parts of Africa; and HIV-2, which is chiefly found in West African patients. HIV-2, discovered in 1986, appears to be less virulent than HIV-1 and may also have a longer latency period.

HUMAN PAPILLOMAVIRUS (HPV). The most common sexually transmitted virus, HPV causes genital warts and cervical cancer.

HUMOR. A theoretical liquid contained in the human body once thought to be responsible for ill health.

HYDROCARBONS. Any organic chemical compound containing hydrogen (H) and carbon (C).

HYDROCEPHALUS. Abnormal accumulation of cerebrospinal fluid within the cavities inside the brain.

HYGIENE. Any practice or set or practices that maintains good health and prevents the spread of disease.

HYPERAROUSAL. A state of increased emotional tension and anxiety, often including jitteriness and being easily startled.

HYPEREMESIS. Severe vomiting during pregnancy. Hyperemesis appears to increase a woman's risk of postpartum depression.

HYPERLIPIDEMIA. Abnormally high levels of lipids in the blood.

HYPERPLASTIC OBESITY. Excessive weight gain in childhood, characterized by an increase in the number of fat cells.

HYPERSENSITIVITY. The state where even a tiny amount of allergen can cause the airways to constrict and bring on an asthmatic attack.

HYPERTENSION. Abnormally high arterial blood pressure, which if left untreated can lead to heart disease and stroke.

HYPERTROPHIC OBESITY. Excessive weight gain in adulthood, characterized by expansion of pre-existing fat cells.

HYPERVIGILANCE. A condition of abnormally intense watchfulness or wariness. Hypervigilance is one of the most common symptoms of PTSD.

HYPOTHERMIA. Development of a subnormal body temperature.

I

IATROGENIC. Caused by a medical procedure.

IDEAL WEIGHT. Weight corresponding to the lowest death rate for individuals of a specific height, gender, and age.

IMMEDIATE HYPERSENSITIVITY REACTIONS. Allergic reactions that are mediated by mast cells and occur within minutes of allergen contact.

IMMUNE GLOBULIN. A preparation of antibodies that can be given before exposure for short-term protection against hepatitis A and for persons who have already been exposed to hepatitis A virus. Immune globulin must be given within two weeks after exposure to hepatitis A virus for maximum protection.

IMMUNE SYSTEM. The system of specialized organs, lymph nodes, and blood cells throughout the body, which work together to prevent foreign invaders (bacteria, viruses, fungi, etc.) from taking hold and growing.

IMMUNIZATION. Administering a vaccine that stimulates the body to create antibodies to a specific disease (immunity) without causing symptoms of the disease.

IMMUNOASSAY. A laboratory test that uses an antigen-antibody response to determine the presence of a bacterium or other substance in a patient sample.

IMMUNOCOMPROMISED. To have a poor immune system due to disease or medication. Immunocompromised persons are at risk for developing infections because they cannot fight off microorganisms as can healthy persons.

IMMUNOGLOBULIN (IG). A protein molecule made by B cells that neutralizes specific disease–causing substances and organisms. Also called "antibody." Immunoglobulins are divided into five classes: IgA, IgD, IgE, IgG, and IgM.

IMMUNOGLOBULIN E (IGE). Antibodies produced in the lungs, skin, and mucous membranes that are responsible for allergic reactions.

IMMUNOGLOBULIN G (IGG). A group of antibodies against certain viral infections that circulate in the bloodstream. One type of IgG is specific against the mumps paramyxovirus.

IMMUNOSUPPRESSED. Suppression of the immune system by medications during the treatment of diseases such as cancer or following an organ transplantation.

IMMUNOSUPPRESSIVE THERAPY. Medical treatment in which the immune system is purposefully thwarted. Such treatment is necessary, for example, to prevent organ rejection in transplant cases.

IMMUNOTHERAPY. Treatment of cancer by stimulating the body's immune defense system.

IMPLANTATION. The process in which the fertilized egg embeds itself in the wall of the uterus.

INALIENABLE RIGHTS. Privileges to which all humans are entitled, just because they are human. These are unlike legal rights, which can be taken away and may not be equal for everyone.

INATTENTION BLINDNESS. Commonly used when describing distracted driving, particularly while talking on a cell phone, this describes a driver's ability to see something but be delayed in recognizing or reacting to the information as a result of the cognitive distraction created by another activity.

INCIDENCE. The number of new cases of a specific disease within a specific time period within a specific population.

INCUBATION PERIOD. The time between when an individual becomes infected with a disease-causing agent and when symptoms begin to appear.

INFECTIOUS DISEASE. A disease caused by a microorganism; may or may not be communicable. A non-communicable disease would be one spread through food or environmental sources.

INFIBULATION. A procedure that closes the labia majora to prevent sexual intercourse, leaving only a small opening for the passage of urine and menstrual blood.

INFLAMMATION. Pain, redness, swelling, and heat that usually develop in response to injury or illness.

INFLAMMATORY BOWEL DISEASE (IBD). Disease in which the lining of the intestine becomes inflamed.

INFLUENZA. A disease caused by viruses that infect the respiratory tract.

INSECTICIDES. Any substance used to kill insects.

INSOMNIA. Prolonged or abnormal inability to obtain adequate sleep.

INTERNALLY DISPLACED PERSONS (IDPS). The official term for individuals pushed from their homes as a result of persecution, violence, or natural disaster. IDPs are persons displaced within the boundaries of their native country.

INTERPERSONAL VIOLENCE. Violence that occurs between two individuals, such as domestic partners, family members, or two unrelated strangers.

INTERVENTION. In public health, any plan, policy, or activity intended to encourage behaviors conducive to good health or discourage behaviors harmful to health. Interventions may include treatments, prevention strategies, screening programs, diagnostic tests, different health care settings, and educational materials or programs.

INTOXICATION. The mental, physical, or emotional state produced by a substance.

INTRACEREBRAL HEMORRHAGE. A cause of some strokes in which vessels within the brain begin bleeding.

INTUSSUSCEPTION. A type of bowel blockage that results from one portion of the bowel sliding into another. It is more common in children than adults.

ION. An electrically charged particle.

IONIZE. to transform a molecule or atom—a neutral particle—into an ion—a particle with a positive or negative charge.

IONIZING RADIATION. Radiation that produces ions.

INTELLIGENCE QUOTIENT (IQ). The comparison of an individual's mental age to his/her true or chronological age multiplied by 100.

IRIS. The colored ring just behind the cornea and in front of the lens that controls the amount of light sent to the retina.

ISCHEMIA. Loss of blood supply to a tissue or organ resulting from the blockage of a blood vessel.

J

JARISCH–HERXHEIMER REACTION. A rare reaction to the dead bacteria in the blood stream following antibiotic treatment.

JARISCH-HERXHEIMER REACTION. A temporary reaction to penicillin treatment for syphilis that includes fever, chills, and worsening of the skin rash or chancre.

JAUNDICE. A yellowish discoloration of the skin and whites of the eyes caused by increased levels of bile pigments from the liver in the patient's blood.

K

KAPOSI'S SARCOMA. A cancer of the connective tissue that produces painless purplish red (in people with light skin) or brown (in people with dark skin) blotches on the skin. It is a major diagnostic marker of AIDS.

KARYOTYPE. A photomicrograph (picture taken through a microscope) of a person's 46 chromosomes, lined up in 23 pairs, that is used to identify some types of genetic disorders.

KOPLIK'S SPOTS. Tiny spots occurring inside the mouth, especially on the inside of the cheek. These spots consist of minuscule white dots (like grains of salt or sand) set onto a reddened bump. Unique to measles.

L

LABIA MAJORA. The outer fatty folds of the vulva; sometimes also called the "lips" surrounding the vagina.

LACTOSE. A sugar found in milk that provides energy.

LARYNX. The part of the airway lying between the pharynx and the trachea.

LATRINE. A type of toilet, often one used by a number of individuals.

LDL CHOLESTEROL. Low-density lipoprotein cholesterol is the primary cholesterol molecule. High levels of LDL increase the risk of coronary heart disease. LDL is nicknamed "bad cholesterol."

LEARNED HELPLESSNESS. The tendency to give up on solving a problem when efforts appear to bring no results.

LEARNING DISABILITIES. An impairment of the cognitive processes of understanding and using spoken and written language that results in difficulties with one or more academic skill sets (e.g., reading, writing, mathematics).

LEAVENING. Yeast or other agents used for rising bread.

LEGIONELLOSIS. A disease caused by infection with a Legionella bacterium.

LEISHMAN-DONOVAN BODY. A body of a (trypanosomatid) protozoa at a particular and characteristic stage in its life cycle; the infectious (trypanosomatid) protozoa can cause leishmaniasis, and is relatively easy to identify at that stage.

LEISHMANIASIS. An infection of the respiratory tract transmitted by the female sandfly.

LEPTIN. A peptide hormone produced by fat cells that acts on the hypothalamus to suppress appetite and burn stored fat.

LESION. Any visible, local abnormality of the tissues of the skin, such as a wound, sore, rash, or boil.

LETHARGY. The state of being sluggish.

LIFE EXPECTANCY. Indicates the average age an individual in a given population can expect to live. This figure is often further categorized by gender and age group. Factors contributing to life expectancy include income, education, access to adequate healthcare, dietary habits, hygiene, and sanitation.

LIFE SPAN. The total number of years an organism can expect to live from birth to death.

LIPODYSTROPHY. The medical term for redistribution of body fat in response to HAART, insulin injections in diabetics, or rare hereditary disorders.

LISTERIOSIS. Illness caused by food contaminated with the bacterium *Listeria monocytogenes*.

LOCAL AUTHORITY. In the United Kingdom, administrative bodies responsible for policy and programs at the town, city, county, or other local area. The term has somewhat different meanings in England, Wales, Scotland, and Northern Ireland.

LOEFFLER'S MEDIUM. A special substance used to grow diphtheria bacilli to confirm a diagnosis.

LUES MALIGNA. Areas of ulcerated and dying skin tissue that may occur with secondary syphilis, most frequently in HIV-positive patients.

LUMBAR PUNCTURE (LP). A medical test in which a very narrow needle is inserted into a specific space between the vertebrae of the lower back in order to obtain a sample of CSF for examination. It is also known as a spinal tap.

LUMEN. The inner cavity or canal of a tube-shaped organ, such as the bowel.

LYME DISEASE. An acute disease that is usually marked by skin rash, fever, fatigue, and chills. Left untreated, it may cause heart and nervous system damage.

LYMPH NODES. Small, bean-shaped masses of tissue scattered along the lymphatic system that act as filters and immune monitors, removing fluids, bacteria, or cancer cells that travel through the lymph system.

LYMPH/LYMPHATIC. One of the three body fluids that is transparent and a slightly yellow liquid that is collected from the capillary walls into the tissues and circulates back to the blood supply.

LYMPHATIC SYSTEM. The circulatory system that drains and circulates fluid containing nutrients, waste products, and immune cells, from between cells, organs, and other tissue spaces.

LYMPHOCYTE. Any of a group of white blood cells of crucial importance to the immune system's production of a tailor-made defense against specific invading organisms.

LYMPHOMA. A group of cancers in which the cells of tissue usually found in the lymph nodes or spleen multiply abnormally.

LYSSAVIRUS. A genus of viruses that includes the rabies virus and related viruses that infect insects as well as mammals.

M

MACROPHAGE. A cell of the immune system that engulfs and digests foreign invaders such as bacteria and viruses in an attempt to stop them from causing disease within the body.

MACULA. The central part of the retina where the rods and cones are densest.

MAGNETIC RESONANCE IMAGING (MRI). MRI is diagnostic radiography using electromagnetic energy to create an image of the central nervous system (CNS), blood system, and musculoskeletal system.

MAINSTREAM SMOKE. The tobacco smoke exhaled by a smoker

MAJOR TRANQUILIZERS. The family of drugs that includes the psychotropic or neuroleptic drugs, sometimes used to help autistic people. They carry significant risk of side effects, including Parkinsonism and movement disorders, and should be prescribed with caution.

MALABSORPTION SYNDROME. A condition characterized by indigestion, bloating, diarrhea, loss of appetite, and weakness, caused by poor absorption of nutrients from food as a result of HIV infection itself, giardiasis or other opportunistic infections of the digestive tract, or certain surgical procedures involving the stomach or intestines.

MALARIA. A serious disease prevalent in the tropics. It is caused by parasites and produces severe fever and sometimes complications affecting the kidneys, liver, brain, and blood. It is spread by the Anopheles mosquito and can be fatal.

MALIGNANT. A general term for cells and the tumors they form that can invade and destroy other tissues and organs.

MALIGNANT MESOTHELIOMA. Malignant mesothelioma is a rare form of cancer that develops from transformed cells originating in the mesothelium, the protective lining that covers many of the internal organs of the body. It is usually caused by exposure to asbestos. The most common anatomical site for the development of mesothelioma is the pleura (the outer lining of the lungs and internal chest wall), but it can also arise in the peritoneum (the lining of the abdominal cavity), and the pericardium (the sac that surrounds the heart), or the tunica vaginalis (a sac that surrounds the testis).

MANTOUX TEST. Another name for the PPD test.

MARXIST. Refers generally to people sharing social and/or economic viewpoints with German philosopher Karl Marx. Marxists follow in Marx'ss footsteps in criticizing capitalism as a disproportionately unfair and undesirable system of wealth distribution. Marxists favor socialism, which advocates for equal distribution of wealth, work, and power across a population.

MAST CELLS. A type of immune system cell that displays immunoglobulin E (IgE) on its cell surface and participates in allergic reactions by releasing histamine and other chemicals from intracellular granules. The lining of the nasal passages and eyelids are particularly rich in mast cells.

MEASLES. An acute and highly contagious viral disease marked by distinct red spots followed by a rash that occurs primarily in children.

MEDIA. Substance which contains all the nutrients necessary for bacteria to grow in a culture.

MEDICAID. A joint state and federal program for providing medical care for low-income children and families.

MEDICALLY NEEDY. A term that describes a group whose coverage is optional with the states because of high medical expenses. These persons meet category requirements of Medicaid (they are children or parents or elderly or disabled), but their income is too high to qualify them for coverage as categorically needy.

MEDICARE. The U.S. government healthcare system for those aged 65 and over.

MEDITATION. Technique of concentration for relaxing the mind and body.

MEFLOQUINE. An antimalarial drug that was developed by the U.S. Army in the early 1980s. By the early 2000s, malaria resistance to this drug had become a problem in some parts of Asia (especially Thailand and Cambodia).

MELANIN. A naturally-occurring pigment found in human skin, hair, and eyes. Melanin determines skin color and reacts to UV rays to make skin appear tanned.

MELANOMA. A type of skin cancer. Melanoma is the most dangerous of the various types of skin cancer.

MELATONIN. A hormone involved in regulation of circadian rhythms.

MENIERE'S DISEASE. The combination of vertigo and decreased hearing caused by abnormalities in the inner ear.

MENINGES. A series of membranous layers of connective tissue that protect the central nervous system (brain and spinal cord). Damage or infection to the meninges, such as in meningitis, can cause serious neurological damage and even death.

MENINGITIS. Inflammation of the membranes covering the brain and spinal cord called the meninges.

META-ANALYSIS. A method of contrasting and combining results from different studies in order to identify patterns among study results, sources of disagreement among those results, or other significant relationships among the various studies.

METABOLIC ACTIVITY. The sum of the chemical processes in the body that are necessary to maintain life.

METABOLIC BONE DISEASE. Weakening of bones due to a deficiency of certain minerals, especially calcium.

METABOLIC EQUIVALENT OF TASK; MET. The energy cost of a physical activity, measured as a multiple of the resting metabolic rate, which is defined as 3.5 milliliters of oxygen consumed per kilogram (kg) of body weight per minute, equivalent to 1 kilocalorie per kg per hour.

METASTASIS. The spread of cancer from one part of the body to another.

METHAMPHETAMINE (METH, METHADRINE, "SPEED"). A highly addictive medication that is used to treat attention deficit disorder and obesity, but is widely abused as a stimulant.

MIASM. In homeopathy, an inherited weakness or predisposition to disease. The syphilitic miasm is considered to be one of the most powerful.

MIASMA. A theoretical agent in the air that causes disease and is produced by the decay of dead organisms.

MICROBE. Any type of living organism made up of no cells, a single cell, or a cluster of cells. Bacteria, viruses, algae, eukaryotes, protozoa, and fungi are all common microbes.

MICROCEPHALY. An abnormally small head.

MICROFILARIAE. The larvae and infective form of filarial worms.

MICROFINANCE. The process of loaning a small amount of money for the purposes of starting or developing a small business, as a means of growing local economies and providing new economic opportunities.

MICRONUTRIENT. A substance needed in small amounts to allow for normal growth and development. Common examples of micronutrients include vitamins, such as vitamin C and vitamin D, and minerals, such as iron and zinc.

MICROORGANISM. A microscopic organism made up of one cell or a small cluster of cells. There are many different types of microorganisms and they can be helpful or benign to human health, however, some microorganisms like certain bacteria and fungi can be dangerous to human health.

MIGRATION. Movement of an individual or group of individuals from one geographic region to another geographic region within a single nation or across international boundaries.

MILIARY TUBERCULOSIS. The form of TB in which the bacillus spreads through all body tissues and organs, producing many thousands of tiny tubercular lesions. It is often fatal unless promptly treated.

MINERAL. an inorganic substance found in the earth that is necessary in small quantities for the body to maintain a health. Examples include zinc, copper, iron.

MIRACIDIUM. The form of the schistosome worm that infects freshwater snails.

MISCARRIAGE. Spontaneous pregnancy loss.

MITIGATION. A general term for attempts to prevent disasters or reduce their impact.

MMR VACCINE. The standard measles, mumps, and rubella (MMR) vaccine that is given to prevent measles, mumps and rubella (German measles). The MMR vaccine is now given in two dosages. The first should be given at 12-15 months of age. The second vaccination should be given at 4-6 years. There are some exceptions depending on a person's health condition.

MONOGAMY. Being married to only one person or having only one sexual partner at a time.

MONOMER. A molecule that can be bound to other similar molecules in order to make a polymer.

MONONUCLEAR PHAGOCYTE. A type of cell of the human immune system that ingests bacteria, viruses, and other foreign matter, thus removing potentially harmful substances from the bloodstream. These substances are usually then digested within the phagocyte.

MONOUNSATURATED FAT. Fats that contain one double or triple carbon bond per molecule; examples include canola oil and olive oil.

MORGELLONS DISEASE. A mysterious medical condition first described in the seventeenth century featuring the sensation of itching and/or crawling on the skin, where no cause can be found medically. Some Morgellons patients have additional health side effects or conditions and many show an inflammatory response though no cause can be located. Despite being described for hundreds of years, Morgellons Disease has not yet been recognized by any official medical body in the United States.

MOTOR NEURON. A type of cell in the central nervous system that controls the movement of muscles either directly or indirectly.

MOTOR SKILLS. Controlled movement of muscle groups. Fine motor skills involve tasks that require dexterity of small muscles, such as buttoning a shirt. Tasks such as walking or throwing a ball involve the use of gross motor skills.

MUCOUS MEMBRANES. The inner tissue that covers or lines body cavities or canals open to the outside, such as nose and mouth. These membranes secrete mucus and absorb water and salts.

MULTIPLE SCLEROSIS. A progressive disease of brain and nerve tissue.

MUMPS. An acute and highly contagious viral illness that usually occurs in childhood.

MUTAGENIC. Having a tendency to cause genetic mutations.

MYASTHENIA GRAVIS. A muscle weakness that occurs because the body makes antibodies to the natural chemical that facilitates transmission of impulses between the nerve and the muscle.

MYCOBACTERIA. A group of bacteria that includes *Mycobacterium tuberculosis*, the bacterium that causes tuberculosis, and other forms that cause related illnesses.

MYOCARDITIS. Inflammation of the heart tissue.

MYOCARDIUM. The medical term for the specialized involuntary muscle tissue found in the walls of the heart.

N

NALTREXONE. A medication originally developed to treat addiction to heroin or morphine that is also used to treat alcoholism. It works by reducing the craving for alcohol rather than by producing vomiting or other unpleasant reactions.

NARCOLEPSY. A condition characterized by brief attacks of deep sleep.

NASAL SCRAPING. Pathological material obtained for clinical study by scratching the inner surface of the nose with a clinical instrument.

NASOPHARYNGEAL. Referring to the passage connecting the nasal cavity behind the nose to the top of the throat behind the soft palate.

NASOPHARYNX. The breathing tube continuous with the nose.

NATIONAL HEALTH EDUCATION STANDARDS (NHES). A set of guidelines that serve as a framework for an effective school health education program.

NATIONAL SCHOOL LUNCH PROGRAM. A program of the U.S. government designed to provide low-cost nutritional meals to students from families who are at or slightly above the national poverty levels.

NATURAL SELECTION. The process by which certain biological traits become either more or less common in the population of a given species as a result of the different rates of reproduction of individuals bearing those traits.

NECROSIS. A form of cell injury that results in the death of living tissue. Tissue necrosis is a common symptom of septicemic plague.

NEED-BASED ASSISTANCE. Financial or other type of aid to a person or a family that is determined entirely by that person's or family's needs.

NEMATODE. Round worms.

NEO-MALTHUSIAN. Refers generally to people with the same general opinions or worries as eighteenth-century Reverand Thomas Malthus, who is considered to be the founder of demographic studies. Neo-Malthusians, like Malthus himself, tend to be concerned about uncurbed population expansion and favor population control programs, including birth control for population control purposes.

NEURAL TUBE. A structure in the human embryo that is the forerunner of the brain and spinal cord. Neural tube defects are responsible for such congenital abnormalities as anencephaly and spina bifida.

NEUROLOGIC. Pertaining to the nervous system.

NEURON. A nerve cell.

NEUROPATHY. Damage to a nerve or group of nerves, resulting in lost or diminished ability to move, feel, or function.

NEUROSYPHILIS. Syphilis of the central nervous system.

NEUROTOXICANT. A substance that is man-made or introduced to an environment by man and is poisonous to the human nervous system. Toxicants are similar to toxins except that they are artificially produced or introduced, where toxins are naturally-occurring.

NEUROTRANSMITTERS. Chemicals within the nervous system that transmit information from or between nerve cells.

NICOTINE. A substance found in tobacco and other plants of the nightshade family (Solanaceae) that acts as a stimulant. Nicotine is highly addictive.

NITROGEN DIOXIDE. With the chemical formula NO_2 (where N stands for nitrogen, and O for oxygen), a reddish-brown toxic gas that is one of several nitrogen oxides.

NOCICEPTOR. A neuron that is capable of sensing pain.

NODULES. A small mass of tissue in the form of a protuberance or a knot that is solid and can be detected by touch.

NON-NUCLEOSIDE REVERSE TRANSCRIPTASE INHIBITORS. The newest class of antiretroviral drugs that work by inhibiting the reverse transcriptase enzyme necessary for HIV replication.

NON-STAPLE FOODS. Food that is not a dominant portion of a population's standard diet. Examples for the United States include carbonated beverages, snack foods, and chocolate.

NONPOTABLE. Not safe to drink.

NORMAL WEIGHT. A BMI of less than 25.0.

NOROVIRUS. Norwalk virus; a large family of RNA viruses that are the most common cause of illness from contaminated food.

NOSOCOMIAL INFECTIONS. Infections that were not present before the patient came to a hospital but were acquired by a patient while there.

NOSODE. A homeopathic remedy made from microbes, pus, or other disease material. Syphilinum is a nosode made from a diluted solution of killed *T. pallidum*.

NUCLEIC ACIDS. The cellular molecules DNA and RNA that act as coded instructions for the production of proteins and are copied for transmission of inherited traits.

NUCLEOSIDE ANALOGUES. The first group of effective anti-retroviral medications. They work by interfering with the AIDS virus' synthesis of DNA.

NULLIPARITY. The condition of being nulliparous, or not bearing offspring.

O

OBESITY. Excessive weight due to accumulation of fat, usually defined as a body mass index (BMI) of 30 or above or body weight greater than 30% above normal on standard height-weight tables.

OBSESSIVE-COMPULSIVE DISORDER (OCD). An anxiety disorder in which a person cannot prevent himself from dwelling on unwanted thoughts, acting on urges, or performing repetitive rituals, such as washing one's hands or checking to make sure lights have been turned off.

OFF-LABEL USE. The practice of prescribing a medication for an indication, age group, dosage level, or method of administration unapproved (or not yet approved) by the Food and Drug Administration.

OMEGA-3 FATTY ACIDS. A class of fatty acids which lowers the level of cholesterol in the blood. Omega-3 fatty acids are also essential for the growth and development of the brain and nerve tissue.

ONCOGENE. A gene that causes normal cell growth, but if mutated or expressed at high levels, encourages normal cells to change into cancerous cells.

ONE HEALTH. A movement based on the concept of individuals from a wide variety of disciplines to obtain the maximum level of health possible for individuals of all species.

OOCYTE. An immature female egg.

OPHTHALMIA. Inflammation of the eye. Usually severe and affecting the conjunctiva. Trachoma is sometimes called Egyptian ophthalmia.

OPIATE BLOCKERS. A type of drug that blocks the effects of natural opiates in the system. This makes some people, including some people with autism, appear more responsive to their environment.

OPPORTUNISTIC INFECTION. An infection caused by an organism that does not cause disease in a person with a healthy immune system.

OPTIC NERVE. The nerve that carries visual messages from the retina to the brain.

ORAL REHYDRATION SOLUTION (ORS). A liquid preparation developed by the World Health Organization that can decrease fluid loss in persons with diarrhea. Originally developed to be prepared with materials available in the home, commercial preparations have recently come into use.

ORCHITIS. Inflammation or swelling of the scrotal sac containing the testicles.

OSTEOPOROSIS. A disease characterized by low bone mass and structural deterioration of bone tissue, leading to bone fragility.

OTOSCLEROSIS. A disease that scars and limits the motion of the small conducting bones in the middle ear.

OVARY. The female organ in which eggs (ova) are stored and mature.

OVERWEIGHT. A BMI between 25.0 and 30.0.

OVULATION. The release of an egg (ovum) from the ovary.

OVUM (PLURAL: OVA). The reproductive cell of the female, which contains genetic information and participates in the act of fertilization. Also popularly called the egg.

OXYGEN FREE RADICALS. Reactive molecules containing oxygen and can cause cell damage.

OXYTOCIN. A hormone that stimulates contractions during child labor and the production of breast milk.

P

PACEMAKER. A surgically implanted electronic device that sends out electrical impulses to regulate a slow or erratic heartbeat.

PANCREAS. A gland near the liver and stomach that secretes digestive fluid into the intestine and the hormones insulin and glucagon into the bloodstream.

PANDEMIC. The occurrence of a disease that in a short time infects a large percentage of the population over a wide geographical area.

PANIC ATTACK. A time-limited period of intense fear accompanied by physical and cognitive symptoms. Panic attacks may be unexpected or triggered by specific internal or external cues.

PAP TEST. A screening test for cervical cancer devised by Giorgios Papanikolaou (1883–1962) in the 1940s.

PAPULES. Firm bumps on the skin.

PARALYSIS. The inability to voluntarily move.

PARAMYXOVIRUS. A genus of viruses that includes the causative agent of mumps.

PARASITE. An organism that lives in or with another organism, called the host, in parasitism, a type of association characterized by the parasite obtaining benefits from the host, such as food, and the host being injured as a result.

PARASITOID. A parasite whose presence on or in an animal ultimately causes the death of that animal.

PARAVETERINARIAN. A person who assists a veterinarian in working with nonhuman animals.

PARENT-TEEN DRIVING CONTRACTS. A contract drawn up and signed by a parent and prospective teenager driver, detailing the rules and responsibilities for the teenage driver. These contracts usually include what is considered safe driving behavior, prohibited or unsafe driving behaviors, and consequences for violating the contract. Such a contract helps the teenager feel more adult, while making the responsibilities of driving clear and carefully outlining what is expected of them. When using such a contract, it is important for parents to set the example by exhibiting the safe driving behaviors that they expect from their teenage driver.

PARENTERAL NUTRITION. Feeding a patient intravenously, thus bypassing normal eating and digestive processes.

PARKINSON'S DISEASE. A progressive disorder of the nervous system that affects your movement. It develops gradually, sometimes starting with a barely noticeable tremor in just one hand. But while tremor may be the most well-known sign of Parkinson's disease, the disorder also commonly causes stiffness or slowing of movement.

PARKINSONISM. A neurological disorder that includes a fine tremor, muscular weakness and rigidity, and an altered way of walking.

PAROTITIS. Inflammation and swelling of the salivary glands.

PARTICIPANT OBSERVATION. A type of qualitative research in which the observer or researcher becomes involved with a specific group of individuals, such as a religious congregation, extended family, or other small group over an extended period of time, and participates in the life of the group as well as making direct observations of the group members.

PASSIVE IMMUNIZATION. Treatment that provides immunity through the transfer of antibodies obtained from an immune individual.

PASTEURIZATION. The process of applying heat, usually to milk or cheese, for the purpose of killing, or retarding the development of, pathogenic bacteria.

PASTIA'S LINES. Red lines in the folds of the skin, especially in the armpit and groin, that are characteristic of scarlet fever.

PATHOGEN. Any microorganism, virus, or other substance that causes disease in another organism.

PEDOPHILE. A person who sexually abuses children.

PELVIC INFLAMMATORY DISEASE (PID). An inflammation of the tubes leading from a woman's ovaries to the uterus (the Fallopian tubes), caused by a bacterial infection. PID is a leading cause of fertility problems in women.

PENICILLIN. An antibiotic that is used to treat bacterial infections.

PERFORMANCE-BASED OBJECTIVE. An objective that is measured by some type of action and defined by the results of that action.

PERIODONTAL. Pertaining to the gums.

PESTICIDES. Chemicals used to kill insects.

PETECHIAE. Pinpoint size red spots caused by hemorrhaging under the skin.

pH. A measurement of the acidity or alkalinity of a fluid. A neutral fluid, neither acid nor alkali, has a pH of 7.

PHAGOCYTOSIS. The "ingestion" of a piece of matter by a cell.

PHENYLKETONURIA (PKU). An enzyme deficiency present at birth that disrupts metabolism and causes brain damage. This rare inherited defect may be linked to the development of autism.

PHOTODYNAMIC THERAPY (PDT). A treatment for tumors in which a light-sensitive dye is injected into the blood (or skin) to be taken up selectively by the tumors. Light of a specific wavelength is then applied to the affected area to kill the tumors.

PHOTOPHOBIA. Abnormal sensitivity to light.

PHTHALATES. Toxic chemical that may be present in toys and may lead to development dangers.

PHYSICAL ACTIVITY. Any activity that involves moving the body and burning calories.

PHYSICAL FITNESS. A combination of muscle strength, cardiovascular health, and flexibility that is usually attributed to regular exercise and good nutrition.

PIA MATER. The innermost layer of the meninges.

PISTON. The plunger that slides up and down the inside barrel of a syringe.

PLACENTA. The organ that develops in the uterus during pregnancy that links the blood supplies of the mother and baby.

PLAGUE. A highly infectious disease that can be fatal if not treated promptly. The bacteria that cause plague mainly infect rats, mice, squirrels, and other wild rodents. The disease is passed to people through fleas. Infected people can then spread the disease to other people.

PLAQUE. A thin, sticky, colorless film of bacteria that forms on teeth; or, a mass of material made up of fat, cholesterol, calcium, and other substances found in the blood. It can stick to the walls of arteries, partially or totally blocking blood flow.

PLASMID. A small loop of genetic material that is not part of a chromosome and can be easily transferred between bacteria.

PLATELETS. Circulating blood cells that are crucial to the mechanism of clotting.

PLEURAL EFFUSION. Pleural effusion is excess fluid that accumulates between the two pleural layers, the fluid-filled space that surrounds the lungs. Excessive amounts of such fluid can impair breathing by limiting the expansion of the lungs during ventilation.

PLEURAL PLAQUES. Pleural plaques are localized scars (fibrosis) consisting of collagen fiber deposits that form as a result of exposure to asbestos. They are the most common manifestation of exposure to asbestos. Normally, pleural plaque is found on the inside of the diaphragm, but in very rare cases it also can be found near the ribcage. Pleural plaques themselves are not associated with any symptoms. However, many people who develop pleural plaques also develop pleural effusion, asbestosis, malignant mesothelioma and other conditions associated with asbestos inhalation.

PNEUMOCOCCAL. Infection by the bacterium *Streptococcus pneumoniae* that causes acute pneumonia.

PNEUMONIA. Inflammation of the lungs, usually caused by infection with a bacterium, virus, or fungus.

PNEUMOTHORAX. Air inside the chest cavity that may cause the lung to collapse. It is both a complication of pulmonary tuberculosis and a means of treatment designed to allow an infected lung to rest and heal.

POLYCARBONATE PLASTICS. With a variety of household and industrial uses, these plastics are clear, hard, and incredibly durable. These plastics are subject to breakdown and chemical degradation under high temperatures.

POLYCHLORINATED BIPHENYLS. Any compound derived from biphenyl and containing chlorine (Cl), which is considered an hazardous environmental pollutant; with the abbreviation PCBs.

POLYMER. A natural or synthetic substance composed of multiple monomers.

POLYSOMNOGRAPHY. Monitoring of respiratory, cardiac, brain, muscular, and ocular function simultaneously during sleep. This form of monitoring is often used to diagnose sleep apnea.

POLYUNSATURATED FAT. Fats that contain two or more double or triple carbon bonds per molecule; examples include fish, safflower, sunflower, corn, and soybean oils.

POST–TRAUMATIC STRESS DISORDER (PTSD). Also known as rape trauma syndrome, it is a mental health disorder that describes a range of symptoms often experienced by someone who has undergone a severely traumatic event.

POST-EXPOSURE PROPHYLAXIS (PEP). A four-week course of antiretroviral drugs given to people immediately following exposure to HIV infection from rape, unprotected sex, needlestick injuries, or sharing needles.

POST-HERPETIC NEURALGIA (PHN). Long-lasting nerve pain caused by herpes zoster.

POST-TRAUMATIC STRESS DISORDER (PTSD). A psychological response to a highly stressful event; typically characterized by depression, anxiety, flashbacks, nightmares, and avoidance of reminders of the traumatic experience.

POSTPARTUM. Following childbirth.

POTABLE. Safe for drinking.

POVERTY LEVEL. A minimum amount of income for an individual or family that allows adequate lifestyle in any particular country, state, or region.

POX. A pus-filled bump on the skin.

PREGNANCY CATEGORY. A system of classifying drugs according to their established risks for use during pregnancy. Category A: Controlled human studies have demonstrated no fetal risk. Category B: Animal studies indicate no fetal risk, but no human studies; or adverse effects in animals, but not in well-controlled human studies. Category C: No adequate human or animal studies; or adverse fetal effects in animal studies, but no available human data. Category D: Evidence of fetal risk, but benefits outweigh risks. Category X: Evidence of fetal risk. Risks outweigh any benefits.

PREPUCE. The fold of tissue covering the clitoris in females and the tip of the penis in males.

PRESENTEEISM. A term used to describe inefficiency or poor quality of work from employees who can come to work but are hampered by physical or mental illness.

PREVALENCE. The total number of cases of a disease at any one time in a region.

PRIMARY ENFORCEMENT. A law in which a police officer can pull over and ticket a driver for, without any other cause.

PRIMARY HEALTH CARE. A level of health care that is necessary for an individual to maintain good health that normally involves preventive education and treatment and early diagnosis and treatment of possible health and medical problems.

PRION. An infectious agent composed of a protein that has been folded in an abnormal manner. Prions are believed to be responsible for various neurodegenerative diseases, including bovine spongiform encephalitis (mad cow disease).

PROBIOTICS. Food supplements containing live bacteria or other microbes intended to improve or restore the normal balance of microorganisms in the digestive tract.

PROCAINE PENICILLIN. An injectable form of penicillin that contains an anesthetic to reduce the pain of the injection.

PROCESS ADDICTION. Addiction to certain mood-altering behaviors, such as eating, gambling, sexual activity, overwork, and shopping.

PROCTOSCOPE. An instrument consisting of a thin tube with a light source, used to examine the inside of the rectum.

PRODROME. Early symptoms or warning signs

PROPENSITY. A greater risk for developing a disease.

PROPHYLACTIC. A drug, medical device, or technique intended to prevent (rather than treat) disease. Condoms are sometimes called prophylactics.

PROSPECTIVE PAYMENT SYSTEM (PPS). A method of making medical payments based on a standard developed through the analysis of previous payments for particular types of services

PROSTAGLANDINS. Fatty acids produced by the body that are responsible for inflammation features, such as swelling, pain, stiffness, redness, and warmth as well as being involved in smooth muscle contractions.

PROSTHESIS. A synthetic replacement for a missing part of the body, such as a knee or a hip.

PROTEASE INHIBITORS. The second major category of drug used to treat AIDS that works by suppressing the replication of the HIV virus.

PROTEIN. Chains of amino acids that are essential constituents of all living cells and include structural components, enzymes, hormones, and antibodies.

PROTOZOA. Single–celled microorganisms of the Kingdom Protista, some of which can cause infectious disease in humans.

PROTOZOAN(PLURAL, PROTOZOA). A single-celled, usually microscopic organism that is eukaryotic and, therefore, different from bacteria (prokaryotic).

PROVITAMIN. A substance that the body can convert into a vitamin.

PSYCHIATRIC BOARDING. The practice of holding mentally ill patients in emergency department corridors and waiting areas, because of the lack of hospital beds or other facilities.

PSYCHOACTIVE DRUG. A drug that affects the central nervous system by crossing the blood-brain barrier. These drugs cause alterations in the brain's ability to function normally.

PSYCHOLOGICAL TESTS. Written, verbal, or visual tasks that assess psychological functioning, intelligence, and/or personality traits.

PSYCHOSIS. A serious mental disorder characterized by defective or lost contact with reality often with hallucinations or delusions.

PUBLIC HEALTH ENGLAND. A new agency in the United Kingdom created to carry out the provisions of the white paper, "Healthy Lives, Healthy People." It is currently within the bureaucratic structure of the Department of Health.

PUBLIC SERVICE ANNOUNCEMENTS (PSAS). Media including television or radio commercials, brochures, and posters gained at affecting change on behalf of the public good. PSAs may try to enhance compliance with existing laws, like obeying seat belt or child safety seat laws). PSAs may also attempt to improve consumer behavior in ways that will increase safety—for instance, PSAs discouraging text messaging while driving preceded legislation that made this behavior illegal.

PUERPERAL FEVER. An infection in women who have just undergone childbirth.

PULMONARY. Having to do with the lungs or respiratory system.

PULMONARY EOSINOPHILIA. Swelling of lung tissue as a result of increase production of white blood cells.

PURIFIED PROTEIN DERIVATIVE (PPD). An extract of tubercle bacilli that is injected into the skin to find out whether a person presently has or has ever had tuberculosis.

PYROMANIA. A disorder of impulse control in which a person sets fires either for gratification or to relieve tension. About 90% of persons diagnosed with pyromania are males.

Q

Q-FEVER. A disease marked by high fever, chills, and muscle pain. It is seen in North America, Europe, and parts of Africa. It may be spread by drinking raw milk or by tick bites.

QUALITATIVE RESEARCH. An approach to research that focuses on human behavior and the reasons for it; it is usually based on social interactions, words, or images rather than numbers and statistics. Qualitative research typically uses a small study sample, and the information obtained is regarded as limited to that sample rather than applicable to the general population.

QUANTITATIVE RESEARCH. A quantifiable approach to research in which raw data are collected and turned into usable information by mathematical computation. Quantitative research uses statistics to make generalizations or predictions about a population larger than the study sample.

QUARANTINE. The practice of isolating sick persons or animals, or restricting travel or passage in order to prevent the spread of a contagious disease. The English word comes from the Italian word for forty, the number of days customary for quarantining ships visiting Italian ports during the medieval plague epidemics.

QUININE. One of the first treatments for malaria, a natural product made from the bark of the Cinchona tree. It was popular until being superseded by chloroquine in the 1940s. In the wake of widespread chloroquine resistance, however, it became popular again. Quinine, or its close relative quinidine, can be given intravenously to treat severe *Falciparum* malaria.

R

RABIES. A rare but serious disease caused by a virus carried in saliva. It is transmitted when an infected animal bites a person.

RADIATION THERAPY. Treatment using high-energy radiation from x-ray machines, cobalt, radium, or other sources.

RADIOACTIVE RADIATION. Radiation produced from radioactive substances.

RADIOISOTOPE. An unstable isotope that emits radiation when it decays or returns to a stable state.

RADIOTHERAPY. The use of x rays or radioactive substances to treat disease.

RANDOMIZED CONTROLLED TRIAL (RCT). A study in which subjects are allocated at random to receive one of several clinical interventions.

REASONABLE VOLUME. The number of indigent clients a clinic, nursing home, hospital, or other healthcare facility is required to treat in order to qualify for Hill-Burton grants and loans. The term has been interpreted by courts in specific cases, but never defined specifically by the U.S. Congress.

RECESSIVE INHERITANCE. A pattern of inheritance where both parents carry the gene responsible for a trait or disease (although they seldom show symptoms). Their offspring will have a 25% chance of having the trait or disease. Recessive inheritance is also responsible for disorders such as hemophilia, where the mother carries the affected gene on the X chromosome and passes it to her son.

RECOMMENDED DIETARY ALLOWANCE (RDA). The daily amount of a vitamin the average person needs to maintain good health.

REFERRED PAIN. Pain felt at a site different from the location of the injured or diseased part of the body. Referred pain is due to the fact that nerve signals from several areas of the body may "feed" the same nerve pathway leading to the spinal cord and brain.

REFUGEE CAMP. A rudimentary, makeshift city constructed to house large numbers of refugees, often in the case of war or nationwide violence. These camps are almost exclusively managed and funded by international organizations and charities, particularly branches of the United Nations. Refugee camps provide basic shelter (usually in the form of tents), as well as basic food supplies and emergency medical care. Refugee camps are often plagued by contaminated water, insufficient sanitation, overcrowding, violence (especially against women), and the spread of illness and disease.

REITER'S SYNDROME. A group of symptoms that includes arthritis, inflammation of the urethra, and conjunctivitis, and develops as a late complication of infection with *Shigella flexneri*. The syndrome was first described by a German doctor named Hans Reiter in 1918.

RELAPSE. A recurrence of symptoms after a period of improvement or recovery.

RELATIVE DEPRIVATION. The tendency to base one's criteria for normalcy on comparisons with neighbors and relatives.

REM. Rapid eye movement; a stage of the normal sleep cycle characterized by rapid eye movements, increased forebrain and midbrain activity, and dreaming.

RENAL. Referring to the kidneys.

REPETITIVE STRESS INJURY. An injury that occurs as a result of repeating some physical action over and over again many times in sequence.

REPORTABLE DISEASE. Any disease that is required by law to be reported to government authorities or to such organizations as the CDC or WHO. Reportable diseases are also called notifiable diseases.

RESERVOIR. In epidemiology, any species (including humans) that maintains a specific disease organism in nature.

RESPITE CARE. Temporary care of a patient to provide caregivers with a period of physical, mental, and emotional rest.

RESTLESS LEGS SYNDROME (RLS). A neurological disorder characterized by aching, burning, or creeping sensations in the legs and an urge to move the legs, often resulting in insomnia.

RETINA. The light-sensitive layer of the eye.

RETROVIRUS. A virus that uses its RNA to produce DNA and add that DNA to the genetic material of infected cells.

REVERSE TRANSCRIPTION-POLYMERASE CHAIN REACTION (RT-PCR). A method of polymerase-chain-reaction amplification of nucleic acid sequences that uses RNA as the template for transcribing the corresponding DNA using reverse transcriptase.

REYE'S SYNDROME. A rare, but often fatal, disease that involves the brain, liver, and kidneys. It may brought on by giving salicylates to children (but not adults) who have a viral infection.

RH DISEASE. Illness caused when an Rh-negative woman is pregnant with an Rh-positive fetus, and her body produces antibodies against the fetus's blood.

RH IMMUNE GLOBULIN (RHOGAM). A vaccine given to a woman after an abortion, miscarriage, or prenatal tests in order to prevent sensitization to Rh disease. Sensitization to the disease occurs when the blood of a woman who is Rh positive is exposed to the blood of a previous fetus, which was Rh negative.

RH NEGATIVE. Lacking the Rh factor, which is a genetically determined antigen on red blood cells that produce immune responses.

RHABDOVIRUS. A type of virus named for its rod- or bullet-like shape. The rabies virus belongs to a family of viruses called Rhabdoviridae.

RHEUMATIC FEVER. A heart disease that is a complication of a strep infection.

RHEUMATOID ARTHRITIS. An autoimmune disease characterized by inflammation and degeneration of connective tissue in multiple joints at a young age. It also can affect additional organ systems.

RHINORRHEA. A name for the common cold.

RHINOVIRUS. A virus that infects the upper respiratory system and causes the common cold.

RHYTHM METHOD. The oldest method of contraception with a very high failure rate, in which partners periodically refrain from having sex during ovulation. Ovulation is predicted on the basis of a woman's previous menstrual cycle.

RING-FENCED FINANCING. Financing for a particular project that is protected from use for any purpose than that for which it was specifically designated.

RISK. The probability that exposure to a hazard will have a negative consequence. There are mathematical equations and computer programs that can be used to calculate risk in specific situations.

RISK ASSESSMENT. A procedure by which a health worker and an individual review one' current medical status with the goal of accurately estimating future chances of developing a particular medical condition and reviewing ways of changing that probability.

RISK FACTOR. A substance or condition that increases the probability of developing a particular medical condition.

ROENTGEN EQUIVALENT IN MAN. Short for roentgen equivalent in man, it is a dose equivalent radiation. One rem is equal to 0.01 Sievert (Sv).

ROSE SPOTS. A pinkish rash across the trunk or abdomen that is a classic sign of typhoid fever.

ROSEOLA. A viral infection that typically affects infants and young children. Its common symptoms include a skin rash and fever.

RUBELLA. A contagious viral disease that is milder than typical measles but is damaging to the fetus when it occurs early in pregnancy. Also called German measles.

S

SAFETY-NET PROVIDERS. Healthcare providers who offer services to patients regardless of their ability to pay; and who have a patient mix with a substantial share of uninsured, Medicaid, or otherwise vulnerable patients.

SALMONELLOSIS. Severe diarrhea caused by food contaminated with bacteria of the genus *Salmonella*.

SANITARIAN. A person who has been trained in the sanitary sciences and is qualified to work in some aspect of that field.

SATURATED FAT. Fat molecules that contain only single carbon bonds; examples include whole milk, cream, palm and coconut oils, and solid fats such as cheese, butter, and meat.

SCLERA. The tough, fibrous, white outer protective covering that surrounds the eye.

SCORCHED EARTH. A military strategy that includes confiscating or destroying the civilian food supply as well as destroying other resources that might be useful to the enemy.

SECONDARY OR OPPORTUNISTIC INFECTION. An infection by a microbe that occurs because the body is weakened by a primary infection caused by a different kind of microbe.

SEDENTARY. Inactivity and lack of exercise; a lifestyle that is a major risk factor for becoming overweight or obese and developing chronic diseases.

SEIZURE. A sudden attack, spasm, or convulsion.

SELECTIVE PRESSURE. Influence exerted by an antibiotic or other factor on natural selection to promote the survival of one group of organisms over another.

SELECTIVE SEROTONIN REUPTAKE INHIBITORS (SSRIS). A class of antidepressants that works by blocking the reabsorption of serotonin in the brain, raising the levels of serotonin.

SELF-DELIVERANCE. Another term for assisted suicide, more commonly used in Great Britain than in the United States.

SELF-DIRECTED VIOLENCE. Suicidal or self-harm acts or thoughts.

SEMEN. The thick whitish liquid released from the penis during sexual intercourse. It contains sperm and other secretions.

SENESCENCE. The state or process of aging.

SEPARATE-BUT-EQUAL. A now illegal doctrine that posits that individuals of different race, class, ethnicity, or other traits may be treated equally even if services are provided in physically separate facilities, such as schools or hospitals.

SEPSIS. Presence of various pus-forming and other pathogenic organisms, or their toxins, in the blood or tissues.

SEPTICEMIA. The presence of disease organisms and their toxins in the bloodstream.

SEQUENCING. The process of discovering the sequence of amino acids in a protein or nucleotides in a DNA molecule.

SEROCONVERSION. The development of detectable specific antibodies in a patient's blood serum as a result of infection or immunization.

SEROTONIN. A neurotransmitter located primarily in the brain, blood serum, and stomach membrane.

SEX-LINKED GENETIC DISORDER. A disease or disorder caused by a gene mutation located on the X (female) or Y (male) chromosome.

SEXUAL ABUSE. Sexual activity forced upon an individual by use of threats or other fear tactics, or incurred by an individual who is physically unable to refuse.

SEXUAL ASSAULT NURSE EXAMINER (SANE). A registered nurse who is trained to collect and document evidence from a sexual assault victim, to evaluate and treat for sexually transmitted diseases (STDs) and pregnancy, and to refer victims to follow-up medical care and counseling.

SEXUAL TOURISM. The practice of traveling to other countries for the purpose of paid sexual encounters.

SEXUAL VIOLENCE. Violence between two or more individuals that involves non-consensual sexual acts with or without physical contact.

SHEEP BLOOD AGAR PLATE. A petri dish filled with a nutrient gel containing red blood cells that is used to detect the presence of streptococcal bacteria in a throat culture. Streptococcal bacteria will lyse or break open red blood cells, leaving a clear spot around the bacterial colony.

SHELTER IN PLACE. A phrase used to describe remaining indoors in a safe location during an emergency rather than evacuating the area.

SHIGA TOXIN-PRODUCING E. COLI (STEC). Strains of the common, normally harmless, intestinal bacterium *Escherichia coli* that can contaminate food with Shiga toxin; *E. coli* O157:H7 is the most commonly identified STEC in North America.

SHINGLES. Also known as "herpes zoster,"it is a viral infection that causes a painful rash. The virus that causes shingles also causes chickenpox.

SHOCK. An abnormal condition resulting from low blood volume due to hemorrhage or dehydration. Signs of shock include rapid pulse and breathing, and cool, moist, pale skin.

SICKLE CELL DISEASE. An inherited disorder characterized by a genetic flaw in hemoglobin production. (Hemoglobin is the substance within red blood cells that enables them to transport oxygen.) The hemoglobin that is produced has a kink in its structure that forces the red blood cells to take on a sickle shape, inhibiting their circulation and causing pain. This disorder primarily affects people of African descent.

SIDESTREAM SMOKE. The smoke emitted from burning tobacco (not exhaled by a smoker).

SIEVERT. Abbreviated Sv, it is a unit of dose equivalent radiation in the International System of Units (SI). One Sv is equal to 100 rem, or 100,000 millirem (mrem).

SIGMOIDOSCOPY. A medical procedure that allows a doctor to examine the interior lining of the lower part of the colon and rectum. It provides a less-complete view of the colon than a colonoscopy does.

SINOATRIAL NODE (SAN). The heart's natural pacemaker, a group of cells located in the wall of the right atrium (upper chamber) of the heart near the entry of the superior vena cava, a major vein that carries deoxygenated blood from the upper part of the body to the heart.

SLASH-AND-BURN. An agricultural practice that involves the cutting and burning of trees in a forested area to create new fields. It quickly results in soil depletion followed by soil erosion.

SMALLPOX. A highly contagious viral disease characterized by fever, weakness, and skin eruption with pustules that form scabs that slough off, leaving scars.

SMEAR. A specimen prepared for microscopic study by spreading the material across a slide and treating it with a specific stain.

SOCIOECONOMIC STATUS. Perceived status of an individual, family or community based on average income, education level, and social status.

SORE. An open wound, bruise, or lesion on the skin.

SPACE DISASTER. Events that follow accidents that occur in space or as the result of space materials, such as the collision of an asteroid with the surface of the Earth.

SPERM. The reproductive cell of the male, which contains genetic information and participates in the act of fertilization of an ovum.

SPERMATOGENESIS. The process by which sperm develop to become mature sperm, capable of fertilizing an ovum.

SPILLOVER. In epidemiology, the sporadic transmission of a disease agent from a reservoir species to a non-reservoir species.

SPINA BIFIDA. A congenital defect in which part of the vertebrae fail to develop completely, leaving a portion of the spinal cord exposed.

SPIROCHETE. Any of a family of spiral- or coil-shaped bacteria known as Spirochetae. *L. interrogans* is a spirochete, as well as are the organisms that cause syphilis and relapsing fever.

SPIROMETRY. A test using an instrument called a spirometer that shows how difficult it is for an asthmatic individual to breathe. It is used to determine the severity of asthma and to see how well it is responding to treatment.

SPIRULINA. A nutritional supplement made from two species of blue-green algae belonging to the genus *Arthrospira*.

SPORADIC. Rare and occasional in occurrence. Listeriosis in humans is a sporadic disease.

SPORE. A dormant form assumed by some bacteria, such as anthrax, that enable the bacterium to survive high temperatures, dryness, and lack of nourishment for long periods of time. Under proper conditions, the spore may revert to the actively multiplying form of the bacteria.

SPUTUM. Secretions produced in the lung and coughed up. A sign of illness, sputum is routinely used as a specimen for culturing the tubercle bacillus in the laboratory.

STAKEHOLDER. An individual or organization with an interest in or concern for some specific topic or problem.

STANDARD PRECAUTIONS. A set of minimum infection prevention practices used in all types of patient care, regardless of suspected or confirmed infection status of any patients, in any setting where healthcare is delivered.

STAPHYLOCOCCAL INFECTION. An infection caused by the organism *Staphylococcus Aureus*. Infection by this agent is common and is often resistant to antibiotics.

STATE CHILDREN'S HEALTH INSURANCE PROGRAM; SCHIP; CHIP. A state-administered health insurance program for lower- and middle-income children who are without private health insurance and whose family incomes are above the Medicaid eligibility limits.

STATINS. A group of medications given to lower blood cholesterol levels that work by inhibiting an enzyme involved in cholesterol formation. Statins are also known as HMG-CoA reductase inhibitors.

STERILE. Free from living microorganisms.

STERILIZATION. Any procedure that kills all micro-organisms in and on a product.

STIGMA. A mark or characteristic trait of a disease or defect; by extension, a cause for reproach or a stain on one's reputation.

STIMULANTS. A class of drugs, including Ritalin, used to treat people with autism. They may make children calmer and better able to concentrate, but they also may limit growth or have other side effects.

STIMULUS. A factor capable of eliciting a response in a nerve.

STOOL. Passage of fecal material; a bowel movement.

STRABISMUS. An improper muscle balance of the ocular muscles resulting in crossed or divergent eyes.

STRAWBERRY TONGUE. A sign of scarlet fever in which the tongue appears to have a red coating with large, raised bumps.

STREET DRUG. A substance purchased from a drug dealer; may be a legal substance, sold illicitly (without a prescription, and not for medical use), or it may be a substance that is illegal to possess.

STRESS HARDINESS. A personality characteristic that enables persons to stay healthy in stressful circumstances. It includes belief in one's ability to influence the situation; commitment to or full engagement with one's activities; and a positive view of change.

STRESS MANAGEMENT. A category of popularized programs and techniques intended to help people deal more effectively with stress.

STRESS TEST. An electrocardiogram recorded before, during, and after a period of increasingly strenuous cardiovascular exercise, usually on a treadmill or stationary bicycle.

STRESSOR. A stimulus, or event, that provokes a stress response in an organism. Stressors can be categorized as acute or chronic and as external or internal to the organism.

STROKE. Irreversible damage to the brain caused by insufficient blood flow to the brain as the result of a blocked artery. Damage can include loss of speech or vision, paralysis, cognitive impairment, and death.

STROMA. A term used to describe the supportive tissue surrounding a particular structure. An example is that tissue which surrounds and supports the actually functional lung tissue.

STUNTING. A height more than two standard deviations from the median height for the age in the reference population.

SUBARACHNOID HEMORRHAGE. A cause of some strokes in which arteries on the surface of the brain begin bleeding.

SUBCUTANEOUS. The area directly beneath the skin.

SUICIDE GESTURE. Attempted suicide characterized by a low-lethality method, low level of intent or planning, and little physical damage; sometimes called pseudocide.

SUICIDE MAGNET. A bridge, tall building, or geographic location that acquires a reputation for attracting people who want to commit suicide and attempt it.

SULFADOXONE/PYRIMETHAMINE (FANSIDAR). An antimalarial drug developed in the 1960s. It was the first drug tried in some parts of the world where chloroquine resistance is widespread. It has been associated with severe allergic reactions due to its sulfa component.

SULFONAMIDES. A class of synthetic drugs used to prevent certain types of bacteria from reproducing.

SUN PROTECTION FACTOR (SPF). A numerical value assigned to sunscreen and sunblock products to communicate the product's ability to protect against UV-B rays. The higher the number, the greater the protection.

SUNBURN. The inflammation and redness of the skin caused by prolonged exposure to the sun.

SUPERBUG. An informal term for a bacterium that has become resistant to many different antibiotics. Bacteria that are resistant to several different drugs are also called multidrug-resistant or MDR bacteria.

SUPPLEMENTAL SECURITY INCOME (SSI). A federal entitlement program that provides cash assistance to low-income blind, disabled, and elderly people. In most states, people receiving SSI benefits are eligible for Medicaid.

SURFACE PLASMON RESONANCE (SPR). Describes the use of light to cause the oscillation of valence electrons in a solid. SPR can be used to measure absorption of material.

SURGICAL HAND ANTISEPSIS. An antiseptic handwash or handrub in preparation for surgery that follows a carefully prescribed sequence of steps. Also known as surgical hand preparation or presurgical hand preparation.

SURVEILLANCE. In epidemiology, the monitoring and reporting of cases of contagious disease in order to establish patterns of its spread to prevent or minimize the development of epidemics and pandemics.

SWEATSHOP. According to the United States Department of Labor, a workplace is considered a sweatshop if it violates two or more basic labor laws, including (but not limited to): child labor, fire safety, minimum wage, or overtime pay.

SYLVATIC. Pertaining to or living in the woods or forested areas. The form of yellow fever transmitted by mosquitoes to rainforest monkeys is called sylvatic yellow fever.

SYMBIOTIC. Having to do with a close physical association between individuals of two different species.

SYNDEMIC. A combination of two or more diseases in a given population in which there is a positive biological interaction between the two diseases that intensifies their negative effects on health.

SYSTEMATIC REVIEW. A summary of the medical literature that uses explicit methods to perform a comprehensive literature search and critical appraisal of individual studies, and also uses appropriate statistical techniques to combine these valid studies.

SYSTEMIC. Relating to the complete body of an organism.

SYSTEMIC LUPUS ERYTHEMATOSUS (SLE). A chronic, inflammatory, autoimmune disorder in which the individual's immune system attacks, injures, and destroys the body's own organs and tissues. It may affect many organ systems, including the skin, joints, lungs, heart, and kidneys.

SYSTEMIC NAME. The official chemical name of a compound.

T

T CELLS. Immune system white blood cells that have highly specific antigen receptors on their surfaces. Some T cells stimulate other immune system cells to produce and release antibodies.

T-LYMPHOCYTE. A type of white blood cell, also known as a T-helper cell, a T_h cell, an effector T cell, or a CD4+ T cell, whose numbers in a blood sample can be used to monitor the progression of HIV infection.

TABES DORSALIS. A progressive deterioration of the spinal cord and spinal nerves that is associated with tertiary syphilis.

TANNING. The usually intentional process of prolonged exposure to UV rays—either from the sun or special light bulbs—in order to darken one's skin.

TARGET HEART RATE. The heart rate, in beats per minute (bpm), that should be maintained during cardiovascular exercise by an individual of a given age.

TARTAR. A hardened yellow or brown mineral deposit from unremoved plaque; also called "calculus."

TAURINE. An amino acid that is important in the development of brain tissue. Taurine is a key component of bile which is needed to digest fats.

TD. Tetanus and diphtheria vaccine.

TECTONIC PLATES. A rigid rocky plate within the lithosphere that moves horizontally below the Earth's surface.

TEMPERATURE INVERSION. A weather condition in which cooler air near the ground has a layer of warmer air above it, in contrast to the normal pattern of air temperature decreasing steadily with altitude. Temperature inversions have been implicated in several instance of smog-related disasters.

TENESMUS. Ineffective spasms of the rectum or bladder accompanied by the desire to evacuate the rectum or pass urine but without being able to do so. Tenesmus is a characteristic feature of bacillary dysentery.

TERATOGEN. Any drug, chemical, maternal disease, or exposure that can cause physical or functional defects in an exposed embryo or fetus.

TETRALOGY OF FALLOT. A congenital heart condition characterized by four separate anatomical abnormalities in the baby's heart. It is named for Arthur Fallot (1850–1911), a French physician who described it in detail in 1888.

THERMOSETTING PLASTIC. A polymer that, once formed, can not be reheated, melted, or reformed. Also known as a resin.

THROMBUS. A blood clot that forms inside an intact blood vessel and remains there.

TISSUE PLASMINOGEN ACTIVATOR (TPA). A substance that is sometimes given to patients within three hours of a stroke to dissolve blood clots within the brain.

TOLERANCE. The requirement for higher doses of a substance or more frequent engagement in an activity to achieve the same effect.

TOMOGRAPHY. Any of a number of medical imaging procedures that image sections of a body with the use of various types of penetrating waves, such as x rays.

TOPICAL. Referring to a type of medication applied directly to the skin or outside of the body.

TOXICANT. Any toxic chemical produced by human activity, as distinct from natural toxins.

TOXICITY. The quality of being or the degree to which a substance is poisonous.

TOXICOLOGY. The branch of medicine that deals with the effects, detection, and treatment of poisons.

TOXINS. Any type of poison made by humans or introduced into the environment by human activity, such as insecticides.

TOXOID. A preparation made from inactivated exotoxin, used in immunization.

TOXOPLASMA GONDII. A very common parasite that is a leading cause of death from food contamination; although it infects large numbers of people, T. gondii is usually dangerous only in immunocompromised patients and newly infected pregnant women.

TRACHEOTOMY. A surgical procedure in which a hole is cut through the neck to open a direct airway through an incision in the trachea (windpipe).

TRAJECTORY. The path of an object in motion.

TRANS FAT. Fat that is produced by hydrogenation during food processing; trans fats increase bad cholesterol and decrease good cholesterol.

TRANSIENT ISCHEMIC ATTACK (TIA). A brief stroke lasting from a few minutes to 24 hours. TIAs are sometimes called mini-strokes.

TRANSLATIONAL SCIENCE. A term used in the health sciences to describe the transfer and application of laboratory science to bedside clinical practice or population-based public health interventions.

TRANSLOCATION. The rearrangement or exchange of segments of chromosomes that does not alter the total number of chromosomes, but sometimes results in a genetic disorder or disease.

TRAUMA. A severe injury or shock to a person's body or mind.

TRAVELERS' DIARRHEA. An illness due to infection from a bacteria or parasite that occurs in persons traveling to areas where there is a high frequency of the illness. The disease is usually spread by contaminated food or water.

TREPONEMA PALLIDUM. The spirochete bacterium that causes syphilis.

TRIAGE. A method for determining the priority of patient treatment during a disaster or mass casualty event according to the severity of the injuries.

TRICARE. A healthcare program provided by the federal government to active military personnel and their dependents and to retired personnel.

TRIGLYCERIDES. Neutral fats; lipids formed from glycerol and fatty acids that circulate in the blood as lipoprotein. Elevated triglyceride levels contribute to the development of cardiovascular disease.

TRIHALOMETHANES (THMS). a group of organic chemicals that often occur in drinking water that has been treated through chlorination. THMs are categorized by the Environmental Protection Agency as probable human carcinogens. The THMs are chloroform, bromodichloromethane, dibromochloromethane, and bromoform. The most common THM is chloroform.

TRIMESTER. One-third (or 13 weeks) of a pregnancy. A woman's pregnancy is therefore divided into the first trimester, second trimester, and third/final trimester

TRISOMY. A chromosomal disorder in which there are three copies of a chromosome in each body cell instead of the normal two copies. The most common trisomies are trisomy 21 (Down syndrome) and trisomy 18 (Edwards syndrome).

TROPHOZOITE. The active feeding stage of a protozoal parasite, as distinct from its encysted stage.

TUBERCULOMA. A tumor-like mass in the brain that sometimes develops as a complication of tuberculosis meningitis.

TUBERCULOSIS. An infectious disease that primarily infects the lungs. Tuberculosis can cause weight lost, chest pain, fever, and death. Tuberculosis is caused by various strains of bacteria and is passed from one person to another through the air.

TUBEROUS SCLEROSIS. A genetic disease that causes skin problems, seizures, and mental retardation. Autism occurs more often in individuals with tuberous sclerosis.

TUMOR. An abnormal growth resulting from a cell that lost its normal growth control restraints and started multiplying uncontrollably.

TYPE 1 DIABETES. A chronic immune system disorder in which the pancreas does not produce sufficient amounts of insulin, a hormone that enables cells to use glucose for energy. Also called juvenile diabetes, it must be treated with insulin injections.

TYPE 2 DIABETES. Sometimes called adult-onset diabetes, this disease prevents the body from properly using glucose (sugar).

TYPHOID FEVER. An infectious disease caused by *Salmonelli typhi* bacterium and characterized by a lingering fever, diarrhea, feelings of exhaustion and depression, and rose-colored spots on the chest and abdomen. The disease is spread through poor sanitation.

TZANCK PREPARATION. A procedure in which skin cells from a blister are stained and examined under the microscope.

U

ULCERATION. An area of pitting and irritation.

ULTRA HIGH TEMPERATURE (UHT) PROCESSING. Procedure in food processing where a product is heated, for a short time, to a higher temperature than those used in pasteurization. Result of UHT processing is near sterilization of the food product.

ULTRASOUND. A technique that uses high-frequency sound waves for medical diagnosis and treatment by creating images of internal organs.

ULTRAVIOLET (UV) RAYS. A term describing the sun's rays and encompassing both UV-A and UV-B rays. In small doses, these rays help the human body create vitamin D, which is needed for many bodily processes. In large doses, these rays can lead to health problems including sunburn, cataracts, blindness, immune system suppression, premature aging, and cancer.

UMBILICUS. The medical term for the navel or belly button.

UNDERSERVED POPULATION. A group of individuals who receive fewer services than would normally be considered necessary for a normaly lifestyle.

UREA. Chemical formed during the body's metabolism of nitrogen and normally excreted by the kidney. Urea levels rise in the blood when kidney failure occurs.

UROLOGIST. Physician specializing in male reproductive and urinary systems.

V

VACCINATION. Injection of a killed or weakened microbe in order to stimulate the immune system against the microbe, thereby preventing disease. Vaccinations, or "immunizations," work by stimulating the immune system so that it will recognize invading bacteria and viruses, and produce substances (antibodies) to destroy or disable them. Vaccinations therefore prepare the immune system to ward off a disease.

VACCINE. A prepartation containing killed or weakened microorganisms used to build immunity against infection from that microorganism.

VALACYCLOVIR. An oral antiviral drug that blocks the replication of the varicella zoster virus.

VASODILATOR. A class of drugs that widen the blood vessels, in turn decreasing resistance to blood flow and lowering blood pressure.

VATA. One of the three main constitutional types found under Ayurvedic principles. Keeping one's particular constitution in balance is considered important in maintaining health.

VECTOR. A carrier organism (such as a fly or mosquito) that delivers a virus (or other agent of infection) to a host.

VENEREAL DISEASE. Another term for sexually transmitted disease.

VENTRICULAR FIBRILLATION. Uncoordinated contraction of the muscle in the ventricles (lower chambers) of the heart.

VENTRICULAR TACHYCARDIA. An abnormally rapid heartbeat originating in one of the lower chambers of the heart. It can lead to ventricular fibrillation.

VESICANT. The scientific name for a toxic chemical that causes blistering of the skin, mucous membranes, and respiratory tract.

VESICLE. A bump on the skin filled with fluid.

VIRAL LOAD. A measure of the severity of HIV infection, calculated by estimating the number of copies of the virus in a milliliter of blood.

VIRULENCE. The degree of a disease organism's ability to produce illness, as indicated by the mortality rate and/or the organism's ability to invade the host's tissues.

VIRUS. a parasitic microorganism that is smaller than a bacterium and has no independent metabolic activity. It is able to replicate only within a cell of a living plant or animal host.

A tiny, disease-causing particle that can reproduce only in living cells.

VITAL EVENT. An occurrence for which a certificate is typically issued. Examples of vital events include births, deaths, marriages, and adoptions.

VITAMIN. A nutrient that the body needs in small amounts to remain healthy but that the body cannot manufacture for itself and must acquire through diet.

VOLATILE ORGANIC CHEMICALS. Any organic chemicals with a high vapor pressure at ordinary, room-temperatures.

VULVA. The external female genital organs, including the labia majora, labia minora, clitoris, and vestibule of the vagina.

W

WASTEWATER TREATMENT. the process by which human waste or sewage is filtered, disinfected, and purified, making it safe to reintroduce into the environment.

WASTING. Weight more than two standard deviations below that of the median weight for the reference population.

WASTING SYNDROME. A combination of weight loss and change in composition of body tissues that occurs in patients with HIV infection. Typically, the patient's body loses lean muscle tissue and replaces it with fat as well as losing weight overall.

WATERBORNE DISEASE. An illness caused by ingesting water contaminated with some type of pathogen.

WAVELENGTH. The distance between two adjacent peaks or troughs of a wave.

WESTERN BLOT. A procedure that uses electrical current passed through a gel containing a sample of tissue extract in order to break down the proteins in the sample and detect the presence of antibodies for a specific disease. The Western blot method is used in HIV testing to confirm the results of an initial screening test.

WHITE NOISE. Sound that contains a mixture of many frequencies and amplitudes, often used to mask competing unpleasant or distracting noises.

WHOOPING COUGH. An infectious disease, also called pertussis, especially afflicting children, that is caused by a bacterium and is marked by a convulsive, spasmodic cough, sometimes followed by a shrill intake of breath.

WINDOW PERIOD. The period of time between a person's getting infected with HIV and the point at which antibodies against the virus can be detected in a blood sample.

WITHDRAWAL. The unpleasant, sometimes life-threatening physiological changes that occur due to the discontinuation of some drugs after prolonged regular use.

WORKPLACE VIOLENCE. Violence that occurs at the workplace of the perpetrator and/or victim.

WOUND. Any injury that breaks the skin, including cuts, scratches, and puncture wounds.

X

X RAYS. High-energy radiation used in high doses, either to diagnose or treat disease.

XEROPHTHALMIA. A drying of the cornea and conjunctiva.

Y

YELLOW FEVER. An infectious disease caused by a virus. The disease, which is spread by mosquitoes, is most common in Central and South America and Central Africa. Symptoms include high fever, jaundice (yellow eyes and skin) and dark-colored vomit, a sign of internal bleeding. Yellow fever can be fatal.

Z

ZOONOSIS (PLURAL, ZOONOSES). Any disease that can be transmitted from animals to people or people to animals.

ZOONOTIC DISEASES. Diseases caused by infectious agents that can be transmitted between (or are shared by) animals and humans. This can include transmission through the bite of an insect, such as a mosquito.

ZOSTER. A viral disease, also known as shingles or zona, that is characterized by a painful rash and can afflict anyone who has had chickenpox.

ZYGOTE. The result of the sperm successfully fertilizing the ovum. The zygote is a single cell that contains the genetic material of both the mother and the father.

INDEX

The index is alphabetized using a word-by-word system. References to individual volumes are listed before colons; numbers following a colon refer to specific page numbers within that particular volume. **Boldface** references indicate main topical essays. Photographs and illustration references are highlighted with an *italicized* page number. Tables are also indicated with the page number followed by a lowercase, italicized *t*.

A

A. fumigatus, 1:370

AARP, **1:1–2**

Ablative pain management procedures, 2:682

Abnormal heart rhythms, 1:229–230, 232

Abnormal pain, 2:680, 681, 683

Abortion, **1:2–6**
  birth defects issues, 1:108
  costs, 1:217
  following genetic testing and counseling, 1:381

Absenteeism, workplace, 2:982

Abstinence, sexual, 1:216, 2:781, 807, 808, 849

Acamprosate, 1:41

Acanthamebiasis, 1:292, 295, 2:691

Access to health care
  American legislation, history, 1:453–454
  community mental health centers, 1:202
  essential medicines, 1:327, 328–329
  federally qualified health centers, 1:341–342
  global public health, 1:393
  health policy, 1:422, 454
  human rights, 1:460
  LGBT populations, 1:548
  migrant workers, U.S., 1:341, 2:601
  poverty, 2:740
  refugees, 2:773
  vaccinations, 1:393, 402
  vulnerable populations, 2:980–983

Accreditation, health departments, 2:746–747

ACE inhibitors, 1:435, 475

Acetaminophen
  children's dosages, 1:175

flu treatment, 1:509
  pain relief, 2:681

Acetone, 1:151, 152

Acetyl cholinesterase (enzyme), 1:512, 513

Acetylcholine, 1:512

Acid rain, 1:35

Acid reflux, 1:82

Acquired immune deficiency syndrome. *See* AIDS

Acrodermatitis chronica atrophicans, 1:560

Acrylamide, **1:7–8**

Action on Smoking and Health, 2:928

Activated charcoal, 1:155–156, 2:596, 723

Acupressure
  influenza, 1:509
  pain relief, 2:681
  PTSD treatment, 2:737
  weight control, 2:669

Acupuncture
  allergy treatment, 1:52
  asthma, 1:86–87
  diabetes, 1:247
  heart disease, 1:437
  infection treatments, 2:884
  influenza, 1:509
  pain relief, 2:681
  veterinary medicine, 2:962, 963
  weight control, 2:669

Acute chemical poisoning, 1:151, 153, 154, 155

Acute meningitis, 2:582, 586, 587

Acute pain, 2:679–680, 683

Acute retroviral syndrome, 1:23–24

Acute rheumatic fever, 1:293

Acute stress, 2:886, 888, 889, 890

Acyclovir, 1:452, 2:716

Addams, Jane, 1:164, 2:999

Addiction, **1:8–14,** 2:595, 899. *See also* Alcoholism; Substance abuse and dependence
  causes and symptoms, 1:10–11, 2:901–902
  costs, 1:9, 13, 2:905
  cross-addiction, 1:13, 37
  diagnosis, 1:11
  painkillers, 2:681
  prevention, 1:13
  progression, 1:9–10, 10–11
  risk factors, 1:10, 2:904
  smoking, 1:9, 2:871, 872, 874
  treatment, 1:11–12, 38, 40–42, 2:596, 874

Adenine, 2:976

Adenosine, 2:813, 863

Adjustment disorders, 2:888, 891

Adler, Robert S., 1:214

Administration of public health. *See* Public health administration

Adrenaline
  anaphylaxis treatment, 1:52
  smoking release, 2:871
  stress, 2:888

Adult-onset asthma, 1:81–82

Adult-onset diabetes, 1:169, 243, 244
  management, 1:245–246, 247
  overweight and obesity, 1:169, 243, 2:663
  risk factors, 1:244

Advance directives, organ donation, 2:676, 677

Advertising. *See* Public service advertising

Aedes aegypti/albopictus mosquito, 1:233

Aerobic exercise, 1:438, *2:701*
  recommendations, 2:700, 702, 704–705
  types, 2:700, 701, 702–703

Anticonvulsant drugs
    essential medicines, 1:327
    fetal development and birth defects, 1:104
    pain relief, 2:681
Antidepressant medications
    addiction treatments, 1:12, 2:596
    pain relief, 2:681
    postpartum depression, 2:785–786
    post-traumatic stress disorder treatment, 2:736–737
    sleep effects, 2:864
    sodium effects, 2:880
    suicide patients, 2:911, 912
    weight loss, 2:668
Antidiabetic agents, 1:246
Antidiarrheal medications, 1:269, 361, 2:799, 852
Antidotes, essential medicines, 1:327
Antifungal medications, 1:371
Antigen-capture enzyme-linked immunosorbent assay (ELISA) test, 1:282, 546
Antihistamines
    allergic reactions actions, *1:45*
    allergy treatments, 1:51, 52, 53, 2:616
    bug bite treatments, 1:98–99
    cold treatments, 1:193–194
Antihypertensive medications, 1:475–476
Anti-infective medicines, 1:327
Anti-inflammatory drugs
    asthma treatments, 1:84–85
    essential medicines, 1:327
Antileukotrienes, 1:51
Antimalarial drugs, 2:567, 568
Antimicrobial agents, 1:70, 264, 265, 266, 354, 2:814
Antimicrobial resistance, 1:69, **70–74,** 264, 294, 489, 2:688, 814
Antimigraine medicines, 1:327
Antineoplastic agents
    birth defects, 1:104
    essential medicines, 1:327
Antioxidants
    detoxification uses, 1:154, 155
    diet and nutrition, 1:437–438, 2:650, 828
    food additives, 1:353, 354
    synthetic, 1:153
    vitamins and nutritional supplements, 1:18, 52, 437, 2:977
Antiplatelets, 1:435
Antiprotozoal medications, 1:270
Antipsychotic drugs

birth defects, 1:104
mental health resources, 1:206
methamphetamine users, 2:596
Antiretroviral drug therapy, 1:22, 26–27, 29, 30–31
Antiseptic cleaning agents, 1:406
Anti-smoking groups, 2:928
Antitoxins, 1:250, 359
Antiviral medications
    cytomegalovirus (testing), 1:226–227
    hepatitis, 1:446
    herpes, 1:452
    influenzas, 1:95, 400, 401, 509
    shingles, 2:856–857
Anxiety and pain, 2:679
Anxiety disorders, 1:102
    children's mental health, 1:173
    eating disorders links, 1:275, 276
    environmental disasters, 1:304
    following female genital mutilation, 1:346
    post-traumatic stress disorder, 1:102, 2:732–738
    sexual assault, 2:844
    stress vs., 2:888, 891
    treatment, 2:736
    women's mental health, 2:996
AOA Foundation, 2:973
APEX-PH. *See* Assessment Protocol for Excellence in Public Health (APEX-PH)
Appendicitis, 1:323, 324, 515
Appert, Nicolas, 2:698
Appetite suppressants, 2:668
Applied epidemiology, 1:314
Applied sociology, 2:877
Aqueous crystalline penicillin G, 2:921
Arboviruses, 1:233, 235, 298
    dengue fever, 1:233–236
    encephalitis, 1:297, 298
Archaeocins (antibiotics), 1:73
Armed Forces Health Surveillance Center, 1:295
Armenian Genocide (1915), 1:339
Arnott, Neil, 1:470
Aromatherapy
    asthma treatment, 1:87
    influenza, 1:509
    stress and anxiety treatment, 1:285, 2:737, 891
Arrhythmia, 1:430, 431
    Lyme disease, 1:560
    treatments, 1:437
Arson, 1:303
Arteriosclerosis. *See* Atherosclerosis

Arthritis
    joint replacement, 1:526, 527
    Lyme disease, 1:558, 560
    osteoarthritis, 2:835
    rates, 2:700
    Reiter's syndrome, 1:268, 271
    stress effects, 2:890
Artificial colors, 1:152, 353, 354, 355, 356
Artificial flavors, 1:353, 354–355, 2:880
Artificial insemination processes, 1:501
Artificial joint replacement, 1:525–527
Artificial sweeteners, 1:152, 354
Asbestos, 1:75, *75,* 76, 78, 113
    smoking and, 1:77, 310
    workplace monitoring, 2:672
Asbestosis, **1:75–78,** 113, 2:999
    prevention, 1:77–78
    public health response, 1:76–77
    symptoms, diagnosis, and treatment, 1:76
Ascariasis, 1:441, 2:691, 692
Ascorbic acid. *See* Vitamin C
Aseptic meningitis, 2:727
Ashkenazi Jewish populations, 1:375, 377–378, 381
Asia
    human trafficking, 1:463, 464
    malaria, 2:565, *566,* 567
    maternal mortality, 2:619–620
    smoking, 2:928
    suicide rates, 2:907, 966
    tuberculosis, 2:937
Asian Americans
    cancer, 2:608
    immunizations, 2:609
    infant mortality, 2:608
    life expectancy, 2:792
    mental health care, 1:203
Asian flu (1957), 1:399, 508, 2:687
Aspartame, 1:152
Asperger syndrome, 1:88, 90, 102
Aspergillosis, 1:370, 372, 2:614, 616, 1009
Aspiration pneumonia, 2:715
Aspirin, 1:194, 436, 439
    cardiovascular health, 2:898
    pain relief, 2:681
    Reye's syndrome, 1:451, 508, 509
    stroke treatment, 2:896
Assertive community treatment (ACT), 1:204
Assessment Protocol for Excellence in Public Health (APEX-PH), **1:78–79,** 2:612

Child poverty, 2:740, 741, 741t, 742

Child Protective Services, 1:158, 160, 162

Child safety seats, 1:140–143

Child sexual assault, 1:160, 2:843, 845, 905

Childbirth
    breastfeeding effects following, 1:485
    education, 2:780–781
    following female genital mutilation, 1:346, 347
    maternal mortality, 2:619–620, 997
    neonatal tetanus, 2:925
    postpartum depression, 2:784–786
    refugees, 2:773

Childhood Autism Rating Scale (CARS), 1:90

Childhood disintegrative disorder, 1:88, 90, 102

Childhood obesity, **1:167–172**
    effects on adult fat ratios, 2:669
    infant nutrition, 1:485, 488
    rates, 1:167, 2:653–654, 661
    side effects, 2:663
    treatment, 2:667, 669–670

Childproofing, 1:177

Children's health, **1:172–179**. *See also* Parent-child relationships; School health
    AIDS, 1:21, 23, 26
    air pollution effects, 1:35
    alcohol abuse, 1:9, 37, 173, 2:904, 905
    allergies, 1:44, 46–47, 49, 53, 54
    antibiotics use, 1:266
    asthma, 1:81, 85, 86, 87
    autism, 1:88–92, 102, 174–175, 176
    automobile accidents, 1:143
    behavioral health issues, 1:102
    bullying, 1:120, 121, *121,* 122–123, 123–125, 2:965, 966
    burns, 1:126
    car seats, 1:140–143, 2:795, 795t
    childhood illnesses, 1:175–176
    cold medications, 1:194
    essential medicines, 1:327
    handwashing, *1:407*
    height and weight, 2:662
    hepatitis, 1:443, 444, 446
    hunger and undernutrition, 1:465–466, 467, 468
    immune systems and infectious disease, 1:178, 493–494, 496, 497, 2:570
    immunization and vaccinations, 1:172–173, 189, 248, 293, 294, 402, 403, 444, 477–483, 509–510, 2:572, 802, 926, *957,* 958–959

influenza, 1:397–398, 509–510

mental health, 1:173, 176, 202–203, 205, 2:733

nutrition, 1:169–171, 483–488, 2:655–656, 825t, 826, 979

physical activity, 2:701

physical safety, 1:176–177, 178, 209–210, 212–213

pneumonia, 2:713, 714, 718

poison dangers, 2:719, *721,* 722, 723

rotavirus, 2:798–800

sleep, 2:862t, 863

smoking and secondhand smoke, 1:9, 2:803, 830, *831,* 832, 873, 875

stroke, 2:893, 895, 898

suicide, 2:906, 908

sun exposure, *2:914,* 915–916

tracking initiatives, 2:620

traumatic brain injury, 1:207, 208

tuberculosis, 2:940

vision, 2:971, 972, 973

whooping cough, 2:991–992

China
    anti-sparrow campaign (1958-62), 1:302–303
    crime and punishment, 2:581
    hunger and famine, 1:303, 337, 339
    Japan-China war (1937-45), 1:302
    migrant workers, 2:599
    plague, 2:686, 707
    population policy, 2:731
    poverty and reduction, 2:740
    product recalls, 2:581
    severe acute respiratory syndrome (SARS), 2:839–840
    sex education, 2:810
    suicide, 2:907, 966
    tuberculosis, 2:937
    veterinary medicine, 2:963
    water, 2:987

Chinese medicine, 1:18
    allergy treatments, 1:52, 53
    asthma, 1:86
    cold treatments, 1:194
    detoxification, 1:155, 313
    dysentery, 1:270
    heart disease, 1:437
    Lyme disease, 1:562
    malaria, 2:567
    rubella, 2:802
    shingles, 2:857
    syphilis, 2:921

Chinese skullcap, 1:53

CHIPs. *See* Community health improvement process (CHIP)

Chiron Corporation, 1:387–388

Chlamydia psittaci, 2:695–696, 714

Chlamydia trachomatis, 2:847, 929, 930, 969

Chlamydial infection, 2:744, 810, 847

Chlamydiosis. *See* Parrot fever

Chloasma, 2:778

Chloracne, 1:311

Chloramines, 1:181

Chlorinated hydrocarbons, pollution, 1:33

Chlorination, **1:179–181,** 185–186, 263, 331, 391, 2:648, 816

Chlorine, in drinking water, 1:179–181, 262, 331, 2:816

Chlorine dioxide, 1:303–304

Chlorofluorocarbons, pollution, 1:36

Chloroform, 2:860

Chloroquine, 2:567, 694

Chlorpheniramine, 1:51

Choking agents, 1:310

Choking hazards, 1:177, 212, 487

Cholecalciferol, 2:914

Cholecystitis, 2:948

Cholera, **1:181–187,** 2:815
    African disease transmission, 1:294
    historical global outbreaks, 2:686–687
    historical UK outbreaks, 1:184, 261, 315, 329, 391, 470, 2:598, 687
    historical U.S. outbreaks, 1:80
    history of discovery, 1:184, 2:598
    outbreaks, 2010-2011, *1:182,* 2:946
    prevention, 1:186
    public health, 1:182–183, 185–186
    treatment, 1:185
    vaccination, 1:186, 2:958
    water chlorination, 1:180

Cholesterol
    heart disease, 1:433, 435, 437, 439, 473, 2:792
    men's health, 2:589–590
    minority health, 2:610
    niacin effects, 2:979
    physical activity effects, 2:703
    stress, 2:889

Choline, 1:202

Chorionic villus sampling (CVS), 1:106, 378–379, 380, 382, 2:776t, 780

Choroidal hemorrhage, 2:970

Chromosomal abnormalities
    Epstein-Barr infection, 1:320
    genetic testing, 1:375, 376–377, 378–379, 383, 2:776t
    sex chromosomes, 1:105, 377, 379

Chromosomal translocation, 1:379

Chromosome mapping, 1:387

Chronic beryllium disease, 2:999

Chronic bronchitis, 2:873

Chronic chemical poisoning, 1:151, 153–154, 156

Chronic constipation, 1:516

Chronic fatigue syndrome, 1:560, 561

Chronic meningitis, 2:582

Chronic myelogenous leukemia, 1:379

Chronic obstructive pulmonary disease (COPD)
    asbestosis and, 1:77
    black lung disease, 1:114
    bronchitis and emphysema, 2:873
    gender differences, 1:19

Chronic pain, 2:680, 683

Chronic wasting disease, 1:117, 221

Cigar smoking, 2:830, 871, 873

Cigarette smoking. See Smoking

Cigarette taxes, 2:875, 928

Cimex lectularius (bedbug), 1:97

Ciprofloxacin, 1:68, 294

Circadian rhythms, 2:863, 866

Circumcision, 1:177, 178, 178, 2:592

Circumcision, female. See Female genital mutilation

Cirrhosis
    alcohol abuse, 1:448
    hepatitis, 1:443, 444, 446, 447, 448

Cities. See Healthy cities; Urban air pollution

Civil War, 2:603

Civilian Health and Medical Program of the Uniformed Services (CHAMPUS), 2:603

Clarithromycin, 1:68, 69

Clarity of vision, 2:968

Clean Air Act (1970), 1:36, 308, 2:641

Clean Air Act (UK; 1956), 1:301–302

Cleaners, household, 1:152, 156, 309, 313, 471, 2:721, 721–722

Cleavers (herb), 2:884

Cleft lip, 1:104, 105

Cleft palate, 1:103, 105, 348

Clemastine, 1:51

Climate change, 1:50
    emissions causes, 1:35
    food contamination, 1:364
    global public health, 1:394, 2:741
    zoonoses, 2:1010

Clinical dieticians, 2:651

Clinical trials
    epidemiological, 1:316
    pharmaceutical, 2:982

polio vaccine, 2:726
    TB vaccine, 2:943
    vitamins, 2:979

Clinton, Bill, 1:166

Clitoridectomy, 1:343, 344, 345, 346

Clomiphene citrate, 1:501, 503

Clostridium, 1:70, 72, **187–191**, 293, 358, 365, 2:816

Clostridium difficile, 1:70, 72, 187, 188, 189, 190, 293

Clostridium tetani, 1:187, 188–189, 2:816, 925

Clozapine, 2:911

Clubfoot, 1:105

CMV. See Cytomegalovirus

Coal dust, 1:113, 114–115, 2:999

Coal-related pollution, 1:33, 35, 36

Coalworkers' pneumoconiosis (CWP), 1:35, 113–115, 2:999

Cobalt-60, 2:770

Cocaine, 2:894, 900, 901, 902

Coccidioidomycosis, 1:370, 372

Cochlear implants, 1:429

Cochleitis, 1:428

Cochrane, Archie, 1:333–334

Cochrane Library, 1:334, 335

Codes of ethics, 1:331–332, 381, 2:678

Coenzyme Q10, 18, 52, 437, 2:650

Cognitive-behavioral therapies
    drug use and addiction, 2:596
    obesity, 1:170
    post-traumatic stress disorder, 2:736
    sleep, 2:866
    stress, 2:891
    substance abuse, 2:904

Cognitive degeneration, stroke, 2:897

Coil embolization, 2:896

Cold and heat
    discredited treatments, 2:921
    pain relief, 2:681–682, 857

Cold-induced asthma, 1:83

Cold sores, 1:318, 450, 451

Cold War
    biological weapons, 1:302, 2:869
    refugee statute interpretation and manipulation, 2:772

Colds. See Common cold

Colic, 1:486, 487

Colitis, 1:514, 515, 516, 517

College students
    drinking habits, 1:275
    eating disorders, 1:275
    norovirus outbreaks, 2:644

Collier, R. John, 1:65

Colon and rectal cancer, 1:135, 138, 516

genetic testing, 1:378, 380
    prevention, 1:517
    screening, 2:744

Colonialism, disease spread, 2:760
    smallpox, 2:687, 870
    syphilis, 2:917

Colonic cleansing, 1:313, 2:694

Colonography tests, 1:517

Colonoscopy, 1:517, 2:693

Color additives
    cosmetics, 1:356
    food, 1:152, 353, 354, 355, 356

Color blindness, 2:969

Colorado tick fever, 1:298

Colposcopy, 1:458

Combustion, pollution, 1:32–34, 35, 144

Commissioned Corps, United States Public Health Service, 2:955–956

Commissioners. See Health commissioners

Common cold, **1:191–195**, 493, 496
    antibiotics precautions, 1:68
    asthma and, 1:82
    bacterial infections following, 1:192–193, 195
    causes and symptoms, 1:192–193, 193
    description, 1:192
    homeopathic treatments, 1:56
    prevention, 1:194, 195
    treatment, 1:192, 193–194

Commonwealth Fund, 2:983

Communicable disease. See Infectious disease

Communication problems. See Hearing loss; Language problems; Languages spoken

Communications. See also Publications
    management-employee, 2:1002
    public health officials, 2:748–749

Community-acquired C. diff infections, 1:188

Community-acquired fungal infections, 1:372

Community-acquired MRSA (CA-MRSA), 1:69, 71

Community and Migrant Health Center programs, 1:341

Community Assessment for Public Health Emergency Response (CASPER) Toolkit, 2:634

Community development workers, **1:195–197**

Community dieticians, 2:651, 653

Community health, **1:197–198**
    elderly services, 2:574

Counter pulsation, 1:436

Counting technique (therapy), 2:737

"Cowpox," 2:867, 870, 957

Coxiella burnetii, 2:757–758

Coxsackie viruses, 1:404

CPR

    carbon monoxide poisoning, 1:145

    stroke, 2:897

Creutzfeldt-Jakob disease, 1:115–116, 117–118, **220–224,** 297, 302

Cribs, consumer safety, 1:212, 213, 214

Criminal behavior

    driving under the influence, 1:39, 254, 2:795, 796t, 797, 904–905

    environmental crimes, 1:303–304

    sexual assault, 2:842–846, 899

    substance abuse factor, 2:899–900

    suicide, 2:905–906, 907

    trauma witnessing or experiencing, 2:732–733, 735–736, 889

    violent crime, reports, 2:966

Critical Access Hospitals, 2:804

Crohn's disease, 1:514, 515, 516, 517

Cromolyn sodium, 1:51

Cross-addiction, 1:13, 37

Cross-linking theory, 1:16

Crowns, dental, 1:239

Crude death rate (CDR), 1:15

Cruise ship illnesses, 2:642, 643t, 644, 648

Cryotherapy, 1:458

Cryptococcosis, 1:372

Cryptosporidiosis, 2:691, 692

    dysentery, 1:268, 269, 270, 272

    susceptibility, 1:29

Cryptosporidium, 1:180, 268, 358

CT scans. *See* Computed tomography (CT) scans

Curricula, health education, 1:417, 2:824–825, 826–827

Cushing's syndrome, 1:474

Cutaneous anthrax, 1:64, 65

Cutaneous diphtheria, 1:249, 250

Cutaneous listeriosis, 1:554

Cutting boards, 1:366, 367

Cyanamide, 2:580

Cyanide, 1:303, 2:720

Cyanurotriamide. *See* Melamine

Cyberbullying, 1:120, 121–122, 124, 2:966

Cyberknifes, 2:771

Cycles of abuse, 1:158, 161, 163, 256, 257

Cycles of poverty, 1:166, 2:741

Cyclophotocoagulation, 2:970

Cyclospora cayetanensis, 1:358

Cystic fibrosis

    genetic causes, 1:105, 377, 381

    pneumonia risks, 2:713

Cytokines, 1:52, 2:863

Cytomegalovirus, 1:105, **224–227,** 450

D

da Rocha Lima, Henrique, 2:950

Daily living skills, fetal alcohol syndrome, 1:349, 350

Dairies, 2:696–697, 697

Dandruff, 1:372

Danube River, 1:303

Darfur, Sudan, 1:461

Dark Winter (terror scenario), 2:870

Databases

    chemical exposures, 2:672

    environmental health data, 1:307

    health departments' collected data, 1:415, 2:748

    medical research and reviews, 1:334, 335

    noroviruses, 2:645, 646

    occupational safety, 2:672

    organ donation, 2:675–676

    toxic substances, 1:310, 312

"Date rape" drugs, 2:723

Datura (hallucinogenic), 2:721

Davey, Humphrey, 1:179

Day care centers. *See* Child care centers

DDT, 1:97, 2:568, 687, 950

Deafness. *See* Hearing loss

Death. *See* Causes of death; Mortality and morbidity

Debridement, burns, 1:128

Debt, personal, 1:283, 284t, 285

Debt cancellation, 2:606

DEC2 (gene), 2:863

Decibels, 2:638

Decompression surgery, 2:682

Decongestant medications, 1:51, 193–194, 2:616

Deep vein thrombosis, 2:897, 932–933, 934

Deepwater Horizon oil spill (2010), 1:301

Deer ticks, disease transmission, 1:493, 558, 559, 561, 2:692, 1010, 1011, 1012

Defibrillation, *1:229,* **229–233**

Deficiency diseases (nutrition)

    scurvy, *2:828,* 828–830, 975

tracking, and fortification programs, 1:362, 363–364

Deforestation, 1:338

Dehydration

    campylobacteriosis, 1:131, 132

    cholera, 1:183–184, 185

    dysentery, norovirus, and rotavirus, 1:269, 270, 271, 2:645, 798, 799, 852, 934

    food poisoning, 1:359

Dehydroepiandrosterone (DHEA), 1:18

Delusional infestation, 1:505–506, 2:596

Demeclocycline, 1:66

Dementia

    aging, 1:17, 2:835–836

    AIDS dementia complex, 1:24–25, 25–26, 28, 30

    alcoholism, 1:11

    traumatic brain injury history, 1:207

Dementia paralytica, 2:918

Democratic Republic of Congo

    Ebola virus, 1:279, 281

    typhoid fever, 2:946

Demographic factors, public health, 1:330

Demography, 2:791, 877

Dengue fever, **1:233–236,** *234*

Dengue shock syndrome, 1:235

Denial, 2:903

Dental dams, 2:808

Dental health, **1:236–241,** *238,* 330, 331

    hygiene, 1:469, 471, 489

    infection control, 1:489

    methamphetamine users, 2:596, 597

    screening, 2:744

Dental schools, 1:237

Dental sealants, 1:240

Department of Education Organizing Act (1979), 1:241

Department of Health, Education, and Welfare, 1:241

Department of Health and Human Services, **1:241–242.** *See also* United States Public Health Service

    cardiovascular disease policy, 2:881, 898

    child abuse, 1:158

    Health Resources and Services Administration, 1:198, 421, 2:955

    Healthy People program, 1:425, 484–485, 2:834–835

    milk pasteurization, 2:699

    National Survey on Drug Use and Health, 1:101–102, 2:901, 904–905

    Office for Human Research Protections, 2:982

DMG (dimethylglycine), 1:91

DNA (deoxyribonucleic acid), 1:222
- birth defects, 1:105
- cancer, 1:133, 134
- creation, 2:977
- forensic medical examination, 2:844–845
- gene tests, 1:376, 378, 383
- genetically modified food, 1:384, 385
- genomics, 1:387, 388
- microbial, 1:70, 2:941
- radiation damage, 1:518, 521–522

Docosahexaenoic acid, 2:783

Doctor-patient relationships
- evidence-based medical practice, 1:334
- geriatric care, 1:552
- prescriptions and safety, 2:681
- risk assessments, 2:793
- rural ratios, 2:803
- sexual identity, 1:548, 549–550
- stress treatment, 2:890–891

Dogs
- fungal infections, 2:788, 790
- seeing-eye, 2:973
- veterinary medicine, *2:962*
- zoonoses, 2:1010

Domagk, Gerhard J. P., 1:265

Domesday Book (1086), 2:877

Domestic abuse, 1:121, **256–258,** 2:965, 967
- alcohol and drug abuse, 1:13, 39
- postpartum depression, 2:785
- post-traumatic stress disorder, 2:732
- traumatic brain injuries, 1:208, 210

Donora smog, Pennsylvania (1948), 1:301

Dopamine
- addiction role, 1:10
- stress, 2:888

Double burden of diseases, 1:393

Douching, 2:850

Down syndrome
- causes and symptoms, 1:103, 105, 106
- genetic testing, 1:375, 379–380, 2:776*t*

Doxycycline, 1:185, 325, 547, 2:674, 757, 921

Dr. P.H. (doctor of public health) degree, 1:316

Dracunculiasis infection, **1:258–261,** *259*

Drills, emergency preparedness, 1:289

Drinking and driving, 1:39, 254, 2:795, 796*t*, 797, 904–905

Drinking water, **1:261–264,** 471, 985. *See also* Sanitation
- acrylamide levels, 1:7, 8
- asthma, 1:86
- chemical poisoning, 1:151, 262, 303
- chlorination, 1:179–181, 262, 263, 331, 2:816
- cholera, 1:182–183, 185–186, 261–262, 2:686
- E. coli, 1:322, 323
- fluoride, 1:240, 330, 331
- improved sources, 2:816–817, 986–987
- infectious disease potential, 1:60, 62, 263, 2:598, 599, 1010
- nonprofit organizations, 1:180, 2:740
- poverty populations, 2:740
- radiation, 1:262, 2:816
- safety and infections, 1:30, 262, 394–395, 2:985–986
- safety standards, 1:262, 329
- travel health, 2:935–936
- typhoid fever, 2:946, 949, 986

Driver fatigue, 2:862, 863

Driver training, 1:253, 255

Driver vision, 2:972

Driving distracted, 1:251–255, 2:795

Driving under the influence (DUI), 1:39, 254, 2:795, 796*t*, 797, 904–905

Drought events, 1:338, 467

Drowning, 1:177

Drug abuse and dependence. *See* Addiction; Substance abuse and dependence

Drug allergies, 1:44, 48, 68, 69, 2:960

Drug delivery systems
- nicotine patch, *2:872,* 874
- pain relief, 2:682

Drug development. *See* Pharmaceutical development

Drug efficacy, essential medicines, 1:327, 328

Drug enforcement agencies, 1:530, 2:594, 681

Drug interaction risks
- antibiotics, 1:535
- avoidance, 2:650
- children's health, 1:175–176
- glaucoma, 2:970
- heart disease medications, 1:439–440
- poisoning, 2:719, 722
- stimulants and antidepressants, 2:595
- vaccines, 2:961
- vitamins, 2:979

Drug overdoses, 1:152, 153, 156, 2:719, 720, 721, 722, 902–903

Drug prescription labeling
- accidents, poisonings, 2:719, 720
- regulations, 1:266, 2:978

Drug resistance, **1:264–267,** 493
- antibiotics precautions, 1:68, 70–71, 264, 294, 489, 2:814
- antimicrobial, 1:69, 70–74, 264, 265–266, 294, 489, 2:688, 814
- mycobacteria, 2:626, 936–937, 939, 940, 942, 943
- pandemic potential, 2:688

Drug tests, 1:530–531

Drug use education and prevention, 2:596–597, 745, 827, 905

Drunk driving, 1:39, 254, 2:795, 796*t*, 797, 904–905

"Drunkorexia," 1:275

DTaP vaccine, 1:172, 189, 251, 479, 2:926, 927, 959, 993

Duchenne muscular dystrophy, 1:105, 379

Duck itch, 2:822

Durkheim, Emile, 2:877

Dysentery, **1:267–273,** 358, 851. *See also* Amebiasis
- bacillary, 1:267, 268–269, 270, 271, 2:850–853
- prevention, 1:272
- treatment, 1:269–271
- water chlorination, 1:180

Dyspareunia, 1:498

Dyspepsia, 1:515

Dysphagia, 2:897

E

E. bieneusi, 1:292

E. coli. *See* Escherichia coli

E. histolytica, 1:59, *59,* 60, 61, 267, 268, 271, 272, 358, 2:691

Ear, anatomy, 1:427, 428, 2:639

Ear infections, 1:428, 429, 2:783, 830

Ear wax, 1:427, 428

Early menopause, 1:500

Early-onset puberty, 1:111

Earth, 2:985

Earthquakes, 1:300, 2:632, 635, 946

Eastern equine encephalitis, 1:297, 298, 299

Eating disorders, 1:102, **273–278,** 2:996–997
- children, 1:170, 173, 2:669
- LGBT populations, 1:549
- prevention, 1:277–278
- rates, 1:273, 2:654, 996–997

Encephalitis *(continued)*
measles, 2:570, 571
mumps, 2:621
parasite infection, 1:352
rabies, 2:763
treatment, 1:298
typhus, 2:952
West Nile, 2:987, 989, 990
Encephalitozoon cuniculi, 1:292
Encephalitozoon hellem, 1:292
Encephalomyelitis, 1:297
Endangered Species Act (1973), 1:308
Endarterectomy, 2:896
Endemic typhus, 2:951, 952–953
Enders, John F., 2:569
Endocarditis, 1:437
listeriosis, 1:555, 556
Q fever, 2:757, 758
staph infections, 2:883
Endocrine disruptors, 1:110, 311
Endodontists, 1:237, 239
Endometriosis, 1:499, 501
Endoparasites, 2:690
Endophthalmitis, 2:970
Endoscope tests, 1:517, 2:693
"Energy gap," 1:168
Energy medicine/work, 1:55, *56,* 2:737
Engineering. *See* Public health engineers
English as a second language
populations, 1:419, 420, 2:599, 601
Entamoeba dispar, 1:59
Entamoeba histolytica, 1:59, *59,* 60, 61,
267, 268, 271, 272, 358, 2:691
Enteritis, 1:187–188, 515
Enterococcus faecalis, 1:71–72
Enterocytozoon bieneusi, 1:292
Enterohemolysin, 1:325
Enterohemorrhagic E. coli, 1:323,
324–325
Enteroinvasive E. coli, 1:323, 324, 325
Enteropathogenic E. coli, 1:323, 324, 325
Enterotoxigenic E. coli, 1:323, 324, 325
Enterovirus 71, 293
Enteroviruses, 1:404, 2:584, 586, 725
Entry inhibitors, 1:27
Environmental cleanup, 1:312–313
Environmental degradation
air pollution, 1:32–36
climate change, 1:35, 50, 2:741
medical waste, 2:577–580
Environmental disasters, **1:300–305**
Environmental engineering, 2:751
Environmental epidemiology, 1:306
Environmental health, **1:305–307**

animal habitat changes and disease,
1:294, 2:1010, 1011
birth defects, 1:103, 105, 151–152,
153, 301
cancer, 1:134, 135, 151, 152–153,
306, 2:591
chemical poisoning, 1:151–152,
153–154, 300–303
diabetes, 1:244
eating disorders, 1:275
health inspection, 1:418–419
hygiene, 1:471
infertility, 1:499, 2:592
military personnel exposures,
2:604–605
public health organizations' focus,
1:80, 304, 305–306
sick building syndrome, 2:859–861
urban health issues, 1:305
Environmental Protection Agency
(EPA), 1:36, 308, **308–309**
asbestos, 1:76–77
Bisphenol A classification, 1:110,
112
chlorination standards, 1:180–181
drinking water standards, 1:262,
2:985
genetically modified food, 1:385
history, 1:301, 308
lung cancer reports, 2:832
medical waste policy, 2:577, 579
noise pollution, 2:638, 641
pesticide poisoning data and
programs, 1:513, 514
pesticides regulation, 1:366
sick building syndrome, 2:859
Environmental smoke. *See* Secondhand
smoke
Environmental toxins, **1:309–314**
Environmental Working Group, 1:110
Enzyme-linked immunosorbent assays
(ELISA), 1:50, 325, 411, 2:646, 799
Ephedra, 1:53, 86
Epidemic Intelligence Service, 1:316
Epidemic typhus, 2:950, 951–952
Epidemic yellow fever, 2:1005
Epidemiological transition, 1:552
Epidemiology, **1:314–318.** *See also*
Infection control
Centers for Disease Control and
Prevention, 1:147, 315, 316
education and field outlook, 1:316
emerging diseases, 1:292–296,
490–491
environmental, 1:306
epidemic/pandemic paths, 2:688

global public health, 1:393
history, 1:184, 261–262, 314–315,
329, 391, 2:687
psychiatric, 1:202
specialties, 1:315
vulnerable populations, 2:982
Epidermis burns, 1:126, *127*
Epididymitis, 2:592
Epiglottis, 2:712, 713
Epiglottitis, 1:402
Epilepsy, 2:865, 898
Epinephrine. *See* Adrenaline
Epizootics, 2:707–708
Epoetin alfa, 1:27
Epoxy resins, 1:109
Epstein, Anthony, 1:318
Epstein-Barr virus, **1:318–322,** *319,* 450
Erectile dysfunction, 1:439–440, 2:592
Erosion, 1:338
Erythema infectiosum, 1:293
Erythema migrans, 1:559, *559*
Erythromycin, 1:68, 69, 71, 132, 185,
2:716, 993
Erythrosine (Red No. 3), 1:356
Escape-related coping, 2:891
Escherich, Theodor, 1:322
Escherichia coli, 1:72, 266, **322–327,**
323, 358, 365, 493, 2:934
genomics, 1:388
prevention and precautions,
1:325–326
strains, 1:323–324
zoonoses, 2:1011
Esophageal atresia, 1:103
Esophageal cancer, 2:873
Esophageal damage, Chagas disease,
1:148, 149
Esophageal disorders, and pneumonia,
2:713
Esophagitis, 1:515
Essential fatty acids. *See* Omega-3 fatty
acids
Essential medicines, **1:327–329**
Essential oils, 2:790
Estelle v. Gamble (1976), 1:219
Estrogen
birth control pills, 1:216–217, 2:783
endocrine disruptors, 1:110
heart disease, 2:996
postpartum levels, 2:784
Estrogen replacement therapy, 1:17
Ethanol, 1:311
Ethics and legal issues of public health,
1:329–332
emergency preparedness, 1:290

F

I

J

M

Index

Milk *(continued)*

pasteurization, 1:118, 119, 365, 2:696–697, 699, 758

sodium, 2:880

unpasteurized, 1:118, 119, 554, 557, 2:697, 699, 757, 812

Vitamin D fortification, 1:362, 2:977

Milk thistle, 1:155, 2:568

Millennium Development Goals, **2:605–607,** *606,* 740

morbidity and mortality, 2:620

poverty, 2:605, 607, 741–742

tuberculosis, 2:937

water safety, 1:263

Millennium Summit (2000), 2:605

"Million Hearts" program, 2:881, 898

Minamata disease, 1:302

Mind/body medicine

asthma, 1:86–87

men's health, 2:590

reflexology, *1:56*

shingles, 2:857

Mine Safety and Health Administration, 1:114

Minerals (nutrition), 1:17, 2:650, 656–657. *See also* specific minerals

food sources, *2:978*

nutritional guidelines, 2:879, 978

sodium, 2:878–881

Miners' asthma, 1:113–115

Mini-strokes, 2:893, 894

Mining accidents, 1:114, 2:1001

Minocycline, 2:757

Minority health, **2:607–612.** *See also* Racial and ethnic differences

disease rates, 2:607–609

infant mortality rates, 2:608, 609, 610, 619

population shifts, 2:610–611

U.S. Public Health Service, 2:955

Miscarriage, 2:996

amniocentesis and CVS risks, 1:382

chromosome analysis, 1:378–379

fetal alcohol syndrome, 1:350

listeriosis, 1:553, 554

rubella, 2:801, 802

stress, 2:890

Misoprostol, 1:4

Mites, 2:951

Mitigation, emergencies, 1:288

Mobilizing for Action through Planning and Partnerships (MAPP), 1:79, 416, **2:612–613**

Mold, **2:613–618,** *614*

allergies, 2:614, 615, 616

cleaning methods, 2:615

crops, and famine, 1:338

discovery of penicillin, 1:265

disease treatment, 2:615–616

food contamination, 1:358, 521

household toxin, 1:311, 313, 2:614, 617, 860

Molecular testing, tuberculosis, 2:941

Monitoring the Future survey, 2:594

Monoamine oxidase inhibitors (MAOIs), 2:736–737

Monogamy, 2:809, 849–850

Monongahela virus, 1:410

Mononucleosis

Epstein-Barr virus, 1:318, 319–320, 321, 450

infected demographics, 1:320

prevention, 1:321–322

symptoms, 1:224, 320

Monosodium glutamate (MSG), 1:152, 355–356, 2:880

Morbidity. *See* Mortality and morbidity

Morgellens disease, 1:505–506

"Morning after" pill, 1:216

Morning sickness (pregnancy), 2:776, 996

Mortality and morbidity, **2:618–620**

Mosquito-borne diseases

dengue fever, 1:233–236

encephalitis, 1:297–298, 299

filariasis, 1:351–353

malaria, 2:565–568, 690–691

tularemia, 2:944

West Nile virus, 2:987–991, *988*

yellow fever, 2:1005–1009

Mosquito repellents, 2:990–991

Mothers Against Drunk Driving (MADD), 2:905

Mouth cancer, 2:873

Mouth-to-mouth resuscitation

carbon monoxide poisoning, 1:145

stroke, 2:897

MRSA. *See* Methicillin-resistant Staphylococcus aureus (MRSA)

Mucocutaneous leishmaniasis, 1:537–538, 539

Multibaccillary leprosy, 1:541, 542

Multidrug resistant tuberculosis (MDR-TB), 1:71, 72, 293, 493, 2:626, 688, 936–937, 939, 940, 942, 943

Multidrug therapy, leprosy, 1:542

Multifetal pregnancy reduction, 1:3

Multiple births, 1:502

Multiple personality disorder, 1:163

Multiple sclerosis

Epstein-Barr virus, 1:318

Lyme disease compared, 1:560

Multnomah County (Oregon) Sheriff's Office, 2:597

Mumps, 1:481, 493, **2:620–624,** *621*

causes and symptoms, 2:621–622

infertility following, 1:498

treatment, 2:622–623

vaccination, 1:481–482, 2:570, 621, 623–624

vaccine avoidance, and disease effects, 1:293, 294, 2:621, 624

Murine typhus, 2:951

Muscle

body composition, 2:666

declines, aging, 1:15, 2:834

declines, AIDS, 1:30

Muscle dysmorphic disorder, 1:273, 274

Muscular dystrophy, 1:380

Mussolini, Benito, 1:302

Mustard gas, 1:302, 309

Mutual masturbation, 2:808

Myasthenia gravis, 1:69

Mycobacterium, **2:624–627,** 940, 942–943

Mycobacterium avium complex, 2:625, 940

Mycobacterium kansasii, 2:625

Mycobacterium leprae, 1:540–541, 543, 2:624, 625

Mycobacterium lepromatosis, 2:625

Mycobacterium marinum, 2:625

Mycobacterium tuberculosis, 1:71, 266, 478, 2:624–625, 936, 937, 939, 940, 942–943

Mycobacterium ulcerans, 2:625

Mycoplasma pneumoniae, 2:715, 716, 717

Mycotoxins, 2:614

Myocardial infarction, 1:430, 431, 432t, 433, 436, 473, 591. *See also* Heart disease

prevention initiatives, 2:881, 898

risks, 2:705

sodium, 2:881

stress, 2:889

symptoms, 1:433, 436, 2:804

treatment, 1:436

Myocardial ischemia, 1:430

Myocarditis, 1:249, 250

leptospirosis, 1:547

Q fever, 2:757

Myocardium, 1:229–230, 430

Myopia (nearsightedness), 2:968

MyPlate (food guide), 2:650, *655,* 670

Myrobalan fruit, 1:270

N

Paroxysmal stage, whooping cough, 2:992

Parrot fever, 1:293, **2:695–696**

"Partial-birth" abortion, 1:3–4, 5

Parvovirus B19, 293

Passenger safety
distracted driving, 1:253
driving under the influence, 2:796*t*
laws, 1:142–143, 2:794

Passive immunization, 2:765

Passive smoking. *See* Secondhand smoke

Pasteur, Louis, 1:63, 264–265, 315, 391, 2:697, 698

Pasteurella bacteria, 1:492, 2:685

Pasteurization, 1:118, 119, 365, **2:696–700**
L. monocytogenes, 1:555
steam, 1:325
unpasteurized foods, 1:360, 554, 557
unpasteurized milk, 1:118, 119, 554, 557, 2:697, 699, 757, 812

Patient autonomy, 1:381

Patient Protection and Affordable Care Act (2010), 1:422
AARP support, 1:2
federally qualified health centers, 1:342
preventive medicine, 2:744–745
Ready Reserve Corps, 2:955–956

Paucibacillary leprosy, 1:541, 542

Peanut allergies, 1:44, 46, 48

Pedestrian safety, 1:177

Pediatric antibiotics, 1:69

Pediculosis. *See* Lice

Pedigrees, 1:381

Pedophilia, 1:161

Peebles, Thomas C., 2:569

Peer-counseling, post-traumatic stress disorder, 2:736

Peer pressure
children's health, 1:173
substance abuse, 2:905

Pelvic adhesions, 1:499, 501

Pelvic inflammatory disease, 1:500, 2:847, 850

Penicillin, 1:67
allergies, 1:44, 68
discovery, 1:265, 2:917
scarlet fever, 2:819–820
syphilis, 2:921

Penile cancer
circumcision and, 1:178, 2:592
human papillomavirus, 1:455, 456, 481

Penis anatomy, infertility, 1:498

Peppermint, 1:401, 2:857

Peptic ulcer, 1:514, 515

Pepto-Bismol, 2:853, 934

Perception of pain. *See* Pain

Perception of stress, 1:283, 2:734, 888, 890–891, 891–892

Perchloroethylene, 1:151

Percutaneous Coronary Intervention (PCI), 1:436, 437

Perforation of the intestine, 2:948

Perforation of the large bowel, 1:323, 324

Performance indicators, education, 1:417, 2:825

Perianal ulcers, 1:60

Pericarditis
extrapulmonary tuberculosis, 2:940
Q fever, 2:757

Pericardium, 1:430

Periodic limb movement disorder, 2:864, 865

Periodontal disease, 1:237, 239, 2:744

Periodontitis, 1:237

Periontitis, 1:515, 2:948

Peripheral acting adrenergic antagonists, 1:475, 476

Peripheral iridotomy, 2:970

Peripheral vision, 2:968–969, 971

Peroxyacetyl nitrate, pollution, 1:34

Personal debt, 1:283, 284*t*, 285

Personal hygiene. *See* Hygiene

Personal safety precautions, 2:844

Personalities
post-traumatic stress disorder development factors, 2:734
stress management differences, 1:283, 2:886, 889, 890–891, 891–892
suicide risks, 2:911–912

Personality disorders, 1:163

Pertussis. *See* Diphtheria, Tetanus, and Pertussis (DTaP) vaccine; Tdap vaccine; Whooping cough

Pervasive developmental disorder, 1:88, 102, 173, 174, 176

Pest control, 1:98, 99, 100, 506. *See also* Infestations

Pesticide poisoning. *See* Insecticide poisoning

Pesticides
chemical poisoning, 1:152, 153, 311, 357, 358, 512–514
child labor laws, 1:167
drinking water, 1:262
as environmental toxin, 1:309

industrial disasters, 1:301
Lyme disease links, 1:294
regulation, 1:366

Petechiae, 1:410

Pets
allergies, 1:44, 54
bites and infectious disease, 1:492
contaminated foods, 2:581
emerging diseases, 1:294, 295
exotics, and diseases, 1:294, 492
fungal infections, 2:788, 790
leptospirosis, 1:544, 545, 547
plague, 2:708–709
rabies risks, 2:763, 765, 766, 1011–1012
Salmonella, 2:812, 813
toxoplasmosis, 2:691
veterinary medicine, 2:962
zoonoses, 2:1010

Peyronie's disease, 2:592

Pfeiffer, Richard Johannes, 1:402

Phage therapy, 1:72–73

Phantom limb pain, 2:680

Pharmaceutical development
antimicrobial agents, 1:266
epidemiological work, 1:316
orders of prohibition, 1:73
prioritizing, 1:73
vitamin supplements, 2:978

Pharmacoepidemiologists, 1:315

Pharmacogenetic testing, 1:379

Pharyngeal diphtheria, 1:249

Phencyclidine, 2:900, 902

Phenylketonuria (PKU), 1:105, 106, 175, 377

Philanthropic organizations, health care, 2:983

Phimosis, 1:178

Phosgene gas, 1:302, 309, 310

Phosphorus-32, 2:770

Photodynamic therapy, 1:457

Photons, 2:767, 769, 770

Photosensitivity, 1:68

Phthalates, 1:110, 212

Physical abuse, 1:158, 159, 162, 256, 257, 2:837, 965–966. *See also* Child abuse; Domestic abuse

Physical activity, **2:700–706**. *See also* Exercise
lack, and heart disease, 1:433, 439, 2:703, 704, 792, 834
national promotion, 2:745
overweight and obesity, 1:168, 169, 171, 2:662, 669, 670, 700, 704
physical education, 2:826–827

Sodium *(continued)*

    heart disease, 2:880, 881

    hypernatremia and hyponatremia, 2:880

    hypertension, 1:438, 476

    sources/food additives, 1:353, 354–355, 359, 2:879–880

Soil bacteria, 1:187–188, 385, 544, 2:816

Soil erosion, 1:338

Soil fungi, 1:369, 372, 2:788, 816

Soil-transmitted helminthiasis, 1:441–442, 2:691–692

Solar flares, 2:633

Soldiers, treatment, 1:460–461

Solid foods (infants), 1:368, 486–487

Solid Waste Disposal Act (1965), 1:308

Solid waste removal, 2:816

Solvents, pollution, 1:35, 36, 309

Soman nerve gas, 1:311

Somatic experiencing, 2:737

Soper, George A., 2:947

Sound levels, 1:427, 428, 429

    laws, 2:641

    noise pollution, 2:638–641

Sound therapy, *1:57*

Soundproofing, 2:641

South American blastomycosis, 1:370

South American yellow fever, 2:1005, 1006

South Korea, 1:95, 2:966

Southeast Asia, AIDS rates, 1:20, 21

Space disasters, 2:633

Spanish flu pandemic (1918-19), 1:508, 2:687, 760

Spanking, 1:158, 161

Sparrows, 1:302–303

Speech impairment, stroke, 2:893, 895, 897

Speech therapy

    children, 1:176

    hearing loss, 1:429

    stroke, 2:896, 897

Spending, tracking, 1:285

Sperm injection processes, 1:106, *499,* 502, 504

Sperm production and count, 1:498, 500–501, 501, 2:592

Spermicides, 1:215, 216, 2:781

Sphygmomanometer, 1:474

Spice (synthetic marijuana), *1:529,* 529–531

Spillover, animal diseases, 1:294

Spina bifida, 1:103, *104,* 105, 106, 107

    folic acid as prevention, 2:780

genetic testing, 1:380

Spinach, *2:600, 977*

Spinal polio, 2:727, 728

Spinal taps

    encephalitis, 1:298

    listeriosis, 1:555

    meningitis testing, 2:585–585

    polio, 2:727

    rabies testing, 2:764

Spinal tuberculosis, 2:940

Spirometry (asthma test), 1:83–84, 2:672

Spirulina, 1:340

Spleen

    Epstein-Barr virus, 1:320

    malaria, 2:565

    mononucleosis, 1:320, 321

    stress processes, 2:888

    typhoid fever, 2:948

Spock, Dr. Benjamin, 1:174

Spongiform encephalopathies. *See* Bovine spongiform encephalopathy; Creutzfeldt-Jakob disease; Gerstmann-Straussler-Scheinker disease; Kuru

Spontaneous generation theory, 2:698

Sporadic Creutzfeldt-Jakob disease, 1:221, 223, 224

Sporadic encephalitis, 1:297

Sports activities, 2:701–702

Sports anorexia, 1:273, 274

Sports injuries, 1:207–208, 209, 210

Sprouts, contamination, 1:359, *2:811*

St. Augustine, 2:907

St. Louis encephalitis, 1:297, 298

Stabilizing agents (food), 1:355

Stalin, Josef, 1:339

Stalking, 1:256, 257, 2:843

Standard precautions, 1:471, 2:633

Staphylococcal infections, **2:882–885**

    causes and symptoms, 2:882, 883–884

    drug resistance, 2:688

    infection control, 1:489

Staphylococcal scalded skin syndrome, 2:882, 883

Staphylococcus aureus, 1:293, 358, 360, 365, 2:882

    antimicrobial resistance, 1:69, 71, 72, 489

    infections, *2:882,* 882–883

Staphylococcus epidermidis, 2:883

Staphylococcus pneumoniae, 2:717

Staphylococcus saprophyticus, 2:883

State and local-level public health. *See* Community health; Community health assessment; Community health improvement process (CHIP);

Community mental health; Health departments; Occupational health

State Associations of Local Boards of Health (SALBOH), 2:630

State Children's Health Insurance Program (SCHIP), 1:205

State epidemiology, 1:315

State laws

    genetically modified foods, 1:386

    physician-assisted suicide, 2:909

    school nutrition, 2:826

    smoking bans, 2:832–833, 874–875

    traffic, 2:794

    workers' compensation, 2:1001

Status of women, 1:166, 392, 2:740, 741

Stem-cell transplantation, 1:137, 138

Steptoe, Patrick Christopher, 1:500

Stereotactic radiosurgery, 2:771

Sterilization birth control methods, 1:216, 217, 2:781

Steroid hormones, 2:888

Steroid injections, 1:215

Stinging nettle, 1:52, 53

Stomach cancer, 1:318, 321

Stomach flu. *See* Gastroenteritis

Stop TB Partnership, 2:942

Stranger danger, 1:177

Strangulation, product safety concerns, 1:212

"Strawberry tongue," 2:819

Strep throat

    bacteria, 1:293

    vs. scarlet fever, 2:819

Streptococcus pneumoniae, 1:266, 482, 494, 2:584, 717, 718

Streptomycin, 2:945

Stress, **2:885–892**, 886t. *See also* Post-traumatic stress disorder (PTSD)

    asthma, 1:81, 83

    blood pressure, 1:473, 474, 476

    child abuse links, 1:160–161

    children's health, 1:173

    cognitive influence, 1:283, 285, 2:886

    diabetes, 1:247

    domestic abuse, 1:256

    eating disorders, 1:275, 2:890

    eating habits, 1:168–169, 170, 2:667, 890

    economic/financial, 1:282–285, 284t, 2:885, 886t

    heart disease risks, 1:434, 438, 439

    intestinal disorders, 1:517, 518, 2:890

    LGBT populations, 1:548, 549